REVIEW OF
Clinical
Anesthesia

SIXTH EDITION

REVIEW OF
Clinical
Anesthesia

Edited By

Neil Roy Connelly, MD

Professor of Anesthesiology
Tufts University School of Medicine
Boston, Massachusetts
Director of Anesthesiology Research
Department of Anesthesiology
Baystate Medical Center
Springfield, Massachusetts

David G. Silverman, MD

Professor and Director of Clinical Research
Department of Anesthesiology
Yale University School of Medicine
Medical Director of Pre-Admission Testing
Yale–New Haven Hospital
New Haven, Connecticut

 Wolters Kluwer | Lippincott Williams & Wilkins
Health

Philadelphia • Baltimore • New York • London
Buenos Aires • Hong Kong • Sydney • Tokyo

Acquisitions Editor: Brian Brown
Product Manager: Nicole Dernoski
Production Project Manager: Priscilla Crater
Senior Manufacturing Manager: Benjamin Rivera
Marketing Manager: Lisa Lawrence
Design Coordinator: Stephen Druding
Production Service: Aptara, Inc.

ISBN 978-1-4511-8372-6

© 2013 by LIPPINCOTT WILLIAMS & WILKINS, a WOLTERS KLUWER business
Two Commerce Square
2001 Market Street
Philadelphia, PA 19103
LWW.com

Printed in The United States of America

Care has been taken to confirm the accuracy of the information presented and to describe generally accepted practices. However, the authors, editors, and publisher are not responsible for errors or omissions or for any consequences from application of the information in this book and make no warranty, expressed or implied, with respect to the currency, completeness, or accuracy of the contents of the publication. Application of the information in a particular situation remains the professional responsibility of the practitioner.

The authors, editors, and publisher have exerted every effort to ensure that drug selection and dosage set forth in this text are in accordance with current recommendations and practice at the time of publication. However, in view of ongoing research, changes in government regulations, and the constant flow of information relating to drug therapy and drug reactions, the reader is urged to check the package insert for each drug for any change in indications and dosage and for added warnings and precautions. This is particularly important when the recommended agent is a new or infrequently employed drug.

Some drugs and medical devices presented in the publication have Food and Drug Administration (FDA) clearance for limited use in restricted research settings. It is the responsibility of the health care provider to ascertain the FDA status of each drug or device planned for use in their clinical practice.

To purchase additional copies of this book, call our customer service department at (800) 638-3030 or fax orders to (301) 223-2320. International customers should call (301) 223-2300.

Visit Lippincott Williams & Wilkins on the Internet at LWW.com. Lippincott Williams & Wilkins customer service representatives are available from 8:30 am to 6 pm, EST.

10 9 8 7 6

THIS BOOK IS DEDICATED TO OUR WIVES,
ANN GIANCASPRO CONNELLY AND SALLY KNIFFIN,
TO OUR CHILDREN,
KEVIN MATTHEW AND ELLEN ALEKSANDRA CONNELLY
AND TYLER AND CHARLOTTE SILVERMAN,
AND TO THE LATE MARY M. CONNELLY, ARTHUR SILVERMAN, HENRIETTA
SILVERMAN, AND BROTHER ROY MOONEY, F.M.S.

CONTRIBUTING AUTHORS

Adam C. Adler, MD, MS
Resident in Anesthesiology
Department of Anesthesiology
Baystate Medical Center
Springfield, Massachusetts

Neil Roy Connelly, MD
Director of Anesthesiology Research
Baystate Medical Center
Springfield, Massachusetts
Professor of Anesthesiology
Tufts University School of Medicine
Boston, Massachusetts

Kamel Ghandour, MD
Assistant Chief of Anesthesia
St. Barnabas Hospital
New York, New York

Matthew Harris, DO
Chief Resident in Anesthesiology
Department of Anesthesiology
Baystate Medical Center
Springfield, Massachusetts

Alexander Hotinsky, MD
Director of Anesthesia Education
St. Barnabas Hospital
New York, New York

Maria-Karnina Iskandar, MD
Department of Anesthesiology
Baystate Medical Center
Springfield, Massachusetts
Assistant Professor of Anesthesiology
Tufts University School of Medicine
Boston, Massachusetts

Vanita K. Jain, DO
Resident in Anesthesiology
Department of Anesthesiology
Baystate Medical Center
Springfield, Massachusetts

Ryan R. Joyce, MD
Baystate Medical Center
Springfield, Massachusetts
Instructor of Anesthesiology
Tufts University School of Medicine
Boston, Massachusetts

Lorraine Kerchum, DO
Resident in Anesthesiology
Department of Anesthesiology
Baystate Medical Center
Springfield, Massachusetts

Brian Kiessling, MD
Chairman of Anesthesia
Munson Medical Center
Traverse City, Michigan

Tanya Lucas, MD
Co-Director of Obstetric Anesthesiology
UMass Memorial Medical Center
Assistant Professor of Anesthesiology
University of Massachusetts Medical School
Worcester, Massachusetts

Brian Martin, MD
Department of Anesthesiology
Baystate Medical Center
Springfield, Massachusetts
Instructor of Anesthesiology
Tufts University School of Medicine
Boston, Massachusetts

Pankaj Mehta, MD
Department of Anesthesiology and Pain Management
Baystate Medical Center
Springfield, Massachusetts
Instructor of Anesthesiology
Tufts University School of Medicine
Boston, Massachusetts

Todd Payne, DO
Resident in Anesthesiology
Department of Anesthesiology
Baystate Medical Center
Springfield, Massachusetts

Karthik Raghunathan, MD, MPH
Assistant Professor
Duke University Medical Center
Department of Anesthesiology
Anesthesiology Services
Durham VA Medical Center
Durham, North Carolina

Jonathan Ross, MD, PhD
Department of Anesthesiology
Baystate Medical Center
Springfield, Massachusetts
Instructor of Anesthesiology
Tufts University School of Medicine
Boston, Massachusetts

Stelian Serban, MD
Department of Anesthesiology
Section Chief, Pain Division
Mount Sinai Medical Center
New York City, New York

Naveed A. Tahir, MD
Department of Anesthesiology
Baystate Medical Center
Springfield, Massachusetts
Instructor of Anesthesiology
Tufts University School of Medicine
Boston, Massachusetts

One of the best ways to judge a book is by the company it keeps. Thus, even before it hits the bookstore shelves, *Review of Clinical Anesthesia* is a "winner." This totally revised work, which parallels the new (seventh) edition of *Clinical Anesthesia,* enjoys a distinguished position on a website along with *Clinical Anesthesia* and other significant texts in the field of anesthesiology.

As stated in the introductions to the previous editions of this review book, the amount of information related to our specialty appears to be growing exponentially; even a carefully honed text such as *Clinical Anesthesia* can seem quite imposing. At times, the reader would like to pause and see what he or she has learned or should learn. These factors were the impetus behind the development of *Review of Clinical Anesthesia.* In its simplest form, the multiple-choice questions in this text can be used as a means of self-assessment before taking a written examination. However, we feel that this book may be of even greater benefit if it is incorporated throughout one's studies; a pretest will help the novice as well as the expert focus his or her reading; a posttest will allow one to assess self-mastery of most relevant material.

The sixth edition of this text has benefited from the extensive updating of the parent text, *Clinical Anesthesia.* This has led to our revision of the material in virtually every chapter, as well as to the addition of several new chapters. As was the case in recent editions, each answer includes a heading and a page number that refer the reader to a section in *Clinical Anesthesia.* This information can be used to direct the reader to a more extensive discussion of the subject matter addressed in the question.

Neil Roy Connelly, MD
David G. Silverman, MD

ACKNOWLEDGMENTS

The generation of the questions in this text could not have been accomplished without the dedicated efforts of the secretarial staffs of our respective institutions. We appreciate the efforts of the members of the staff at Kluwer-Lippincott Williams & Wilkins, who were vital to the organization and completion of this text. We would like to acknowledge the swift and excellent assistance of Nicole Dernoski. We also wish to thank the editors and authors of *Clinical Anesthesia* for, once again, providing us with such a fine source of material. Their careful attention to detail and relevance have facilitated our efforts. We also would like to express our appreciation to our coauthors, whose assiduous efforts have enabled us to assemble a detailed yet cohesive series of questions and answers. Mostly, we would like to thank our families, who waited patiently as we waded through pages of text in search of the questions.

CONTENTS

Introduction to Anesthesiology

CHAPTER 1

The History of Anesthesia

1. Ancient Egyptian pictographs display nerve compression to possibly produce regional anesthesia during surgery of which body part?

   A. The foot
   B. The hand
   C. The nose
   D. The genitals
   E. The ear

2. In the 17th century, Marco Aurelio Severino reported using what substance to create anesthesia at a surgical site?

   A. Heated coal
   B. Liquid mercury
   C. Snow
   D. Gold
   E. Iron shavings

3. During the 1st century, a soporific sponge was used to provide pain relief during surgery. What ingredient(s) were boiled together and cooked into this sponge?

   A. Black cohosh, garlic, and holy water
   B. Eye of newt, leg of toad, and skin of fish
   C. Fentanyl, midazolam, and ketamine
   D. Poppies, black nightshade, and mandrake leaves
   E. Ginseng, cinnamon, and vitamin D

4. Nitrous oxide has the ability to produce lightheadedness. Some thrill seekers intentionally expose themselves to nitrous oxide as a diversion. Who is credited with first preparing nitrous oxide by heating ammonium nitrate with iron filings?

   A. Dr. Thomas Beddoes
   B. Mr. Joseph Priestley
   C. Dr. Humphry Davy
   D. Dr. Horace Wells
   E. Dr. Valerius Cordus

5. Who is credited with the earliest documented use of diethyl ether for painless surgery?

   A. Dr. Crawford W. Long
   B. Dr. Henry Hill Hickman
   C. Dr. William T.G. Morton
   D. Dr. Horace Wells
   E. Dr. Charles T. Jackson

6. In 1845, an anesthetist gave a public demonstration of nitrous oxide at the Massachusetts General Hospital. Even though the patient was unaware, he still cried out during the surgery. This anesthetist thus became the first in modern anesthesia to hear a surgeon say, "Give him more gas!" Who was this man?

   A. Dr. Crawford W. Long
   B. Dr. Henry Hill Hickman
   C. Dr. William T.G. Morton
   D. Dr. Horace Wells
   E. Dr. Charles T. Jackson

7. On October 16, 1846, there was a public demonstration of ether at the Massachusetts General Hospital. The man who demonstrated this not only established ether as an effective anesthetic, he also managed to firmly establish in surgeons' minds that "the anesthetist is always late!" Who was the anesthetist?

   A. Dr. Crawford W. Long
   B. Dr. Henry Hill Hickman
   C. Dr. William T.G. Morton
   D. Dr. Horace Wells
   E. Dr. Charles T. Jackson

8. Who published the use of chloroform for anesthesia during labor and childbirth in the *Lancet* in 1847?

   A. Dr. James Young Simpson
   B. Dr. Virginia Apgar
   C. Dr. William Morton
   D. Dr. Joseph Clover
   E. Queen Victoria

9. Which notable advancement in the field of anesthesiology can be credited primarily to work done by American surgeon Dr. Joseph O'Dwyer in the mid-1880s?

    A. Tracheal intubation
    B. Central venous cannulation
    C. Direct laryngoscopy
    D. Brachial plexus conduction block
    E. Anesthetic record

10. Which pioneer in the field of anesthesiology can be credited with the development of the cuffed endotracheal tube?

    A. Dr. Ralph Waters
    B. Dr. Joseph O'Dwyer
    C. Dr. Arthur Guedel
    D. Dr. Elmer McKesson
    E. Ivan Magill

11. When Dr. Ralph Waters intentionally ventilated only one lung, what airway instrument did Dr. Arthur Guedel propose?

    A. The fiberoptic bronchoscope
    B. The elastic intubating stylet
    C. Nasal endobronchial tubes
    D. Double-cuffed single-lumen tubes
    E. Double-lumen endobronchial tubes

12. Dr. Roger Bullard became frustrated by failed attempts to visualize the larynx of a patient with Pierre-Robin syndrome. He then developed a laryngoscope called the:

    A. Wu-scope
    B. Bullard scope
    C. Combi laryngoscope
    D. LMA camerascope
    E. Anesthesia kaleidoscope

13. With his radical thinking, Dr. Archie Brain made what contribution to airway management?

    A. Patil face mask
    B. Laryngeal mask airway
    C. Wu-scope
    D. Flexible fiberoptic bronchoscope
    E. Bullard laryngoscope

14. Dr. Elmer McKesson is credited with the innovation of which of the following features of modern-day anesthesia machines?

    A. Oxygen fail-safe valve
    B. Flow-ratio system
    C. Oxygen flush valve
    D. Variable bypass vaporizers
    E. Partial rebreathing circuits

15. In 1907, the Draeger "Pulmotor" was introduced as the first of which device?

    A. Cardiopulmonary bypass pump
    B. Intermittent positive pressure ventilator
    C. Mechanical infusion pump
    D. Mechanical operating room table
    E. Agent specific vaporizer

16. During World War II, British aviation researchers began research on devices to improve the supply of oxygen that was provided to pilots flying at high altitude in unpressurized aircraft. This research led to perhaps the most important technologic advance ever made in monitoring the well-being and safety of patients during anesthesia. What is this monitoring system?

    A. Continuous capnography
    B. Electrocardiography
    C. Mass spectrometry
    D. Oxygen sensors
    E. Pulse oximetry

17. Trichloroethylene, a nonexplosive volatile anesthetic, releases what compound when it is warmed in the presence of soda lime?

    A. Compound X
    B. Compound A
    C. Factor X
    D. Phosgene
    E. Ethyl chloride

18. What anesthetic, although popular in the mid-20th century, was abandoned after it was learned that dose-related nephrotoxicity was associated with its prolonged use?

    A. Chloroform
    B. Methoxyflurane
    C. Ether
    D. Enflurane
    E. Halothane

19. The cardiovascular effects of which drug became widely appreciated only after a series of fatalities among military casualties during World War II?

    A. Curare
    B. Thiopental
    C. Fentanyl
    D. Halothane
    E. Cyclopropane

20. What medication introduced in the late 20th century suppresses pharyngeal reflexes, produces anesthesia rapidly, has antiemetic properties, allows patients to awaken promptly, and has popularized total intravenous anesthetic techniques?

    A. Ketamine
    B. Propofol
    C. Meperidine
    D. Chlorpromazine
    E. Droperidol

21. Oncologists identified the antiemetic properties of what medication when dealing with intracranial edema from tumors?

    A. Antihistamines
    B. Propofol
    C. Droperidol
    D. Corticosteroids
    E. Promethazine

22. Dr. Leonard Corning is remembered for coining the term "spinal anesthesia" and for performing a neuraxial block on a patient to treat an addiction to what?

    A. Masturbation
    B. Opium
    C. Gambling
    D. Work
    E. Cocaine

23. Dr. Bier and Dr. Hildebrandt performed a successful spinal anesthetic when Dr. Hildebrandt did not feel pain after his legs were hit with a hammer and his testicles were pulled. How did these physicians celebrate their success?

    A. Wine and cigars
    B. Going out to the opera and then a "cabaret"
    C. By visiting an opium den in Kiel, Germany
    D. With more hammers

24. Who described a continuous spinal anesthetic technique around 1940?

    A. Dr. Heinrich Quincke
    B. Dr. August Bier
    C. Dr. Theodor Tuffier
    D. Dr. William Lemmon
    E. Dr. Richard Hall

25. What anesthesia technique was described by Dr. Achille Dogliott in 1931?

    A. Intravenous regional anesthesia of the arm
    B. Loss of resistance to identify the epidural space
    C. Blind nasotracheal intubation
    D. Cervical spinal anesthesia
    E. Regional block of the ankle

26. Who first described the technique of intravenous regional anesthesia in 1908?

    A. Dr. Harvey Cushing
    B. Dr. August Bier
    C. Dr. Carl Koller
    D. Dr. Leonard Corning
    E. Dr. Hcinrich Braun

27. Who created the first clinic for the treatment of chronic pain in the United States?

    A. Dr. Emery Rovenstine
    B. Dr. Frederick Cotton
    C. Dr. John Snow
    D. Dr. John Booka
    E. Dr. Ambrose Bierce

28. Dr. Jean Baptiste Denis first attempted blood transfusion in 1667. His patient received blood from:

    A. A slave
    B. A cow
    C. A lamb
    D. Dr. Denis himself
    E. A horse

29. This person is credited with advancing American anesthesiology professional societies in the early 20th century. He edited the precursor journal to *Anesthesia and Analgesia*, acted as an ambassador to Europe for American anesthesiology, and founded the International Anesthesia Research Society (IARS). Who was this person?

    A. Dr. Harvey Cushing
    B. Dr. Benjamin Franklin
    C. Dr. Francis McMechan
    D. Dr. Karl Landsteiner
    E. Dr. Carl Gauss

30. Dr. Ralph Waters became frustrated by the low-quality training of anesthesia providers, established the first postanesthetic recovery rooms, and he became the first American professor of anesthesiology. Where was he a professor?

    A. Saint Louis University Hospital
    B. Yale-New Haven Hospital
    C. Fairfield University
    D. University of Wisconsin-Madison Hospital
    E. Baystate Medical Center-Tufts University

31. Which of the following statements regarding the history of cocaine as an anesthetic is FALSE?

    A. Cocaine was the first effective local anesthetic.
    B. Its utility as a local anesthetic was first introduced to the medical community by Dr. Carl Koller in 1884.
    C. Cocaine was the agent used in the first successful spinal anesthetic.
    D. Although its local anesthetic actions were well recognized, cocaine was not used in surgical procedures until 1911.
    E. Reports of central nervous system and cardiac system toxicity were not appreciated until the 1940s.

32. Which of the following is not explosive?

    A. Chloroform
    B. Ether
    C. Cyclopropane
    D. Halothane

ANSWERS

1. B. Ancient Egyptian pictographs from approximately 3,000 BC display images of nerve compression during upper extremity surgery. One pictograph shows a brachial plexus being compressed, and another shows antecubital fossa nerve compression; both surgeries were presumably done on alert patients and done on the hand. (See page 4: Physical and Psychological Anesthesia.)

2. C. People have long recognized that cold temperatures produce insensibility to pain. Remarkably, in the Middle Ages, people attempted to apply the property of cold to perform surgery as an early form of cryoanesthesia. (See page 4: Physical and Psychological Anesthesia.)

3. D. In the 1st century, mandragora was recognized to produce analgesia. Historically, a soporific sponge was used to produce an acceptable level of surgical analgesia. This sponge had various recipe forms depending on the producer; however, all of them included mandrake leaves, black nightshade, and poppies boiled together to form a sponge that was administered to a patient after reconstitution in hot water. (See page 4: Early Analgesics and Soporifics.)

4. B. Nitrous oxide was first prepared in 1773 by the British clergyman and scientist Joseph Priestley. Priestley prepared several other gases during his investigations, the most notable being isolated oxygen. Davy and Wells performed later observations and experiments with nitrous oxide, and Valerius Cordus is credited with having distilled diethyl ether (sweet oil of vitriol) in the 16th century. (See page 5: Inhaled Anesthetics.)

5. A. Although Dr. William Morton has been credited with introducing diethyl ether as a successful anesthetic in the public arena on October 16, 1846, Dr. Crawford W. Long of Athens, Georgia, has the distinction of the first documented successful use of ether in the surgical setting. Dr. Long first administered ether preoperatively on March 30, 1842, but he neglected to make his findings known until 1849, long after Dr. Morton's demonstration. (See page 6: Public Demonstration of Ether Anesthesia.)

6. D. Dr. Horace Wells has the distinction of being the first person in the history of modern anesthesia to have a patient cry out and move during his public demonstration of nitrous oxide. Although the patient did not recall the surgery, Dr. Wells undoubtedly had to listen to the surgeon complain about the patient not holding still during the surgery. Modern anesthetists in the 21st century no longer have this problem, of course. (See page 5: Almost Discovery.)

7. C. On "ether day," October 16, 1846, Dr. William Morton gave a public display of ether for surgical anesthesia to Edward Abbott. The surgeon was Dr. John Warren. Dr. Warren will always be remembered as the first modern surgeon to complain in public that the anesthetist was late. (See page 6: Public Demonstration of Ether Anesthesia.)

8. A. Although Dr. Simpson, an accomplished obstetrician in Edinburgh, Scotland, had been a champion of the use of ether and chloroform anesthesia for labor and childbirth, the relief of obstetric pain had long been discouraged on prevailing religious grounds. It was not until Dr. John Snow, an English contemporary of Dr. Simpson, administered chloroform to a laboring Queen Victoria that widespread acceptance of obstetric anesthesia came into being. As head of the Church of England, the queen's endorsement of the practice ended the debate as to the appropriateness of such anesthetics. (See page 6: Chloroform and Obstetrics.)

9. A. Although Scottish surgeon William Macewen first performed elective oral–tracheal intubation in 1878, it was the work of American surgeon Dr. Joseph O'Dwyer that popularized the technique. In 1885, Dr. O'Dwyer developed a set of metal laryngeal tubes, which he inserted blindly between the vocal cords of children with diphtheritic crises as an alternative to hasty tracheotomies. Three years later, he developed a rigid endotracheal tube with a conical tip, which allowed positive-pressure endotracheal ventilation to be used during thoracic procedures. (See page 7: Tracheal Intubation.)

10. C. In 1926, Dr. Arthur Guedel began a series of experiments that led to the introduction of the cuffed endotracheal tube. His goal was to combine tracheal anesthesia with the closed-circuit technique recently refined by Dr. Ralph Waters. To showcase the utility of these new tubes, Dr. Guedel performed a series of demonstrations with his own dog, "Airway," who he anesthetized and submerged underwater while using the cuffed endotracheal tube. (See page 7: Tracheal Intubation.)

11. D. Dr. Ralph Waters described a bronchial intubation and hypothesized that intentional endobronchial intubation could facilitate surgery on the opposite lung. He related this to Dr. Arthur Guedel, leading to the design of the single-lumen, double-cuff modification of the emerging cuffed airway tube. Later, Dr. Frank Robertshaw popularized the double-lumen endobronchial tube. Since then, there have been several modifications and new techniques described for lung isolation; however, the basic reasoning remains the same. (See page 7: Tracheal Intubation.)

12. B. Dr. Roger Bullard developed the Bullard laryngoscope in response to frustration with the acute angle observed in a patient with Pierre-Robin syndrome. This laryngoscope incorporated fiberoptic bundles that lie beside a curved blade and allowed the user to observe the larynx lying at 90 degrees from the mouth. (See page 9: Advanced Airway Devices.)

13. B. Dr. Archie Brain produced and made popular the laryngeal mask airway after he realized that it was an effective means of ventilating and delivering anesthetics to a patient. Shigeto Ikeda developed the first flexible fiberoptic bronchoscope. Dr. Roger Bullard developed the Bullard laryngoscope to "see around the corner" of the airway. The Wu-scope was later developed to improve on the idea of the Bullard laryngoscope. The Patil Face Mask, developed by Dr. Vijay Patil, was developed to oxygenate the anesthetized patient while a flexible fiberoptic bronchoscope is used to intubate the airway. All of these innovations were prompted by the need to manage patients with challenging, difficult airways. (See page 9: Advanced Airway Devices.)

14. C. Dr. Elmer McKesson, one of the first specialists in anesthesiology in the United States, developed a series of gas machines. Because of concerns over inflammable anesthetics, Dr. McKesson popularized anesthetic inductions with 100% nitrous oxide, with titration of small volumes of oxygen as the anesthetic progressed. Dr. McKesson developed the oxygen flush valve to add oxygen quickly to the system in the event that the resultant cyanosis became too profound. (See page 9: Early Anesthesia Delivery Systems.)

15. B. Mine rescue workers and firefighters were provided with early forms of positive-pressure mechanical ventilators to help resuscitating injured patients. Draeger produced the first marketed device, the "Pulmotor," in 1907. Afterward, the European polio epidemic inspired further refinements in mechanical ventilation. (See page 10: Ventilators.)

16. E. Takuo Aoyagi, a Japanese engineer developed pulse oximetry, which was described by Dr. Severinghaus as "the most important technologic monitoring advance in the history of anesthesia." His work was a refinement of earlier investigations performed by Glen Millikan, an American physiologist, which pertained to oximetric sensors for fighter pilots during World War II. (See page 12: Electrocardiography, Pulse Oximetry, and Capnography.)

17. D. Trichloroethylene was a widely used nonexplosive volatile anesthetic. However, it was found to be toxic to multiple organ systems when administered for prolonged periods or at high concentrations. When the gas is heated in the presence of soda lime, it produces phosgene as a by-product. When phosgene is inhaled, it reacts with water in the lungs to form hydrochloric acid and carbon monoxide, with resultant pulmonary edema. Phosgene was used extensively during World War I as a choking agent. Among the chemicals used in the war, phosgene was responsible for the majority of deaths. (See page 13: Inhaled Anesthetics.)

18. B. Over a protracted period, methoxyflurane use leads to increased serum fluoride concentrations and nephrotoxicity. Before this was discovered, methoxyflurane was a very popular volatile anesthetic in the 1960s. (See page 13: Inhaled Anesthetics.)

19. B. Thiopental was synthesized in 1932 by Tabern and Volwiler of the Abbott Company and was first administered to a patient at the University of Wisconsin in March 1934. The cardiovascular depressive effects of thiopental were widely appreciated only after its use led to fatalities among civilians and soldiers during World War II. After these experiences, fluid replacement therapy was used more aggressively, and thiopental was administered with greater caution. (See page 14: Intravenous Anesthetics.)

20. B. Propofol combined with variable-duration paralytics and faster-acting narcotics made total intravenous anesthesia techniques more accessible. Propofol's antiemetic property, along with a ceiling context-sensitive half-life, makes it a popular anesthetic agent. (See page 14: Intravenous Anesthetics.)

21. D. Corticosteroids decrease intracranial edema in patients with mass lesions and tumors. They also reduce nausea. (See page 18: Antiemetics.)

22. A. Dr. Corning assessed the effects of cocaine injected into the lumbar neuraxial space. He attempted to perform a therapeutic neuraxial block on a man who was "addicted to masturbation." Since, Dr. Corning did not describe an escape of fluid, we can assume that an epidural injection of cocaine was performed. We do not know if the patient was "cured" of his addiction. (See page 19: Regional Anesthesia.)

23. A. The first clearly defined spinal anesthetic involved the release of a large volume of cerebrospinal fluid (CSF) through large-bore needles. The observation of CSF as an end point is still used in modern spinal anesthesia. This led to the first described postdural puncture headache. Drs. Bier and Hildebrandt erroneously attributed the violent headaches to their celebratory wine and cigars. (See page 19: Regional Anesthesia.)

24. D. Dr. William Lemmon described the use of a malleable silver needle to puncture the dura. Local anesthetic was introduced as needed through a hole in the operating table mattress. Later, Dr. Waldo Edwards and Dr. Robert Hingson described the same technique for continuous caudal anesthesia in obstetric patients. (See page 19: Regional Anesthesia.)

25. B. Dr. Achille Dogliotti of Turin, Italy wrote a classic study that made the epidural technique well known. Dr. Dogliotti identified the epidural space by the still used loss-of-resistance technique. (See page 19: Regional Anesthesia.)

26. B. Intravenous regional anesthesia was first reported in 1908 by Dr. August Bier, who used a technique in which procaine was injected into a vein of the upper limb between two tourniquets. The technique was not widely used in the clinical setting until 1963, when Dr. Mackinnon Holmes modified the block by exsanguination before applying a single proximal cuff. (See page 19: Regional Anesthesia.)

27. **A.**   Dr. Emery Rovenstine continued the work of Dr. Gaton Labat and his colleagues. At the Bellevue Hospital in New York City, he used invasive techniques to lyse sensory nerves and to inject local anesthetics in an attempt to treat chronic pain. This association of physicians focused on pain management was the first of its kind in North America. (See page 19: Regional Anesthesia.)

28. **C.**   Amazingly, Dr. Jean Denis, the court physician to Louis XIV, first transfused blood from a lamb into a patient, who benefited from the transfusion. It is reported that the following attempts at interspecies were not successful. Transfusion of blood in humans was banned for religious reasons for more than 100 years in Western Europe. (See page 23: Transfusion Medicine.)

29. **C.**   Dr. Francis McMechan retired from active anesthesia practice in Cincinnati in 1915 because of severe rheumatoid arthritis. Afterward, he dedicated himself to editing the precursor to the anesthesiology journal *Anesthesia and Analgesia* (at the time, it was called *Current Researches in Anesthesia and Analgesia*). In addition, he helped establish an international society for anesthesia research (the IARS) while acting as an ambassador in Europe for American anesthesiology. One by-product of his efforts was the establishment of the International College of Anesthetists, which certified early anesthesiologists and helped raise the standards of anesthesiology quality in the early 20th century. (See page 23: Organized Anesthesiology.)

30. **D.**   Dr. Ralph Waters became the first American academic professor of anesthesiology at the University of Wisconsin-Madison medical school in 1927, where he established an anesthesiology residency-training program. Dr. Waters attracted motivated and talented people to the department, and he fostered many of the qualities that are common in modern academic anesthesiology departments. International experts at the time visited this department and were influenced by it. (See page 23: Organized Anesthesiology.)

31. **E.**   The anesthetic properties of cocaine, an extract of the coca leaf, had been known for centuries before its formal introduction in 1884 by Dr. Carl Koller. Soon thereafter, cocaine gained widespread acceptance as an anesthetic agent for surgical procedures involving the mucous membranes, such as the eyes, mouth, nose, larynx, trachea, and rectum. Dr. Leonard Corning also used cocaine for the first successful spinal anesthetic in 1885. Reports of central nervous system and cardiovascular toxicity were reported soon after the first reports of cocaine use. (See page 19: Regional Anesthesia.)

32. **D.**   Both ether and chloroform were known to be flammable gases and to be explosion hazards. Cyclopropane (also called trimethylene) is an explosive, colorless gas first used in 1934 as a volatile general anesthetic. Both induction and emergence from cyclopropane anesthesia were reported to be usually rapid and smooth, but because it is flammable and could be a source of explosion in the operating area, nonflammable gases replaced it. (See page 13: Inhaled Anesthetics.)

Scope of Practice

1. Accreditation from The Joint Commission lasts for how many years?

   A. 1
   B. 2
   C. 3
   D. 4
   E. 5

2. The main goal of a managed care organization (MCO) is to attempt to manage what aspects of the health care system?

   A. Number of facilities in a geographic area
   B. Utilization of services within a patient population
   C. Outline of the best management for each particular condition
   D. Ensuring that physicians are managed to improve physician income
   E. Being a division of the National Institutes of Health whose goal is the development of universal coverage

3. All of the following factors are the benefits of an anesthesia preoperative clinic EXCEPT:

   A. Increase in the efficiency of operating rooms
   B. Financial savings for the institution
   C. Centralization of pertinent information, including consults, financial data, and diagnostic and laboratory information
   D. Patient and family education on the process, surgery, and postsurgical considerations
   E. Ability to schedule presurgical evaluation at the last minute because of the streamlined process of the clinic

4. All of the following facts are true EXCEPT:

   A. Standard of care is the conduct and skill of a prudent practitioner that can be expected by a reasonable patient.
   B. Courts have traditionally relied on medical experts knowledgeable about the point in question to give opinions as to what the standard of care is.
   C. A less objective way of determining the standard of care is to review the published standards of care, guidelines, practice parameters, and protocols established by the American Society of Anesthesiology.
   D. The standard of care is what a jury says it is.
   E. Expert witnesses can establish the standard of care.

5. Which of the following statements regarding "claims-made" insurance is FALSE?

   A. Policies cover all malpractice claims made while the insurance is being paid.
   B. Premium rates are relatively low during the first year of practice.
   C. Tail coverage is a hidden expense with claims-made policies.
   D. Claims-made policies are more expensive for insurance companies because they have a longer period in which they are exposed to possible claims.
   E. It is critical that the individual practitioner verifies that he or she is thoroughly covered when relocating to another place of employment.

6. Establishing standards of care, practice parameters, and guidelines in anesthesia practice afford individuals all of the following benefits EXCEPT:

   A. Improvement in quality of care
   B. Providing the basis for legal defense in malpractice cases
   C. Guiding thought processes through difficult clinical scenarios
   D. Fulfilling legal mandates
   E. Many protocols are established to improve efficiency and reduce costs

7. After a critical adverse event occurs, which of the following should be implemented?

   A. Limit the number of consultants involved.
   B. Involve the risk management department in the hospital only if a suit is filed.
   C. Record any additions or alterations of the facts in the chart as amendments.
   D. Chart the event, including the facts of the events and speculations regarding the cause of the incident.
   E. Never disclose medical judgment or performance errors to the victim or survivors.

8. Computer scheduling of cases has advantages over handwritten systems in all of the following ways EXCEPT:

   A. Historical precedents of time for procedures can prevent overbooking.
   B. It can result in a decrease of staff overtime costs.
   C. It can easily generate reports and statistics for future use.
   D. It can reduce personal bias in scheduling cases.
   E. Computerized scheduling only benefits large institutions.

9. All of the following regarding the Health Insurance Portability and Accountability Act (HIPAA) of 1996 are true EXCEPT:

   A. Attention is focused on protected health information.
   B. A "privacy officer" must be appointed for each practice group.
   C. Patient charts must be locked away overnight.
   D. A fax containing patient information does not need any special handling.
   E. Patient names must not be used on any information board if there is any chance that anyone not directly involved in their care could see them.

10. Which of the following regarding antitrust considerations is TRUE?

    A. Antitrust laws are concerned with the preservation of competition in a defined marketplace.
    B. Antitrust laws involve the rights of individuals to engage in business.
    C. The Sherman Antitrust Act is approximately 50 years old.
    D. The per se rule is the most frequently applied rule when judging violations.
    E. The *rule of reason* involves the ability to obtain a certificate of need for necessary equipment.

11. Which of the following is TRUE regarding operating room management?

    A. Anesthesiologists should develop a leading role among other operating room personnel.
    B. Block scheduling appears to be the most efficient manner for scheduling surgical cases and should be used exclusively in the creation of the operating room schedule.
    C. Prudent drug selection combined with appropriate anesthesia technique rarely results in dollar savings.
    D. Sharing the responsibility of "running the floor" among all the anesthesiologists is an efficient way to manage the operating room schedule because all anesthesiologists will come to appreciate the nuances of the day-to-day schedule.
    E. In a 2002 survey, over 95% of respondents stated that an anesthesiologist was designated as the Clinical Director of the OR.

12. In dealing with an adverse event, all of the following are recommended EXCEPT:

    A. Establish an "adverse event protocol" in the department in the policies and procedures manual.
    B. It is not necessary to sequester involved equipment for evaluation.
    C. Establish an "incident supervisor" whose responsibility is to help prevent continuation or reoccurrence of incidents, investigating incidents, and ensuring documentation while the original anesthesiologists focus on caring for the patient.
    D. The chief of anesthesiology, facility administrator, risk manager, and anesthesiologist's insurance company should be notified in a timely manner.
    E. Full disclosure of the events as they are best known is currently believed to be the best presentation.

ANSWERS

1. C. Full accreditation from The Joint Commission lasts for 3 years. (See page 32: Establishing Standards of Practice and Understanding the Standard of Care.)

2. B. MCOs are companies that provide health care for large populations. Their main goal is to attempt to control costs through providing appropriate care, negotiating for the lowest prices on services, and restricting access to more expensive services such as operative procedures. (See page 47: Evolving Practice Arrangements.)

3. E. The anesthesia preoperative clinic allows the running of a more efficient operating room schedule. It reduces last-minute cancellations, shotgun ordering of laboratory work, and unnecessary preoperative specialty consultation. Early identification of certain problems requiring special care on the day of surgery (e.g., blocks, pulmonary artery catheters) leads to fewer unanticipated delays. All relevant patient information can be centralized to one location. However, all of these benefits are optimized when the patient is seen relatively early in relation to the day of surgery. Early recognition of patients requiring further workup allows time for another patient to fill the vacant block in the schedule. (See page 55: Preoperative Clinic.)

4. C. The standard of care is the conduct and skill of a prudent practitioner that can be expected by a reasonable patient. Expert witnesses can define it. This was traditionally the method of establishing the standard of care. The problem with this method was that both parties could have expert witnesses, which can support the two opposing sides, thereby making the process subjective. The more objective way of determining the standard of care is reviewing the published standards of care, guidelines, practice parameters, and protocols established by a national organization such as the American Society of Anesthesiologists. The above two methods are the two main sources for information that a jury has available to them to establish the standard of care. (See page 32: Establishing Standards of Practice and Understanding the Standard of Care.)

5. D. The two primary types of malpractice insurance are occurrence and claims-made insurance. An "occurrence" insurance policy means that if the policy was in force at the time of the occurrence of an incident resulting in a claim, whenever that claim might be filed, the practitioner would be covered. "Claims-made" insurance only covers claims that are filed while the insurance is in force. This kind of insurance is relatively inexpensive during the first year because claims typically take some time to be filed. However, if the physician simply discontinues a claims-made policy (e.g., by changing insurers or leaving a given practice) and a claim is filed the next year, there will be no insurance coverage. Therefore, the physician leaving a claims-made policy must secure "tail coverage" for claims filed after the physician is no longer primarily covered by that insurance policy. It is critical that the individual practitioner is absolutely certain through personal verification that he or she is thoroughly covered at the time of any transition. A practitioner arriving in a new location must verify with confirmation in writing (often called a "binder") that malpractice liability insurance coverage is in force before there is any patient contact. (See page 38: Malpractice Insurance.)

6. D. Standards of care, practice guidelines, and parameters have been increasingly used over the past few decades. The impetus for their increased use centers primarily on the improvement of quality of care for patients. American Society of Anesthesiologists (ASA) Monitoring Standards of Care is an excellent example of standard of care guidelines, and the ASA Difficult Airway Algorithm is an outstanding example of practice guidelines. These guidelines, if followed, typically improve patient outcomes and cost effectiveness by reducing unnecessary tests and ineffective treatments. Since experts in the field usually develop these standards, they constitute a powerful legal defense in light of a malpractice suit. Practicing outside the standards of the specialty requires one to justify one's actions and decisions. Standards of care, practice parameters, and practice guidelines are not legally mandated. Many protocols are devised to fast-track patients through the medical care system, especially when an elective procedure is involved, in as little time as possible, thus minimizing costs. (See page 32: Establishing Standards of Practice and Understanding the Standard of Care.)

7. C. After the identification of a critical event, help should be called to minimize the sequelae of the event. Consultants may be helpful and should be called without hesitation. If permanent injury occurs, early involvement of the anesthesia department, hospital administration, risk management department, and insurance company is essential. Charting of the event is critical. Only facts should be included in the chart. No speculation regarding the cause or who is to blame should be recorded. Any change to the chart's original documentation should be recorded as an amendment and labeled as such, with an indication regarding why such an amendment was necessary. There is a relatively recent movement in medical risk management advocating immediate full disclosure to the victim or survivors, including "confessions" of medical judgment and performance errors with attendant sincere apologies. (See page 38: Malpractice Insurance.)

8. E. Computer scheduling programs are powerful tools in operating room management and will likely benefit every OR regardless of size. When historical times for procedures are input into the system, the program can prevent optimistic bookings by surgeons and can prevent operating room time from running long and thus requiring payment of overtime. Inputting this type of data can allow the program to generate reports and statistics that will aid in future planning. The program can examine the schedule and determine whether any staff or equipment double booking has occurred, which may not be obvious on a standard ledger schedule. Computer programs require a large commitment to training and data entry. Computerization can also eliminate personal bias in the scheduling of case time. (See page 55: Computerization.)

9. D. HIPAA requires that attention be focused on protected health information. Each practice group must designate and appoint a "privacy officer." HIPAA provisions require that patient charts must be locked away overnight. Telephone calls and faxes must be handled with special care if they contain identifiable patient information. Patients' names may not be used on an information board (e.g., at the OR desk or in PACU) if there is any chance that anyone not directly involved in their care could see them. (See page 50: HIPAA.)

10. A. The Sherman Antitrust Act is more than 100 years old. Antitrust laws do not involve the right of individuals to engage in business but rather are solely concerned with the preservation of competition within a defined marketplace. The per se rule, which is rarely applied, makes conduct that obviously limits competition illegal. Another type of violation is the *rule of reason,* which involves a careful analysis of the market and that state of competition. (See page 44: Antitrust Considerations.)

11. A. The role of anesthesiologists in operating room management has changed dramatically in the past few years. The current emphasis on cost containment and efficiency necessitates anesthesiologists' involvement in operating room management. Anesthesiologists are in the best position to see the "big picture," both overall and on any given day. They are best qualified to provide leadership in the operating room because they spend a large portion of their time in the operating room. Surgeons, on the other hand, have commitments to their offices and sometimes to multiple facilities.

Block scheduling may work in some facilities that have a large number of surgeons who book far in advance and have very specific office and operating room schedules. However, some degree of open scheduling is necessary, depending on the number of add-on emergencies at a particular facility. Most large institutions use a combination of block scheduling and open scheduling.

Prudent drug selection combined with appropriate technique may produce substantial savings. Reducing fresh gas flow from 5 L/min to 2 L/min can save approximately $10 million per year in the United States.

Delineating the responsibility of "running the floor" to a selected few members of the department provides more consistency in decision making and application of the operating room policies. It helps individuals become very familiar with the nuances of managing the operating room schedule in real time. An individual's personality affects his or her ability in managing difficult surgeons in a consistent and fair manner.

The American Association of Clinical Directors in 2002 reported that 71% of survey respondents stated that an anesthesiologist was designated as the Clinical Director of the OR. (See page 51: Operating Room Management.)

12. B. It is important to establish an adverse event protocol in the department's policies and procedures manual. When a critical incident occurs, call for help. Establish an "incident supervisor" whose responsibility is to help prevent continuation or reoccurrence of the incident, investigate the incident, and ensure documentation while the original and helping anesthesiologists focus on caring for the patient. Consultants may be helpful and should be called without hesitation. The chief of anesthesiology, facility administrator, risk manager, and anesthesiologist's insurance company should be notified in a timely manner. If the surgeon is involved, he or she should notify the family first, but the anesthesiologist and others (risk managers, legal counsel, or insurance loss control officer) might appropriately be included. Full disclosure of the events as they are best known is currently believed to be the best presentation. Any attempt to conceal or shade the truth will only confound an already difficult situation.

There is a new movement in medical risk management advocating immediate full disclosure to the victim, including "confessions" of medical judgment and performance errors with attendant apologies. All discussions with the patient and family should be carefully documented in the medical record. Judgments about causes or responsibilities should not be made. One should never change an existing entry in the medical record. Only the facts, as they are known, should be stated.

After an adverse event, all involved equipment must be sequestered and not touched until such time as it is certain that it was not involved in the incident. (See page 39: Response to an Adverse Event.)

Occupational Health

1. Which of the following substances found in latex gloves is responsible for the majority of generalized allergic reactions?

   A. Preservatives
   B. Polyisoprenes
   C. Protein content
   D. Accelerators
   E. Powder

2. Which of the following statements concerning tuberculosis (TB) is FALSE?

   A. It is transmitted by bacilli carried on airborne particles.
   B. Using any face mask will prevent infection.
   C. Patients with HIV are at increased risk for infection.
   D. If surgery is required, bacterial filters (high-efficiency particulate filters) should be used on the anesthetic breathing circuit for patients with TB.
   E. Elective surgery should be postponed for infected patients.

3. Airborne precautions are an effective preventive measure against which of the following infectious agents?

   A. Cytomegalovirus (CMV)
   B. Tuberculosis (TB)
   C. Herpes simplex
   D. Herpetic whitlow
   E. All of the above

4. Signs of substance abuse inside the hospital include all of the following EXCEPT:

   A. Signing out large quantities of narcotics
   B. Refusing breaks
   C. Volunteering to relieve others and taking extra calls
   D. Disappearing between cases
   E. Their postoperative patients frequently are oversedated with opioids

5. All of the following statements about radiation exposure are true EXCEPT:

   A. The risk of exposure is not influenced by age or gender.
   B. Radiation exposure is inversely proportional to the square of the distance from the source.
   C. The magnitude of radiation absorbed by the individual is a function of total radiation intensity and time.
   D. The lead aprons and thyroid collars commonly worn leave many sites exposed to radiation.

6. Which of the following statements is TRUE regarding studies of anesthetic trends in the operating room and effects on fertility and childbearing?

   A. Scavenging anesthetic does not lower levels in operating rooms.
   B. It is difficult to quantify the levels of anesthetic in an operating room.
   C. There is a slight increase in the relative risk of congenital anomalies in the children of female physicians who work in operating rooms.
   D. Levels of anesthetic exposure are correlated with reproductive outcome.

7. Which of the following statements about methyl methacrylate is FALSE?

   A. Reported risks from repeated occupational exposure to methyl methacrylate include skin irritation, allergic reactions, and asthma.
   B. The Occupational Safety and Health Administration (OSHA) has established an 8-hour, time-weighted allowable exposure of 100 ppm of methyl methacrylate.
   C. Airborne concentrations greater than 170 ppm have been associated with chronic lung, liver, and kidney damage.
   D. When used properly, scavenging devices for venting methyl methacrylate vapor decrease the peak environmental concentration of vapor by only 25%.
   E. When methyl methacrylate is prepared in the operating room to cement prostheses to bone, concentrations of up to 280 ppm have been measured.

8. Which of the following statements regarding latex allergy is FALSE?

   A. The prevalence in anesthesia personnel is about 15%.
   B. Sensitivity to latex cannot be reversed simply by avoiding latex-containing compounds.
   C. Type IV reaction (T cell mediated) is the most severe allergic reaction seen with a latex allergy.
   D. Contact dermatitis accounts for the majority of reactions resulting from wearing latex gloves.
   E. Type I immediate hypersensitivity reactions may manifest by a localized contact dermatitis.

9. Which of the following statements concerning influenza viruses is FALSE?

   A. They are spread by coughing, sneezing, or talking via small particle aerosols.
   B. Vaccination with inactivated virus confers immunity for life.
   C. General anesthesia results in no increase of respiratory morbidity in asymptomatic patients infected with influenza virus.
   D. The flu vaccine changes yearly.
   E. The vaccine is based on viral strains.

10. Which of the following forms of hepatitis is primarily transmitted by blood?

    A. B, C, and D
    B. A, B, and C
    C. B and E
    D. E
    E. A and E

11. Which of the following form(s) of hepatitis can lead to a chronic carrier state?

    A. B, C, and D
    B. A, B, and C
    C. B and E
    D. E
    E. A and E

12. Which of the following statements is FALSE?

    A. Respiratory syncytial virus (RSV) can be recovered for up to 6 hours on contaminated environmental surfaces.
    B. Severe acute respiratory syndrome (SARS) is spread by close person-to-person contact.
    C. Transmission of cytomegalovirus (CMV) occurs through person-to-person contact but not by contact with contaminated urine or blood.
    D. Rubella infection can be associated with congenital malformations and fetal death if it is contracted during the first trimester of pregnancy.
    E. Severe acute respiratory syndrome (SARS) is spread by large respiratory droplets.

13. Which of the following statements concerning hepatitis B is FALSE?

    A. Contaminated dry blood on an environmental surface may be infectious for up to 1 day.
    B. Routine vaccination has reduced the risk of occupationally acquired hepatitis B virus (HBV) infection.
    C. The presence of hepatitis B surface antigen (HbSa) in serum indicates active viral replication in hepatocytes.
    D. The rate of transmission is significantly lower after mucosal contact with infected oral secretions than after percutaneous blood exposure.
    E. Risk of transmission is higher if the patient is positive for HbSa.

14. Which of the following has not been documented as a means for transmission of the human immunodeficiency virus (HIV)?

    A. Sexual contact
    B. Blood
    C. Perinatal transmission
    D. Tears

15. Which of the following statements is TRUE?

    A. The magnitude of radiation absorbed is a function of the distance from the source of radiation and the use of radiation shielding, but not of total exposure intensity.
    B. Radiation exposure is proportional to the square of the distance from the source.
    C. Radiation exposure becomes minimal at a distance greater than 36 inches from the source.
    D. Wearing a thyroid collar in addition to a lead apron protects virtually all vulnerable sites.

16. Which of the following statements is TRUE regarding cancer?

    A. Lymphoid malignancies are an occupational hazard for anesthesiologists.
    B. Male anesthesiologists have a higher risk of malignancy than female anesthesiologists.
    C. There is no difference in overall mortality from cancer in female anesthesiologists compared to internists.
    D. Men exposed to trace concentrations of anesthetic gases have higher cancer rates than those not exposed.

ANSWERS

1. C. Latex is a complex substance that contains polyisoprenes, lipids, phospholipids, and proteins. Numerous additional substances, including preservatives, accelerators, antioxidants, vulcanizing compounds, and lubricating agents, are added to latex gloves. The protein content is responsible for causing the majority of allergic reactions. These reactions are exacerbated by the presence of powder that enhances the potential of latex particles to aerosolize and spread to the respiratory system of personnel and to environmental surfaces during donning and removing gloves. (See page 62: Physical Hazards: Allergic Reactions.)

2. B. Use of a special mask that is fitted to the person wearing it and that is capable of filtering particles 1 to 5 mm in diameter is required to protect health care workers from patients with active TB. (See page 69: Infectious Hazards: Tuberculosis.)

3. B. Preventive measures for the listed infectious agents are as follows: CMV, standard precautions; TB, airborne precautions and isoniazid or ethambutol for purified protein derivative conversion; herpes simplex, standard precautions and contact precautions if disseminated disease is present. (See page 69: Table 3-4, OSHA Standards, Standard Precautions, and Transmission-based Precautions.)

4. E. Signing out large quantities of narcotics, refusing breaks, volunteering to relieve others, disappearing between cases, weight loss, pale skin, pinpoint pupils, and taking extra calls are all signs of substance abuse. Addicts also have unusual changes in behavior, have sloppy charts, and want to work alone to divert narcotics for personal use. They are difficult to find between cases. Their patients often complain of pain in the recovery room. (See page 79: Table 3-7, Emotional Considerations: Substance Use, Abuse, and Addiction.)

5. A. The magnitude of radiation absorbed by individuals is a function of three variables: (1) total radiation exposure, intensity, and time; (2) distance from the source of radiation; and (3) the use of radiation shielding. Unfortunately, the lead aprons and thyroid collars commonly worn leave exposed many vulnerable sites, such as the long bones of the extremities, the cranium, the skin of the face, and the eyes. Since radiation exposure is inversely proportional to the square of the distance from the source, increasing this distance is more universally protective. The risks associated with radiation vary considerably depending on age, gender, and specific organ site exposure. (See page 62: Physical Hazards: Radiation.)

6. C. The use of scavenging techniques lowers the environmental anesthetic levels in operating rooms. Review of existing epidemiologic studies suggests a slight increase in the relative risk of spontaneous abortion and congenital anomalies in the children of female physicians working in operating rooms. Although it is easy to quantify the levels of anesthetic in an operating room, it is harder to assess the effects of other factors such as stress, fatigue, and alterations in work schedule. Levels of anesthetic exposure have not correlated with reproductive outcome. (See page 62: Physical Hazards: Anesthetic Gases.)

7. D. When methyl methacrylate is prepared in the operating room to cement prostheses to bone, concentrations of up to 280 ppm have been measured. Scavenging devices for venting the vapor can decrease peak concentrations by 75%. OSHA has established an 8-hour, time-weighted average allowable exposure of 100 ppm. Airborne concentrations greater than 170 ppm have been associated with chronic lung, liver, and kidney damage. Reported risks from occupational exposure include allergic reactions and asthma, dermatitis, eye irritation, headache, and neurologic signs, which may occur at levels below the OSHA cutoffs. (See page 62: Physical Hazards: Chemicals.)

8. C. Irritant or contact dermatitis accounts for the majority of reactions resulting from wearing latex-containing gloves. The prevalence of latex sensitivity among anesthesiologists is 15%. Type I immediate hypersensitivity reactions may manifest by a localized contact dermatitis or a generalized systemic response. True allergic reactions present as type IV (T-cell–mediated contact dermatitis) and the more severe type I (immunoglobulin E–mediated anaphylactic) reactions. Sensitivity cannot be reversed. (See page 62: Physical Hazards: Allergic Reactions.)

9. B. Influenza viruses are easily transmitted by small particle aerosols (sneezing, coughing, or talking). General anesthesia results in no increase in respiratory morbidity in asymptomatic patients infected with influenza virus. Antigenic variation of influenza viruses occurs over time, so new viral strains (usually two type A and one type B) are selected for inclusion in each year's vaccine. Since the virus has antigenic variation from year to year, immunity is not for life. (See page 69: Infectious Hazards: Respiratory Viruses: Influenza Viruses.)

10. A. Hepatitis A is primarily transmitted by the fecal–oral route. Hepatitis B, C, and D are transmitted by blood. Hepatitis E is enterically transmitted. (See page 69: Infectious Hazards: Viral Hepatitis.)

11. A. Hepatitis B, C, and D can progress to chronic hepatitis and a chronic carrier state. (See page 69: Infectious Hazards: Viral Hepatitis.)

12. C. RSV can be recovered for up to 6 hours on contaminated environmental surfaces. SARS is spread by close person-to-person contact, large respiratory droplets, and possibly airborne transmission. Transmission of CMV occurs through person-to-person contact and contact with contaminated urine or blood. Rubella infection may be associated with congenital malformations and fetal death if it is contracted during the first trimester of pregnancy. (See page 69: Infectious Hazards.)

13. A. HBV may be infectious for at least 1 week in dried blood on environmental surfaces. The rate of transmission is lower after mucosal contact with infected oral secretions than after percutaneous blood exposure. Routine vaccinations, use of safety devices, and postexposure prophylaxis have significantly reduced the risk of occupationally acquired HBV infection. The presence of HbSa in serum indicates active viral replication in hepatocytes and increases the risk of transmission. (See page 69: Infectious Hazards: Viral Hepatitis.)

14. D. HIV may be transmitted by sexual contact, exposure to contaminated blood, and perinatally. It can be found in saliva, tears, and urine, but these body fluids have not been implicated in viral transmission. (See page 69: Infectious Hazards: Pathogenic Human Retroviruses.)

15. C. Radiation exposure is inversely proportional to the square of the distance from the source. Lead aprons and thyroid collars leave many vulnerable sites exposed, such as the long bones of the extremities, the cranium, the skin on the face, and the eyes. The magnitude of radiation absorbed by operating room personnel is a function of the distance from the source of radiation, the use of radiation shielding, and total exposure intensity. Radiation exposure becomes minimal at a distance greater than 36 inches from the source. (See page 62: Physical Hazards: Radiation.)

16. C. Although a 1968 report concluded that male anesthesiologists had an increased risk of malignancies of the lymphoid and reticuloendothelial tissues, data from a subsequent prospective study by the same group contradicted the original findings and found no evidence that lymphoid malignancies were an occupational hazard for anesthesiologists. A 1974 ASA-sponsored study (*vide supra*) found no differences in cancer rates between men exposed and those not exposed to trace concentrations of anesthetic gases. There was a 1.3- to 2-fold increase in the occurrence of various forms of cancer among exposed women, predominantly from an increase in leukemia and lymphoma. The subsequent re-analysis of these data confirmed an increase in relative risk of cancer in exposed women (RR—1.4) but attributed the increase solely to cervical cancer (RR—2.8). ASA-sponsored study of anesthesiologists, covering the period from 1976 to 1995, used data on cause of death from the National Death Index. The mortality risks of a cohort of 40,242 anesthesiologists were compared with a matched cohort of internists. There was no difference between the two groups in overall mortality risk or mortality from cancer. (See page 62: Physical Hazards: Cancer).

CHAPTER 4

Anesthetic Risk, Quality Improvement, and Liability

1. All the following statements are true EXCEPT:

    A. The duty that the anesthesiologist owes the patient is to be a prudent and reasonable physician.
    B. Obtaining informed consent is a responsibility that all physicians have to their patients.
    C. Punitive damages are intended to punish the physician for negligence.
    D. Causation refers to the fact that a reasonably close causal relation exists between the anesthesiologist's acts and the resultant injury.
    E. General damages are actual damages that are a consequence of the injury, such as medical expenses.

2. The court establishes "standard of care" through all of these EXCEPT:

    A. Factual witness
    B. Expert witness
    C. Published societal guidelines
    D. Textbooks
    E. Written hospital policies

3. Which of the following statements concerning risk management and quality improvement is TRUE?

    A. Quality improvement is broadly oriented toward reducing the liability exposure of the organization.
    B. Quality improvement is concerned with patient safety, but risk management is not.
    C. Risk management's exclusive goal is the reduction of institutional liability by maintenance and improvement of patient care.
    D. Risk management involves professional liability, contracts, employee safety, and public safety.
    E. Quality improvement is concerned primarily with liability exposure of the institution.

4. All of the following statements concerning record keeping are true EXCEPT:

    A. Good records can form a strong defense in the face of malpractice litigation.
    B. Change of anesthetic personnel should be documented.

    C. The anesthesiologist's report of a catastrophic event need not be consistent with concurrent records because inconsistencies are easy to defend.
    D. A record-keeping error should be crossed out yet remain legible.
    E. Catastrophic events should be documented in narrative form in the patient's progress notes.

5. The National Practitioner Data Bank (NPDB) requires input from all of the following EXCEPT:

    A. Medical malpractice payment
    B. Licensing actions by medical boards
    C. Patient safety foundations
    D. Clinical privilege actions by hospitals
    E. Actions taken by the Drug Enforcement Agency (DEA)

6. Which statement about continuous quality improvement (CQI) is FALSE?

    A. The focus of CQI is not on blame but rather on identification of the causes of undesirable outcomes.
    B. CQI continually tries to identify random errors and prevent them from recurring.
    C. CQI assumes that the operator is just one part of a complex system.
    D. After areas in need of improvement are identified by CQI programs, outcomes are measured and documented.
    E. CQI is instituted from the bottom up, not from the administrators down.

7. Pay for performance:

    A. Is a program that pays physicians for the hours they work rather than for services
    B. Is a program that provides money to hospitals that service Medicare and Medicaid patients
    C. Is a program that provides monetary incentives for implementation of safe practices
    D. Has been a part of quality improvement since its inception
    E. Is a program that ranks doctors' abilities and pays them according to their rankings

8. For a malpractice suit against a physician to succeed, the patient/plaintiff must prove all of the following EXCEPT:

   A. Breach of duty
   B. Loss of income
   C. Causation
   D. Duty
   E. Damages

9. Considering the cause of lawsuits against anesthesiologists, which of the following statements is FALSE?

   A. Lawsuits regarding death and brain damage injury are usually attributed to airway management problems.
   B. Ulnar nerve injury often occurs despite apparently adequate positioning.
   C. Anesthesia is a high-risk endeavor because of the use of complex equipment and potent drugs.
   D. The leading injury for suits against anesthesiologists is brain damage.
   E. Relatively few adverse outcomes end up in a malpractice suit.

10. When a plaintiff's attorney files a complaint, the anesthesiologist should take certain actions EXCEPT:

    A. Gather all pertinent records including billing statements.
    B. Cooperate fully with the attorney provided by the insurer.
    C. Discuss the case with all involved operating room personnel.
    D. Refrain from making alterations to the chart.
    E. Make a detailed account of all events.

11. If a physician is deposed by a plaintiff's attorney, the physician should do which of the following?

    A. Never attempt to change his or her image by dressing conservatively.
    B. Volunteer all information he or she has about the case.
    C. Not spend too much time preparing so the responses do not seem to be rehearsed.
    D. Rely on his or her attorney for assistance when preparing.
    E. Ask for a settlement offer.

12. Concerning Jehovah's Witnesses and blood transfusions, which of the following statements is TRUE?

    A. Physicians are obligated to treat all patients who apply for treatment, even if they refuse to have a blood transfusion.
    B. Parents of a minor child may legally prevent that child from receiving blood.
    C. Any agreement regarding transfusion of a Jehovah's Witness patient should be documented in the medical record.
    D. **All** Jehovah's Witnesses will accept an autotransfusion if their blood has left their body via continuous tubing.
    E. All Jehovah's Witnesses have identical belief regarding blood transfusions.

13. When considering the National Practitioner Data Bank (NPDB), which of the following statements is FALSE?

    A. After a report is submitted to the NPDB, the physician may dispute the input.
    B. Creation of the NPDB has encouraged physicians to settle nuisance suits because their names are not added to the database.
    C. A practitioner may query the NPDB about his or her file at any time.
    D. The NPDB is a nationwide information system.
    E. It is the obligation of the HOSPITAL risk management DEPARTMENT to make reports and inquiries to the NPDB.

14. Considering quality improvement programs, which of the following statements is TRUE?

    A. "Pay for performance" falls outside the domain of quality improvement.
    B. Critical incidents are events that cause or have the potential to cause patient injury if they are not noticed and corrected in a timely manner.
    C. Quality improvement outcome studies are easily applied to the field of anesthesia because it has a high rate of catastrophic outcomes.
    D. Sentinel events are events with poor outcomes that are directly related to operator actions.
    E. Quality is a concept that is easily defined in medical practice.

ANSWERS

1. E. In most general terms, the duty that the anesthesiologist owes to the patient is to adhere to the "standard of care" for the patient's treatment. Since it is virtually impossible to delineate specific standards for all aspects of medical practice, the courts have created the concept of the "reasonable and prudent physician." One of the general duties of the physician is obtaining informed consent for procedures. The requirement that the consent be "informed" is somewhat more opaque. The definition of *causation* is that a reasonably close causal relation exists between the anesthesiologist's acts and the resultant injury. Breach of duty is the failure of an anesthesiologist to fulfill his or her duty. The court will try to find that the anesthesiologist either did something that should not have been done or failed to do something that should have been done by a prudent and reasonable physician. General damages are those such as pain and suffering that directly result from the injury. Special damages are actual damages that are a consequence of the injury, such as medical expenses, loss of income, and funeral expenses. Punitive damages are intended to punish the physician for negligence that was reckless, wanton, fraudulent, or willful. (See page 99: Professional Liability.)

2. A. In most general terms, the duty that the anesthesiologist owes to the patient is to adhere to the "standard of care" for the treatment of the patient. Since medical practice usually includes issues beyond the comprehension of lay jurors and judges, the court establishes a standard of care for a particular case by the testimony of "expert witnesses." These witnesses differ from factual witnesses mainly in that they are allowed to give opinions. When a physician is called to court as the defendant in a malpractice suit, he or she becomes a factual witness. The standard of care may also be determined from published societal guidelines, written policies of a hospital or department, and textbooks and monographs. (See page 100: Standard of Care.)

3. D. Risk management and quality improvement programs work hand in hand to minimize liability and maximize quality of patient care. The two programs overlap their focus on patient safety. A hospital risk management program is broadly oriented toward reducing the liability exposure of the organization. This includes not only professional liability (and therefore patient safety), but also contracts, employee safety, public safety, and any other liability exposure of the institution. The main goals of quality improvement programs are the maintenance and improvement of the quality of patient care. (See page 91: Risk Management.)

4. C. Good records can form a strong defense if they are adequate, and inadequate records can be disastrous. The anesthetic record itself should be accurate, complete, and as neat as possible. In addition to the patient's vital signs recorded every 5 minutes, special attention should be paid to ensure that the American Society of Anesthesiologists classification, monitors used, fluids administered, and doses and times of drugs given are accurately charted. All respiratory variables that are monitored should be documented. It is important to note that when a change of anesthesia personnel occurs during the conduct of a case. If a critical incident occurs during the conduct of an anesthetic regimen, the anesthesiologist should document in *narrative form* in the patient's progress notes what happened, which drugs were used, what the time sequence was, and who was present. A catastrophic intra-anesthetic event cannot be summarized adequately in a small amount of space on the usual anesthetic record. The report should be as consistent as possible with concurrent records such as those pertaining to the anesthetic, the operating room, the recovery room, and cardiac arrest. (See page 91: Risk Management in Anesthesia.)

5. C. The NPDB is a nationwide information system that theoretically allows licensing boards and hospitals a means of detecting adverse information about physicians. The NPDB requires input from five sources: Medical malpractice payments, licensing actions by medical boards, clinical privilege actions by hospitals and professional societies, actions by the DEA, and Medicare and Medicaid exclusions. (See page 96: National Practitioner Data Bank.)

6. B. CQI takes a systems approach to identifying and improving quality. A CQI program may focus on undesirable outcomes as a way to identify opportunities for improvement in the structure and process of care. The focus is not on blame but rather on identification of the causes of undesirable outcomes. CQI assumes that the operator is just one part of a complex system. Random errors are inherently difficult to prevent, and programs focused in this direction are misguided. System errors, however, should be controllable, and strategies to minimize them should be within reach. After areas for improvement have been identified, their current status is measured and documented. If a change is identified that should lead to improvement, it is implemented. It is a process that is instituted from the bottom up by those who are actually involved in the process to be improved rather than from the top down by administrators. (See page 97: Quality Improvement and Patient Safety in Anesthesia.)

7. C. A relatively recent development related to quality improvement is P4P, or "pay for performance." P4P programs provide monetary incentives for implementation of safe practices, measuring performance, and achieving performance goals. This is a recent and evolving trend. (See page 98: Pay for Performance.)

8. B. "Malpractice" is a lay term that refers to professional negligence pursued in the legal system of civil laws. A successful malpractice suit must prove four things: (1) Duty, that the anesthesiologist owed the patient a duty; (2) breach of duty, that the anesthesiologist failed to fulfill his or her duty; (3) causation, that a reasonably close causal relationship exists between the anesthesiologist's acts and the resultant injury; and (4) damages, that actual damage resulted because of a breach in the standard of care. (See page 99: The Tort System.)

9. D. The leading causes of lawsuits against anesthesiologists are death (22%), nerve damage (21%), and brain damage (10%). The causes of death and brain damage are predominantly problems with airway management. In the past, ulnar nerve injury was the most common cause of nerve damage claims, and it often occurs despite apparent adequate positioning. In the 1990s, spinal cord injury led the list. Anesthesia is a high-risk endeavor for many reasons. The anesthesiologist is likely to be the target of a lawsuit if an untoward outcome occurs because the physician–patient relationship is usually tenuous at best. (See page 100: Causes of Anesthesia-related Lawsuits.)

10. C. A lawsuit begins when the patient/plaintiff's attorney files a complaint. The anesthesiologist needs assistance in answering the complaint. Specific actions that should be taken at this point include the following: (1) Do not discuss the case with anyone, including colleagues who may have been involved, operating personnel, or friends; (2) never alter any records; (3) gather all pertinent records, including copies of the anesthetic record, billing statements, and any correspondence concerning the case; (4) make notes recording all events recalled about the case; and (5) cooperate fully with the attorneys provided by the insurer. (See page 101: What to Do When Sued.)

11. D. After a complaint has been filed, the malpractice suit moves on to the discovery phase. A deposition is the second mechanism of discovery. The plaintiff's attorney deposes the anesthesiologist, and the anesthesiologist must be constantly aware that what is said during the deposition carries as much weight as what is said in court. It is important to be factually prepared for the deposition. Review of notes, anesthetic records, and medical records is necessary. The physician should dress conservatively and professionally. Information should never be volunteered. The physician should rely on his or her attorney for assistance when preparing for a deposition. (See page 101: What to Do When Sued.)

12. C. The religious beliefs of Jehovah's Witnesses preclude them from receiving blood or blood products. Physicians are not obligated to treat all patients who apply for treatment. A physician has the right to refuse to care for a patient in an elective situation if the patient unacceptably limits the physician's ability to provide optimal care. Together, the physician and patient may decide to limit the physician's obligation to adhere to the patient's religious beliefs. Any agreement should be documented clearly in the medical record. It is true that some patients will not allow any blood that has left the body to be infused, but others will accept transfusion if the blood remains in constant contact with the body via tubing. Parents of a minor child may not legally prevent that child from receiving blood. (See page 96: Special Circumstances: "Do Not Attempt Resuscitation" and Jehovah's Witnesses.)

13. B. The NPDB is a nationwide information system that theoretically allows licensing boards and hospitals a means of detecting adverse information about physicians. A practitioner may query the NPDB any time about his or her file. After a report has been submitted, the physician is notified and may dispute the input. The existence of the NPDB reporting requirements has made physicians reluctant to allow settlement of nuisance suits because doing so would cause their names to be added to the data bank. It is usually the obligation of the hospital risk management department to make reports and inquiries to the NPDB. (See page 96: National Practitioner Data Bank.)

14. B. Quality is a concept that has continued to elude precise definition in medical practice. It is generally accepted that attention to quality will improve patient safety and satisfaction. Quality improvement programs are generally guided by requirements of The Joint Commission (formerly the Joint Commission on Accreditation of Healthcare Organizations [JCAHO]). However, adverse outcomes are relatively rare in anesthesia practices, making measurement of improvement difficult. To complement outcome measurements, anesthesia quality improvement programs may focus on critical incidents and sentinel events. Critical incidents are events that cause or have the potential to cause patient injury if they are not noticed and corrected in a timely manner. Sentinel events are single, isolated events that may indicate a systematic problem. "Pay for performance" is an evolving trend in quality improvement programs. (See page 97: Quality Improvement and Patient Safety in Anesthesia.)

Scientific Foundations of Anesthesia

CHAPTER 5

Mechanisms of Anesthesia and Consciousness

1. For volatile anesthetics, potency is proportional to:

   A. Lipid solubility
   B. Vapor pressure
   C. Critical temperature
   D. Minimum alveolar concentration (MAC)
   E. None of the above

2. The Meyer–Overton rule:

   A. Correlates the potency of anesthetic gases with their solubility in oil
   B. Suggests the anesthetic target site to be hydrophilic in nature
   C. Is contradicted by the unitary theory of anesthesia
   D. Applies only to liquids
   E. Applies only to gases that never exist in the liquid state

3. In humans, the definition of minimum alveolar concentration (MAC) is:

   A. The alveolar partial pressure of a gas at which 50% of humans will not mount a sympathetic response.
   B. The alveolar partial pressure of a gas at which 50% of humans will not respond to a surgical incision.
   C. The alveolar partial pressure of a gas at which 30% of humans will not respond to a surgical incision.
   D. The alveolar partial pressure of a gas at which 50% of subjects remain unresponsive to verbal stimuli.
   E. The alveolar partial pressure of a gas at which 50% of subjects will follow a simple command.

4. General anesthesia results from interruption of nervous system activity at all of the following levels, EXCEPT:

   A. Cerebral cortex
   B. Spinal cord
   C. Brainstem
   D. Peripheral sensory receptors
   E. Thalamic centers

5. Which of the following statements is FALSE?

   A. γ-Aminobutyric acid (GABA) is an excitatory neurotransmitter.
   B. Volatile anesthetics modulate GABA receptor function.
   C. Benzodiazepines act at GABA receptors.
   D. Barbiturates and etomidate act at GABA receptors.
   E. GABA mediated effects involve chloride influx.

6. General anesthetics have been shown to inhibit excitatory synaptic transmission in all of the following centers, EXCEPT:

   A. Sympathetic ganglia
   B. Olfactory cortex
   C. Hippocampus
   D. Spinal cord
   E. Locus ceruleus

7. Important features of minimum alveolar concentration (MAC) include all of the following, EXCEPT:

   A. MAC represents the average response of a whole population of subjects rather than the response of a single subject.
   B. MAC can only be directly applied to anesthetic gases.
   C. MAC does not reflect the end-tidal concentration at which there is loss of response to verbal stimuli.
   D. The MAC end point in a MAC determination is relative rather than quantal.
   E. Monitors do not reliably measure awareness.

ANSWERS

1. A. In its simplest incarnation, the lipid theory of anesthesia postulates that anesthetics dissolve in the lipid bilayers of biologic membranes and produce anesthesia when they reach a critical concentration in the membrane. Consistent with this hypothesis, the membrane/gas partition coefficients of anesthetic gases in pure lipid bilayers correlate strongly with anesthetic potency. (See page 110: Lipid Theories of Anesthesia.)

2. A. More than 100 years ago, Meyer and Overton independently observed that the potency of gases as anesthetics was strongly correlated with their solubility in olive oil. Since a wide variety of structurally unrelated compounds obey the Meyer–Overton rule, it has been reasoned that all anesthetics are likely to act at the same molecular site. This idea is referred to as the *Unitary Theory of Anesthesia*. It has also been argued that since solubility in a specific solvent strongly correlates with anesthetic potency, the solvent showing the strongest correlation between anesthetic solubility and potency is likely to most closely mimic the chemical and physical properties of the anesthetic target site in the CNS. Based on this reasoning, the anesthetic target site was assumed to be hydrophobic in nature. Since olive oil/gas partition coefficients can be determined for gases and volatile liquids, but not for liquid anesthetics, attempts have been made to correlate anesthetic potency with solvent/water partition coefficients. (See page 109: The Meyer–Overton Rule.)

3. B. MAC, or minimum alveolar concentration, is defined as the alveolar partial pressure of a gas at which 50% of humans do not respond to a surgical incision. In animals, MAC is defined as the alveolar partial pressure of a gas at which 50% of animals do not respond to a noxious stimulus, such as tail clamp, or at which they lose their righting reflex. (See page 109: How Is Anesthesia Measured?)

4. D. Several lines of evidence indicate that the spinal cord is the main site at which anesthetics act to inhibit movement in response to noxious stimulation. This is, of course, the end point used in most measurements of anesthetic potency. Some studies suggest not only that anesthetic action at the spinal cord underlies MAC, but also that anesthetic action on the brain may actually sensitize the cord to noxious stimuli. Also, several in vitro electrophysiologic studies have demonstrated inhibition of excitatory synaptic transmission in the spinal cord by volatile anesthetics, arguing that they act, at least in part, directly on spinal neurons. Recent work has revealed that neurons in the mesencephalic locomotor region may be responsible for supraspinal augmentation of locomotor circuits in the spinal cord at concentrations below 1 MAC. Different anesthetics inhibit the sensory neurons in the dorsal horn or motor neurons in the ventral horn. The thalamus has been postulated as a likely target for anesthetic ablation of consciousness but the precise mechanisms remains unclear. (See page 122: Where in the Central Nervous System Do Anesthetics Work?)

5. A. GABA is the most important inhibitory neurotransmitter in the mammalian CNS. GABA-activated ion channels (GABA$_A$ receptors) mediate the postsynaptic response to synaptically released GABA by selectively allowing chloride ions to enter and thereby hyperpolarize neurons. The function of GABA$_A$ receptors is modulated by a wide variety of pharmacologic agents including convulsants, anticonvulsants, sedatives, anxiolytics, and anesthetics. Barbiturates, benzodiazepines, propofol, etomidate, and volatile anesthetics all have been shown to modulate GABA receptor function. (See page 116: Anesthetic Effects on Ligand-gated Ion Channels: GABA-activated Ion Channels.)

6. E. Synaptic transmission is widely considered to be the most likely subcellular site of general anesthetic action. General anesthetics inhibit excitatory synaptic transmission in a variety of preparations, including sympathetic ganglia, olfactory cortex, hippocampus, and spinal cord. (See page 112: How Do Anesthetics Interfere with the Electrophysiologic Function of the Nervous System? Synaptic Function.)

7. D. MAC is defined as the alveolar partial pressure of a gas at which 50% of humans do not respond to a surgical incision. In animals, MAC is defined as the alveolar partial pressure of a gas at which 50% of animals do not respond to a noxious stimulus, such as tail clamp, or at which they lose their righting reflex. The MAC concept has several important limitations, particularly when trying to relate MAC values to anesthetic potency observed in vitro. First, the end point in a MAC determination is quantal: A subject is either anesthetized or unanesthetized; he or she cannot be partially anesthetized. Furthermore, MAC represents the average response of a whole population of subjects rather than the response of a single subject. Another limitation of MAC measurements is that they can only be directly applied to anesthetic gases. Parenteral anesthetics (barbiturates, neurosteroids, propofol) cannot be assigned a MAC value, making it difficult to compare the potency of parenteral and volatile anesthetics. A further limitation of MAC is that it is highly dependent on the anesthetic end point used to define it. For example, if loss of response to verbal commands is used as an anesthetic end point, the MAC values obtained (MAC-awake) will be much lower than classic MAC values based on response to a noxious stimulus. The most popular of the anesthetic depth monitors converts spontaneous electroencephalogram waveforms into a single value that correlates with anesthetic depth for some general anesthetics. To date, these monitors have not been shown to be more effective at preventing awareness during anesthesia. (See page 109: How Is Anesthesia Measured?)

Genomic Basis of Perioperative Medicine

Match the following genetic terms with the appropriate definitions:

1. Mutation
2. Polymorphism
3. Indels
4. Haplotypes
5. Allele

A. DNA sequence alternatives
B. Insertion or deletion of one or more nucleotides
C. Nucleotide polymorphisms inherited in blocks
D. Rare genetic variants
E. Widespread DNA sequence variations

6. The term used to refer to nearby single nucleotide polymorphisms on a chromosome that are inherited in blocks is:

   A. Alleles
   B. Haplotypes
   C. Polymorphic mutations
   D. Indels
   E. Phenotype

7. One of the most common inherited prothrombotic risk factors is a point mutation in which factor?

   A. Factor II
   B. Factor V
   C. Factor VII
   D. Factor XI
   E. Factor XII

8. After cardiac surgery, what is the incidence of significant neurologic morbidity (ranging from focal stroke to coma)?

   A. 0.1% to 0.2%
   B. 1% to 3%
   C. 10% to 15%
   D. 20% to 30%
   E. >40%

9. Malignant hyperthermia follows what pattern of inheritance?

   A. Autosomal dominant
   B. Autosomal recessive
   C. X-linked dominant
   D. X-linked recessive
   E. It is not an inherited disease

10. A point mutation in the gene encoding for which receptor has been shown to render the patient insensitive to the immobilizing actions of both etomidate and propofol?

    A. β_2 subunit of the $GABA_A$ receptor
    B. α_{2A}-adrenergic receptor
    C. NMDA receptor
    D. β_3 subunit of the $GABA_A$ receptor
    E. $5-HT_3$ receptor

11. What is a "knockout" animal?

    A. An animal that misexpresses an additional gene
    B. An animal that overexpresses an additional gene
    C. A kangaroo with boxing gloves
    D. An animal with a nonfunctional gene
    E. An animal with a gene predisposing to sleep

12. Our understanding of pain has been increased by mice with knockout genes for:

    A. Substance P
    B. Opioid transmitters
    C. Nerve growth factors
    D. All of the above
    E. None of the above

13. Numerous clinical trials attempting to block single inflammatory mediators in patients with sepsis have been largely unsuccessful. Which of the following best explains the lack of success?

    A. Large tertiary care centers have a low incidence of septic shock.
    B. There is a lack of clinical investigators with an interest in septic shock.
    C. The genes themselves are distorted by septic shock.
    D. Cascades of biologic pathways interact in complex and redundant ways making the standard "single gene" paradigm insufficient to adequately describe the tissue response to severe systemic stimuli.
    E. The specimens become contaminated by toxins.

ANSWERS

1. D.

2. E.

3. B.

4. C.

5. A. *Perioperative genomics* applies functional genomics into clinical practice. Physicians need to understand the patterns of human genome variation and its methods of study. *Mutations* are rare genetic variations that have been identified with more than 1,500 disorders. *Polymorphism* refers to widespread population-based DNA variations. *Indels* are insertions and deletions of nucleotides. Single nucleotide polymorphisms inherited in blocks are referred to as haplotypes. *Alleles* are DNA sequence alternatives that contribute to either mutant variants or polymorphism within a population. (See page 132: Overview of Human Genetic Variation.)

6. B. Haplotypes are inherited in blocks, and an analysis of these can be useful in discovering diseased genes. An indel is an insertion or deletion of one or more nucleotides. (See page 132: Overview of Human Genetic Variation.)

7. B. A point mutation in coagulation factor V results in resistance to activated protein C and is commonly known as factor V Leiden. This factor has been associated with thromboses in the postoperative setting. (See page 137: Predictive Biomarkers for Perioperative Adverse Cardiac Events.)

8. B. The incidence of coma and focal stroke after cardiac surgery is approximately 1% to 3%. More subtle deficits occur in up to 69% of patients. This variability in neurologic deficit is poorly explained by risk factors related to the procedure. The role of apolipoprotein E genotypes in relation to modulating the inflammatory response, extent of aortic atheroma, and cerebral blood flow and autoregulation may explain the observed associations with poor neurologic outcomes. (See page 143: Predictive Biomarkers of Adverse Perioperative Neurological Outcomes.)

9. A. Malignant hyperthermia is a rare autosomal dominant genetic disease of skeletal muscle calcium metabolism. Susceptibility to malignant hyperthermia has been linked to the ryanodine receptor gene locus on chromosome 19. (See page 145: Genetics of Malignant Hyperthermia.)

10. D. A point mutation in the gene encoding the β_3 subunit of the $GABA_A$ receptor previously known to render the receptor insensitive to etomidate and propofol in vitro, was validated in vivo by creating a knockout mouse strain that proved also essentially insensitive to the immobilizing actions of etomidate and propofol. (See page 146: Genetic Variability and Response to Anesthetic Agents.)

11. D. "Knockout" animals are created by inserting a vector with a disrupted gene into an animal. Typically, a mouse is used. The goal is to achieve two nonfunctioning alleles so that a gene is not expressed. This is done to study specific functions of specific genes. Animals that misexpress or overexpress a gene are termed "transgenic." (See page 146: Genetic Variability and Response to Anesthetic Agents.)

12. D. Multiple genes appear to mediate sensitivity to noxious stimuli and chronically painful exposure. Various knockout mice missing functional genes for neurotrophins, nerve growth factors, substance P, opioid transmitters, and nonopioid transmitters and their receptors have significantly contributed to our knowledge of pain processing. (See page 146: Genetic Variability and Response to Pain.)

13. D. At the cell level, various cascades and pathways are triggered when an organism is stressed. These pathways are often interrelated and work to both increase and suppress gene expression. Since negative and positive feedback occur in a complex manner, attempts to study the expression of a single gene (products such as tumor necrosis factor-α) have been difficult. (See page 148: Functional Genomics of Injury.)

CHAPTER 7

Basic Principles of Clinical Pharmacology

1. Which of the following statements concerning passage of drugs across membranes is FALSE?

    A. Small lipophilic drugs can passively diffuse across cell membranes.
    B. The walls of most capillaries do not allow passage of water-soluble drugs.
    C. Active transport is able to shuttle proteins against their concentration gradient.
    D. Thiopental easily crosses cell membranes.
    E. The capillaries of the central nervous system (CNS) do not allow passive transport of water-soluble drugs.

2. Which of the following statements about drug distribution to the central nervous system (CNS) is FALSE?

    A. Equilibration in the brain and muscle does not occur simultaneously.
    B. Diffusion of water-soluble drugs into the brain is severely restricted.
    C. For more polar compounds, the rate of entry into the brain is proportional to their lipid solubility.
    D. Distribution of highly lipid-soluble drugs into the CNS is directly proportional to cerebral blood flow.
    E. Recovery from a single dose of thiopental depends primarily on hepatic elimination.

3. Elimination half-life:

    A. Is not influenced by drug distribution
    B. Is not influenced by drug elimination
    C. Is the time it takes the amount of drug in the vessel-rich group to decrease by 50%
    D. Is not influenced by age
    E. Is the time it takes the amount of drug in the body to decrease by 50%

4. Which statement about drug elimination is FALSE?

    A. Elimination can occur by excretion of unchanged drug.
    B. Metabolism is a step in some drug clearance.
    C. The liver and kidney are the most important organs in drug elimination.
    D. The liver eliminates drugs primarily by excretion.
    E. The kidney primarily excretes water-soluble, polar compounds.

5. Which of the following statements concerning the volume of drug distribution and clearance is TRUE?

    A. The smaller the volume of distribution, the longer the half-time of elimination.
    B. The calculated volume of steady-state distribution can exceed the actual volume of the body.
    C. The volume of distribution is equal to the total amount of drug present divided by plasma volume and vessel-rich group volume.
    D. The volume of distribution provides information regarding the tissues into which the drug distributes and the concentration in those tissues.
    E. The volume of distribution cannot be as small as the plasma volume.

6. If 10 mg of drug is present and the plasma concentration is 2 mg/L, then the volume of distribution (V_d) is _____ L.

    A. 5
    B. 50
    C. 500
    D. 20
    E. 0.2

7. Which statement regarding altered hepatic and/or renal function is FALSE?

    A. Drug doses must be altered in patients with decreased hepatic and renal function.
    B. Liver disease decreases drugs' clearance.
    C. Acute renal failure requires a change in drug doses.
    D. Patients compensate for chronic renal failure, so drug doses should not be changed in these patients.
    E. Age decreases renal function.

8. Which of the following statements is FALSE?

    A. Cytochrome P450 (CYP) accounts for 45% of all drug metabolism.
    B. CYP are found in liver, lung, and kidneys.
    C. CYP are involved in secretion of hormones, cholesterol, and prostaglandins.
    D. Phase 2 biotransformations occur via CYP system.
    E. CYP system protects the organism against various toxins.

9. Which of the following statements concerning hepatic clearance is FALSE?

   A. If the extraction ratio (and intrinsic clearance) is very high, then total hepatic clearance will be proportional to hepatic blood flow.
   B. Clearance of drugs with low extraction ratios occurs relatively independent of the amount of hepatic blood flow.
   C. Intrinsic clearance is the amount of blood that bypasses the liver, not allowing for drug clearance.
   D. The hepatic extraction ratio is the fraction of the drug removed from the blood passing through the liver.
   E. Clearance of lidocaine is reduced in patients with congestive cardiac failure in proportion to the decrease in hepatic blood flow.

10. Which of the following statements concerning renal clearance is FALSE?

   A. Normally, only unbound drugs can pass through the glomerular membrane into the renal tubule.
   B. Active transport makes renal elimination more efficient.
   C. Highly lipophilic drugs, such as thiopental, undergo virtually no renal clearance of the parent molecule.
   D. Changes in renal drug clearance are proportional to changes in creatinine clearance.
   E. Passive elimination of drugs by glomerular filtration is very efficient.

11. Which of the following statements about pharmacokinetics is FALSE?

   A. The initial bolus of drug is not instantaneously mixed and equilibrated with the entire volume of tissue that will eventually take up the drug.
   B. The lungs and kidneys are part of the vessel-poor group.
   C. When the tissue concentrations of a drug are high enough, the decrease in plasma drug concentration becomes solely dependent on drug elimination.
   D. Elimination only slightly contributes to the initial drop in plasma concentration.
   E. Hypovolemia may increase the incidence of drug toxicity.

12. What is the half-time of elimination for a drug that undergoes first-order elimination with a rate constant of 0.1 minute?

   A. 10 minutes
   B. 100 minutes
   C. 0.1 minutes
   D. 6.93 minutes
   E. 693 minutes

13. What is mean residence time (MRT)?

   A. The time it takes a drug to reach its steady state after starting an infusion.
   B. The time a drug molecule spends in the vessel-rich group of tissues.
   C. The average time a drug molecule spends in the body before being eliminated.
   D. The average time a drug molecule spends in the renal cells before being excreted.
   E. The average time it takes a drug to reach its volume of distribution.

14. Which statement regarding target-controlled infusions (TCI) is TRUE?

   A. All studies have shown an advantage with TCI.
   B. They require the physician to calculate the volume of distribution for each drug and patient.
   C. The mathematical principles governing TCI are actually exquisitely complex.
   D. It is primarily influenced by elimination.
   E. The physician must program a target plasma concentration of the drug into the pump.

15. Which of the following statements regarding genetic variation in drug metabolism is TRUE?

   A. Drug metabolism varies substantially among individuals because of variability in the genes.
   B. For most enzymes, there is usually only one bioactive isoform.
   C. Individual subjects' rates of metabolism have a multimodal distribution.
   D. The resulting distribution of individual rates of metabolism is known as *unimodal.*
   E. The vast majority of drug-metabolizing enzymes do not exhibit genetic polymorphism.

16. FALSE statements about agonists and antagonists include all of the following EXCEPT:

   A. Competitive antagonists bind irreversibly to receptors.
   B. Competitive antagonists do not change the maximum possible effect that can be elicited by an agonist.
   C. Noncompetitive antagonists bind reversibly to receptors.
   D. Noncompetitive antagonists change the maximum effect elicited by an agonist.
   E. Agonists that differ in potency but bind to the same receptors will have nonparallel concentration–response curves.

ANSWERS

1. B. Since biologic membranes are lipid bilayers composed of a lipophilic core sandwiched between two hydrophilic layers, only small lipophilic drugs can passively diffuse across the membrane down its concentration gradient. In order for water-soluble drugs to passively diffuse across the membrane down its concentration gradient, transmembrane proteins that form a hydrophilic channel are required. Because of the abundance of these nonspecific hydrophilic channels in the capillary endothelium of all organs except for the central nervous system, where the blood–brain barrier capillary endothelial cells have very limited numbers of transmembrane hydrophilic channels, ***passive transport*** of drugs from the intravascular space into the interstitium of various organs is limited by blood flow, not by the lipid solubility of the drug. Hydrophilic drugs can only enter the central nervous system after binding to drug-specific transmembrane proteins that actively transport the hydrophilic drug across the capillary endothelium into the central nervous system interstitium. (See page 157: Pharmacokinetic Principles Drug Absorption and Routes of Administration.)

2. E. Although the rate of initial drug delivery may be dependent on the relative blood flow of the organ, the rate of drug equilibration by the tissue is dependent on the ratio of blood flow to tissue content. Therefore, drug uptake rapidly approaches equilibrium in the highly perfused, but low volume brain, kidneys, and lungs in a matter of minutes, whereas drug transfer to the less well-perfused, intermediate volume muscle tissue may take hours to approach equilibrium, and drug transfer to the poorly perfused, large cellular volumes of adipose tissue does not equilibrate for days. Highly lipophilic drugs such as thiopental and propofol rapidly begin to diffuse into the highly perfused brain tissue usually less than a minute after intravenous injection. Because of the low tissue volume but high perfusion of the brain, the drug concentration in the cerebral arterial blood rapidly equilibrates, usually within three minutes, with the concentration in the brain tissue. (See page 159: Drug Distribution.)

3. E. The elimination half-life is the time during which the amount of drug in the body decreases by 50%. Although this parameter appears to be a simple summary of the physiology of drug elimination, it is actually a complex parameter, influenced by the distribution and the elimination of the drug, as follows:

$$t_{1/2\beta} = \frac{\ln 2}{k_\beta} = 0.693 \times \frac{V_d}{Cl_E}$$

Therefore, when a physiologic or pathologic perturbation changes the elimination half-life of a drug, it is not a simple reflection of the change in the body's ability to metabolize or eliminate the drug. For example, the elimination half-life of thiopental is prolonged in the elderly; however, the elimination clearance is unchanged and the volume of

distribution is increased. Therefore, elderly patients need dosing strategies that accommodate for the change in the distribution of the drug rather than a decreased metabolism of the drug. In contrast, in patients with renal insufficiency, the increase in the elimination half-life of pancuronium is due to a simple decrease in renal elimination of the drug and the volume of distribution is unchanged. (See page 165: Elimination Half-life.)

4. D. *Elimination clearance* (drug clearance) is the theoretical volume of blood from which drug is completely and irreversibly removed in a unit of time. Elimination clearance has the units of flow (volume per time). *Total* drug clearance can be calculated with pharmacokinetic models of blood concentration versus time data. Drug clearance is often corrected for weight or body surface area, in which case the units are mL/min/kg or mL/min/m², respectively.

Elimination clearance, *Cl*, can be calculated from the declining blood levels observed after an IV injection, as follows:

$$Cl = \frac{dose \ of \ drug \ ad \min istered}{area \ under \ the \ concentration \ versus \ time \ curve}$$

If a drug is rapidly removed from the plasma, its concentration will fall more quickly than the concentration of a drug that is less readily eliminated. *Elimination* is an inclusive term that refers to all the processes that remove drugs from the body. Elimination occurs either by excretion of unchanged drug or by metabolism (biotransformation) and subsequent excretion of metabolites. The liver and kidneys are the most important organs for drug elimination. The liver eliminates drugs primarily by metabolism to less active compounds and, to a lesser extent, by hepatobiliary excretion of drugs or their metabolites. The primary role of the kidneys is the excretion of water-soluble, polar compounds. (See page 159: Drug Elimination.)

5. B. Volume of distribution is a numeric index of the extent of drug distribution that does not have any relationship to the actual volume of any tissue or group of tissues. It may be as small as plasma volume, or, if overall tissue uptake is extensive, the apparent volume of distribution may greatly exceed the actual total volume of the body. In general, lipophilic drugs have larger volumes of distribution than hydrophilic drugs. Since the volume of distribution is a mathematical construct to model the distribution of a drug in the body, the volume of distribution cannot provide any information regarding the actual tissue concentration in any specific real organ in the body. However, this simple mathematical construct provides a useful summary description of the behavior of the drug in the body. (See page 164: Volume of Distribution.)

6. A. If a drug is extensively distributed, then the concentration will be lower relative to the amount of drug present, which equates to a larger volume of distribution. For example, if a total of 10 mg of drug is present and the concentration is 2 mg/L, then the apparent volume of distribution is 5 L. (See page 164: Volume of Distribution.)

7. **D.**   In patients with hepatic disease, the elimination half-life of drugs metabolized or excreted by the liver is often increased because of decreased clearance, and, possibly, increased volume of distribution caused by ascites and altered protein binding. Drug concentration at steady state is inversely proportional to elimination clearance. Therefore, when hepatic drug clearance is reduced, repeated bolus dosing or continuous infusion of such drugs as benzodiazepines, opioids, and barbiturates may result in excessive accumulation of drug as well as excessive and prolonged pharmacologic effects. In patients with renal failure, similar concerns apply to the administration of drugs excreted by the kidneys. It is almost always better to underestimate a patient's dose requirement, observe the response, and give additional drug if necessary. (See page 161: Renal Drug Clearance.)

8. **D.**   Phase I biotransformations. CYP3A4 is the single most important enzyme, accounting for 40% to 45% of all CYP-mediated drug metabolism. CYP are incorporated into the smooth endoplasmic reticulum of hepatocytes and the membranes of the upper intestinal enterocytes in high concentrations. CYP are also found in the lungs, kidneys, and skin, but in much smaller amounts. The CYP system is able to protect the organism from the deleterious effects of accumulation of exogenous compounds because of its two fundamental characteristics—broad substrate specificity and the capability to adapt to exposure to different substances by induction of different CYP isoenzymes. Phase II reactions transform the original drug by conjugating a variety of endogenous compounds to a polar functional group of the drug, making the metabolite even more hydrophilic. (See page 159: Phase I Reactions.)

9. **C.**   Drug elimination by the liver depends on the intrinsic ability of the liver to metabolize the drug (intrinsic clearance, Cl_l), and the amount of drug available to diffuse into the liver. Many types of mathematical models have been developed to attempt to accurately model the relationship between hepatic artery blood flow, portal artery blood flow, intrinsic clearance, and drug binding to plasma proteins. Intrinsic clearance represents the ability of the liver to remove drug from the blood in the absence of any limitations imposed by blood flow or drug binding. For drugs with a high extraction ratio and a high intrinsic clearance, hepatic elimination clearance is directly proportional to hepatic blood flow. Therefore, any manipulation of hepatic blood flow will be directly reflected by a proportional change in hepatic elimination clearance; in states where cardiac output is decreased (e.g., heart failure, shock, spinal anesthesia, *etc.*), high extraction ratio drugs will have a decrease in hepatic elimination, whereas low extraction rate drugs will have minimal change in clearance. (See page 161: Hepatic Drug Clearance.)

10. **E.**   The primary role of the kidneys in drug elimination is to excrete into urine the unchanged, hydrophilic drugs, and the hepatic derived metabolites from Phase I and Phase II reactions of lipophilic drugs. The passive elimination of drugs by passive glomerular filtration is a very inefficient process—any significant degree of binding of the drug to plasma proteins or erythrocytes will decrease the renal clearance below the glomerular filtration rate of 20% of renal blood flow. Since overall renal function is readily estimated by clearance of endogenous creatinine, renal drug clearance, even for drugs eliminated primarily by tubular secretion, is dependent on renal function. Therefore, in patients with acute and chronic causes of decreased renal function, including age, low cardiac output states, and hepatorenal syndrome, drug dosing must be altered in order to avoid accumulation of parent compounds and potentially toxic metabolites (e.g., lidocaine, meperidine, etc.). (See page 161: Renal Drug Clearance.)

11. **B.**   The highly perfused core circulatory components (i.e., vessel-rich group) – the brain, lungs, kidneys and certain muscles – receive the highest relative distribution of cardiac output and therefore are the initial organs to reach equilibrium with plasma drug concentrations. Drug concentrations then equilibrate with the less well-perfused muscles and liver and then, finally, with the relatively poorly perfused splanchnic vasculature, adipose tissue, and bone.

Drug distribution after injection is assumed to be instantaneous, so there are no concentration gradients within the compartment. The concentration can decrease only by elimination of drug from the system. There are two discrete phases in the decline of the plasma concentration. The first phase after injection is characterized by a very rapid decrease in concentration. The initial bolus of drug is not instantaneously mixed and equilibrated with the entire volume of tissue that will eventually take up the drug. The rapid decrease in concentration during this "distribution phase" is largely caused by passage of drug from the plasma into vessel-rich tissues. The distribution phase is followed by a slower decline of the concentration owing to drug elimination. Elimination also begins immediately after injection, but its contribution to the drop in plasma concentration is initially much smaller than the fall in concentration because of drug distribution. When the tissue concentrations of a drug are high enough, the decrease in plasma drug concentration below therapeutic threshold becomes solely dependent on drug elimination from the body. The volume of the central compartment is important in clinical anesthesiology because it is the pharmacokinetic parameter that determines the peak plasma concentration after an IV bolus injection. Hypovolemia, for example, reduces the volume of the central compartment. If doses are not correspondingly reduced, the higher plasma concentrations will increase the incidence of adverse pharmacologic effects. (See page 166: Compartmental Pharmacokinetic Models.)

12. **D.**   The elimination half-life is the time during which the amount of drug in the body decreases by 50%. Although this parameter appears to be a simple summary of the physiology of drug elimination, it is actually a complex

parameter, influenced by the distribution and the elimination of the drug, as follows:

$$t_{1/2\beta} = \frac{\ln 2}{k_\beta} = 0.693 \times \frac{V_d}{Cl_E}$$

Given drug's rate constant of elimination = 0.693 ÷ 0.1 minute = 6.93 minutes. Thus, it would take 6.93 minutes for the concentration to change by a factor of 2 for a drug with a rate constant of 0.1 minute. (See page 165: Elimination Half-life.)

13. C. The main unique parameter of noncompartmental analysis is the Mean Residence Time (MRT), which is the average time a drug molecule spends in the body before being eliminated. The MRT unfortunately suffers from the main failings of the elimination half-life derived from compartmental models—not only does it fail to capture the contribution of extensive distribution versus limited elimination to allow a drug to linger in the body, but both parameters also fail to describe the situation where the drug effect can dissipate by redistribution of drug from the site of action back into blood and then into other, less well-perfused tissues. (See page 168: Noncompartmental [Stochastic] Pharmacokinetic Models.)

14. E. By linking a computer with the appropriate pharmacokinetic model to an infusion pump, it is possible for the physician to enter the desired target plasma concentration of a drug and for the computer to nearly instantaneously calculate the appropriate infusion scheme to achieve this target in a matter of seconds. Since drug accumulates at various rates among the various tissues and organs in the body, the computer continually calculates the current drug concentration and adjusts the infusion pump in order to account for the current status of drug uptake, distribution, and elimination. To maintain the target plasma concentration, a series of infusions of decreasing rate can be used that match the elimination clearance and compensate for drug loss from the central to the peripheral compartments during the initial period of extensive drug distribution and the second period of moderate drug distribution. This manual dosing scheme has been termed the BET scheme, where B is the loading bolus dose, E is the infusion to replace drug removed by elimination clearance, and T is a continuously decreasing infusion that compensates for transfer of drug to the peripheral

tissues (i.e., distribution). Therefore, the computer driven BET scheme can in fact control the infusion pump in order to achieve a steady target concentration. The mathematical principles governing TCI are actually quite simple. TCI performance is influenced by the model chosen. Some studies have shown better control and a more predictable emergence with TCI, whereas others have simply shown no advantage. Pulmonary vasculature is part of the multi-organ system. (See page 180: Target-controlled Infusions.)

15. A. For most enzymes involved in Phase I and Phase II reactions, there are several biologically available isoforms. Drug metabolism varies substantially among individuals because of variability in the genes. For most drugs, individual subjects' rates of metabolism have a unimodal distribution. The resulting multimodal distribution of individual rates of metabolism is known as *polymorphism*. For example, different genotypes result in either normal, low, or (rarely) absent plasma pseudocholinesterase. (See page 161 : Genetic Variations in Drug Metabolism.)

16. D. Drugs that bind to receptors and produce an effect are called *agonists*. Drugs may be capable of producing the same maximal effect (E_{MAX}), although they may differ in concentration that produces the effect (i.e., potency). Agonists that differ in potency but bind to the same receptors will have parallel concentration–response curves. Differences in potency of agonists reflect differences in affinity for the receptor. *Partial agonists* are drugs that are not capable of producing the maximal effect, even at very high concentrations. Compounds that bind to receptors without producing any changes in cellular function are referred to as *antagonists*—antagonists blocking the active binding site(s) inhibit agonist binding to the receptors. *Competitive antagonists* bind reversibly to receptors, and their blocking effect can be overcome by high concentrations of an agonist (i.e., competition). Therefore, competitive antagonists produce a parallel shift in the dose–response curve, but the maximum effect is not altered. *Noncompetitive antagonists* bind irreversibly to receptors. This has the same effect as reducing the number of receptors and shifts the dose–response curve downward and to the right, decreasing both the slope and the maximum effect. (See page 169: Drug–Receptor Interactions: Agonists, Partial Agonists, and Antagonists.)

CHAPTER 8

Electrical and Fire Safety

1. Electrical contact may produce all of the following types of injuries EXCEPT:

   A. Disruption of normal electrical function of the cells
   B. Respiratory paralysis
   C. Muscle relaxation
   D. Cardiac arrhythmias
   E. Altered brain function

2. Injury from macroshock is affected by all of the following EXCEPT:

   A. Skin resistance
   B. Duration of contact with the electrical source
   C. Current density
   D. Capacitance
   E. Amount of current (number of amperes)

3. Which of the following statements regarding grounded electrical systems is FALSE?

   A. The hot wire (black) carries a voltage of 120 V above ground.
   B. A ground wire (green or bare) is not necessary to complete a circuit.
   C. The white wire is neutral.
   D. The circuit breaker prevents macroshock by preventing current flow.
   E. A black wire and a neutral wire are all that are needed to produce the path for the current to flow through a resistance and perform work.

4. An ungrounded electrical system has which of the following properties?

   A. It makes the use of a ground wire obsolete.
   B. The 120-V potential exists only between the two wires in the system.
   C. It eliminates the potential for microshock.
   D. It does not require the presence of an isolation transformer.
   E. An individual who contacts both wires within the isolated system will not complete the circuit.

5. Which of the following statements regarding the line isolation monitor (LIM) is FALSE?

   A. The value on the LIM display indicates that current is actively flowing to ground.
   B. The LIM measures the impedance of current flow to ground that exists in the system.
   C. The LIM is set to alarm at 2 to 5 mA.
   D. The LIM is necessary to identify faulty equipment, which, despite a contact to ground, will function normally in an ungrounded system.
   E. The LIM alarm can be triggered if too many pieces of electrical equipment have been plugged in.

6. Which of the following statements regarding fires in the operating room is FALSE?

   A. Fires in the operating room present just as much danger today as compared with 100 years ago, when patients were anesthetized with flammable anesthetic agents.
   B. A combination of 50% oxygen and 50% nitrous oxide would support combustion as well as 100% oxygen.
   C. An ignition source and an oxidizer are enough to start a fire.
   D. Paper drapes are much easier to ignite and can burn with greater intensity than cloth drapes.
   E. When plastics burn, a variety of injurious compounds can be produced including carbon monoxide, ammonia, hydrogen chloride, and cyanide.

7. All of the following statements regarding fires in the operating room are true EXCEPT:

   A. Major ignition sources for operating room fires are the electrosurgical unit and the laser.
   B. The ends of some fiber-optic light cords can become hot enough to start a fire.
   C. Fires on a patient occur most often during surgery in and around the head and neck, when the patient is receiving supplemental oxygen during monitored anesthesia care.
   D. Fires in or on the patient represent the more common type of operating room fire.
   E. Use of nitrous oxide anesthetic during laparoscopic surgery in the abdomen would not support combustion.

8. In regards to responding to an operating room fire, which of the following statements is TRUE?

   A. The operating room sprinkler systems effectively respond to the majority of fires.
   B. If an endotracheal tube is on fire, it should be removed immediately and then extinguished.
   C. If the paper drapes are burning, water or saline will likely douse the fire effectively.
   D. Common acronyms for responding to a fire include "RACE" and "PASS."
   E. The newer "nonflammable" volatile anesthetics are not potential fire hazards.

9. In regards to electrosurgery and patient monitoring devices, which of the following is NOT affected by the electrosurgical unit (ESU)?

   A. Pacemaker
   B. Temperature probe monitoring
   C. Automatic implantable cardioverter-defibrillator (AICD)
   D. ECG monitoring
   E. Pulse oximetry

10. Any substance that permits the flow of electrons is called a/an:

    A. Conductor
    B. Insulator
    C. Capacitance
    D. Circuit
    E. Impedance

11. The presence of a substance opposing the flow of electrons is:

    A. Impedance
    B. Alternating current
    C. Capacitance
    D. Insulation
    E. Conduction

12. Which of the following statements pertaining to microshock is FALSE?

    A. Equipment ground wire can protect against microshock.
    B. Wearing rubber gloves when caring for an electrically susceptible patient offers no protection from the patient receiving a microshock.
    C. Patients with a pacing wire or those who have a central venous or pulmonary artery catheter are at risk for microshock.
    D. A nerve stimulator coming into contact with an electrically susceptible patient could lead to microshock.
    E. Microshock can lead to cardiac arrhythmia such as ventricular fibrillation.

ANSWERS

1. C. Electrical contact may result in flow of current through an individual. First, the electrical current may disrupt the normal electrical function of cells. Depending on the magnitude, it can cause muscle contraction (not muscle relaxation), changes in brain function, respiratory paralysis, and disruption of normal heart function leading to ventricular fibrillation. Depending on the path taken, the flow of current through tissue will produce heat if the resistance to flow is high. (See page 191: Electrical Shock Hazards: Source of Shocks.)

2. D. The severity of an electrical shock is determined by the amount of current (number of amperes) and the duration of the current flow. Injury from electricity is influenced by skin resistance, duration of contact with the electrical source, and current density. High skin resistance decreases the transfer of electricity and thus is protective. Contact time results in more current flow and thus more energy transferred, which produces more tissue damage in high-resistance tissues. Furthermore, prolonging the exposure to current flow increases the risk of inducing ventricular fibrillation during a vulnerable period of the cardiac cycle. Current density describes the surface area onto which the current is transferred. The quantity of injury is inversely related to the surface area and is directly related to the quantity of current transferred through that surface area. This is the reason that small voltages applied to a small surface area of a vulnerable tissue results in injury (e.g., ventricular fibrillation with current down a pacing wire). Capacitance refers to the storage of current in two conductive materials separated by an insulatory layer. It does not play a role in the magnitude of injury, although capacitance can store current, which can result in injury even when an item is unplugged. (See page 190: Principles of Electricity: Capacitance and page 191: Electrical Shock Hazards: Source of Shocks.)

3. D. In a normal grounded circuit, the power company delivers a hot wire with a voltage above ground. Within a house, it is carried by a black wire, which carries a voltage of 120 V above ground potential. The power company also supplies a neutral wire for the current to return to the earth. This is usually a white wire. These two wires are all that are needed to produce the path for the current to flow through a resistance and perform work. A circuit breaker between the hot supply and the receptacle prevents current flow in excess of the wire's capabilities. Exceeding the wire's capabilities results in heat production and a possible fire hazard. Circuit breakers do not prevent macroshock. The ground wire, which is bare or green, acts as a safety feature to prevent shock in the event that the object containing the electricity comes in contact with the hot wire. In these malfunctioning devices, the casing of the object becomes hot and carries the same potential as the hot wire. If someone comes into contact with the case (and if he or she is grounded), he or she will provide a path for current to flow and will be electrocuted. The ground wire acts as a

low-resistance pathway for electrical potentials within the case and thus reduces the flow in the individual. A ground wire is a safety feature, but it is not necessary to complete a circuit. (See page 193: Electrical Power: Grounded.)

4. B. Supplying ungrounded power to the OR requires the use of an isolation transformer. An ungrounded power supply uses an isolation transformer to separate itself from the power company. The isolation transformer creates a power gradient of 120 V between the two wires within the system but no gradient between any of the two wires and the ground. Thus, individuals can contact either wire of an ungrounded system and not complete a circuit. An individual who contacts both wires within the isolated system will complete a circuit and be electrocuted. Isolation transformer systems thus significantly reduce the risk of macroshock in the operating room environment but do not reduce the risk of microshock. A ground wire is still used within an isolation transformer system because it constitutes an additional, alternative safety system. The ground wire is attached to the device's case to provide a low-resistance pathway if the case of the device becomes electrically hot. (See page 197: Electrical Power: Ungrounded.)

5. A. The LIM is a device that monitors the integrity of the isolation of the ungrounded electrical system. Such monitoring is essential in that a first fault to the ground in an isolated system will result in normal function of an electrical device (but will alert that the isolation of the power has been breached). The typical cause of loss of isolation is that the case and the ground wire have become connected. Since the ground is not in the path of the isolated power, no short circuit exists, and the equipment is safe to use and will continue to function. However, if an individual comes into contact with the other limb of the isolated circuit, he or she would then be in contact with both sides of the isolated power (through the ground and the ground wire) and will thus receive a shock. The LIM monitors the impedance to ground of each side of the isolated power. The value measured on the LIM does not mean that current is actually flowing; rather, it indicates how much current would flow in the event of a fault. Normally, the LIM is set to alarm at 2 to 5 mA. In a perfect system, the impedance to ground is infinite, but because alternating current creates capacitance (and this can leak to the ground even with perfect isolation), a buffer of acceptable leak is permitted to prevent alarming secondary to capacitance leakage. If the LIM alarm is triggered, the first thing to do is to check the gauge to determine if it is a true fault. The other possibility is that too many pieces of electrical equipment have been plugged in and the 2-mA limit has been exceeded. The next step is to identify the faulty equipment, which is done by unplugging each piece of equipment until the alarm ceases. If the faulty piece of equipment is not of a life-support nature, it should be removed from the OR. (See page 199: The Line Isolation Monitor.)

6. C. Fires in the operating room are just as much a danger today as they were 100 years ago, when patients were anesthetized with flammable anesthetic agents. Today, the risk of an operating room fire is probably as great as or greater than in the days when ether and cyclopropane were used. This is because of the routine use of potential sources of ignition in an environment rich in flammable materials. For a fire to start, three elements are necessary: a heat or ignition source, fuel, and an oxidizer. The main oxidizers in the operating room are air, oxygen, and nitrous oxide. Oxygen and nitrous oxide function equally well as oxidizers, so a combination of 50% oxygen and 50% nitrous oxide would support combustion as well as 100% oxygen. Fuel for a fire can be found everywhere in the operating room. Paper drapes have largely replaced cloth drapes, and these are much easier to ignite and can burn with greater intensity. Other sources of fuel include gauze dressings, endotracheal tubes, gel mattress pads, and even facial or body hair. When materials, such as plastics burn, a variety of injurious compounds can be produced including carbon monoxide, ammonia, hydrogen chloride, and even cyanide, which can lead to injury by damaging airways and lung tissue and can cause asphyxia. (See page 210: Fire Safety.)

7. E. Major ignition sources for operating room fires are electrosurgical units and lasers. However, the ends of some fiber-optic light cords can also become hot enough to start a fire if they are placed on paper drapes. Operating room fires can be divided into two different types. The more common type of fire occurs in or on the patient. These include endotracheal tube fires; fires during laparoscopy or bronchoscopy; or a fire in the oropharynx, which may occur during a tonsillectomy. The other type of operating room fire is one that is remote from the patient, including an electrical fire in a piece of equipment. Fires on the patient seem to have become the most frequent type of operating room fire. These cases most often occur during surgery in and around the head and neck, when the patient is receiving monitored anesthesia care with supplemental oxygen *via* face mask or a nasal cannula. Laparoscopic surgery in the abdomen is another potential risk for a surgically related fire. Ordinarily, the abdomen is inflated with CO_2, which does not support combustion. However, nitrous oxide administered to the patient as part of the anesthetic can, over 30 minutes, diffuse into the abdominal cavity and attain a concentration that could support combustion. (See page 210: Fire Safety.)

8. D. If a fire does occur, it is important to extinguish it as soon as possible. This is best accomplished by removing the oxidizer from the fire. Therefore, if an endotracheal tube is on fire, disconnecting the anesthetic circuit from the tube or disconnecting the inspiratory limb of the circuit will usually put out the fire immediately. It is not recommended to remove a burning endotracheal tube because this may cause even greater harm to the patient. After the fire has been extinguished, the endotracheal tube can be safely removed, the airway inspected via bronchoscopy, and the patient's trachea reintubated. If the drapes are burning, particularly if they are paper drapes, they must be removed and placed on the floor. Paper drapes are impervious to water, so throwing water or saline on them will do little to extinguish the fire. After the burning drapes have been removed from the patient, the fire can then be extinguished with a fire extinguisher. In most operating room fires, the sprinkler system is not activated. This is because sprinklers are usually not located directly over the operating room table, and operating room fires are seldom hot enough to activate the sprinklers. To use a fire extinguisher effectively, the acronym "PASS" can be helpful. This stands for *pull* the pin to activate the fire extinguisher, *aim* at the base of the fire, *squeeze* the trigger, and *sweep* the extinguisher back and forth across the base of the fire. When responding to a fire, the acronym RACE is useful. This stands for *rescue, alarm, confine,* and *extinguish.* Even the newer, "nonflammable" volatile anesthetics can, under certain circumstances, present fire hazards. For example, sevoflurane is nonflammable in air, but it can serve as a fuel at concentrations as low as 11% in oxygen and 10% in nitrous oxide. Furthermore, sevoflurane and desiccated CO_2 absorbent (either soda lime or Baralyme) can undergo exothermic chemical reactions that have been implicated in several fires that involved the anesthesia breathing circuit. (See page 210: Fire Safety.)

9. B. The high-frequency electrical energy generated by the electrosurgical unit (ESU) interferes with everything from the ECG signal to cardiac output computers and pulse oximeters. The ESU has also caused other problems in patients with pacemakers, including reprogramming and microshock. Furthermore, the use of a unipolar ESU may cause electrical interference that could be interpreted by the AICD as a ventricular tachydysrhythmia. This would trigger a defibrillation pulse to be delivered to the patient and would likely cause an actual episode of ventricular tachycardia or ventricular fibrillation. The patient with an AICD is also at risk for ventricular fibrillation during electroconvulsive therapy. Therefore, the AICD should be disabled by placing a magnet over the device or by use of a specific protocol to shut it off. It is best to consult with someone experienced with the device before starting surgery. The device can be reactivated by reversing the process. Also, an external defibrillator and a noninvasive pacemaker should be in the OR whenever a patient with an AICD is anesthetized. Temperature probe monitoring would not be affected by ESU. (See page 204: Electrosurgery.)

10. A. Any substance that permits the flow of electrons is called a conductor. Current is characterized by electrons flowing through a conductor. If the electron flow is always in the same direction, it is referred to as *direct current* (DC). However, if the electron flow reverses direction at a regular interval, it is termed *alternating current* (AC). Either of these types of current can be pulsed or continuous in nature. (See page 190: Principles of Electricity: Alternating and Direct Currents.)

11. D. An insulator is a substance that opposes the flow of electrons. Therefore, an insulator has a high impedance to electron flow, whereas a conductor has a low impedance to electron flow. (See page 190: Principles of Electricity: Impedance.)

12. B.   Macroshock, which refers to large amounts of current flowing through a person, is dangerous and can cause harm or death. Microshock, which refers to very small amounts of current applied only to an electrically susceptible patient, is also a serious safety concern. An electrically susceptible patient is an individual who has an external conduit that is in direct contact with the heart. This can be a pacing wire or a saline-filled catheter such as a central venous or pulmonary artery catheter. In the case of an electrically susceptible patient, even minute amounts of current (microshock) may cause ventricular fibrillation. The catheter orifice or electrical wire with a very small surface area in contact with the heart produces a relatively large current density at the heart. Even very small amounts of current applied directly to the myocardium will cause ventricular fibrillation. The exact amount of current necessary to cause ventricular fibrillation in this type of patient is unknown. Furthermore, the stray capacitance that is part of any AC-powered electrical instrument may result in significant amounts of charge buildup on the case of the instrument. If an individual simultaneously touches the case of an instrument where this has occurred and the electrically susceptible patient, he or she may unknowingly cause a discharge to the patient that might result in ventricular fibrillation. Therefore, the equipment ground wire constitutes the major source of protection against microshock for the electrically susceptible patient. There are, however, other things that the anesthesiologist can do to reduce the incidence of microshock. One should never simultaneously touch an electrical device and a saline-filled central catheter or external pacing wire. Whenever one is handling a central catheter or pacing wires, it is best to insulate oneself by wearing rubber gloves. Also, one should never let any external current source, such as a nerve stimulator, come into contact with the catheter or wires. (See page 191: Electrical Shock Hazards: Source of Shocks and page 203: Microshock.)

Experimental Design and Statistics

1. If a target population contains several strata of importance, the best method of obtaining a representative population sample is:

    A. Limit sampling
    B. Convenience sampling
    C. Crossover sampling
    D. Random sampling
    E. Double-blind sampling

2. An example of a contemporaneous-parallel control would be:

    A. Each patient could receive the standard drug under identical experimental circumstances at another time.
    B. A group of patients could have been studied previously with the standard drug under similar circumstances.
    C. Another group of patients receiving the standard drug could be studied simultaneously.
    D. Literature reports show the effects of the drug under related but not necessarily identical circumstances.
    E. Each patient could receive the standard drug under nonexperimental conditions simultaneously with the test group.

3. The risks of constructing a rigidly standardized study include all of the following EXCEPT:

    A. A fixed dose may produce excessive numbers of side effects in some patients.
    B. A standardized treatment may be so artificial that it has no broad clinical relevance.
    C. A fixed dose may be therapeutically insufficient in some patients.
    D. A fixed dose makes the research work more difficult.
    E. A fixed dose may not allow an effect or desired end point to be achieved.

4. The best method for random allocation of treatment groups is:

    A. Based on the day of the week
    B. Based on assignment of a previous patient
    C. Using hospital chart numbers
    D. Patient preference
    E. Computer-generated random numbering

5. Which statement about blinding is TRUE?

    A. It can bias a researcher's ability to administer the research protocol.
    B. It causes the researchers to not trust themselves to record the data impartially and dispassionately.
    C. It can be used in case reports.
    D. It masks from the patient and experimenters the experimental group to which the patient is assigned.
    E. It has the names *single blind* and *double blind,* which are often applied consistently but uncommonly in research reports.

6. The most potent scientific tool for evaluating medical treatment is:

    A. A longitudinal prospective study of deliberate intervention with historical controls
    B. A longitudinal prospective study of deliberate intervention with concurrent controls
    C. A longitudinal retrospective study with concurrent case controls
    D. A longitudinal retrospective study with historical controls
    E. A cross-sectional prospective study without controls

7. The error of failing to reject a false null hypothesis is called a/an:

    A. False-positive
    B. Type II error
    C. α error
    D. Zero-order error
    E. Parameter

8. The number of degrees of freedom and the value for each degree of freedom does NOT depend on:

    A. The type of statistical test
    B. The number of subjects
    C. Dividing the standard deviation by the square root of the sample size
    D. The specifics of the statistical hypothesis
    E. The number of experimental groups

9. Variance is the:

    A. Statistical average
    B. Average deviation
    C. Average squared distance
    D. Square root of the average deviation
    E. Square of the standard error

10. The mean ± 3 standard deviation encompasses what percentage of the sample population?

    A. 50
    B. 68
    C. 75
    D. 95
    E. 99

11. A study is performed looking at the difference in postoperative nausea in males and females undergoing laparoscopic cholecystectomy. The category "male or female" is an example of what kind of data?

    A. Ordinal
    B. Dichotomous
    C. Nominal
    D. Discrete interval
    E. Continuous interval

12. All of the following are aspects of enumeration data EXCEPT:

    A. They provide counts of subject responses.
    B. They provide a measure of central location of a binary data.
    C. They are also called categorical binary data.
    D. They provide a measure of central location for continuous data.
    E. They can be used to obtain a ratio of responders to the number of subjects.

13. The most versatile approach for handling comparisons of means between more than two groups or between several measurements in the same group is called a/an:

    A. Paired *t*-test
    B. Chi-square test
    C. Interval data testing
    D. Analysis of variance (ANOVA)
    E. Unpaired *t*-test

14. Identify the slope and *y*-intercept for the following linear regression equation: $y = a + bx$.

    A. *a,b*
    B. *y,a*
    C. *y,b*
    D. *b,a*
    E. *x,y*

15. Systematic differences between the patients receiving each intervention are called:

    A. Selection bias
    B. Performance bias
    C. Attrition bias
    D. Detection bias
    E. Experimenter bias

16. In dichotomous data testing:

    A. The results are often presented as odds ratios.
    B. The chi-square test cannot be used to analyze contingency tables with more than two rows and two columns.
    C. The Fishers exact test and the chi-square test allow comparison of the success rates between two sampled populations of a procedure.

    D. The chi-square test is computationally more complex than Fishers exact test.
    E. Assumptions of sample size and response rate are achieved by this test.

17. The probability of a type II error increases with all of the following EXCEPT:

    A. Small α value
    B. Large sample size
    C. Small difference between experimental conditions
    D. Larger variability in populations being compared
    E. Decreasing the number of subjects

18. All of the following are true of nonparametric statistics EXCEPT:

    A. They are used whenever there are serious concerns about the shape of the data.
    B. They do not require any assumptions about probability distributions of the populations.
    C. They are less able than parametric tests to distinguish between the null and alternative hypotheses if the data are normally distributed.
    D. They are also called "order statistics."
    E. They are the tests of choice for dichotomous data.

19. Which of the following statements is TRUE?

    A. A confidence interval describes how likely it is that the population parameter is estimated by any particular sample statistic such as the mean.
    B. The standard error (SE) is used to describe the dispersion of the sample.
    C. Sample size planning cannot be used as a mechanism for increasing statistical power.
    D. Studies using historical controls obtain the same results as studies with concurrent controls if appropriate strata are selected.
    E. When describing the precision with which the population center is known, the standard deviation (SD) should be used.

For questions 20 to 24, please pick the best answer to the scenario given. Any of the answers may be used once, multiple times, or not at all.

    A. Mode
    B. F ratio
    C. P value
    D. Power
    E. Standard Error

20. Example of a summary statistic.

21. A calculation that requires the knowledge of the study size and standard deviation.

22. Always used in descriptive statistical discussion but rarely in statistical practice.

23. Likelihood of obtaining a risk ratio at least as far from the null of 1.

24. Test statistics on means where there are more than two groups.

ANSWERS

1. D. A sample is a subset of the target population. The best hope for a representative sample of the population would be realized if every subject in the population had the same chance of being in the experiment; this is random sampling. If there are several strata of importance, random sampling from each stratum is appropriate. Convenience sampling is subject to the nuances of the surgical schedule, the goodwill of the referring physician and attending surgeon, and the willingness of the patient to cooperate. At best, a convenience sample is representative of patients at the institution, with no assurance that these patients are similar to greater general patient population. An example of convenience sampling would be in studying new anesthetic drugs in volunteers; these studies typically are performed on "healthy, young students." (See page 220: Sampling.)

2. C. A researcher can obtain comparative data by utilizing two basic tenets of controls: Contemporaneous or historical. Examples of contemporaneous controls include: (1) Each patient receiving the standard drug under identical experimental circumstances at another time (crossover); or (2) another group of patients receiving the standard drug being studied simultaneously (parallel). Historical control examples include: (1) A group of patients studied previously with the standard drug under similar circumstances; or (2) literature reports of the effects of the drug under related (but not necessarily identical) circumstances. If the outcome with an old treatment is not studied simultaneously with the outcome of a new treatment, one cannot know if any differences in results are a consequence of the two treatments, or of unsuspected and unknowable differences between the patients, or of other changes over time in the general medical environment. (See page 220: Control Groups.)

3. D. The risks of constructing a rigidly standardized study do not inherently make the research work more difficult. In contrast, standardizing the treatment groups by fixed doses simplifies the research work. The associated risks to this standardization are: (1) A fixed dose may produce excessive numbers of side effects in some patients, (2) a fixed dose may be therapeutically insufficient in others, and (3) a treatment standardized for an experimental protocol may be so artificial that it has no broad clinical relevance even if it is demonstrated to be superior. The researcher should carefully choose and report the adjustment or individualization of experimental treatments. (See page 220: Experimental Constraints.)

4. E. Experimental groups should be as similar to each other as possible in order to best reflect the target population; if the groups are different, this introduces a bias into the experiment. While randomly allocating subjects of a sample to one or another of the experimental groups requires additional work, this principle prevents selection bias by the researcher, minimizes (but cannot always prevent) the possibility that important differences exist among the experimental groups, and disarms critics' complaints about research methods. Random allocation is most commonly accomplished by computer-generated random numbers. Failure to conceal random allocation leads to biases in the results of clinical studies. (See page 221: Random Allocation of Treatment Groups.)

5. D. Blinding refers to the masking of the patient and experimenters to the experimental group to which the subject has been or will be assigned. In clinical trials, the necessity for blinding starts even before a patient is enrolled in the research study; this is called the concealment of random allocation. There is good evidence that if the process of random allocation is accessible to view, the referring physicians, the research team members, or both are tempted to manipulate the entrance of specific patients into the study to influence their assignment to a specific treatment group; they do so having formed a personal opinion about the relative merits of the treatment groups and desiring to get the "best" for someone they favor. This creates bias in the experimental groups. A researcher's knowledge of the treatment assignment can bias his or her ability to administer the research protocol and to observe and record data faithfully; this is true for clinical, animal, and in vitro research. If the treatment group is known, those who observe data cannot trust themselves to record the data impartially and dispassionately. (See page 221: Blinding.)

6. B. The randomized, controlled clinical trial is the most potent scientific tool for evaluating medical treatment and is a longitudinal, prospective study of deliberate intervention with concurrent controls. Longitudinal studies are the study of changes over time, whereas the cross-sectional studies describe a phenomenon at a certain point in time. A prospective (cohort) study would be one in which a group of patients undergoing neurologic surgery was divided into two groups, given two different opioids (remifentanil or fentanyl), and followed for the development of a perioperative myocardial infarction. In a retrospective (case-control) study, patients who suffered a perioperative myocardial infarction would be identified from hospital records; a group of subjects of similar age, gender, and disease who did not suffer a perioperative myocardial infarction also would be chosen, and the two groups would then be compared for the relative use of the two opioids (remifentanil or fentanyl). Studies of deliberate intervention are further subdivided into those with concurrent controls and those with historical controls. Concurrent controls are either a simultaneous parallel control group or a self-control study; historical controls include previous studies and literature reports. Randomization into treatment groups is relied on to equally weigh the subjects' baseline attributes that could predispose or protect the subjects from the outcome of interest. (See page 221: Types of Research Design.)

7. B. Since statistics deal with probabilities rather than certainties, there is a chance that the decision concerning the null hypothesis is erroneous. The error of wrongly rejecting the null hypothesis (false-positive result) is called the type I or α error. The error of failing to reject a false null hypothesis (false-negative result) is called a type II or β error. A parameter is a number describing a variable of a population. (See page 224: Logic of Proof.)

8. C.   Some additional parameters of theoretical probability distributions have been given the special name *degrees of freedom* and are represented by Latin letters such as *m, n,* and *s*. Associated with the formula for computing a test statistic is a rule for assigning integer values to the one or more parameters called degrees of freedom. The number of degrees of freedom and the value for each degree of freedom depends on the number of subjects, the number of experimental groups, the specifics of the statistical hypothesis, and the type of statistical test. (See page 225: Inferential Statistics.)

9. C.   The concept of describing the spread of a set of numbers by calculating the average distance from each number to the center of the numbers applies to both samples and populations; this average squared distance is called the variance. (See page 223: Spread or Variability.)

10. E.   Most biologic observations appear to come from populations with normal or Gaussian distributions. By accepting this assumption of a normal distribution, further meaning can be given to the sample summary statistics that have been calculated. This involves the use of the expression $\bar{x} \pm \kappa \times s$, where k = 1, 2, 3, and so on. If the population from which the sample is taken is unimodal and roughly symmetric, then the bounds for 1, 2, and 3 encompasses roughly 68%, 95%, and 99% of the sample and population members. (See page 223: Spread or Variability.)

11. B.   Putting observations into two or more discrete categories derives *categorical variables*. Dichotomous data allow only two possible variables (i.e., male versus female). Ordinal data have three or more categories that can be logically ranked or ordered (i.e., ASA physical status). Whereas discrete interval data can have only integer values (e.g., age in years), continuous interval data are measured on a continuum and can be decimal fractions (e.g., temperature of 37.1°C). A nominal variable can be placed into a category that has no logical ordering (e.g., eye color). (See page 222: Data Structure and page 223: Table 9-2: Data Types.)

12. D.   Categorical binary data, also called *enumeration data*, provide counts of subject responses. Given a sample of subjects of whom some have a certain characteristic (e.g., death, female gender), a ratio of responders to the number of subjects can be easily calculated as $P = x/n$; this ratio or rate can be expressed as a decimal fraction or as a percentage. It should be clear that this is a measure of central location of binary data in the same way that μ is a measure of central location for continuous data. (See page 228: Confidence Intervals on Proportions.)

13. D.   The most versatile approach for handling comparisons of means between more than two groups or between several measurements in the same group is called ANOVA (ANalysis Of VAriance). Analysis of variance consists of rules for creating test statistics on means when there are more than two groups. These test statistics are called *F ratios*. As with the *t*-test, the *F*-test statistic is a ratio; in general terms, the numerator expresses the variability of the mean values of the groups, whereas the denominator expresses the average variability or difference of each sample value from the mean of all sample values. The currently available nonparametric tests are not used more commonly because they do not adapt well to complex statistical models and they are less able than parametric tests to distinguish between the null and alternative hypotheses if the data are normally distributed. (See page 228: Analysis of Variance.)

14. D.   In the simplest type of experiment, a straight line (linear relationship) is assumed between two variables: One (y), the response or dependent variable, is considered a function of the other (x), the explanatory or independent variable. This is expressed as the linear regression equation $y = a + bx$; the parameters of the regression equation are a and b. The parameter b is the slope of the straight line relating x and y; for each 1-unit change in x, there is a b-unit change in y. The parameter a is the intercept (value of y when x equals 0). (See page 229: Simple Linear Regression.)

15. A.   Selection bias is systematic difference(s) between the patients receiving each intervention. Performance bias is systematic differences in care being given to study patients other than the preplanned interventions being evaluated. Attrition bias is systematic differences in the withdrawal of patients from each of the two intervention groups. Detection bias is systematic differences in the ascertainment and recording of outcomes. Experimenter bias occurs when the outcome of the experiment tends to be biased toward a result expected by the human experimenter. (See page 232: Systematic Reviews and Meta-Analyses.)

16. C.   A variety of statistical techniques allow a comparison of success rate. These include Fishers exact test and (Pearson's) chi-square test. The chi-square test offers the advantage of being computationally simpler, and it can also analyze contingency tables with more than two rows and two columns. However, certain assumptions of sample size and response rate are not achieved by this test. The results of such experiments are often presented as rate ratios. (See page 229: Hypothesis Testing.)

17. B.   The error of failing to reject a false null hypothesis (false-negative) is called a type II or β error. The power of a test is $1 - \beta$. The probability of a type II error depends on four factors. Unfortunately, the smaller the α, the greater the chance of a false-negative conclusion; this fact keeps the experimenter from automatically choosing a very small α. Second, the more variability there is in the populations being compared, the greater the chance of a type II error. This is analogous to listening to a noisy radio broadcast: The more static there is, the harder it will be to discriminate between words. Third, increasing the number of subjects lowers the probability of a type II error. The fourth and most important factor is the magnitude of the difference between the two experimental conditions. The probability of a type II error goes from very high, when only a small difference exists, to extremely low, when the two conditions produce large differences in population parameters. (See page 224: Logic of Proof.)

18. **E.**   Statistical tests that do not require any assumptions about probability distributions of the populations are known as nonparametric tests; they can be used whenever there is very serious concern about the shape of the data. Nonparametric statistics are also the tests of choice for ordinal data. The basic concept behind nonparametric statistics is the ability to rank or order the observations; nonparametric tests are also called *order statistics*. The currently available nonparametric tests are not used more commonly because they do not adapt well to complex statistical models, and they are less able than parametric tests to distinguish between the null and alternative hypotheses if the data are normally distributed. (See page 228: Robustness and Nonparametric Tests.)

19. **A.**   A confidence interval describes how likely it is that the population parameter is estimated by any particular sample statistic such as the mean. The four options for decreasing type II error (increasing statistical power) are to increase the α, reduce the population variability, make the sample bigger, and make the difference between the conditions greater. Under most circumstances, only the sample size can be varied; thus, sample size planning has become an important part of research design for controlled clinical trials. When describing the spread, scatter, or dispersion of the sample, the standard deviation should be used; when describing the precision with which the population center is known, the SE should be used. Historical controls indicate a favorable outcome for a new therapy more often than concurrent controls (i.e., parallel control group or self-control). If the outcome with an old treatment is not studied simultaneously with the outcome of a new treat-

ment, one cannot know whether any differences in results are a consequence of the two treatments, of unsuspected and unknowable differences between the patients, or of other changes over time in the general medical environment. (See page 225: Sample Size Calculations and page 227: Confidence Intervals.)

20. **A.**   Although the results of a particular experiment may be presented by repeatedly showing the entire set of numbers, there are concise ways of summarizing the information content of the set into a few numbers. These numbers are called *sample* or *summary statistics*. The three most common summary statistics are the mean, median, and mode. (See page 223: Central Location.)

21. **E.**   For a sample of interval data taken from a normally distributed population for which population, for which CIs are to be chosen for, the precision factor is called the *standard error of the mean* and is obtained by dividing SD by the square root of the sample size or
$$SE = \frac{SD}{\sqrt{n}} = \sqrt{\sum_{i=1}^{n}(x_i - \bar{x})^2 / n(n-1)}.$$ (See page 227: Confidence Intervals.)

22. **A.**   The mode is the most popular number of a sample, that is, the number that occurs most frequently. The mode is always mentioned in discussions of descriptive statistics, but it is rarely used in statistical practice. (See page 223: Central Location.)

23. **C.**   The P value is the probability of getting a risk ratio at least as far from the null value of 1. (See page 226: Table 9-6.)

24. **B.**   Analysis of variance consists of rules for creating test statistics on means when there are more than two groups. These test statistics are called *F ratios*, after Ronald Fisher; the critical values for the *F*-test statistic are taken from the *F* probability distribution that Fisher derived. (See page 228: Analysis of Variance.)

CHAPTER

10

Cardiac Anatomy and Physiology

1. Regarding the cardiac cycle, which of the following is FALSE?

   A. Left ventricle (LV) systole has three phases.
   B. Isovolumic contraction occurs after mitral valve closure.
   C. The decrease in ejection fraction (EF) is proportional to the decrease in LV function.
   D. Isovolumic contraction occurs in both the LV and right ventricle (RV).
   E. Diastasis allows free blood flow through the left atrium (LA).

2. Which statement regarding coronary blood supply is FALSE?

   A. The left anterior descending, left circumflex, and right coronary arteries supply blood to the LV.
   B. Most coronary blood flow to the LV myocardium occurs during systole.
   C. A "right dominant" coronary circulation occurs when the right coronary artery supplies blood to the posterior descending coronary artery and is observed in approximately 80% of patients.
   D. Right atrial (RA), LA, and RV coronary perfusion occurs during both systole and diastole.
   E. Branches of the left circumflex coronary artery are the major sources of blood supply to the left atrium.

3. Each of the following is a characteristic of cardiac and skeletal muscle fibers EXCEPT:

   A. Both sarcolemma contain Na^+ channels.
   B. Impulses reach the myocytes through "T transverse tubules."
   C. Mitochondria are highly abundant in both types of fibers.
   D. Actin and myosin are the contractile proteins.
   E. They use transporter enzymes to regulate intracellular ion concentrations.

4. The heart normally extracts between 75% and 80% of arterial O_2 content, by far the greatest O_2 extraction of all the body's organs. In regards to O_2 demand and consumption by the heart, all of the following statements are true EXCEPT:

   A. Cardiac O_2 extraction dramatically increases to near maximal during exercise.
   B. The primary mechanism by which myocardium meets its O_2 demand through enhanced O_2 delivery.
   C. Coronary blood flow and myocardial O_2 consumption increase four- to fivefold during strenuous physical exercise.
   D. Heart rate is the primary determinant of myocardial O_2 demand in the intact heart.
   E. Myocardial O_2 consumption is a major determinant of coronary blood flow.

5. In regards to coronary physiology, which of the following statements is FALSE?

   A. The two major determinants of coronary blood flow are perfusion pressure and vascular resistance.
   B. Blood supply to the LV is directly dependent on the difference between the aortic pressure and LV end-diastolic pressure (coronary perfusion pressure), and inversely related to the vascular resistance to flow, which varies to the fourth power of the radius of the vessel.
   C. Resting coronary blood flow in the adult is approximately 25 mL/min (0.1 mL/min/g) or 10% of total cardiac output.
   D. The LV subendocardium is exposed to a higher wall pressure than the subepicardial layer during systole.
   E. In the presence of coronary artery stenoses, pressure-overload hypertrophy, or pronounced tachycardia, the subendocardial layer of the LV is more susceptible to ischemia.

6. The pressure–volume diagram, which plots continuous LV pressure and volume against one another, is useful for analysis of LV systolic and diastolic function. Based on the relationship between LV pressure and volume, all of the following statements are true EXCEPT:

   A. When LV pressure is greater than aorta pressure, the aortic valve opens.
   B. The aortic valve closes when LV pressure drops below aortic pressure.
   C. When LA pressure falls below LV pressure during iso-volumic relaxation, the mitral valve opens.
   D. The normal EDV and ESV are approximately 120 and 40 mL, respectively.
   E. Stroke volume is 80 mL and ejection fraction is 67% in the normal heart.

7. In regards to LV systolic function, which of the following statements is FALSE?

   A. LV hypertrophy is an important adaptation response to chronic increases in LV afterload that reduces LV wall stress by increasing wall thickness.
   B. Cardiac output and ejection fraction are most often used to quantify LV systolic function.
   C. Contractility may decline at heart rates greater than 175 beats/min.
   D. End-diastolic volume is most often used to define LV afterload.
   E. A commonly used clinical estimate of LV afterload is systemic vascular resistance, which equals $((MAP - RAP) \times 80)/CO$, where MAP, RAP, and CO are mean arterial pressure, right atrial pressure, and cardiac output respectively.

8. Which of the following statements regarding cardiac myocytes is FALSE?

   A. The contractile apparatus is composed of myosin, actin, tropomyosin, and the three-protein troponin complex.
   B. Troponin I alone is a strong inhibitor of actin–myosin binding, and when combined with tropomyosin, the troponin I–tropomyosin complex becomes a weak inhibitor of actin–myosin binding.
   C. Actin is the major component of the thin filament.
   D. Tropomyosin is one of two major inhibitors of actin–myosin interaction.
   E. Thick filaments are composed of myosin and its binding protein as well as titin.

9. Which of the following statements regarding the LA is FALSE?

   A. When compared to the LV, the LA is more susceptible to acute increases in afterload because the LA has thinner walls and less muscle mass.
   B. LA contractile dysfunction occurs as the chamber dilates in response to reduced LV compliance and increased pressure.
   C. The LA acts as a contractile chamber, a reservoir, and a conduit and its function is crucial to LV performance.
   D. Exercise enhances LA contractility and reduces its reservoir function.
   E. Under normal conditions, LA emptying fraction is dependent on LA contractility and preload.

10. Common cause(s) of left ventricular diastolic dysfunction include all of the following EXCEPT:

    A. Ventricular remodeling after infarction
    B. Only extremes of age (i.e., >80 years of age but not at >60 years of age)
    C. Volume-overload hypertrophy
    D. Pericardial diseases
    E. Pressure-overload hypertrophy

11. In regards to the gross anatomy of the heart and its valvular structures, which of the following statements is FALSE?

    A. The mitral valve opens in response to a positive pressure gradient between the LA and LV that occurs during the late phase of relaxation.
    B. The tricuspid valve is composed of anterior, posterior, and septal leaflets.
    C. The LV more easily decompensates with acute increases in afterload than the RV.
    D. The RV is able to produce less than 20% of the total pressure–volume (stroke) work produced by the LV.
    E. The atrial and ventricular myocardia are continuously interwoven and cannot be separated into distinct "layers."

12. **Which of the following statements about** the heart's electrical activity is FALSE?

    A. The initial SA node depolarization is rapidly transmitted across the RA to the AV node by the anterior, middle, and posterior internodal pathways.
    B. Atrial depolarization normally is directed solely to the RV and the LV through the AV node.
    C. Supraventricular tachyarrhythmias can result due to accessory pathways that bypass the AV node and establish abnormal conduction between the atria and ventricles.
    D. AV node conduction is relatively fast compared with the pathways proximal and distal to it.
    E. The heart's cartilaginous skeleton electrically isolates the atria from ventricles.

13. Which of the following statements pertaining to the pericardium is FALSE?

    A. The pericardium separates the heart from other structures in the mediastinum.
    B. The fluid in the pericardium consists of plasma ultra-filtrate, lymph, and myocardial interstitial fluid.
    C. Pericardial restraint is equally apparent throughout the heart's atria and ventricles.
    D. The pericardium equally restrains the RV and the LV, playing a crucial role in ventricular interdependence.
    E. Pericardial fluid facilitates cardiac movement.

14. Which of the following statements regarding heart failure with normal ejection fraction (HFNEF) is FALSE?

    A. Response to medical therapy does not predict prognosis in patients with HFNEF.
    B. A possible cause of HFNEF includes an abnormal coupling between the LV and the arterial circulation.
    C. LV diastolic dysfunction is a primary cause of HFNEF.
    D. The severity and response to medical therapy are key factors that establish exercise tolerance.
    E. Nearly one-half of patients with CHF have normal LV EF.

ANSWERS

1. D. LV systole is commonly divided into three phases: isovolumic contraction, rapid ejection, and slower ejection. Closure of both the tricuspid and mitral valves occurs when RV and LV pressures exceed the corresponding atrial pressure and causes the source of the first heart sound (S_1). Isovolumic contraction is the interval between closure of the mitral valve and the opening of the aortic valve. True isovolumic contraction does not occur in the RV because of the sequential nature of inflow followed by outflow during RV contraction. The normal LV end-diastolic volume is about 120 mL. The average ejected stroke volume is 80 mL, and the normal EF is approximately 67%. A decrease in EF below 40% is typically observed when the myocardium is affected by ischemia, infarction, or cardiomyopathic disease processes (e.g., myocarditis, amyloid infiltration). After left atrial and LV pressures have equalized, the mitral valve remains open, and pulmonary venous return continues to flow through the LA into the LV. This phase of diastole is known as diastasis, during which the LA functions as a conduit. Tachycardia progressively shortens and may completely eliminate this phase of diastole. Diastasis accounts for no more than 5% of total LV end-diastolic volume under normal circumstances. (See page 248: The Cardiac Cycle.)

2. B. Most coronary blood flow to the LV myocardium occurs during diastole (not systole) because during diastole aortic blood pressure is greater than LV pressure. Blood is supplied to the LV by the left anterior descending, left circumflex, and right coronary arteries (LAD, LCCA, and RCA, respectively). The "dominance" of the coronary circulation is determined by which major coronary artery feeds the posterior descending coronary artery (PDA). A "right dominant" circulation occurs when the RCA supplies blood to the PDA and is found in approximately 80% of patients. A "left dominant" circulation, which occurs in the remaining 20% of patients, is when the PDA is supplied by the LCCA. Coronary perfusion to the RA, LA, and RV occurs during both systole and diastole because the aortic blood pressure always exceeds the pressure within each of these chambers. In regards to the LA, branches of the LCCA are the major sources of its blood supply, and therefore, occlusion of the LCCA often causes left atrial contractile dysfunction, whereas an acutely occluded LAD can lead to a compensatory increase in left atrial contractility. Branches of both the RCA and the LCCA supply blood to the right atrium. (See page 241: Gross Anatomy-Coronary Blood Supply.)

3. C. The sarcolemma is the external membrane of the cardiac muscle cell, and it contains ion channels (e.g., Na^+, K^+, Ca^{2+}), ion pumps and exchangers (e.g., Na^+-K^+ ATPase, Ca^{2+}-ATPase, Na^+-Ca^{2+} or -H^+ exchangers), G-protein coupled and other receptors (e.g., β_1-adrenergic, adenosine, opioid), and transporter enzymes. These regulate intracellular ion concentrations, facilitate signal transduction, and provide metabolic substrates required for energy production. The contractile proteins are actin and myosin. Transverse ("T") tubules are deep invaginations of the sarcolemma that penetrate the internal structure of the myocyte at regular intervals, ensuring rapid and uniform transmission of the depolarizing impulses that initiate contraction to be simultaneously distributed throughout the cell. Unlike the skeletal muscle cell, the cardiac myocyte is densely packed with mitochondria, which are responsible for generation of the large quantities of high-energy phosphates (e.g., adenosine triphosphate) that are required for the heart's phasic cycle of contraction and relaxation. The sarcomere is the fundamental contractile unit of cardiac muscle. (See page 245: Cardiac Myocyte Anatomy and Function-Ultrastructure.)

4. A. Cardiac O_2 extraction is near maximal under resting conditions and cannot be substantially increased during exercise. Therefore, enhanced O_2 delivery is the primary mechanism by which myocardium meets its O_2 demand, which is proportional to coronary blood flow when hemoglobin concentration is constant. Furthermore, during strenuous physical exercise, coronary blood flow and myocardial O_2 consumption increase four- to fivefold. The primary determinant of myocardial O_2 demand in the intact heart is heart rate, but increases in myocardial contractility, preload, and afterload are also associated with elevations in myocardial O_2 demand. A major determinant of coronary blood flow is myocardial O_2 consumption. For example, coronary vascular resistance is greater in the rested, perfused heart than in the contracting heart, which indicates that coronary blood flow increases in response to a higher rate of O_2 consumption. (See page 244: Coronary Physiology.)

5. C. Resting coronary blood flow in the adult is approximately 250 mL/min (1 mL/min/g) or 5% (not 10%) of total cardiac output (approximately 70 mL/beat × 70 beats/min). Blood supply to the LV is directly dependent on the difference between the aortic pressure and LV end-diastolic pressure (coronary perfusion pressure) and inversely related to the vascular resistance to flow, which varies to the fourth power of the radius of the vessel (Poiseuille's law). Perfusion pressure and vascular resistance are two major determinants of coronary blood flow. Coronary perfusion pressure changes in response to aortic, intramyocardial, and coronary venous pressures, but the variable resistance produced by coronary vascular smooth muscle is the major factor that regulates coronary blood flow. During systole, the LV subendocardium is exposed to a higher wall pressure than the subepicardial layer. Also, the systolic intraventricular pressure may be higher than the peak LV systolic pressure. Because of these differences in tissue pressure, the subendocardial layer is more susceptible to ischemia in the presence of coronary artery stenoses, pressure-overload hypertrophy, or pronounced tachycardia. (See page 244; Coronary Physiology.)

6. C.   Continuous LV pressure and volume plotted against each other is useful for analysis of LV systolic and diastolic function. The LV pressure–volume diagram proceeds in a counterclockwise direction over time. End-diastole initiates the cardiac cycle, and it is followed by isovolumic contraction, in which a rapid increase in LV pressure occurs without change in LV volume. When LV pressure is greater than aorta pressure, the aortic valve opens, and ejection of blood from the LV into the proximal great vessels causes a sudden decline in LV volume. The aortic valve closes when LV pressure drops below aortic pressure. When LV pressure falls below LA pressure (not when LA pressure falls below LV pressure) during isovolumic relaxation, the mitral valve opens and LV filling occurs, thereby increasing LV volume during the remainder of diastole concomitant with small increases in LV pressure. The lower right and upper left corners of the pressure–volume diagram identify the LV end-diastolic and end-systolic volumes (EDV and ESV, respectively). The normal EDV and ESV are approximately 120 and 40 mL, respectively. Thus, stroke volume (EDV − ESV) is 80 mL and ejection fraction (SV/EDV) is 67% in the normal heart. (See page 250: The Pressure–Volume Diagram and page 250: Figure 11.)

7. D.   EDV is most often used to define LV preload (not afterload) because this volume of blood is directly related to LV end-diastolic wall stress. LV hypertrophy is an important adaptation response to chronic increases in LV afterload that reduces LV wall stress by increasing wall thickness; however, this compensatory response also increases myocardial oxygen demand and reduces LV compliance. Consequently, the hypertrophied LV is more susceptible to myocardial ischemia and diastolic dysfunction. Cardiac output and ejection fraction are most often used to quantify LV systolic function. In regards to LV contractility, heart rates greater than 175 beats/min may lead to decline in contractility because LV relaxation abnormalities begin to develop as a result of insufficient Ca^{2+} uptake from the contractile apparatus and because the duration of LV diastole becomes too brief to allow adequate LV filling. Therefore, tachyarrhythmias or rapid pacing may cause profound hypotension or hemodynamic collapse. Systemic vascular resistance is the most commonly used clinical estimate of LV afterload calculated as ((MAP − RAP) × 80)/CO, where MAP, RAP, and CO are mean arterial, right atrial pressures, and cardiac output, respectively, and 80 is a constant that converts mm Hg·min^{-1}·L^{-1} to dynes·sec·cm^{-5}. (See page 250: Factors that Determine Systolic Function.)

8. B.   The contractile apparatus of the cardiac monocyte is composed of myosin, actin, tropomyosin, and the three-protein troponin complex. Actin is a major component of the thin filament while thick filaments are composed of myosin and its binding protein as well as titin. Tropomyosin is one of two major inhibitors of actin–myosin interaction. Furthermore, troponin I alone weakly inhibits the interaction between actin and myosin, but when combined with tropomyosin, the troponin I–tropomyosin complex becomes a major inhibitor (not weak) of actin–myosin binding. (See page 245: Cardiac Myocyte Anatomy and Function-Contractile Apparatus.)

9. D.   The LA acts as a contractile chamber, a reservoir (storage of blood before mitral valve opening), and a conduit, and its function is vital to LV performance. Under normal conditions, LA emptying fraction is dependent on LA contractility and preload. When compared to the LV, the LA is more susceptible to acute increases in afterload because the LA has thinner walls and less muscle mass. LA contractile dysfunction occurs as the chamber dilates in response to reduced LV compliance and increased pressure. Exercise enhances not only LA contractility but also LA reservoir function. (See page 255: Factors that Determine Diastolic Function-Atrial Function.)

10. B.   Common causes of left ventricular diastolic dysfunction include the following: Age >60; acute myocardial ischemia (supply or demand); myocardial stunning, hibernation, or infarction; ventricular remodeling after infarction; pressure-overload hypertrophy (e.g., aortic stenosis, hypertension); volume-overload hypertrophy (e.g., aortic or mitral regurgitation); hypertrophic obstructive cardiomyopathy; dilated cardiomyopathy; restrictive cardiomyopathy (e.g., amyloidosis, hemochromatosis); and pericardial diseases (e.g., tamponade, constrictive pericarditis). (See page 256: Table 2—Common Causes of Left Ventricular Diastolic Dysfunction.)

11. C.   The mitral valve opens in response to a positive pressure gradient between the LA and LV that occurs during the late phase of relaxation. Untwisting and elastic recoil of the LV as the chamber relaxes further facilitates this process. Closure of the leaflets occurs during early systole as retrograde blood flow moves toward the valve. The tricuspid valve is composed of anterior, posterior, and septal leaflets, and provides unidirectional movement of blood from the RA and RV. Furthermore, the RV more easily decompensates with acute increases in afterload compared to the LV because the RV is able to produce less than 20% of the total pressure–volume (stroke) work than the thicker, more muscular LV. However, the RV is highly compliant and is able to accommodate to acute changes in intraventricular volume to a greater degree than the LV. The atrial and ventricular myocardia are continuously interwoven, and thus, they cannot be separated into distinct "layers." (See page 240: Gross Anatomy-Architecture and Valve Structure.)

12. D.   The initial SA node depolarization is quickly transmitted across the RA to the AV node by the anterior, middle (Wenckebach), and posterior (Thorel) internodal pathways. Also, through Bachmann's bundle (a branch of the anterior internodal pathway), the SA node depolarization is transmitted to the LA through the atrial septum. The heart's cartilaginous skeleton electrically isolates the atria from the ventricles. As a result, atrial depolarization is directed solely to the RV and the LV through the AV node. Since AV node conduction is relatively slow compared with the pathways proximal and distal to it, the AV node is responsible for the sequential contraction pattern of the atria and the ventricles. Therefore, supraventricular tachyarrhythmias can result due to accessory pathways that bypass the AV node and establish abnormal conduction between the atria and ventricles. (See page 240: Gross Anatomy-Impulse Conduction.)

13. C. The pericardial restraint is most apparent in the atria and RV because they have thinner walls than the LV. The pericardium not only separates the heart from other structures in the mediastinum but also limits the heart's displacement through its diaphragmatic and great vessel attachments. The fluid in the pericardium, which is made up of plasma ultrafiltrate, lymph, and myocardial interstitial fluid, facilitates cardiac movement. Furthermore, the pericardium equally restrains the RV and the LV playing a crucial role in ventricular interdependence. Consequently,

an acute increase in RV pressure and volume leads to increased pressure within the pericardium resulting in compression of the LV, reducing its effective compliance and impairing its filling. (See page 255: Factors that Determine Diastolic Function-Pericardium.)

14. A. Heart failure with normal ejection fraction (HFNEF), also known as diastolic heart failure, can be caused by delayed LV relaxation, reduced compliance, and abnormal coupling between the LV and the arterial circulation. Therefore, LV diastolic dysfunction is a primary cause of HFNEF, and the severity and response to medical therapy are key factors that establish exercise tolerance and may predict prognosis. Nearly one-half of patients with CHF have normal LV EF. (See page 255: Factors that Determine Diastolic Function.)

CHAPTER
11

Respiratory Function in Anesthesia

1. Which of the following statements regarding lung compliance is FALSE?

   A. Diseases that decrease lung compliance typically result in increased respiratory rates.
   B. Spontaneous respiratory rate is a poor indicator of lung compliance.
   C. Continuous positive airway pressure (CPAP) improves lung compliance and therefore lowers the work of breathing in patients with reduced compliance.
   D. Diseases that increase lung compliance typically result in increased functional residual capacity (FRC).
   E. Significant increases in lung compliance may require the use of the ventilatory muscles to exhale actively.

2. Which of the following statements regarding ventilation–perfusion (V/Q) matching is TRUE?

   A. West zone 1 can be best characterized as physiologic shunt.
   B. West zone 1 can be increased by increasing pulmonary artery pressure (Ppa).
   C. West zone 3 occurs above the level of the third rib in the sitting position.
   D. West zone 3 has Ppa > Pulmonary venous pressure (Ppv) > Alveolar pressure (Pa) and therefore has perfusion in excess of ventilation.
   E. In West zone 1, pulmonary capillary wedge pressure (PCWP) is transmitted to the alveoli promoting alveolar collapse, resulting in no ventilation of this area.

3. Functional residual capacity (FRC):

   A. Is the maximal volume that can be exhaled in a single breath.
   B. Is increased by mechanical factors such as obesity and pregnancy.
   C. Can be used to quantify the degree of pulmonary restriction.
   D. Is significantly increased in the supine position.
   E. Is markedly reduced in patients with chronic obstructive pulmonary disease (COPD).

4. Which of the following tests is most useful and cost-effective in screening overall pulmonary function?

   A. The flow–volume loop
   B. The CO_2 diffusing capacity of the lungs (DLCO)
   C. The maximum voluntary ventilation
   D. Spirometry measurements
   E. Blood gas analysis

5. Which of the following statements regarding postoperative pulmonary function is TRUE?

   A. The changes in postoperative pulmonary function are primarily obstructive.
   B. Postoperative spontaneous ventilation is characterized by the absence of sighs.
   C. Thoracic operations have a more severe impact on functional residual capacity (FRC) than nonlaparoscopic upper abdominal operations.
   D. The normal postoperative respiratory rate is 12 to 13 breaths/min.
   E. Intracranial procedures typically decrease FRC by 40% to 50%.

6. The maximum benefit from preoperative smoking cessation occurs at approximately:

   A. 24 hours
   B. 2 days
   C. 2 weeks
   D. 4 weeks
   E. 8 weeks

7. Which of the following statements regarding cigarette smoking and lung disease is FALSE?

   A. Smoke increases mucus production and decreases ciliary motility.
   B. Smoking leads to a decrease in proteolytic enzymes in the lung that directly cause damage to lung parenchyma.
   C. Patients with chronic obstructive pulmonary disease (COPD) who smoke have up to a six fold greater risk of developing postoperative pneumonia than nonsmokers.
   D. Normalization of mucociliary activity requires at least 2 to 3 weeks of abstinence from smoking.
   E. Smokers' relative risk of postoperative pulmonary complications is doubled even in the absence of clinical pulmonary disease and abnormal pulmonary function test results.

8. All of the following strategies reduce the risk of postoperative pulmonary complications EXCEPT:

   A. Intraoperative inhalational anesthetic
   B. Postoperative pain management
   C. Incentive spirometry
   D. Stir-up regimens
   E. Intermittent continuous positive airway pressure (CPAP) by mask

9. When diaphragm function is impaired in patients with cervical spinal cord transection, which of the following act as primary inspiratory muscles?

   A. Intercostal muscles
   B. Cervical strap muscles
   C. Abdominal muscles
   D. Intervertebral muscles of the shoulder girdle
   E. Sternocleidomastoid muscles

10. Which is the last airway component that is incapable of gas exchange?

    A. Respiratory bronchiole
    B. Terminal bronchiole
    C. Alveolar ducts
    D. Mainstem bronchi
    E. Alveolar sacs

11. Which of the following statements regarding type 1 cells is FALSE?

    A. They contain extremely thin cytoplasmic extensions that provide surface for gas exchange.
    B. They are highly differentiated.
    C. They cover 80% of the alveolar surface.
    D. They are very resistant to injury.
    E. They are metabolically limited.

12. Which of the following primarily limits the depth of inspiration?

    A. Pneumotaxic center
    B. Apneustic center
    C. Ventral respiratory group
    D. Dorsal respiratory group
    E. Reticular activating system

13. Which of the following does not cause absolute or true shunt?

    A. Acute lobar atelectasis
    B. Extensive acute lung injury
    C. Advanced pulmonary edema
    D. Pulmonary embolus
    E. Consolidated pneumonia

14. Which of the following statements is FALSE about the CO_2 diffusing capacity of the lungs (DLCO)?

    A. Decreased hemoglobin concentration decreases the DLCO.
    B. DLCO values increase two to three times normal during exercise.
    C. DLCO is decreased in obstructive disease states.
    D. Decreased alveolar PCO_2 increases DLCO.
    E. Low DLCO is related to loss of lung volume or capillary bed perfusion.

15. Which of the following is not a component of the alveolar wall?

    A. Thin capillary epithelial cell
    B. Basement membrane
    C. Pulmonary capillary endothelial cell
    D. Surfactant lining layer
    E. Schwann cell

16. Which of the following conditions does not favor turbulent flow over laminar flow?

    A. High gas flows
    B. Sharp angles within the tube
    C. Branching in the tube
    D. Increase in the tube's diameter

17. Which of the following statements regarding the trachea is TRUE?

    A. In the supine position, the most likely place for aspirated material to fall is the right lower lobe.
    B. It is totally intrathoracic, with 50% in the superior mediastinum and 50% in the inferior mediastinum.
    C. The tracheal bifurcation is usually at the level of T4.
    D. The trachea's fixed position in the inferior mediastinum serves as an important reference point.

18. Which of the following statements regarding bronchioles is TRUE?

    A. They are approximately 4 mm in diameter.
    B. They have the highest proportion of smooth muscle in their walls.
    C. They are the last segment of the conducting airways to contain cartilage.
    D. The terminal bronchioles may be involved in terminal gas exchange if they are recruited.

19. Which of the following characteristics regarding gas flow is TRUE?

    A. With laminar gas flow, significant alveolar ventilation can occur, even when tidal volume is less than dead space.
    B. Density is the only physical gas property that is relevant under laminar gas flow conditions.
    C. Helium does not improve gas flow under turbulent conditions.
    D. During turbulent flow, resistance decreases in proportion to flow rate.

20. The Hering–Breuer reflex:

    A. Produces apnea in humans when continuous positive airway pressure (CPAP) reaches 40 cm H_2O.
    B. Is a pulmonary stretch reflex that is primarily generated from the intercostal muscles and the diaphragm.
    C. Is prominent in humans but not lower-order mammals.
    D. Is blocked by bilateral vagotomy.

21. Which of the following does not result in an enhanced CO_2 response (shift of CO_2 response curve upward and to the left)?

    A. Anxiety
    B. Metabolic acidosis
    C. Arterial hypoxemia
    D. Opioid antagonists in the absence of opioids

22. Inspiratory capacity:

    A. Is defined as the greatest volume that can be inhaled from the resting inspiratory level.
    B. Is commonly measured as part of routine pulmonary function testing.
    C. Can be a sensitive indicator of extrathoracic airway obstruction.
    D. Is less sensitive than expiratory measurements to extrathoracic obstruction.

23. Which of the following statements is TRUE?

    A. The direct effect of CO_2 on central chemoreceptors is responsible for more than 80% of the resultant increase in ventilatory response.
    B. A sudden decrease in the pressure of end-tidal CO_2 ($PETCO_2$) in a mechanically ventilated patient in the intensive care unit is most often caused by pulmonary air embolism.
    C. Preoperative pulmonary function testing is important in predicting the likelihood of postoperative pulmonary complications.
    D. Patients having intrathoracic operations are at a slightly lower risk of experiencing postoperative pulmonary complications than patients having upper abdominal operations.

24. With regards to the relationship between the carbon dioxide response curve and PaO_2:

    A. PaO_2 of >100 mm Hg causes the CO_2 response curve to shift left.
    B. PaO_2 of 65 to 100 mm Hg has a small effect on the CO_2 response curve.
    C. PaO_2 of 45 to 65 mm Hg has no effect on the CO_2 response curve.
    D. PaO_2 of <45 mm Hg causes the CO_2 response curve to shift right.

25. As $PaCO_2$ increases beyond a threshold, it begins to act as a CNS depressant; the equivalent of a 1 MAC anesthetic in CO_2 levels is approximately:

    A. 75 mm Hg
    B. 100 mm Hg
    C. 150 mm Hg
    D. 200 mm Hg
    E. 250 mm Hg

26. Which of the following mechanisms does not involve reflex control of ventilation?

    A. Swallowing
    B. Vomiting
    C. Coughing
    D. Golgi tendon organs
    E. Valsalva maneuver

27. During breath holding, $PaCO_2$ levels change in the following manner:

    A. The apneic anesthetized patient has a $PaCO_2$ rise of approximately 12 mm Hg in the first minute and 6 mm Hg each minute thereafter.
    B. Hyperventilation in an awake patient will usually not result in an apneic period.
    C. It is more effective for swimmers to hyperventilate with room air than 100% O_2 prior to underwater swimming.
    D. An awake person will feel "compelled" to breathe at a $PaCO_2$ of 40 mm Hg.
    E. With larger lung volumes, CO_2 concentration in the lung will increase more rapidly during breath holding.

28. With regards to a flow–volume loop, which of the following is true?

    A. Flow is on the x axis.
    B. The data obtained are superior to imaging the lung for preoperative screenings.
    C. The subject generates a complete forced expiration followed by a maximal forced inhalation.
    D. Flow is plotted on the abscissa.
    E. The principal use is in the diagnosis and categorization of small airway disease.

29. Which of the following is NOT true of patients with obstructive pulmonary disease?

    A. High alveolar concentrations of most potent inhalational anesthetics will blunt airway reflexes and reflex bronchoconstriction.
    B. Administration of opioids will decrease airway reactivity.
    C. Spontaneous ventilation during GA in patients with severe obstructive disease is more likely to result in hypocapnia than in patients with normal pulmonary function.
    D. Peak airway pressures should be kept below 40 cm H_2O.
    E. Deep extubation is suggested in young, asthmatic patients.

30. Chemoreceptors involved in the control of respiration include all of the following EXCEPT:

    A. Carotid bodies
    B. Aortic bodies
    C. Inferolateral medulla near CN IX and X
    D. Lewy bodies

ANSWERS

1. B. When lung compliance is small, larger changes in intrapleural pressure are needed to create the same tidal volume (Vt) (i.e., one has to inhale harder to force the same volume of gas into the lungs). Thus, patients with low lung compliance typically breathe with a smaller Vt at more rapid rates. Spontaneous ventilatory rate is one of the most sensitive indices of lung compliance. CPAP shifts the vertical line to the right, allowing the patient to breathe on a steeper and more favorable portion of the volume–pressure curve. This results in a slower ventilatory rate with a larger Vt. Patients with diseases that increase lung compliance have larger than normal FRCs (gas trapping) and pressure–volume curves that are shifted to the left and steeper. These patients expend less elastic work to inspire, but elastic recoil is reduced significantly. COPD and acute asthma are the most common examples of diseases with high lung compliance. If lung compliance and FRC are sufficiently high (elastic recoil is minimal), the patient must use the ventilatory muscles to expire actively. (See page 266: Elastic Work.)

2. D. Zone 1 receives ventilation in the absence of perfusion and creates alveolar dead space ventilation. Normally, zone 1 areas exist only to a limited extent. However, in conditions of decreased Ppa, such as hypovolemic shock, zone 1 enlarges. Since Pa is approximately equal to atmospheric pressure, Ppa in zone 1 is subatmospheric but necessarily greater than Ppv (Pa > Ppa > Ppv). Pa that is transmitted to the pulmonary capillaries promotes their collapse, with a consequent theoretical blood flow of zero to this lung region. Thus, zone 1 receives ventilation in the absence of perfusion and creates alveolar dead space ventilation. Zone 3 occurs in the most gravity-dependent areas of the lung, where Ppa > Ppv > Pa and blood flow is primarily governed by the Ppa to Ppv difference. Since gravity also increases Ppv, the pulmonary capillaries become distended. Thus, perfusion in zone 3 is lush, resulting in capillary perfusion in excess of ventilation, or physiologic shunt. The pressure difference between Ppa and Pa determines blood flow in zone 2. Ppv has little influence. Well-matched ventilation and perfusion occur in zone 2, which contains the majority of alveoli. (See page 274: Distribution of Blood Flow.)

3. C. FRC is the volume of gas remaining in the lungs at passive end expiration. Residual volume is the gas remaining within the lungs at the end of forced maximal expiration. The FRC may also be used to quantify the degree of pulmonary restriction. Disease processes that reduce FRC and lung compliance include acute lung injury, pulmonary edema, pulmonary fibrotic processes, and atelectasis. Mechanical factors also reduce FRC (e.g., pregnancy, obesity, and pleural effusion). The FRC decreases 10% when a healthy subject lies down. Ventilatory muscle weakness and paralysis also decrease FRC. In contrast, patients with COPD have excessively compliant lungs that recoil less forcibly. Their lungs retain an abnormally large volume at the end of passive expiration, a phenomenon called gas trapping. (See page 278: Lung Volumes and Capacities.)

4. D. Although we have a host of pulmonary function tests from which to choose, spirometry is the most useful, cost-effective, and most commonly used test. (See page 281: Practical Application of PFT's.)

5. B. The changes in pulmonary function that occur postoperatively are primarily restrictive, with proportional decreases in all lung volumes and no change in airway resistance. This defect is generated by abdominal contents that impinge on and prevent normal movement of the diaphragm and an abnormal respiratory pattern that is shallow, rapid, and devoid of sighs. Whereas the normal resting respiratory rate for adults is 12 breaths/min, postoperative patients usually breathe approximately 20 breaths/min. The operative site is one of the single most important determinants of the degree of pulmonary restriction and the risk of postoperative pulmonary complications. Nonlaparoscopic upper abdominal operations cause the most profound restrictive defect, precipitating a 40% to 50% decrease in FRC compared with preoperative levels when conventional postoperative analgesia is used. Lower abdominal and thoracic operations cause the next most severe change in pulmonary function, with decreases in FRC to 30% of preoperative levels. Most other operative sites, including intracranial, have approximately the same effect on FRC, with reductions to 15% to 20% of preoperative levels. (See page 284: Postoperative Pulmonary Function.)

6. E. Patients who smoke should be advised to stop smoking 2 months before elective operations to maximize the effect of smoking cessation or for at least 4 weeks to gain some benefit from improved mucociliary function. Normalization of mucociliary function requires 2 to 3 weeks of abstinence from smoking, during which time sputum increases. Several months of smoking abstinence are required to return sputum clearance to normal. If patients cannot stop smoking for these periods of time, they probably should be advised to stop smoking for at least 24 hours before the operation so that carboxyhemoglobin levels will approach normal. Smokers who decrease but do not stop cigarette consumption without the aid of nicotine replacement therapy continue to acquire equal amounts of nicotine from fewer cigarettes by changing their technique of smoking to maximize nicotine intake. (See page 283: Effects of Cigarette Smoking on Pulmonary Function.)

7. B. Smoking affects pulmonary function in many ways. The irritant smoke decreases ciliary motility and increases sputum production. Thus, these patients have a high volume of sputum and decreased ability to clear it effectively. As smoking habits persist, airway reactivity and the development of obstructive disease become problematic. Studies of the pathogenesis of COPD suggest that smoking results in an excess of pulmonary proteolytic enzymes that directly cause damage to the lung parenchyma. Exposure to smoke increases synthesis and release of elastolytic enzymes from the alveolar macrophages (cells instrumental in the genesis of COPD resulting from smoking).

Smoking is one of the main and most prevalent risk factors associated with postoperative morbidity. Patients with COPD who smoke have a two- to sixfold risk of developing postoperative pneumonia compared with nonsmokers. Furthermore, smokers' relative risk of postoperative pulmonary complications is doubled, even if they do not have evidence of clinical pulmonary disease or abnormal pulmonary function. Normalization of mucociliary function requires 2 to 3 weeks of abstinence from smoking, during which time sputum increases. (See page 283: Effects of Cigarette Smoking on Pulmonary Function.)

8. A.   There are several strategies by which it is possible to reduce the risk of postoperative pulmonary complications, including use of lung-expanding therapies after surgery, choice of analgesia, and cessation of smoking. After upper abdominal operations, which are associated with the highest incidence of postoperative pulmonary complications, functional residual capacity (FRC) recovers over 3 to 7 days. With the use of intermittent CPAP by mask, FRC recovers within 72 hours. Patients use incentive spirometers correctly only 10% of the time unless therapy is supervised. Stir-up regimens are as effective as incentive spirometry at preventing postoperative pulmonary complications and are less expensive than supervised incentive spirometry, so they are preferred over incentive spirometry therapy. The choice of anesthetic technique for intraoperative anesthesia does not change the risk of postoperative pulmonary complications, but the choice of postoperative analgesia strongly influences the risk of these complications. The advent of postoperative epidural analgesia, particularly for abdominal and thoracic operations, has markedly decreased the risk of postoperative pulmonary complications and appears to contribute to decreased length of stay in the hospital postoperatively. (See page 284: Postoperative Pulmonary Complications.)

9. B.   The ventilatory muscles include the diaphragm, intercostal muscles, abdominal muscles, cervical strap muscles, sternocleidomastoid muscles, and large back and intervertebral muscles of the shoulder girdle. During breathing, the diaphragm performs most of the muscle work. Work contribution from the intercostal muscles is minor. With an increase in work, the cervical strap muscles help elevate the sternum and upper portions of the chest. The cervical strap muscles, active even during breathing at rest, are the most important inspiratory accessory muscles. When diaphragm function is impaired, as in patients with cervical spinal cord transaction, they can become the primary inspiratory muscles. During periods of maximal work, the large back and paravertebral muscles of the shoulder girdle contribute to ventilatory effort. The abdominal wall muscles are the most powerful muscles of expiration. (See page 264: Functional Anatomy of the Lungs.)

10. B.   The airway generation beyond the trachea is composed of the right and left mainstem bronchi. Further generations consist of bronchioles, of which the final generation is termed the terminal bronchiole; this is the last airway component incapable of gas exchange. The respiratory bronchiole, which follows the terminal bronchiole, is the first site in the tracheobronchial tree where gas exchange occurs. In adults, two or three generations of respiratory bronchioles lead to alveolar ducts, of which there are four to five generations, each with multiple openings into alveolar sacs. (See page 264: Lung Structures.)

11. D.   Type 1 alveolar cells cover approximately 80% of the alveolar surface. Type 1 cells contain flattened nuclei and extremely thin cytoplasmic extensions that provide the surface for gas exchange. They are highly differentiated and metabolically limited, which makes them highly susceptible to injury. (See page 264: Lung Structures.)

12. A.   The primary function of the pneumotaxic center is to limit the depth of inspiration. When maximally activated, the pneumotaxic center secondarily increases ventilatory frequency. However, it performs no pacemaking function and has no intrinsic rhythmicity. The dorsal respiratory group is the source of elementary ventilatory rhythmicity and serves as the pacemaker for the respiratory system. The ventral respiratory group serves as the expiratory coordinating center. With activation, the apneustic center sends impulses to inspiratory dorsal respiratory group neurons and is designed to sustain inspiration. (See page 269: Generation of Ventilatory Pattern.)

13. D.   Physiologic shunt occurs in a lung that is perfused but poorly ventilated. Physiologic shunt is the portion of the total cardiac output that returns to the left heart and systemic circulation without receiving oxygen in the lung. Diseases that cause absolute or true shunt include acute lobar atelectasis, extensive acute lung injury, advanced pulmonary edema, and consolidated pneumonia. Physiologic dead space ventilation applies to areas of the lung that are ventilated but poorly perfused as in pulmonary embolus. (See page 277: Physiologic Shunt.)

14. D.   DLCO collectively measures all of the factors that affect the diffusion of gas across the alveolar capillary membrane. DLCO values may increase to two or three times normal during exercise. Decreased hemoglobin concentration decreases DLCO. An increased $PaCO_2$ increases DLCO. Low DLCO is more closely related to loss of lung volume or capillary bed perfusion. DLCO is decreased in all obstructive disease states. (See page 280: Carbon Monoxide Diffusing Capacity.)

15. E.   The alveolar–capillary interface is well designed to facilitate gas exchange. The alveolar wall consists of a thin capillary epithelial cell, basement membrane, pulmonary capillary endothelial cell, and surfactant lining layer. Schwann cells are the principal glia of the peripheral nervous system. (See page 264: Lung Structures.)

16. D.   Four conditions that change laminar flow to turbulent flow are high gas flows, sharp angles within the tube, branching in the tube, and a decrease in the tube's diameter. During laminar flow, resistance is inversely proportional to the gas flow rate. During turbulent flow, resistance increases significantly in proportion to the flow rate. (See page 268: Turbulent Flow.)

17. C. The diameter of the right bronchus is generally greater than that of the left. In adults, whereas the right bronchus leaves the trachea at approximately 25 degrees from the tracheal axis, the angle of the left bronchus is approximately 45 degrees. Thus, inadvertent endobronchial intubation or aspiration of foreign material is more likely to occur in the right lung than in the left. Furthermore, the right upper lobe bronchus dives almost directly posterior at approximately 90 degrees from the right main bronchus. Foreign bodies and fluid aspirated by a supine subject usually fall into the right upper lobe. In adults, the trachea is a fibromuscular tube approximately 10 to 12 cm long with an outside diameter of approximately 20 mm. The trachea enters the superior mediastinum and bifurcates at the sternal angle (the lower border of the fourth thoracic vertebral body). Normally, half of the trachea is intrathoracic, and the other half is extrathoracic. Both ends of the trachea are attached to mobile structures. Thus, the carina can move superiorly as much as 5 cm from its normal resting position. (See page 265: Conductive Airways.)

18. B. The bronchioles typically have diameters of 1 mm. They are devoid of cartilaginous support and have the highest proportion of smooth muscle in their walls. There are approximately three to four bronchiolar generations. The final bronchiolar generation is the terminal bronchiole, which is the last airway component that is not directly involved in gas exchange. (See page 265: Conductive Airways.)

19. A. A clinical implication of laminar flow in the airways is that significant alveolar ventilation can occur even when the tidal volume is less than anatomic dead space. This phenomenon is important in high-frequency ventilation. Viscosity is the only physical gas property that is relevant under conditions of laminar flow. Helium has a low density, but its viscosity is close to that of air. Therefore, helium will not improve gas flow that is laminar. Flow is usually turbulent when there is critical airway narrowing or abnormally high airway resistance, thus making low-density helium therapy useful. Resistance during laminar flow is inversely proportional to gas flow rate. Conversely, during turbulent flow, resistance increases in proportion to the flow rate. (See page 268: Resistance to Gas Flow.)

20. D. The Golgi tendon organs (tendon spindles), which occur in series arrangements within ventilatory muscles, facilitate proprioception. Whereas the intercostal muscles are rich in tendon spindles, the diaphragm has a limited number. Thus, the pulmonary stretch reflex primarily involves the intercostal muscles but not the diaphragm. When the lungs are full and the chest wall is stretched, these receptors send signals to the brainstem, further inhibiting inspiration. In 1868, Hering and Breuer reported that lightly anesthetized, spontaneously breathing animals cease or decrease ventilatory effort during sustained lung distention. This response was blocked by bilateral vagotomy. The Hering–Breuer reflex is prominent in lower-order mammals, such as rabbits, but is only weakly present in humans. This reflex is sufficiently active in lower mammals, such that 5 cm H_2O CPAP induces apnea. In humans, however, the reflex is only weakly present, as evidenced by the fact that humans continue to breathe spontaneously with CPAP in excess of 40 cm H_2O. This inflation reflex is associated with inspiratory muscle inhibition, as documented by marked reductions in the electrical activity of both the phrenic nerve and the diaphragmatic muscle itself. The second component of the Hering–Breuer reflex, the deflation reflex, produces increased ventilatory muscle activity after sustained lung deflation. (See page 270: Reflex Control of Ventilation.)

21. D. Three clinical states result in a left shift or a steepened slope of the CO_2 response curve. These same three situations are the only causes of true hyperventilation (i.e., an increase in minute ventilation such that the decreased $PaCO_2$ creates respiratory alkalemia). The three causes of hyperventilation (enhanced CO_2 response) are arterial hypoxemia, metabolic acidemia, and central etiologic factors. Examples of central etiologic factors that cause hyperventilation include drug administration, intracranial hypertension, hepatic cirrhosis, and nonspecific arousal states such as anxiety and fear. Aminophylline, salicylates, and norepinephrine stimulate ventilation independent of peripheral chemoreceptors. Opioid antagonists, given in the absence of opioids, do not stimulate ventilation. However, when they are given after opioid administration, they do reverse the effects of opioids on the CO_2 response curve. (See page 272: Quantitative Aspects of Chemical Control of Breathing.)

22. B. The inspiratory capacity is the largest volume of gas that can be inspired from the resting expiratory level and is frequently decreased in the presence of significant extrathoracic airway obstruction. This measurement is one of the few simple tests that can detect extrathoracic airway obstruction. Most routine pulmonary function tests measure only exhaled flows and volumes, which are relatively unaffected by extrathoracic obstruction unless it is severe. Changes in the absolute volume of inspiratory capacity usually parallel changes in vital capacity. Expiratory reserve volume is not of great diagnostic value. (See page 278: Lung Volumes and Capacities.)

23. D. Although the central response is the major factor in the regulation of breathing by CO_2, CO_2 has little direct stimulating effect on these chemosensitive areas. These receptors are primarily sensitive to changes in H^+ concentration. CO_2 has a potent but indirect effect by reacting with water to form carbonic acid, which dissociates into H^+ and bicarbonate ions. The $PETCO_2$ in ventilated patients varies linearly with the dead space (Vd) to tidal volume (Vt) ratio (Vd/Vt) and correlates poorly with $PaCO_2$. Monitoring $PETCO_2$ gives far more information about ventilatory efficiency or Vd than it does about the absolute value of $PaCO_2$. Anesthesiologists commonly measure $PETCO_2$ to detect venous air embolism during anesthesia. A lowered cardiac output alone, in the absence of venous air embolism, may sufficiently decrease pulmonary perfusion so that Vd increases and $PETCO_2$ decreases. Thus, a depressed $PETCO_2$ is a sensitive but nonspecific monitor, and in mechanically ventilated patients is most likely due to decreased pulmonary perfusion.

The goals one hopes to achieve through preoperative pulmonary function testing are to predict the likelihood of pulmonary complications, obtain quantitative baseline information concerning pulmonary function, and identify patients who may benefit from therapy to improve pulmonary function preoperatively. For patients who will have lung resection, pulmonary function testing provides some predictive benefit. However, for other patients, the overwhelming evidence suggests that preoperative pulmonary function testing does not predict or assign risk for postoperative pulmonary complications. The operative site is the single most important determinant of both the degree of pulmonary restriction and postoperative pulmonary complications. Nonlaparoscopic upper abdominal operations increase the risk of postoperative pulmonary complications by at least twofold. Lower abdominal and intrathoracic operations are associated with slightly lower risk but still higher risk than extremity, intracranial, and head and neck operations. (See page 271: Central Chemoreceptors: Assessment of Physiologic Dead Space; page 284: Postoperative Pulmonary Complications; and page 281: Preoperative Pulmonary Assessment.)

24. B.   Once PaO_2 exceeds 100 mm Hg, it no longer influences the carbon dioxide response curve. When the PaO_2 is between 65 and 100 mm Hg, its effect on the carbon dioxide response curve is small. However, when PaO_2 falls to less than 65 mm Hg, the carbon dioxide response curve shifts to the left and its slope increases, probably as a result of increased ventilatory drive stimulated by the peripheral chemoreceptors. (See page 272: Quantitative Aspects of Chemical Control of Breathing.)

25. D.   Increasing the $PaCO_2$ to higher than 100 mm Hg allows carbon dioxide to act as a ventilatory and CNS depressant, the origin of the term "carbon dioxide narcosis," with 1 minimum alveolar concentration (MAC) being approximately 200 mm Hg. (See page 272: Quantitative Aspects of Chemical Control of Breathing.)

26. E.   During swallowing, inspiration ceases momentarily; it is usually followed by a single large breath, and briefly increases ventilation. Vomiting significantly modifies normal ventilatory activity; input into the respiratory centers occurs from both cranial and spinal cord nerves. Coughing results from stimulation of the tracheal subepithelium, especially along the posterior tracheal wall and carina. An effective cough requires deep inspiration and then forced exhalation against a momentarily closed glottis to increase intrathoracic pressure, thus allowing an expulsive expiratory maneuver. Proprioception in the pulmonary system, the qualitative knowledge of the gas volume within the lungs, probably arises from smooth muscle spindle receptors. Clinical conditions in which pulmonary airway stretch receptors are stimulated include pulmonary edema and atelectasis. Golgi tendon organs (tendon spindles), which are arranged in series within ventilatory muscles, facilitate proprioception. The pulmonary stretch reflex primarily involves the intercostal muscles but not the diaphragm. When the lungs are full and the chest wall is stretched, these receptors send signals to the brainstem that inhibit further inspiration. (See page 270: Reflex Control of Ventilation.)

27. B.   After 1 minute of breath holding under these circumstances, PaO_2 decreases to ~65 to 70 mm Hg and $PaCO_2$ increases by ~12 mm Hg. In the absence of supplemental oxygen and hyperventilation, the "breakpoint" at which normal people are compelled to breathe is remarkably constant at a $PaCO_2$ of 50 mm Hg. With smaller lung volumes, the same amount of carbon dioxide is emptied into a smaller volume during the apneic period, thus increasing the carbon dioxide concentration more rapidly than occurs with larger lung volumes. The rate of rise of $PaCO_2$ in apneic anesthetized patients is 12 mm Hg during the first minute and 3.5 mm Hg/min thereafter, significantly lower than in the awake state. During underwater swimming after poolside hyperventilation, the urge to breathe is first stimulated by a rising $PaCO_2$. Since an increased arterial carbon dioxide tension provides the stimulus to inspire, swimmers who hyperventilate with room air before swimming long distances frequently lose consciousness from arterial hypoxemia before the $PaCO_2$ is sufficiently increased to stimulate the "need" to breathe. Hyperventilation is rarely followed by an apneic period in awake humans, despite a markedly depressed $PaCO_2$. However, minute ventilation may decrease significantly. (See page 272: Breath-Holding.)

28. C.   The flow–volume loop graphically demonstrates the flow generated during a forced expiratory maneuver followed by a forced inspiratory maneuver, plotted against the volume of gas expired. The subject forcefully exhales completely, then immediately forcefully inhales to vital capacity. The expired and inspired volumes are plotted on the abscissa (X-axis) and flow is plotted on the ordinate (Y-axis). Flow–volume loops were formerly useful in the diagnosis of large airway and extrathoracic airway obstruction prior to the availability of precise imaging techniques. It is rare that flow–volume loops are useful for preoperative pulmonary evaluation in the modern era of imaging. (See page 280: Flow–Volume Loops.)

29. C.   Patients with marked obstructive pulmonary disease are at increased risk for both intraoperative and postoperative pulmonary complications. High alveolar concentrations of most potent inhalational anesthetics will blunt airway reflexes and reflex bronchoconstriction but require a fairly robust cardiovascular system. Adjunctive intravenous administration of opioids and lidocaine prior to airway instrumentation will decrease airway reactivity by deepening anesthesia. Spontaneous ventilation during general anesthesia in patients with severe obstructive disease is more likely to result in hypercapnia than in patients with normal pulmonary function. Tidal volume and inspiratory flows should be adjusted to keep peak airway pressure less than 40 cm H_2O. For some patients with obstructive disease (e.g., the young asthmatic), many advocate tracheal extubation during deep anesthesia at the conclusion of the operation. (See page 282: Anesthesia and Obstructive Pulmonary Disease.)

30. D.   The peripheral chemoreceptors are composed of the carotid and aortic bodies. The carotid bodies, located at the bifurcation of the common carotid artery, have predominantly ventilatory effects. The aortic bodies, which are scattered about the aortic arch and its branches, have predominantly circulatory effects. The chemosensitive areas of the brainstem are in the inferolateral aspects of the medulla near the origin of cranial nerves IX and X. (See page 271: Chemical Control of Ventilation.)

CHAPTER 12

The Allergic Response

1. The humoral defense system includes all the following EXCEPT:

   A. Antibodies
   B. Cytokines
   C. Complement
   D. Lymphocytes
   E. Circulating proteins

2. Which type of T-cell does not require specific antigen stimulation to initiate its function?

   A. Cytotoxic
   B. Lymphotrophic
   C. Suppressor
   D. Helper
   E. Killer

3. Which of the following statements regarding antibodies is TRUE?

   A. Each antibody has two heavy chains and one light chain.
   B. The Fab segment binds the antigen.
   C. The light chain is responsible for the unique biologic properties of the different classes of immunoglobulins.
   D. There are six major classes of antibodies in humans.
   E. The light chain determines the structure and function of each molecule.

4. The attachment of an antibody or complement fragment to the surface of foreign cells is called:

   A. Immunogenicity
   B. Hepatogenicity
   C. Opsonization
   D. Lymphotropism
   E. Lymphokinesis

5. Which kind of cells regulate immune responses by presenting antigens to result in microbicidal function?

   A. Eosinophils
   B. Basophils
   C. Neutrophils
   D. Mast cells
   E. Macrophages

6. Complement can be activated by all of the following EXCEPT:

   A. Immunoglobulin G (IgG)
   B. Plasmin
   C. Killer T-cells
   D. Endotoxin
   E. The alternate pathway

7. True statements concerning the secondary treatment of anaphylaxis include all of the following EXCEPT:

   A. Bicarbonate should be given to treat severe acidemia.
   B. Corticosteroids require 12 to 24 hours to work.
   C. Corticosteroids are recommended for IgE-mediated reactions.
   D. Antihistamines inhibit histamine release.
   E. Catecholamines, such as epinephrine, can be used if bronchospasm is present.

8. Which of the following tests is used to determine basophil activation?

   A. Skin testing
   B. The leukocyte histamine release test
   C. Enzyme-linked immunosorbent assay (ELISA)
   D. The radioallergosorbent test
   E. The protamine test

9. Most of the allergic reactions evoked by intravenous drugs occur within how many minutes of administration?

   A. 5
   B. 10 to 20
   C. 30 to 45
   D. 45 to 60
   E. >60

10. With regard to latex allergy, all of the following patients are at increased risk for anaphylaxis EXCEPT:

   A. Health care workers
   B. Children with spina bifida
   C. Patients with urogenital abnormalities
   D. Patients with penicillin allergy
   E. Patients allergic to bananas

11. Which of the following statements regarding chemical mediators of inflammation is FALSE?

    A. Leukotrienes are derived from arachidonic acid metabolism of phospholipid membranes.
    B. Prostaglandins are potent mast cell mediators.
    C. Prostaglandin D_2 produces bronchospasm.
    D. Kinins are synthesized by lymphocytes.
    E. Prostaglandin D_2 produces vasodilation.

12. Which of the following statements regarding anaphylactic reactions is TRUE?

    A. There is more than 60% loss of intracellular fluid during anaphylactic reactions.
    B. Inhalational anesthetics are the bronchodilators of choice after anaphylaxis.
    C. Corticosteroids are important in attenuating the late-phase reactions that occur 1 to 2 hours after anaphylaxis.
    D. Phenylephrine is the drug of choice for resuscitation during anaphylactic shock.
    E. Epinephrine causes bronchodilation via β_2 receptors.

13. The following statements regarding perioperative immunologic responses are true, EXCEPT:

    A. Most anesthetic drugs and agents have been reported to produce anaphylactic reactions.
    B. Muscle relaxants are the most common agents responsible for intraoperative allergic reactions.
    C. Although life-threatening allergic reactions are more likely to occur in individuals with a history of allergy, atopy, or asthma, this history is not a reliable predictor whether an allergic reaction will occur.
    D. There is no cross-sensitivity between succinylcholine and the nondepolarizing muscle relaxants.

14. Which of the following statements regarding latex reactions is false?

    A. There is a 24% incidence of contact dermatitis among anesthesiologists.
    B. Patients with an allergy to bananas have antibodies that may cross-react to latex.
    C. A history of atopy is a risk factor for latex sensitization.
    D. Pretreatment always prevents anaphylaxis.

15. Which of the following agents is the initial pharmacologic therapy for the treatment of hypotension during anaphylaxis?

    A. Corticosteroids
    B. Bronchodilators
    C. Phenylephrine
    D. Vasopressin
    E. Epinephrine

ANSWERS

1. D. The host defense systems can be divided into cellular and humoral elements. The humoral system includes complement, cytokines, antibodies, and other circulating proteins. The cellular system defense is mediated by specific lymphocytes of the T-cell series. (See page 288: Basic Immunologic Principles.)

2. E. The thymus of the fetus differentiates immature lymphocytes into thymus-derived cells (T-cells). The two types of regulator T-cells are helper cells and suppressor cells. Helper cells are important for effective cell responses. Suppressor cells inhibit immune function. Killer cells do not require specific antigen stimulation to initiate their function. Cytotoxic T-cells destroy mycobacteria, fungi, and viruses. (See page 288: Basic Immunologic Principles: Thymus-derived Lymphocytes [T-cell] and Bursa-derived Lymphocytes [B-cell].)

3. B. Each antibody has two heavy chains and two light chains that are bound together by disulfide bonds. Whereas the Fab fragment has the ability to bind antigen, the Fc (crystallizable) is responsible for the unique biologic properties of the different classes of immunoglobulins. The five major classes of antibodies in humans are IgG, IgA, IgM, IgD, and IgE. The heavy chain determines the structure and function of each molecule. (See page 288: Basic Immunologic Principles: Antibodies.)

4. C. The attachment of an antibody or complement fragment on the surface of foreign cells is called opsonization, a process that facilitates effector cell killing of foreign cells. Haptens are small molecules that form bonds with either host proteins or cell membranes to form a complete antigen. The ability to act as an antigen is referred to as immunogenicity. (See page 288: Basic Immunologic Principles: Effector Cells and Proteins of the Immune Response Cells.)

5. E. Neutrophils are the first cells to appear in an acute inflammatory reaction. Eosinophils accumulate at sites of parasitic infection, tumor, and allergic reactions. Mast cells are tissue fixed and located in the perivascular spaces of the skin and intestine; when they are activated, they release a broad spectrum of physiologically active mediators. Macrophages regulate immune responses by presenting antigens to result in microbicidal function. Basophils possess IgE receptors on their surfaces and likewise release mediators. (See page 288: Basic Immunologic Principles: Effector Cells and Proteins of the Immune Response Cells.)

6. C. The primary humoral response to antigen and antibody binding is the activation of the complement system. Complement activation can be initiated by IgG or IgM, by plasmin through the classic pathway, by endotoxin, or by drugs through the alternate (properdin) pathway. The major function of the complement system is to recognize bacteria, both directly and indirectly by the attraction of phagocytes, as well as the increased adhesion of phagocytes to antigens and cell lysis through activation of the complement system. T-cells are a component of the cellular immune response system. (See page 288: Basic Immunologic Principles: Effector Cells and Proteins of the Immune Response Cells [Complement].)

7. D. Administration of a histamine (H_1) antagonist may be useful in treating acute anaphylaxis; it does not inhibit H_1 release but competes with H_1 at the receptor sites. Steroids should be considered a secondary treatment in the management of patients with anaphylactic bronchospasm. Steroids require 12 to 24 hours to exert their peak clinical effect. Although the exact corticosteroid dose and preparation are unclear, investigators have recommended 0.25 to 1 g intravenously of hydrocortisone for IgE-mediated reactions. Acidosis frequently accompanies persistent hypotension. Acidemia decreases the effectiveness of administered epinephrine on the myocardium. Therefore, with refractory hypotension and acidemia, sodium bicarbonate should be given as indicated by arterial blood gas evaluation. Catecholamines, such as epinephrine, can be used in patients with persistent hypotension or bronchospasm after initial resuscitation. (See page 292: Anaphylactic reactions: Non–IgE-mediated Reactions [Nonimmunologic Release of Histamine, Treatment Plan, and Secondary Treatment].)

8. B. The histamine test involves incubating the patient's leukocytes with the offending drug and measuring the histamine release as a marker for basophil activation. The radioallergosorbent test allows in vitro detection of specific IgE directed toward particular antigens by linking them to insoluble material to make them immunoabsorbent. ELISA measures antigen-specific antibodies. (See page 297: Perioperative Management of the Patient with Allergies: Evaluation of Patients with Allergic Reactions [Testing for Allergy].)

9. A. More than 90% of the allergic reactions evoked by intravenous drugs occur within 5 minutes of administration. In the anesthetized patient, the most common life-threatening manifestation of an allergic reaction is circulatory collapse, reflecting vasodilation with resulting decreased venous return. (See page 291: Hypersensitivity Responses: Intraoperative Allergic Reactions.)

10. D. Health care workers and children with spina bifida, urogenital abnormalities, or certain food allergies have also been recognized as people at increased risk for anaphylaxis to latex. Brown et al reported a 24% incidence of irritant or contact dermatitis and a 12.5% incidence of latex-specific IgE positivity in anesthesiologists. Of this group, 10% were clinically asymptomatic, although IgE positive. A history of atopy was also a significant risk factor for latex sensitization. Brown et al suggested that these people are in their early stages of sensitization and perhaps, by avoiding latex exposure, their progression to symptomatic disease can be prevented. Patients allergic to bananas, avocados, and kiwis have also been reported to have antibodies that cross-react with latex. Multiple attempts are being made to reduce latex exposure to both health care workers and patients. If latex allergy occurs, then strict avoidance of latex from gloves and other sources needs to be considered. Since latex is such a common environmental antigen, this ongoing effort by suppliers of hospital equipment has significantly reduced the latex exposure over recent years. (See page 297: Perioperative Management of the Patient with Allergies: Agents Implicated in Allergic Reactions: Latex Allergy.)

11. D.   Various leukotrienes are synthesized after mast cell activation from arachidonic acid metabolism of phospholipid cell membranes via the lipoxygenase pathway. Prostaglandins are potent mast cell mediators that produce vasodilation, bronchospasm, pulmonary hypertension, and increased capillary permeability. Prostaglandin D_2, the major metabolite of mast cells, produces bronchospasm and vasodilation. Kinins are synthesized in mast cells and basophils and produce vasodilation, increased capillary permeability, and bronchoconstriction. (See page 292: Anaphylactic Reactions: IgE-mediated Pathophysiology; Kinins.)

12. E.   Epinephrine, not phenylephrine, in conjunction with volume expansion, is the drug of choice during anaphylactic shock because it reverses hypotension (α-adrenergic effects) and causes bronchodilation (β_2 receptor). The route of epinephrine administration and the dose depend on the patient's condition. Inhaled β-adrenergic agents may be included as an adjuvant if bronchospasm is a major feature. Vasopressin is an important drug for refractory shock, including vasodilatory shock associated with anaphylaxis. Inhalation anesthetics are not the bronchodilators of choice for treating bronchospasm after anaphylaxis because they interfere with the body's compensatory response to the cardiovascular collapse associated with anaphylaxis. Up to a 40% loss of intravascular fluid into the interstitial space during reactions has been reported. Since H_1 receptors mediate many of the adverse effects of histamine, the intravenous administration of an H_1 antagonist may be useful in treating acute anaphylaxis. Antihistamines do not inhibit anaphylactic reactions or histamine release, but compete with histamine at receptor sites. Corticosteroids may be important in attenuating the late-phase reactions reported to occur 12 to 24 hours after anaphylaxis. (See page 292: Anaphylactic Reactions: Treatment Plan [Initial Therapy].)

13. D.   Most anesthetic agents administered perioperatively have been reported to produce anaphylactic reactions. Muscle relaxants are the most common agents used that are responsible for evoking intraoperative allergic reactions. There is a cross-sensitivity between succinylcholine and the nondepolarizing muscle relaxants. Life-threatening allergic reactions are more likely to occur in individuals with a history of allergy, atopy, or asthma but do not necessarily predict whether an allergic reaction will occur. (See page 297: Perioperative Management of the Patient with Allergies: Immunologic Mechanisms of Drug Allergy.)

14. D.   There is a 24% incidence of contact dermatitis among anesthesiologists. Patients with an allergy to bananas have antibodies that can cross-react to latex. A history of atopy is a risk factor for latex sensitization. Pretreatment can help to prevent anaphylaxis. (See page 297: Perioperative Management of the Patient with Allergies: Agents Implicated in Allergic Reactions [Latex Allergy].)

15. E.   Epinephrine is the drug of choice when resuscitating patients during anaphylactic shock. α-adrenergic causes vasoconstriction to reverse hypotension; β_2 receptor stimulation bronchodilates and inhibits mediator release by increasing cyclic adenosine monophosphate (cAMP) in mast cells and basophils. The route of epinephrine administration and the dose depend on the patient's condition. Since H_1 receptors mediate many of the adverse effects of histamine, the intravenous administration of an H_1 antagonist may be useful in treating acute anaphylaxis. Antihistamines do not inhibit anaphylactic reactions or histamine release, but compete with histamine at receptor sites. Inhaled β-adrenergic agents may be included as an adjuvant if bronchospasm is a major feature. Despite the unproven usefulness of corticosteroids in treating acute reactions, they are often administered as adjuncts to therapy when refractory bronchospasm or refractory shock occurs after resuscitative therapy. Vasopressin is an important drug for refractory shock, including vasodilatory shock associated with anaphylaxis. (See page 292: Anaphylactic Reactions: Treatment Plan: Initial Treatment.)

CHAPTER
13

Inflammation, Wound Healing, and Infection

1. Which of the following is effective at removing spores?

   A. Alcohol-based rinses and gels
   B. Plain soap and water
   C. Iodine and iodophors
   D. Chlorhexidine
   E. Triclosan

2. The majority of postoperative surgical infections are caused by flora that are:

   A. Endogenous to the patient
   B. Environmental contaminants
   C. Airborne organisms
   D. Spore-forming organisms
   E. Organisms from OR personnel and traffic

3. Which of the following statements is FALSE regarding preoperative antibiotic prophylaxis?

   A. Administration of antibiotics should be done within 1 hour of incision.
   B. Drugs that require infusion over an hour should be completed before incision.
   C. When a tourniquet is used, infusion must be completed before tourniquet inflation.
   D. Depending on half-life, antibiotics should be repeated during long operations.
   E. The most common organisms targeted with antibiotic prophylaxis are gram-positive cocci.

4. Which of the following is not an independent risk factor for methicillin-resistant *Staphylococcus aureus* (MRSA) infection?

   A. Use of drains for more than 24 hours
   B. Increasing number of procedures performed on the patient
   C. Long hospital stay
   D. Use of prophylactic antibiotics for more than 48 hours
   E. Lack of hand hygiene

5. Which of the following is the most critical element for effective wound repair?

   A. Medical comorbidities
   B. Nutrition
   C. Oxygen supply to the wound
   D. Sympathetic nervous system activation
   E. Age of the patient

6. Which of the following phases of wound healing is characterized by erythema and edema of the wound edges?

   A. Proliferation
   B. Remodeling
   C. Inflammation
   D. Hemostasis
   E. Coagulation

7. When the wound environment becomes hypoxic and acidotic with high lactate levels, all of the following are present EXCEPT:

   A. Decreased oxygen supply
   B. Decreased respiratory burst activity
   C. Increased metabolic demand
   D. Aerobic glycolysis by inflammatory cells
   E. Vascular damage and coagulation

8. The proliferative phase of wound healing consists of all of the following EXCEPT:

   A. Maturation
   B. Synthesis of collagen
   C. Neovascularization
   D. Epithelization
   E. Synthesis of connective tissue proteins

9. Which of the following statements is FALSE regarding wound healing?

   A. The proliferative phase normally begins 4 days after injury.
   B. Helical configuration of collagen is primarily responsible for tissue strength.
   C. Local hypoxia is a normal and inevitable result of tissue injury.
   D. Neutrophil function does not depend on a high partial pressure of oxygen.
   E. Inflammatory cell oxidants in wound tissue provide resistance to infection and increase neovascularization.

10. Which of the following statements is FALSE about subcutaneous tissue?

    A. It is a reservoir used to maintain central volume.
    B. It is the major site of thermoregulation.
    C. The rate of wound infection is directly proportional to postoperative subcutaneous wound tissue oxygen tension.
    D. Peripheral vasoconstriction from subcutaneous vascular tone is an impediment to wound healing.
    E. Subcutaneous tissue oxygen tension is significantly higher in patients with good pain control.

11. For an indwelling venous catheter placement, which agent is the BEST antiseptic?

    A. Soap
    B. Alcohol gels
    C. Iodine
    D. Chlorhexidine
    E. Ethanol

12. Which of the following statements involving antisepsis is FALSE?

    A. Wearing masks reduces surgical site infections.
    B. An increased number of operating room personnel is related to an increased incidence of infection.
    C. Putting on a gown and gloves before central venous cannulation is vital to infection control.
    D. Masks and gowns significantly reduce the incidence of epidural abscesses.
    E. The use of epidural catheters is contraindicated in patients with bacteremia.

13. Which of the following factors is NOT an important factor for optimizing wound healing?

    A. Aseptic technique
    B. Prophylactic antibiotics
    C. Perfusion of wound
    D. Oxygenation of wound
    E. Presence of high concentrations of corticosteroids

14. Prolonging the course of prophylactic antibiotics for more than 24 hours increases the likelihood of all of the following EXCEPT:

    A. Effectiveness against infection
    B. Clostridium difficile infection
    C. Sensitization
    D. Antibiotic resistance
    E. Incidence of antibiotic side effects

15. Increased oxygen levels play an important role in all of the following physiologic processes EXCEPT:

    A. Wound healing
    B. Aerobic respiration
    C. Collagen breakdown
    D. Oxidative phosphorylation
    E. Leukocyte-mediated bacterial killing and collagen formation

16. All of the following factors have been shown to decrease wound infections in patients undergoing major abdominal surgery EXCEPT:

    A. Prevention or correction of hypothermia
    B. Intraoperative phenylephrine use
    C. Providing supplemental oxygen postoperatively
    D. Prevention or correction of blood volume deficit
    E. Use of high inspired oxygen intraoperatively

17. Wound oxygen delivery depends upon all of the following factors EXCEPT:

    A. Vascular anatomy
    B. Degree of vasoconstriction
    C. Arterial PO_2
    D. Hemoglobin-bound oxygen
    E. Decreased intercapillary diffusion distances

18. Which of the following regarding the use of gloves in the OR is FALSE?

    A. Wearing gloves during 100% of patient contact with appropriate frequent changing of gloves precludes the need for hand washing.
    B. Gloves should be removed after every intubation.
    C. Gloves provide additional protection against bacterial contamination.
    D. Double gloving is an effective approach to helping minimize contamination.
    E. As with vascular access, gloves should be changed after neuraxial anesthesia.

ANSWERS

1. **B.** The most crucial component of infection prevention is frequent and effective hand hygiene. Plain (not antiseptic) soap and water is generally the least effective method of reducing hand contamination but is very effective at removing spores and therefore should be used when contamination with either *Clostridium difficile* or *Bacillus anthracis* is a concern. Alcohol-based rinses and gels denature proteins, which confers their antimicrobial activity. Antiseptics containing 60% to 95% ethanol with a water base are germicidal and effective against gram-positive and gram-negative bacteria, lipophilic viruses such as herpes simplex, human immunodeficiency, influenza, respiratory syncytial, and vaccinia viruses, and hepatitis B and C viruses. Iodine and iodophors penetrate the cell wall and impair protein synthesis and cell membrane function; they are effective against spore-forming bacteria but are inactive against spores. Chlorhexidine disrupts cytoplasmic membranes and is effective against gram-positive bacteria and lipophilic viruses but not against gram-negative bacteria or spore-forming organisms. (See page 305: Hand Hygiene.)

2. **A.** Most postoperative surgical infections are caused by flora that are endogenous to the patient. Environmental and airborne contaminants may also play a causative role to a lesser extent. As the number of people in the operating suite increases, the patient exposure to airborne organisms increases. (See page 310: Antisepsis.)

3. **B.** Antibiotic prophylaxis has now become standard for surgeries in which there is more than a minimum risk of infection. Ideally, prophylaxis administration should be within 1 hour of incision. For drugs such as vancomycin that require infusion over an hour, it is considered acceptable if the infusion is started before incision. When a tourniquet is used, the infusion must be complete before inflation of the tourniquet. Depending on the drug's half-life, antibiotics should be repeated during long operations or operations with large blood loss. The agent for antibiotic prophylaxis must cover the most likely spectrum of bacteria present in the surgical field with the most commonly used antibiotic being cefazolin, targeted against gram-positive cocci from the skin. (See page 310: Antibiotic Prophylaxis.)

4. **C.** Unfortunately, MRSA is becoming a more common pathogen. Independent risk factors identified for MRSA infection include prolonged use of prophylactic antibiotics, use of drains for more than 24 hours, and increasing number of procedures performed on the patient. Longer hospital stays and geographic regions are not an independent risk factor for MRSA infection. Hand hygiene is among the most effective means of preventing development of MRSA because when they are used properly, alcohol-based gel kills more than 99.9% of all transient pathogens, including MRSA. (See page 310: Antibiotic Prophylaxis.)

5. **C.** Many factors may impair wound healing. Systemic factors such as medical comorbidities, nutrition, sympathetic nervous system activation, and age have substantial effects on the repair process. Although all of these factors are important, perhaps the most critical element is oxygen supply to the wound. Wound hypoxia impairs all of the components of healing. (See page 314: Mechanisms of Wound Repair.)

6. **C.** Wound healing has been described in four separate phases: Hemostasis, inflammation, proliferation, and remodeling. Coagulation is a contributing factor to the hemostasis phase. The initial response to injury is the hemostasis phase, which prevents exsanguination but also widens the area that is no longer perfused. The inflammatory phase is characterized by erythema and edema of the wound edges. The proliferative phase consists of granulation tissue formation and epithelization. The final stage of wound repair is the maturation (and remodeling) phase. (See page 314: The Initial Response to Injury.)

7. **B.** In wounds, the local blood supply is compromised at the same time that metabolic demand is increased. As a result, the wound environment becomes hypoxic and acidotic with high lactate levels. This represents the sum of three effects: (1) Decreased oxygen supply caused by vascular damage and coagulation, (2) increased metabolic demand caused by the heightened cellular response (anaerobic glycolysis), and (3) aerobic glycolysis by inflammatory cells. In activated neutrophils, the respiratory burst, in which oxygen and glucose are converted to superoxide, hydrogen ion, and lactate, accounts for up to 98% of oxygen consumption; in the setting of injury, this activity INCREASES by up to 50fold over baseline. (See page 314: The Initial Response to Injury.)

8. **A.** The proliferative phase normally begins approximately 4 days after injury, concurrent with a waning of the inflammatory phase. It consists of granulation tissue formation and epithelization. Granulation involves neovascularization as well as synthesis of collagen and connective tissue proteins. Maturation is the final stage of wound healing. (See page 314: Mechanisms of Wound Repair.)

9. **D.** The proliferative phase normally begins approximately 4 days after injury. Collagen can only be exported from the cell when it is in a triple helical structure. The helical configuration is primarily responsible for tissue strength. Local hypoxia is a normal and inevitable result of tissue injury. Hypoxia acts as a stimulus to repair but also leads to poor healing and increased susceptibility to infection. The neutrophil is the primary cell responsible for nonspecific immunity, and its function depends on a high partial pressure of oxygen. Oxidants produced by inflammatory cells have a dual role in wound repair. Not only are they central to resistance to infection, but they also play a major role in initiating and directing the healing process

via the respiratory burst, increase in neovascularization, and in collagen deposition. (See page 314: Mechanisms of Wound Repair.)

10. C.   Any reduction in wound partial pressure of oxygen may impair immunity and repair. In surgical patients, the rate of wound infections is inversely proportional, and collagen deposition is directly proportional to postoperative subcutaneous wound tissue oxygen tension. High oxygen tensions (>100 mm Hg) can be reached in wounds only if perfusion is rapid and arterial PO_2 is high. This is because subcutaneous tissue serves a reservoir function, so there is normal flow in excess of nutritional needs. Wound cells consume relatively little oxygen at a normal perfusion rate. Peripheral vasoconstriction is probably the most frequent and clinically the most important impediment to wound oxygenation. Subcutaneous tissue is both a reservoir to maintain central volume and a major site of thermoregulation. Subcutaneous tissue oxygen tension is significantly higher in patients with good pain control than those with poor pain control after arthroscopic knee surgery. (See page 317: Wound Perfusion and Oxygenation.)

11. D.   The ideal hand hygiene agent kills a broad spectrum of bacteria and has antimicrobial activity that lasts for more than 6 hours after application. Soap and water are generally the least effective at reducing hand contamination with bacteria and are associated with an increased risk of skin irritation and drying. Alcohol-based gels denature proteins and are germicidal against bacteria and lipophilic viruses such as herpes, HIV, influenza, and hepatitis. Chlorhexidine is an antiseptic that disrupts cytoplasmic membranes and ultimately leads to precipitation of cellular components; it has substantial skin persistence, so the Centers for Disease Control and Prevention has identified it as the topical agent of choice for central venous catheter placement. It may cause corneal damage if it accidentally comes into contact with the eye, ototoxicity if it comes into contact with middle ear, and potential neurotoxicity if it comes into contact with the brain or meninges. (See page 305: Infection Control: Hand Hygiene.)

12. D.   Masks are almost universally used in operating rooms; their role has long been established in protecting both patients and health care providers, especially when combined with eye protection. A recent study shows a trend toward increased postoperative infectious complications after orthopedic procedures that are associated with an increased number of personnel in the operating room; current recommended practices are that traffic patterns should limit the flow of people through operating rooms. Gowning and gloving should be routine when central venous catheterization is being used. Epidural catheter placement requires a careful aseptic technique such as hand washing, skin preparation, and draping. However, gowning and wearing masks are unlikely to reduce the risk of infection. Hand washing, skin preparation, draping, and maintenance of a sterile field should be carefully observed when placing epidural catheters. Gowning and wearing a mask likely play a smaller role, but are reasonable given the devastating consequences of infection. Epidurals should

probably be avoided in patients known or suspected to have bacteremia. (See page 310: Antisepsis.)

13. E.   Effective hand hygiene and careful surgical technique are fundamental to optimal wound healing. Antibiotic prophylaxis has become the standard for surgeries in which there is more than a minimum risk of infection. Prophylactic antibiotics are given pre- or intraoperatively. At the same time, maintaining oxygenation and perfusion of the wound is important for wound healing. As myofibroblasts contract during scar formation, the collagenous matrix cross-links in the shortened position, which helps to strengthen the matrix and minimize scarring. Contraction is inhibited by the use of high doses of corticosteroids—even if given days after injury. (See page 305: Hand Hygiene, Antisepsis, Antibiotic Prophylaxis, Maturation, and Remodeling.)

14. A.   Prophylactic antibiotics are given pre- or intraoperatively. They should be discontinued by 24 hours after surgery. Prolonging the course of prophylactic antibiotics does not reduce the risk of infection but does increase the risk of adverse consequences of antibiotic administration, including resistance, *Clostridium difficile* infection, and sensitization. (See page 310: Antibiotic Prophylaxis.)

15. C.   Oxygen plays a key role in aerobic respiration and energy production via oxidative phosphorylation. In wound healing, oxygen is required as a cofactor for enzymatic processes and for cell-signaling mechanisms. Oxygen is a rate-limiting component in leukocyte-mediated bacterial killing and collagen formation because specific enzymes require oxygen at a partial pressure of at least 40 mm Hg. Hypoxia leads to poor healing and increased susceptibility to infection. (See page 314: Mechanisms of Wound Repair.)

16. B.   Prevention and correction of hypothermia and blood volume deficits have been shown to decrease wound infections and increase collagen deposition in patients undergoing major abdominal surgery. Preoperative systemic or local warming has also been shown to decrease wound infections, even in clean, low-risk surgeries. While still in some debate, the preponderance of evidence indicates that use of high inspired oxygen intraoperatively, and providing supplemental oxygen postoperatively, in major abdominal surgery patients will reduce the risk of wound infection. Peripheral vasoconstriction is probably the most frequent and clinically most important impediment to wound oxygenation. Subcutaneous tissue is particularly vulnerable to vasoconstriction stimulated by cold, pain, fear, blood volume deficits, and by various pharmacologic agents including nicotine, β-adrenergic antagonists, and α_1-agonists, all commonly present in the perioperative environment. (See page 317: Wound Perfusion and Oxygenation.)

17. D.   Normally, wounds on the extremities and trunk heal more slowly than those on the face. The major difference in these wounds is the degree of tissue perfusion and thus the wound tissue oxygen tension. Wound oxygen delivery depends on the vascular anatomy, the degree of vasoconstriction, and arterial PO_2. The standard teaching that oxygen delivery depends more on hemoglobin-bound oxygen than on arterial PO_2 may be true of working muscle but is not true for wound healing. In muscle, intercapillary distances are small, and oxygen consumption is high. In contrast, intercapillary distances are large, and oxygen consumption is relatively low in subcutaneous tissue. In wounds, where the microvasculature is damaged, diffusion distances are substantially increased. Peripheral vasoconstriction further increases diffusion distance. The driving force of diffusion is partial pressure. Resistance to infection is critically impaired by wound hypoxia and becomes more efficient as partial pressure of oxygen increases to very high levels. This is one mechanism for the proposed benefit of hyperbaric oxygen therapy as an adjunctive treatment for necrotizing infections and chronic refractory osteomyelitis. (See page 317: Wound Perfusion and Oxygenation.)

18. A. Wearing gloves does not reduce the need for hand hygiene. Although gloves provide protection, bacterial flora from patients may be cultured from up to 30% of health care workers who wear gloves during patient contact. Therefore, hand hygiene should be practiced both before putting on gloves and immediately after removal. Moreover, gloves should be removed or changed immediately after each procedure, including vascular access, intubation, and neuraxial anesthesia, because gloves become contaminated by patient contact just as hands do. Double gloving and providing a convenient location for contaminated equipment have been suggested as effective approaches. (See page 305: Hand Hygiene.)

CHAPTER

14

Fluids, Electrolytes, and Acid–Base Physiology

1. A previously healthy patient acutely develops metabolic alkalosis resulting from intravenous diuretic administration. The measured HCO_3 is 36 mEq/L. The arterial blood gas analysis shows:

   A. pH, 7.51; $PaCO_2$, 47; PO_2, 90
   B. pH, 7.42; $PaCO_2$, 52; PO_2, 90
   C. pH, 7.51; $PaCO_2$, 47; PO_2, 110
   D. pH, 7.61; $PaCO_2$, 52; PO_2, 90
   E. pH, 7.51; $PaCO_2$, 40; PO_2, 100

2. Metabolic acidosis with a normal anion gap may be caused by:

   A. Aspirin toxicity
   B. Diabetic ketoacidosis
   C. Chronic diarrhea
   D. Uremia
   E. Lactic acidosis

3. What is the best interpretation of an arterial blood gas analysis of pH, 7.35; $PaCO_2$, 60; PO_2, 80; and HCO_3, 32?

   A. Acute respiratory acidosis
   B. Chronic respiratory acidosis with metabolic compensation
   C. Chronic respiratory acidosis without metabolic compensation
   D. Chronic metabolic alkalosis with respiratory compensation
   E. Acute metabolic alkalosis

4. What is the best interpretation of an arterial blood gas analysis of pH, 7.24; $PaCO_2$, 60; PO_2, 80; and HCO_3, 26?

   A. Acute respiratory acidosis
   B. Chronic respiratory acidosis with appropriate metabolic compensation
   C. Chronic respiratory acidosis with inappropriate metabolic compensation
   D. Chronic metabolic alkalosis with respiratory compensation
   E. Acute metabolic alkalosis

5. What is the best interpretation of an arterial blood gas analysis of pH, 7.50; $PaCO_2$, 30; PO_2, 110; and HCO_3, 22?

   A. Acute respiratory alkalosis
   B. Chronic respiratory alkalosis with metabolic compensation
   C. Acute metabolic acidosis with respiratory compensation
   D. Chronic metabolic alkalosis with respiratory compensation
   E. Chronic metabolic acidosis

6. Total body water is approximately _____% of total body weight.

   A. 10
   B. 20
   C. 40
   D. 60
   E. 80

7. Intracellular volume (ICV) is _____% of total body weight.

   A. 10
   B. 20
   C. 40
   D. 60
   E. 80

8. Plasma volume is approximately _____% of the extracellular volume (ECV).

   A. 10
   B. 20
   C. 30
   D. 40
   E. 50

9. The extracellular concentration of sodium (Na) is approximately _____ mEq/L.

   A. 150
   B. 130
   C. 140
   D. 120
   E. 110

10. The intracellular concentration of potassium (K) is approximately _____ mEq/L.

    A. 110
    B. 130
    C. 150
    D. 4
    E. 10

11. An acute blood loss of 2,000 mL represents _____% of the predicted blood volume in a previously healthy 70-kg man.

    A. 10
    B. 20
    C. 30
    D. 40
    E. 50

12. To achieve a more than transient 2,000-mL restoration of plasma volume (PV) would require infusion of _____ mL of D5W solution.

    A. 2,000
    B. 4,500
    C. 7,000
    D. 14,000
    E. 28,000

13. To achieve a more than transient 2-L restoration of plasma volume using lactated Ringer's solution would require infusion of approximately _____ L.

    A. 10
    B. 15
    C. 30
    D. 45
    E. 50

14. To achieve a more than transient 2-L restoration of plasma volume using 5% albumin would require infusion of _____ L.

    A. 1
    B. 2
    C. 5
    D. 7
    E. 10

15. Reabsorption of filtered water and sodium is enhanced by changes mediated by the hormonal factors, which include all of the following EXCEPT:

    A. Antidiuretic hormone (ADH)
    B. Atrial natriuretic Peptide (ANP)
    C. Aldosterone
    D. Cortisol
    E. Brain natriuretic peptide

16. Chronic gastric losses tend to cause:

    A. Hypochloremic alkalosis
    B. Hyperchloremic alkalosis
    C. Hypochloremic acidosis
    D. Hyperchloremic acidosis
    E. Alkalosis with a normal chloride value

17. Chronic diarrhea tends to produce:

    A. Hypochloremic acidosis
    B. Hypochloremic alkalosis
    C. Hyperchloremic acidosis
    D. Hyperchloremic alkalosis
    E. Alkalosis with a normal chloride value

18. What is the osmolality (mOsm/kg) of plasma that contains 140 mEq/L of Na, 90 mg/dL of glucose, and blood urea nitrogen (BUN) of 11.5 mg/dL?

    A. 280
    B. 290
    C. 300
    D. 310
    E. 320

19. Which of the following formulas accurately expresses Starling law of capillary filtration?

    A. $Q = kA\left[(P_c - P_i) + k\,(\pi_i - \pi_c)\right]$
    B. $Q = kA\left[(P_c - P_i) - k\,(\pi_i - \pi_c)\right]$
    C. $Q = kA\left[(P_c - P_i) - \sigma\,(\pi_i - \pi_c)\right]$
    D. $Q = kA\left[(P_c - P_i) + \sigma\,(\pi_i - \pi_c)\right]$
    E. $Q = kA\left[(P_c - P_i) + (\pi_i - \pi_c)\right]$

20. Which of the following is NOT a typical finding during hypovolemia?

    A. Blood urea nitrogen (BUN) > 20 mg/dL
    B. BUN/serum creatinine > 20 mg/dL
    C. Urinary Na < 20 mEq/L
    D. Urinary osmolality > 400 mOsm/kg
    E. Serum/urine creatinine ratio > 1:40

21. What is the typical daily fluid requirement for a 30-kg child?

    A. 300 mL
    B. 3,000 mL
    C. 1,100 mL
    D. 1,400 mL
    E. 1,700 mL

22. Which of the following statements concerning Na regulation is FALSE?

    A. Aldosterone promotes reabsorption of Na in the kidney.
    B. Aldosterone promotes exchange of Na for potassium and hydrogen.
    C. Stretching of the atria promotes release of atrial natriuretic peptide.
    D. Antidiuretic hormone (ADH) affects serum Na concentration.
    E. Excess ADH results in increased free water excretion.

23. Physiologic consequences of metabolic alkalosis include:

    A. Rightward shift of the oxyhemoglobin dissociation curve
    B. Hyperkalemia
    C. Hypercalcemia
    D. Hypercarbia
    E. Decreased cardiac output

24. TRUE statements concerning the treatment of metabolic acidosis with HCO_3 include:

    A. It improves cardiovascular response to catecholamines.
    B. It is clearly effective in improving outcome.
    C. The appropriate dose is $0.7 \times$ (Body weight in kg) $(24 - HCO_3)$.
    D. It reduces plasma-ionized calcium.
    E. It does not result in changes in pH during lactic acidosis.

25. Respiratory alkalosis and metabolic alkalosis both:

    A. Produce hypokalemia
    B. Decrease cerebral blood flow
    C. Attenuate digoxin toxicity
    D. Produce hypercalcemia
    E. Cause bronchodilation

26. Physiologic and hormonal changes from hypovolemia and decreased cardiac output include:

    A. Increased natriuretic hormone release from the cardiac ventricles.
    B. Increased reabsorption of water from the medullary collecting ducts.
    C. Increased reabsorption of water and Na resulting from increased atrial natriuretic hormone.
    D. Decreased renin release.
    E. Increased sodium reabsorption in response to decreased aldosterone levels.

27. Which of the following statements concerning fluid resuscitation and the brain is TRUE?

    A. The cerebral capillary membrane is highly permeable to sodium.
    B. Changes in serum osmolality provide minimal changes in brain water because of the blood–brain barrier.
    C. Normal saline is superior to albumin in the context of brain injury.
    D. Reducing colloid osmotic pressure produces changes in both cortical water content and ICP.
    E. Reducing plasma osmolality reduces ICP.

28. Which of the following statements concerning abnormal Na^+ concentrations is TRUE?

    A. Absorption of irrigant solution during transurethral resection of the prostate may result in hyponatremia in the presence of a high serum osmolality.
    B. Hypernatremia may result from inappropriate antidiuretic hormone (ADH) secretion.
    C. Mannitol may result in hypernatremia in the presence of a high serum osmolality.
    D. A decrease in plasma sodium leads to a decrease in intracellular brain water.
    E. Acute hyponatremia produces less severe neurologic symptoms than chronic hyponatremia.

29. A TRUE statement concerning hypermagnesemia includes:

    A. Magnesium stimulates the release of catecholamines from adrenergic nerve terminals.
    B. Heart block commonly is noted at 18 mg/dL.
    C. Hypotension is not noted until concentrations are 13 mg/dL.
    D. Magnesium should not be used in patients with pheochromocytoma.
    E. Areflexia often is noted at levels above 7 mg/dL.

30. Which of the following statements concerning diabetes insipidus is TRUE?

    A. DI is caused by osmotically induced intravascular gains of sodium and water.
    B. It is more common after pituitary surgery.
    C. Polyuria is a rare finding.
    D. It often results in hyponatremia.
    E. Central diabetes insipidus is exacerbated by desmopressin.

31. Which of the following statements concerning regulation of serum potassium levels is FALSE?

    A. Aldosterone increases potassium excretion.
    B. Potassium excretion is increased in the presence of nonreabsorbable anions in the renal luminal fluid.
    C. Insulin causes an intracellular shift of potassium.
    D. Exogenous β_2 agonists cause an extracellular shift of potassium.
    E. Acidosis shifts potassium extracellularly.

32. Which of the following statements concerning hypokalemia is FALSE?

    A. The ratio of intracellular to extracellular potassium remains relatively stable with chronic potassium loss.
    B. Hypokalemia is rarely caused by drugs.
    C. As a general rule, a decrease of 1 mEq/L represents a total body deficit of 200 to 300 mEq.
    D. An intracellular shift of potassium may accompany respiratory alkalosis.
    E. Hypothermia may cause acute hypokalemia.

33. Changes associated with hypokalemia include all of the following EXCEPT:

    A. Hyperpolarization of cardiac cells
    B. ST segment depression
    C. Re-entrant arrhythmias
    D. Exacerbation of digitalis toxicity
    E. Right bundle branch block

34. Which of the following statements concerning hyperkalemia is TRUE?

    A. It may be treated with triamterene.
    B. It may result from increases in mineralocorticoid.
    C. It may be treated with angiotensin-converting enzyme (ACE) inhibitors.
    D. Furosemide promotes kaliuresis.
    E. ECG is a sensitive method of detecting hyperkalemia.

35. Effects of hyperkalemia include all the following EXCEPT:

 A. Peaked P waves
 B. Shortened PR interval
 C. Widened QRS complex
 D. Tall, peaked T waves
 E. Sine wave pattern

36. Symptomatic hyperkalemia may be treated with all the following EXCEPT:

 A. Glucose
 B. NaHCO$_3$
 C. Spironolactone
 D. Regular insulin
 E. β_2 agonists

37. TRUE statements about ionized calcium include:

 A. The ionized calcium concentration in the extracellular fluid (ECF) is approximately 10 mM.
 B. Its concentration is increased by increased parathyroid hormone activity.
 C. Its concentration may be increased by hyperphosphatemia.
 D. Its concentration is decreased by acidemia.
 E. Hypophosphatemic hypocalcemia results from increased calcium excretion.

38. The FALSE statement concerning hypocalcemia is:

 A. It may cause increased sensitivity to digitalis.
 B. It does not necessarily occur after transfusion, even if 5 U of blood is infused within 1 hour.
 C. It may cause QT prolongation.
 D. It may cause laryngeal spasm.
 E. It causes neuronal membrane tetany.

39. The TRUE statement about hypercalcemia is:

 A. Severe symptoms are generally noted when the total serum calcium concentration is above 10 mg/dL.
 B. Symptoms include lethargy, anorexia, nausea, and polyuria.
 C. Cardiovascular effects include hypotension.
 D. A patient with hypercalcemia is not helped by infusion of NaCl.
 E. Heart block and cardiac arrest are not associated with hypercalcemia.

40. The FALSE statement about altered phosphate concentrations is:

 A. High concentrations promote deposition of calcium in the bone, soft tissues, and kidneys.
 B. Hypophosphatemia leads to muscle weakness, which may lead to decreased ventilatory strength.
 C. The serum concentration of phosphate decreases in response to acute alkalemia.
 D. Rapid administration of phosphate to a patient with hypocalcemia may precipitate more severe hypocalcemia.
 E. Hypophosphatemia is never caused by renal loss.

41. The TRUE statement concerning hypomagnesemia is:

 A. Symptoms generally develop when the serum magnesium (Mg^{2+}) concentration is below 1 mg/dL.
 B. It causes resistance to digitalis.
 C. Rapid correction of hypermagnesemia may cause symptoms consistent with hypercalcemia.
 D. It predisposes to gastric artery spasm.
 E. Approximately 90% of alcoholic patients admitted to the hospital are hypomagnesemic.

ANSWERS

1. A. This represents metabolic alkalosis with partial respiratory compensation. The rules of thumb for calculating the expected response to metabolic alkalosis are as follows: (1) $PaCO_2$ increases approximately 0.5 to 0.6 mm Hg for each 1 mEq/L increase in HCO_3 and (2) the last two digits of the pH should equal the HCO_3 + 15. Hypercarbia is accompanied by a reduced PaO_2 as given by the alveolar gas equation. (See page 328: Metabolic Alkalosis and page 329: Table 14-3.)

2. C. Metabolic acidosis may be characterized by a high anion gap or a normal anion gap. Metabolic acidosis with a high anion gap results from excess anions such as lactate, ketoacetate, sulfate, salicylate, and other toxic compounds. Metabolic acidosis with a normal anion gap is caused by loss of HCO_3 resulting from diarrhea, biliary drainage, or renal tubular acidosis. (See page 329: Metabolic Acidosis and page 330: Table 14-4.)

3. B. The pH below 7.40 suggests acidosis as the primary event, and the $PaCO_2$ of 60 shows that this patient has respiratory acidosis. The appropriate chronic metabolic compensation is that HCO_3 increases 4 mEq/L for each 10 mm Hg increase in $PaCO_2$, thus bringing the HCO_3 to 32 mEq/L. The pH will return toward normal. (See page 331: Practical Approach to Acid–Base Interpretation and page 332: Table 14-7.)

4. A. The pH 7.24 suggests acidosis as the primary event, and the $PaCO_2$ of 60 shows that this patient has respiratory acidosis. (See page 331: Practical Approach to Acid–Base Interpretation and page 332: Table 14-7.)

5. A. The pH of 7.50 suggests alkalosis as the primary event, and the $PaCO_2$ of 30 shows that this patient has respiratory alkalosis. (See page 331: Practical Approach to Acid–Base Interpretation and page 332: Table 14-7.)

6. D. Total body water (in liters) is equal to approximately 60% of total body weight (in kilograms). The intracellular volume constitutes 40% of total body weight, and the extracellular volume constitutes 20% of body weight. (See page 333: Fluid Management, Physiology, Body Fluid Compartments.)

7. C. Total body water consists of ICV, which constitutes 40% of total body weight (28 L in a 70-kg person), and extracellular volume, which constitutes 20% of body weight (14 L). (See page 333: Fluid Management, Physiology, Body Fluid Compartments.)

8. B. Plasma volume, approximately 3 L, equals about one-fifth (20%) of the ECV. The remainder of the ECV is interstitial fluid. Red blood cell (RBC) volume, approximately 2 L, is part of the intracellular volume. Total blood volume is approximately 5 L (3 L of plasma + 2 L of RBC mass). (See page 333: Body Fluid Compartments.)

9. C. The extracellular fluid contains most of the Na in the body, with equal Na concentrations (~140 mEq/L) in the plasma and interstitium. (See page 333: Body Fluid Compartments.)

10. C. The predominant intracellular cation is K^+, with an intracellular concentration of approximately 150 mEq/L. (See page 333: Body Fluid Compartments.)

11. D. A 2,000-mL blood loss represents approximately 40% of the predicted 5-L blood volume in a previously healthy 70-kg patient. The normal blood volume is approximately 70 mL/kg; the normal plasma volume is three-fifths of this value, or approximately 3 L. (See page 333: Body Fluid Compartments.)

12. E. The volume that is to be infused to achieve a 2 L increase in PV is equal to Expected PV increment × Distribution volume of infusate/Normal PV. The normal PV is 3 L; the distribution volume for D5W is the total body water, which is 42 L (60% of 70 kg). Hence, the equation becomes: 2 L × 42 L/3 L = 28 L. To achieve a 2 L increase in overall intravascular volume, 28 L of D5W would theoretically be required. (See page 333: Body Fluid Compartments.)

13. A. The distribution volume for lactated Ringer's solution is the extracellular fluid, which is 14 L (20% of 70 kg). Hence, the equation for plasma expansion becomes 2 L × 14 L/3 L = 9.3 L. (See page 333: Distribution of Infused Fluids.)

14. B. If 5% albumin, which exerts colloid osmotic pressure similar to plasma, were infused, the infused volume initially would remain in the PV, perhaps attracting additional interstitial fluid intravascularly. Alternatively, 25% human serum albumin, a concentrated colloid, expands PV by approximately 400 mL for each 100 mL infused. (See page 333: Distribution of Infused Fluids.)

15. B. Reabsorption of filtered water and sodium is enhanced by changes mediated by the hormonal factors antidiuretic hormone (ADH), atrial natriuretic peptide (ANP), and aldosterone. Renal water handling has three important components: (1) Delivery of tubular fluid to the diluting segments of the nephron, (2) separation of solute and water in the diluting segment, and (3) variable reabsorption of water in the collecting ducts. In the descending loop of Henle, water is reabsorbed while solute is retained to achieve a final osmolality of tubular fluid of approximately 1,200 mOsm/kg. Two powerful hormonal systems regulate total body sodium. The natriuretic peptides, ANP, brain natriuretic peptide, and C-type natriuretic peptide, defend against sodium overload and the renin–angiotensin–aldosterone axis defends against sodium depletion and hypovolemia. (See page 334: Regulation of Extracellular Fluid Volume.)

16. A. Chronic gastric losses (i.e., vomiting) tend to produce hypochloremic hypokalemic metabolic alkalosis. (See page 328: Metabolic Alkalosis.)

17. C. Chronic diarrhea may produce hyperchloremic metabolic acidosis. (See page 336: Surgical Fluid Requirements.)

18. B. The *osmolarity* of a solution refers to the number of osmotically active particles per *liter* of solvent. O*smolality*, a measurement of the number of osmotically active particles per *kilogram*, can be estimated as follows: Osmolality = ([Na⁺] × 2) + (Glucose/18) + (BUN/2.3), where Na⁺ is expressed in mEq/L and serum glucose and BUN is expressed in mg/dL. Hence, plasma, which contains 140 mEq/L of Na⁺, 90 mg/dL of glucose, and a BUN of 11.5 mg/L, has 280 + 5 + 5 for a total of 290 mmol/kg. The Na⁺ is doubled to account for "matching" anions (e.g., Cl). (See page 338: Colloids, Crystalloids, and Hypertonic Solutions.)

19. D. The filtration rate of fluid from the capillaries into the interstitial space is the net result of a combination of forces, including the gradient from intravascular to interstitial colloid osmotic pressures and the hydrostatic gradient between intravascular and interstitial pressures. The net fluid filtration at any point within a systemic or pulmonary capillary is represented by Starling's law of capillary filtration, as expressed in the equation: $Q = kA \left[(P_c - P_i) + \sigma (\pi_i - \pi_c) \right]$ where Q = fluid filtration, k = capillary filtration coefficient (conductivity of water), A = the area of the capillary membrane, P_c = capillary hydrostatic pressure, P_i = interstitial hydrostatic pressure, σ = reflection coefficient for albumin, π_i = interstitial colloid osmotic pressure, and π_c = capillary colloid osmotic pressure. The reflection coefficient (σ) describes the permeability of capillary membranes to individual solutes. (See page 338: Colloids, Crystalloids, and Hypertonic Solutions.)

20. E. A ratio of BUN to serum Cr exceeding the normal range (10–20) suggests dehydration. In prerenal oliguria, enhanced sodium reabsorption should reduce urinary [Na⁺] to ≤20 mEq/L and enhanced water reabsorption should increase urinary concentration (i.e., urinary osmolality >400, urine/plasma creatinine ratio >40:1). (See page 340: Fluid Status: Assessment and Monitoring.)

21. E. Typical maintenance requirements may be calculated according to formulas for hourly or daily administration. For the first 10 kg of weight, 4 mL/kg/hr or 100 mL/kg/day should be administered. For the 11th to 20th kg, 2 mL/kg/hr or 50 mL/kg/day should be given. For each additional kilogram, 1 mL/kg/hr or 20 mL/kg/day should be administered. Thus, a 30-kg child should receive 1,000 mL + 500 mL + 200 mL = 1,700 mL. (See page 336: Fluid Replacement Therapy and page 336: Table 14-10: Hourly and Daily Maintenance Water Requirements.)

22. E. Increased secretion of ADH results in reabsorption of water by the kidneys and subsequent dilution of the plasma Na⁺; inadequate ADH secretion results in renal free water excretion that, in the absence of adequate water intake, results in hypernatremia. Total body Na is also regulated by aldosterone, which is responsible for renal Na reabsorption in exchange for potassium and hydrogen. Alternatively, stretching of the cardiac atria causes secretion of atrial natriuretic peptide, which increases renal Na excretion. (See page 341: Sodium.)

23. D. Metabolic alkalosis is associated with hypokalemia, ionized hypocalcemia, secondary ventricular arrhythmias, increased digoxin toxicity, and compensatory hypoventilation (hypercarbia). Alkalemia may reduce tissue oxygen availability by shifting the oxyhemoglobin dissociation curve to the left and by decreasing cardiac output. (See page 328: Metabolic Alkalosis.)

24. D. Both evidence and opinion suggests that NaHCO₃ should rarely be used to treat acidemia induced by metabolic acidosis. In critically ill patients with lactic acidosis, there were no important differences between the physiologic effects (other than changes in pH) of 0.9 M NaHCO₃ and 0.9 M sodium chloride. Importantly, NaHCO₃ did not improve the cardiovascular response to catecholamines and actually reduced plasma-ionized calcium. The initial dose of HCO₃ may be calculated as:

$$NaHCO_3(mEq/L) = \frac{Wt(kg) \times 0.3 \times (24\ mEq/L - Actual\ HCO_3)}{2}$$

where 0.3 = the assumed distribution space for bicarbonate. (See page 329: Metabolic Acidosis.)

25. A. Respiratory alkalosis, like metabolic alkalosis, may produce hypokalemia, hypocalcemia, cardiac dysrhythmias, bronchoconstriction, and hypotension, and may potentiate the toxicity of digoxin. In addition, both brain pH and cerebral blood flow are tightly regulated and respond rapidly to changes in systemic pH. Doubling minute ventilation reduces PaCO₂ to 20 mm Hg and halves cerebral blood flow; conversely, halving minute ventilation doubles PaCO₂ and doubles cerebral blood flow. (See page 330: Respiratory Alkalosis.)

26. B. Renal water handling has three important components: (1) Delivery of tubular fluid to the diluting segments of the nephron, (2) separation of solute and water in the diluting segment, and (3) variable reabsorption of water in the collecting ducts. ANP, released from the cardiac atria in response to increased atrial stretch, exerts vasodilatory effects and increases the renal excretion of sodium and water. ANP secretion is decreased during hypovolemia. Acting primarily in the distal tubules, high concentrations of aldosterone cause sodium reabsorption and may reduce urinary excretion of sodium nearly to zero. Hypovolemia produces decreased stretch in the baroreceptors of the aortic arch and carotid body and stretch receptors in the great veins, pulmonary vasculature, and atria result in increased sympathetic tone. Increased sympathetic tone, in combination with decreased renal perfusion, leads to renin release and formation of angiotensin I from angiotensinogen. Angiotensin-converting enzyme (ACE) converts angiotensin I to angiotensin II, which stimulates the adrenal cortex to synthesize and release aldosterone. (See page 334: Regulation of Extracellular Fluid Volume.)

27. C. Since the cerebral capillary membrane, the blood–brain barrier, is highly impermeable to sodium, abrupt changes in serum osmolality produced by changes in serum sodium, produce reciprocal changes in brain water. In anesthetized rabbits, reducing plasma osmolality from 295 to 282 mOsm/kg (which decreases plasma osmotic pressure by ~250 mm Hg) increased cortical water content and ICP; in contrast reducing colloid osmotic pressure from 20 to 7 mm Hg produced no significant change in either variable. Similar independence of brain water and ICP from colloid osmotic pressure has been demonstrated with prolonged hypoalbuminemia and in animals after forebrain ischemia and focal cryogenic injury. There is an apparent increase in mortality in traumatic brain injury patients managed with albumin rather than 0.9% saline during intensive care. (See page 339: Implications of Crystalloid and Colloid Infusions on Intracranial Pressure.)

28. A. Since the blood–brain barrier is poorly permeable to sodium but freely permeable to water, a rapid decrease in plasma [Na^+] promptly increases both extracellular and intracellular brain water. Since the brain rapidly compensates for changes in osmolality, acute hyponatremia produces more severe symptoms than chronic hyponatremia. In anesthesia practice, a common cause of hyponatremia associated with a normal osmolality is the absorption of large volumes of sodium-free irrigating solutions (containing mannitol, glycerine, or sorbitol as the solute) during transurethral resection of the prostate. Neurologic symptoms are minimal if mannitol is used because the agent does not cross the blood–brain barrier and is excreted with water in the urine. In contrast, as glycine or sorbitol is metabolized, hyposmolality will gradually develop and cerebral edema may appear as a late complication, that is, hyposmolality is more important in generating symptoms than hyponatremia per se. Hyponatremia likewise may result from high levels of ADH. (See page 341: Sodium.)

29. E. Normal serum Mg^{2+} ranges between 1.8 and 2.4 mg/dL (0.8–1.2 mmol/L; 1.6–2.4 mEq/L). Therapeutic hypermagnesemia is used to treat patients with premature labor, pre-eclampsia, and eclampsia. Since magnesium blocks the release of catecholamines from adrenergic nerve terminals and the adrenal glands, magnesium has been used to reduce the effects of catecholamine excess in patients with tetanus and pheochromocytoma. Symptoms that develop during hypermagnesemia include: Hyporeflexia and nausea (>5 mg/dL), somnolence, areflexia and ECG changes (>7 mg/dL), heart block, paralysis, and cardiac arrest (>12 mg/dL). (See page 356: Magnesium and page 358: Table 14-23.)

30. B. Hypernatremia produces neurologic symptoms (including stupor, coma, and seizures), hypovolemia, renal insufficiency (occasionally progressing to renal failure), and decreased urinary concentrating ability. Since hyper-natremia frequently results from diabetes insipidus (DI) or osmotically induced losses of sodium and water, many patients are hypovolemic or bear the stigmata of renal disease. Postoperative neurosurgical patients who have undergone pituitary surgery are at particular risk of developing transient or prolonged DI. Polyuria may be present for only a few days within the first week of surgery, may be permanent, or may demonstrate a triphasic sequence: Early DI, return of urinary concentrating ability, then recurrent DI. Treatments include water replacement, desmopressin (DDAVP), vasopressin, and drugs that stimulate ADH release (chlorpropamide, clofibrate, thiazide diuretics). (See page 341: Sodium.)

31. D. Aldosterone increases renal reabsorption of Na^+ and excretion of K^+. Renal excretion of K^+ is also increased by high urinary flow rates and the presence in the renal tubular fluid of nonreabsorbable anions such as carbenicillin and phosphates. An intracellular shift of K^+ is caused by insulin, and β_2 agonists. Metabolic and respiratory acidoses tend to shift potassium out of cells, while metabolic and respiratory alkaloses favor movement into cells. (See page 347: Potassium.)

32. B. Hypokalemia ([K^+] < 3.5 mEq/L) is a frequent complication of treatment with diuretic drugs and occasionally complicates other diseases and treatment regimens. Chronic potassium loss that causes a 1 mEq/L decrease of plasma K^+ is typically associated with a total body deficit of 200 to 300 mEq. However, in contrast to the hyperpolarization that accompanies an acute loss, the ratio of intracellular to extracellular K^+ remains relatively stable during a chronic loss. An intracellular shift of K^+ (and hypokalemia) may accompany respiratory and metabolic alkalosis and severe hypothermia; the changes resolve upon correction of alkalosis and rewarming. (See page 347: Potassium.)

33. E. Acute hypokalemia causes hyperpolarization of the cardiac cell, which may lead to ventricular escape activity, re-entrant arrhythmias, and delayed conduction, with potentiation of digitalis-induced effects. Common signs include first-degree atrioventricular block and ST segment depression. (See page 347: Potassium.)

34. D. A mineralocorticoid deficiency may lead to hyperkalemia. Likewise, administration of a drug (e.g., ACE inhibitor) that reduces the release of aldosterone or opposes the effects of aldosterone (e.g., triamterene or spironolactone) causes an increase in K^+ levels. These effects may be offset by a drug that promotes kaliuresis (e.g., furosemide). They may also be treated with mineralocorticoid supplementation. Although the ECG may provide the first suggestion of hyperkalemia in some patients, and despite the well-described effects of hyperkalemia on cardiac conduction and rhythm, the ECG is an insensitive and nonspecific method of detecting hyperkalemia. (See page 347: Potassium.)

35. A. With progressive hyperkalemia, the electrocardiogram shows tall, peaked T waves followed by a prolonged

PR interval and then a decrease in P-wave height. These changes may progress to widening of the QRS complex. Finally, the QRS complex widens into a pattern resembling a sine wave, as a prelude to asystole. The effects are exacerbated by hyponatremia, hypocalcemia, acidosis, and digitalis toxicity. (See page 347: Potassium.)

36. C.   Serum K^+ concentrations may be acutely lowered by administration of $NaHCO_3$ (50–100 mEq), 5 to 10 U of regular insulin administered intravenously with 50 mL of 50% glucose, β_2-adrenergic agonists, or furosemide (or related diuretics). Acute therapy may also include calcium chloride, which depresses the membrane threshold potential. More delayed forms of therapy include Na polystyrene sulfonate resin (Kayexalate) exchanges. Spironolactone opposes the effects of aldosterone causing an increase in K^+ levels. (See page 347: Potassium.)

37. B.   The concentration of free calcium in the ECF is normally 1 to 1.25 mM. Since calcium is divalent, this corresponds to 2 to 2.5 mEq/L. The remaining 50% of extracellular calcium is protein bound (40%) or chelated (10%). Parathyroid hormone helps regulate the concentration of the physiologically active (ionized) form and increases plasma calcium levels. Calcium may be lowered by increased phosphate. Hyperphosphatemic hypocalcemia results from calcium precipitation and suppression of calcitriol synthesis. Whereas acute acidemia decreases protein-bound calcium (i.e., increases ionized calcium), acute alkalemia increases protein-bound calcium (i.e., decreases ionized calcium). (See page 352: Calcium.)

38. A.   Hypocalcemia causes increased neuronal membrane irritability and tetany, as demonstrated by eliciting the Chvostek or Trousseau sign. It causes Q-T and ST prolongation, T-wave inversion, and insensitivity to digitalis. Hypocalcemia may cause laryngeal spasm after parathyroid removal. In massive transfusion, citrate may produce hypocalcemia by chelating calcium. However, a healthy, normothermic adult with intact hepatic and renal function can adequately metabolize the citrate provided (without becoming hypocalcemic) when 5 U of blood is infused in 1 hour. When citrate clearance is decreased or when blood transfusion rates are rapid (e.g., 0.5–2 mL/ kg/min), severe hypocalcemia can occur. (See page 352: Calcium.)

39. B.   Patients with moderate hypercalcemia (total serum calcium, 11.5–13 mg/dL) may show symptoms of lethargy, anorexia, nausea, and polyuria. Severe hypercalcemia (total serum calcium >13 mg/dL) is associated with severe neuromyopathic symptoms (including muscle weakness, depression, impaired memory, emotional lability, lethargy, stupor, and coma), renal calcium salt precipitation (nephrocalcinosis), and cardiovascular changes (hypertension, arrhythmias, heart block, cardiac arrest, and digitalis sensitivity). General supportive treatment includes hydration, correction of associated electrolyte abnormalities, removal of offending drugs, and dietary calcium restriction. Infusion of 0.9% saline will dilute serum calcium, reverse Na and water depletion, and promote renal excretion. Other treatments include calcitonin, mithramycin, and etidronate disodium (a diphosphonate). (See page 352: Calcium.)

40. E.   The clinical features of hyperphosphatemia relate primarily to the development of hypocalcemia and ectopic calcification. Hyperphosphatemia can promote calcification in vital organs such as the kidneys and myocardium. Neurologic manifestations of hypophosphatemia include paresthesias, encephalopathy, delirium, seizures, and coma. Hematologic abnormalities include dysfunction of erythrocytes, platelets, and leukocytes. Muscle changes include myopathies, with respiratory muscle failure and myocardial dysfunction. Phosphate should be administered cautiously to hypocalcemic patients because of the risk of precipitating more severe hypocalcemia. Acute alkalemia may reduce serum phosphate to 1 to 2 mg/dL. Common in postoperative and traumatized patients, hypophosphatemia (<2.5 mg/dL) is caused by three primary abnormalities in phosphate homeostasis: An intracellular shift, an increase in renal loss, and a decrease in gastrointestinal absorption. (See page 355: Phosphate.)

41. A.   Normal Mg^{2+} levels in the plasma are approximately 1.7 mg/dL. Symptoms of hypomagnesemia occur at levels below 1 mg/dL. The clinical features of hypomagnesemia, similar to those of hypocalcemia, are characterized by increased neuronal irritability, tetany, weakness, lethargy, muscle spasms, paresthesias, and depression. Severe hypomagnesemia may induce cardiovascular abnormalities, including coronary artery spasm, cardiac failure, dysrhythmias, hypotension, and increased myocardial sensitivity to digitalis. Rapid correction of hypomagnesemia may cause symptoms consistent with hypocalcemia. Of alcoholic patients admitted to the hospital, 30% are hypomagnesemic. (See page 356: Magnesium.)

15

Autonomic Nervous System: Physiology and Pharmacology

1. Which of the following statements concerning the sympathetic nervous system (SNS) is TRUE?

   A. The preganglionic fibers originate in the gray column of the 2 lower cervical, 12 thoracic, and first lumbar segments of the spinal cord.
   B. There are 22 paired sympathetic ganglia.
   C. Preganglionic fibers only synapse with postganglionic fibers in ganglia at the level of exit.
   D. Preganglionic fibers may also synapse in a ganglion to fibers that can then traverse to the adrenal gland.
   E. All preganglionic fibers are unmyelinated fibers.

2. Which of the following statements concerning postganglionic fibers of the sympathetic nervous system (SNS) is TRUE?

   A. The postganglionic nerve cell bodies are located only in the paired lateral ganglia.
   B. The celiac and inferior mesenteric ganglia are located along the spinal cord and are considered part of a sympathetic paired ganglion.
   C. Ganglia of the sympathetic chain are almost always located closer to the spinal cord than to the organs they innervate.
   D. Postganglionic myelinated fibers proceed from paired ganglia to the respective organs.
   E. Approximately 25% of the fibers in the average somatic nerve are sympathetic.

3. Which of the following statements concerning the sympathetic nervous system (SNS) is TRUE?

   A. The first four to five thoracic spinal segments generate fibers that converge to form three special paired ganglia.
   B. The middle cervical ganglion also is known as the stellate ganglion.
   C. The stellate ganglion provides sympathetic innervation only to the head, neck, and chest.
   D. The SNS produces discrete, rather than diffuse physiologic responses.
   E. One preganglionic fiber influences one postganglionic neuron.

4. Which of the following statements regarding the parasympathetic nervous system (PNS) is TRUE?

   A. The sacral fibers originate from the white matter of the second, third, and fourth sacral nerves.
   B. Preganglionic fibers are myelinated fibers analogous to those in the sympathetic nervous system (SNS) and terminate in ganglia next to the spinal cord.
   C. The ratio of preganglionic to postganglionic fibers in the PNS is similar to the ratio found in the SNS.
   D. Postganglionic neurons are located in or near the organ to be innervated.
   E. Cranial nerve X has the least innervation of all PNS nerves.

5. All of the following are functions of the autonomic innervation of the heart EXCEPT:

   A. The autonomic nervous system (ANS) changes the heart rate (chronotropism).
   B. The ANS changes the strength of contraction (inotropism).
   C. The ANS modulates coronary blood flow.
   D. There is parasympathetic innervation of the ventricles of the heart.
   E. The vagus affects the sinoatrial (SA) and atrioventricular (AV) nodes.

6. Which of the following statements regarding the autonomic nervous system (ANS), peripheral circulation, and lungs is TRUE?

   A. The sympathetic nervous system (SNS) and parasympathetic nervous system (PNS) are equally important regulators in the peripheral circulation.
   B. The PNS tends to constrict, rather than dilate vessels.
   C. SNS stimulation of the coronary arteries may produce constriction or dilation, depending on the type of receptors which the SNS fiber terminates on.
   D. Vascular tone is predominantly controlled by PNS activity.
   E. SNS stimulation produces bronchoconstriction and pulmonary vasoconstriction.

7. All of the following statements about neurotransmission in the autonomic nervous system (ANS) are true EXCEPT:

   A. The sympathetic nervous system (SNS) and parasympathetic nervous system (PNS) are commonly designated as adrenergic and cholinergic, respectively.

   B. In the PNS, the postganglionic receptors secrete acetylcholine (Ach).

   C. Norepinephrine is the only neurotransmitter of postganglionic SNS sites.

   D. The preganglionic neurotransmitter is Ach in both the PNS and SNS.

   E. Terminations of postganglionic fibers are anatomically and physiologically similar in both the SNS and PNS.

8. Which of the following statements regarding the parasympathetic nervous system (PNS) is TRUE?

   A. In addition to acetylcholinesterase, pseudocholinesterase also plays a significant role in the termination of acetylcholine (Ach).

   B. Acetylcholine is stored in presynaptic vesicles and is released in small amounts called quanta.

   C. After it is released, any nonhydrolyzed Ach undergoes reuptake by the presynaptic membrane.

   D. Drugs that alter calcium release do not affect the release of Ach because its release is calcium independent.

   E. Ach is formed by acetylation of choline by the enzyme acetylcholinesterase.

9. All of the following statements regarding the sympathetic nervous system (SNS) are true EXCEPT:

   A. Epinephrine, norepinephrine, and ATP are mediators of the peripheral SNS.

   B. In the adrenal medulla, the preganglionic neurotransmitter is acetylcholine (Ach).

   C. Chromaffin cells in the adrenal medulla are responsible for the release of epinephrine and norepinephrine.

   D. The massive release of norepinephrine and epinephrine is the "fight or flight" response and lasts approximately 10 times as long as local direct stimulation.

   F. Equal amounts of epinephrine and norepinephrine are released during stimulation of the adrenal medulla.

10. Which of the following statements about catecholamines is TRUE?

    A. Circulating catecholamines are responsible for stimulating receptors in the central nervous system during the "fight or flight" response.

    B. All sympathomimetics are catecholamines, but not all catecholamines are sympathomimetics.

    C. Catecholamine precursors include phenylalanine and tyrosine.

    D. Catecholamines have a direct, not indirect, effect on adrenergic receptors.

    E. Intermediate precursors of catecholamine synthesis have no effect on adrenergic receptors.

11. All of the following statements regarding the autonomic receptors are true EXCEPT:

    A. Acetylcholine (Ach) is the neurotransmitter in the parasympathetic nervous system (PNS), at preganglionic receptors of the sympathetic nervous system (SNS), and at the neuromuscular junction.

    B. Muscarinic receptors in the myocardium are stimulated by Ach and inhibit the release of norepinephrine.

    C. The two subdivisions of cholinergic receptors are muscarinic and nicotinic.

    D. Muscarinic stimulation causes tachycardia, inotropism, bronchodilation, and miosis.

    E. Nicotinic receptors are located in the SNS.

12. Which of the following statements regarding α receptors is TRUE?

    A. The α_1 receptors result in increased vasoconstriction, but not inotropism.

    B. Actions of postsynaptic α_2 receptors include vasodilation, inhibition of insulin release, inhibition of bowel motility, and inhibition of antidiuretic hormone release.

    C. When stimulated, presynaptic α_2 receptors mediate inhibition of epinephrine release into the synaptic cleft.

    D. Coronary vasoconstriction is mediated more by postsynaptic α_1 than α_2 receptors.

    E. Norepinephrine is the most potent venoconstrictor of all the catecholamines.

13. All of the following statements regarding β-adrenergic receptors are true EXCEPT:

    A. The β receptors are found in both the presynaptic and postsynaptic membranes.

    B. Activation of the presynaptic β_2 receptor has the same physiologic response as antagonism of the presynaptic α_2 receptor.

    C. The postsynaptic β_2 receptors respond primarily to circulating epinephrine.

    D. The β_2 receptors are primarily located postsynaptically in the myocardium, sinoatrial node, and ventricular conduction system.

    E. The β_1 receptors are equally sensitive to norepinephrine and epinephrine.

14. Which of the following statements regarding the β receptors in the heart and peripheral vessels is FALSE?

    A. When activated, β_1 and β_2 receptors induce activation of adenylate cyclase.

    B. Increased catecholamine levels in heart failure leads to a larger downregulation of β_2 receptors compared with β_1 receptors.

    C. Whereas the inotropic effect of epinephrine is mediated via β_1 and β_2 receptors, the inotropic effect of norepinephrine is mediated entirely through β_1 receptors.

    D. The postsynaptic β_1 receptors are predominantly found in the myocardium, sinoatrial node, and ventricular conduction system. The β_2 receptors have the same distribution but are presynaptic.

    E. The β_2 receptors approximate 20% to 30% of β receptors in the myocardium.

15. Which of the following statements regarding dopamine receptors is TRUE?

    A. The dopamine-1 receptors are located postsynaptically.
    B. The dopamine-2 receptors are located only presynaptically.
    C. The dopamine receptors have been located in the myocardium and are responsible for increased inotropism.
    D. The dopamine receptors inhibit the release of prolactin in the hypothalamus.
    E. The dopamine receptors located on vascular smooth muscle of the kidneys and mesentery produce regional vasoconstriction.

16. Which of the following statements regarding the baroreceptors is TRUE?

    A. Impulses from the carotid sinus and aortic arch reach the vasomotor center through the hypoglossal and the vagal nerve, respectively.
    B. Increased sensory input from the baroreceptors caused by decreased blood pressure inhibits sympathetic nervous system (SNS) effector traffic.
    C. The Valsalva maneuver can be used to identify patients at risk for autonomic nervous system (ANS) instability.
    D. Dysfunction in the SNS is suspected if prolonged hypertension develops during the forced expiration phase of the Valsalva maneuver.
    E. The presence of "overshoot" in blood pressure at the end of the Valsalva maneuver indicates dysfunction of the sympathetic nervous system (SNS).

17. Which of the following is the principal site of autonomic nervous system (ANS) organization and long-term blood pressure control?

    A. Cerebral cortex
    B. Hypothalamus
    C. Medulla
    D. Pons
    E. Cerebellum

18. In which of the following organs do the preganglionic fibers pass directly without synapsing in a ganglion?

    A. Sweat glands
    B. Adrenal gland
    C. Spleen
    D. Liver
    E. Pancreas

19. Which of the following statements about dobutamine is FALSE?

    A. Dobutamine does not cause norepinephrine release or stimulate dopamine receptors.
    B. Dobutamine is a synthetic catecholamine modified from the classic inodilator isoproterenol.
    C. Dobutamine increases the heart rate more than epinephrine for a given increase in cardiac output.
    D. Dobutamine is a coronary artery constrictor.
    E. Dobutamine is highly controllable, with a half-life of 2 minutes.

20. Which of the following statements is FALSE regarding fenoldopam?

    A. Fenoldopam is a selective dopamine-1 agonist with no α- or β-receptor activity.
    B. Fenoldopam has diuretic properties.
    C. Use of fenoldopam for greater than 12 hours leads to tolerance of its blood pressure lowering effects.
    D. Fenoldopam has an elimination half-life of 5 minutes.
    E. Fenoldopam is a direct renal vasodilator.

21. Which of the following symptoms is not included under clonidine withdrawal syndrome?

    A. Hypertension
    B. Headache
    C. Tachycardia
    D. Somnolence
    E. Sweating

22. All of the following are side effects of α-blockers, EXCEPT:

    A. Hypotension
    B. Orthostatic hypotension
    C. Nasal stuffiness
    D. Mydriasis
    E. Inhibition of ejaculation

23. All of the following are β_1 selective blockers, EXCEPT:

    A. Atenolol
    B. Esmolol
    C. Carvedilol
    D. Metoprolol
    E. Bisoprolol

24. All of the following are interactions of the autonomic nervous system (ANS) with endocrine regulatory systems, EXCEPT:

    A. Release of antidiuretic hormone secondary to changes in plasma osmolality
    B. β-receptor stimulation in the pancreas
    C. Release of renin from the juxtaglomerular apparatus
    D. Adrenal cortical function
    E. Increased insulin secretion with alpha stimulation

25. Which of the following pharmacology statements is TRUE?

    A. Hydralazine relaxes smooth muscle tone via adrenergic receptors.
    B. Milrinone is a phosphodiesterase II inhibitor which facilitates the breakdown of cyclic adenosine monophosphate (cAMP).
    C. Nitroglycerin has no vasodilatory effects on the arterial vasculature.
    D. Sodium nitroprusside is an arterial vasodilator and decreases afterload while maintaining preload.
    E. Undesirable side effects of hydralazine include a reflex tachycardia and a lupus-like syndrome.

26. Which of the following statements regarding adrenergic agonists and sympathomimetics is FALSE?

   A. Clonidine reduces plasma renin activity, as well as levels of norepinephrine and epinephrine.
   B. Dexmedetomidine is a partial α_2 agonist, and clonidine is a more selective α_2 agonist.
   C. Vasopressin acts on cardiac myocytes, vascular smooth muscle, and renal collecting ducts.
   D. The dose for vasopressin in ACLS protocols is 40 units.
   E. Adenosine may be used with caution in patients with Wolff–Parkinson–White and a narrow complex tachycardia.

27. Which of the following statements regarding adrenergic agonists is TRUE?

   A. Isoproterenol is a pure β_1 agonist which increases heart rate and contractility.
   B. With dopamine use, dopamine receptors are the most sensitive, followed by β receptors, then α receptors.
   C. As an inotropic agent, dobutamine is considered more potent than dopamine.
   D. Clinical studies suggest that dopamine is less likely to increase heart rate than dobutamine.
   E. Dopamine vasodilates the pulmonary vasculature and is helpful in treating right heart failure and cor pulmonale.

28. Which of the following statements regarding adrenergic agonists is FALSE?

   A. Norepinephrine is considered the first-line agent for treating hypotension in the septic patient.
   B. Norepinephrine acts on α and β receptors and at low doses can increase cardiac output.
   C. Ephedrine is an α and β agonist.
   D. Phenylephrine increases both venous and arterial constriction and generally does not change cardiac output.
   E. For moderate croup, intravenous (rather than intramuscular) epinephrine is the preferred route of administration.

29. Which of the following statements regarding muscarinic antagonists is TRUE?

   A. Glycopyrrolate is a tertiary amine.
   B. Atropine, like scopolamine, crosses the blood–brain barrier and causes amnesia, sedation, and euphoria.
   C. Scopolamine can cause a paradoxical bradycardia when given in low doses.
   D. Scopolamine, but not atropine, is contraindicated in patients with narrow-angle glaucoma.
   E. Atropine, but not scopolamine, blocks acetylcholine transmission to sweat glands.

30. Which of the following statements regarding anticholinesterases is FALSE?

   A. Most of the anticholinesterases inhibit both acetylcholinesterase and pseudocholinesterase.
   B. Muscarinic activity is evoked at lower concentrations of acetylcholine than are necessary to produce the desired nicotinic effect.
   C. Excess accumulation of acetylcholine at the motor end plate produces a depolarizing block similar to succinylcholine or high doses of nicotine.
   D. Pyridostigmine is a tertiary amine that readily passes through the CNS and can be used to treat atropine poisoning.
   E. Echothiophate may be effective for 2 to 3 weeks after cessation of therapy and cause prolonged duration of action of succinylcholine.

ANSWERS

1. B. The preganglionic fibers originate from T1 to T12 and L1 to L3 in the gray intermediolateral column. These fibers are myelinated nerve axons that leave the spinal cord with the motor fibers to form the white communicating rami. These fibers enter the 22 paired sympathetic ganglia. After entering these ganglia, the fibers may take three possible courses: They may synapse with postganglionic fibers in the ganglion, they may move up and down the SNS to another ganglion, or they may track through the sympathetic chain and exit without synapsing to SNS collateral ganglia. The exception to this rule is the group of myelinated fibers that terminate in the adrenal medulla without first synapsing in a ganglion. Many of the postganglionic fibers pass from the lateral SNS chain back into the spinal nerves to form the gray (unmyelinated) communicating rami at all levels of the spinal cord. They are distributed distally to the sweat glands, pilomotor muscle, and blood vessels of the skin and muscle. (See page 363: Functional Anatomy.)

2. C. Postganglionic neuronal cell bodies of the SNS are located in the paired lateral ganglia or unpaired collateral ganglia. The celiac and inferior mesenteric ganglia are considered to be collateral ganglia. SNS ganglia are located primarily near the spinal cord rather than near the organs they innervate. The postganglionic fibers are unmyelinated. The average somatic nerve has approximately 8% sympathetic fibers. (See page 363: Functional Anatomy.)

3. A. The first four to five thoracic segments' preganglionic fibers form three specialized paired ganglia: The superior cervical, middle cervical, and cervicothoracic ganglia. The latter is known as the stellate ganglion. It is a fusion of the inferior cervical and first thoracic SNS ganglia. This provides sympathetic innervation to the head, neck, upper extremities, heart, and lungs. The response from sympathetic system activation is diffuse. The preganglionic neurons are fewer than the postganglionic neurons. Hence, preganglionic fibers influence a number of postganglionic neurons. (See page 363: Functional Anatomy.)

4. D. The PNS consists of preganglionic and postganglionic neurons. The preganglionic nerve fibers originate in cranial nerves III (oculomotor), VII (facial), IX (glossopharyngeal), and X (vagus). In addition, fibers originate from the intermediolateral horn of the second, third, and fourth sacral nerves. Preganglionic nerve fibers pass directly to the organ that is innervated. Postganglionic neurons are located in or near the organ to be innervated. Therefore, postganglionic innervation is limited, and responses are discrete. Cranial nerve X (vagus) accounts for 75% of the PNS activity. The ratio of postganglionic to preganglionic fibers in many organs appears to be 1:1 to 3:1 compared with the 20:1 found in the SNS system. (See page 363: Functional Anatomy.)

5. D. The heart is well supplied by both the SNS and parasympathetic nervous system (PNS). These fibers are responsible for changing the rate of the heart (chronotropism), changing the strength of contraction (inotropism), and modulating coronary blood flow. PNS innervation is mainly in the SA and AV nodes, and to a lesser extent, the atria. There is no PNS supply to the ventricles. (See page 363: Functional Anatomy.)

6. C. The SNS is the predominant regulator of the peripheral circulation; PNS innervation is minimal. The PNS tends to dilate vessels. The SNS may cause vasodilation or vasoconstriction, depending on receptor activity. Vascular tone is predominantly influenced by the SNS. In the lungs, SNS activity causes bronchodilation and pulmonary vasoconstriction. (See page 363: Functional Anatomy.)

7. C. The SNS and PNS are designated as adrenergic and cholinergic, respectively. In the PNS, Ach is secreted at the postganglionic receptor site. In the SNS, norepinephrine is the main neurotransmitter at postganglionic sites, with the exception of sweat glands. The preganglionic neurotransmitter for both the PNS and SNS is Ach. The postganglionic fibers of the SNS and PNS are anatomically and physiologically similar. The terminals branch out into terminal effector plexuses. One terminal branches to thousands of effector cells. The terminal ending is called a varicosity. Each varicosity contains vesicles within which the neurotransmitter is stored. (See page 363: Functional Anatomy.)

8. B. Ach is formed within the presynaptic membrane by acetylation of choline with acetylcoenzyme. This process is catalyzed by choline acetyltransferase. The active product of this reaction, Ach, is stored in presynaptic vesicles. During the resting state, small amounts of Ach ("quanta") are continually released, resulting in miniature end-plate potentials. Arrival of an action potential causes a release of hundreds of quanta, causing depolarization of an end plate. This release is dependent on calcium influx. Drugs that alter calcium influx may decrease the release of Ach. Ach is removed by rapid hydrolysis by the enzyme acetylcholinesterase. There is no reuptake into the presynaptic membrane. Pseudocholinesterase, or plasma cholinesterase, is an enzyme similar to acetylcholinesterase but does not appear to be physiologically important in the termination of the action of Ach. (See page 363: Functional Anatomy.)

9. E. Epinephrine and norepinephrine are mediators of SNS peripheral activity. Vascular SNS nerve terminals also release adenosine triphosphate (ATP), which is considered a coneurotransmitter with norepinephrine. In the adrenal medulla, Ach is the primary neurotransmitter at the preganglionic site. It causes release of norepinephrine and epinephrine from the chromaffin cells. These cells are considered the postganglionic neurons. Stimulation of the adrenal medulla results in massive release of epinephrine and norepinephrine, which lasts 10 times as long as local direct stimulation. Epinephrine release is greater in proportion to norepinephrine release. (See page 363: Functional Anatomy.)

10. C.   A catecholamine is a compound consisting of a catechol nucleus and amine site chain. Catecholamines and other sympathomimetics (e.g., clonidine) can activate adrenergic receptors. (All clinically useful catecholamines are sympathomimetics, but not all sympathomimetics are catecholamines.) Phenylalanine or tyrosine are taken up into the axoplasm of nerve terminals and synthesized into norepinephrine or epinephrine. Catecholamines may have a direct or indirect effect on receptors. The indirect effect is mediated through the release of stored neurotransmitter. Direct effects are independent of norepinephrine release. Some drugs may have a mixed mode of action. The brain contains both noradrenergic and dopaminergic receptors, but circulating catecholamines do not cross the blood–brain barrier. The catecholamines present in the brain are synthesized there. (See page 363: Functional Anatomy.)

11. D.   Cholinergic receptors are subdivided into muscarinic and nicotinic receptors. The nicotinic receptors are located at the preganglionic receptors of the SNS and PNS and at the neuromuscular junction of striated muscle. Muscarinic receptors are primarily associated with the postganglionic junctions of the PNS. PNS muscarinic stimulation causes bradycardia, decreased inotropism, bronchoconstriction, miosis, salivation, gastrointestinal hypermotility, and increased gastric acid secretion. Muscarinic receptors are also found on the presynaptic membrane of sympathetic nerve terminals in the myocardium, coronary vessels, and peripheral vasculature. These are referred to as adrenergic muscarinic receptors because of their location; however, they are stimulated by Ach. Stimulation of these receptors inhibits release of norepinephrine in a manner similar to α_2-receptor stimulation. (See page 371: Receptors.)

12. E.   The α_1 receptors are believed to have a positive inotropic effect on cardiac tissues in most mammals. Postsynaptic α_2 receptors mediate vasoconstriction, platelet aggregation, inhibition of insulin release, inhibition of bowel motility, stimulation of growth hormone release, and inhibition of antidiuretic hormone release. The α_2 presynaptic receptors mediate inhibition of norepinephrine release, and thus play a significant role in reducing sympathetic outflow. This results in decreases in systemic vascular resistance, cardiac output, and heart rate. In the CNS, these receptors may contribute to analgesia and sedation. Coronary vasoconstriction is mediated more by postsynaptic α_2 receptors than α_1. The α_1 receptors in the epicardial vessels only contribute 5% of the total resistance in the normal coronary circulation. Therefore, α_1 agonists such as phenylephrine probably have minimal effect on coronary resistance. Norepinephrine is the most potent venoconstrictor. (See page 371: Receptors.)

13. D. β_1 and β_2 are the two subtypes of β-adrenergic receptors. There is now evidence of a β_3 receptor as well. The β_1 receptors are located in the myocardium, sinoatrial node,

and ventricular conduction system. They are equally sensitive to circulating norepinephrine and epinephrine, which distinguishes them from β_2 receptors, which are more sensitive to epinephrine than to norepinephrine. The β_1 receptors are located only postsynaptically. The β_2 receptors have the same distribution but are presynaptic. The effects of activation of presynaptic β_2 receptors are diametrically opposed to α_2 presynaptic receptors. The β_2 presynaptic receptors accelerate endogenous norepinephrine release. Antagonism of these receptors results in a physiologic response that is similar to activation of presynaptic α_2 receptors. (See page 371: Receptors.)

14. B.   Activation of all the β receptors leads to activation of adenylate cyclase.

Chronic heart failure leads to downregulation of myocardial β_1 receptors because of high levels of circulating catecholamines. There is no evidence of downregulation of α_1 or β_2 receptors. Whereas the effect of norepinephrine on inotropism in the normal heart is mediated entirely through the postsynaptic β_1 receptor, the inotropic effects of epinephrine are mediated through both the β_1 and β_2 myocardial receptors. The postsynaptic β_1 receptors are distributed predominantly to the myocardium, the sinoatrial node, and the ventricular conduction system. The β_2 receptors have the same distribution but are presynaptic. Activation of the presynaptic β_2 receptor accelerates the release of norepinephrine into the synaptic cleft. The β_2 receptor approximates 20% to 30% of the β receptors in the ventricular myocardium and up to 40% of the β receptors in the atrium. (See page 371: Receptors.)

15. A.   The dopamine receptors are of two types, dopamine-1 and dopamine-2. Whereas the type 1 receptors are located postsynaptically, the type 2 receptors are located both presynaptically and postsynaptically. Dopamine receptors have not been located in the myocardium. They are located in the hypothalamus, where they enhance the release of prolactin. They also are located in the basal ganglia, where they coordinate motor function. Dopamine receptors in the smooth muscle of the kidneys and mesentery produce vasodilation, resulting in increased blood flow to these organs. (See page 371: Receptors.)

16. C.   Impulses from the carotid sinus and aortic arch reach the medullary vasomotor center by the glossopharyngeal and vagus nerves, respectively. Increased sensory traffic from the baroreceptors, caused by increased blood pressure, inhibits SNS effector traffic. The relative increase in vagal tone produces vasodilation, slowing of the heart rate, and a lowering of the blood pressure. Real increases in vagal tone occur when the blood pressure exceeds normal limits. The arterial baroreceptor reflex can best be demonstrated by the Valsalva maneuver. The arterial blood pressure increases momentarily as the intrathoracic blood is forced into the heart (preload). Sustained intrathoracic pressure diminishes venous return, reduces the cardiac output, and decreases the blood pressure. Reflex vasoconstriction and tachycardia ensue. The blood pressure returns to normal with release of the forced expiration but then briefly "overshoots" because of the vasoconstriction and increased venous return. A slowing of the heart rate accompanies the overshoot in pressure. The Valsalva maneuver has been used to identify patients at risk for ANS instability. Dysfunction of the SNS is implicated if exaggerated and prolonged hypotension develops during the forced expiration phase. In addition, the overshoot at the end of the Valsalva maneuver is absent. (See page 378: Autonomic Nervous System Reflexes and Interactions.)

17. B. The cerebral cortex is the highest level of ANS integration. Fainting at the sight of blood is an example of this higher level of somatic and ANS integration. The principal site of ANS organization is the hypothalamus. Long-term blood pressure control, reactions to physical and emotional stress, sleep, and sexual reflexes are regulated through the hypothalamus. The medulla oblongata and pons are the vital centers of acute ANS organization. Together, they integrate momentary hemodynamic adjustments and maintain the sequence and automaticity of ventilation. (See page 378: Autonomic Nervous System Reflexes and Interactions.)

18. B. The efferent sympathetic nervous system (SNS) is referred to as the thoracolumbar nervous system. The preganglionic fibers of the SNS (thoracolumbar division) originate in the intermediolateral gray column of the 12 thoracic (T1–T12) and the first three lumbar segments (L1–L3) of the spinal cord. The myelinated axons of these nerve cells leave the spinal cord with the motor fibers to form the white (myelinated) communicating rami. The rami enter one of the paired 22 sympathetic ganglia at their respective segmental levels. Upon entering the paravertebral ganglia of the lateral sympathetic chain, the preganglionic fiber may follow one of three courses: Synapse with postganglionic fibers in ganglia at the level of exit; course upward or downward in the trunk of the SNS chain to synapse in ganglia at other levels; or track for variable distances through the sympathetic chain and exit without synapsing to terminate in an outlying, unpaired SNS collateral ganglion. The adrenal gland is an exception to the rule. The preganglionic fibers pass directly into the adrenal medulla without synapsing in a ganglion. (See page 363: Functional Anatomy.)

19. D. Dobutamine is a synthetic catecholamine modified from the classic inodilator isoproterenol. It does not cause norepinephrine release or stimulate dopamine receptors. Dobutamine possesses weak α_1 agonism, which can be unmasked by β blockade as a prompt and dramatic increase in blood pressure. Dobutamine increases the heart rate more than epinephrine for a given increase in cardiac output. Dobutamine is a coronary vasodilator, in contrast to dopamine, which is a coronary vasoconstrictor. Dobutamine is highly controllable, with a half-life of 2 minutes. (See page 380: Clinical Autonomic Nervous System Pharmacology.)

20. C. Fenoldopam, a benzazepine derivative, is a selective dopamine-1 agonist with no α- or β-receptor activity. Intravenous fenoldopam has direct natriuretic and diuretic properties and promotes an increase in creatinine clearance.

Fenoldopam has an elimination half-life of 5 minutes. There has been no evidence of tolerance during fenoldopam use to lower blood pressure for up to 24 hours. Fenoldopam is a direct renal vasodilator, so it is useful in cases where the renal arteries have been temporarily clamped, or where renal vasoconstriction is an expected complication. (See page 380: Clinical Autonomic Nervous System Pharmacology.)

21. D. One of the more worrisome complications of chronic clonidine use is a withdrawal syndrome upon acute discontinuation of the drug. This usually occurs about 18 hours after discontinuation. The signs and symptoms are hypertension, tachycardia, insomnia, flushing, headache, apprehension, sweating, and tremulousness. It lasts for 24 to 72 hours and is most likely to occur in patients taking more than 1.2 mg/day of clonidine. The withdrawal syndrome has been noted postoperatively in patients withdrawn from clonidine before surgery. The withdrawal syndrome can be confused with anesthesia emergence symptoms, particularly in patients with uncontrolled hypertension. Absent the availability of the oral route in the surgical patient, withdrawal can be treated with transdermal clonidine, rectal clonidine, or intravenous clonidine. (See page 380: Clinical Autonomic Nervous System Pharmacology.)

22. D. Drugs that bind selectively to α-adrenergic receptors block the action of endogenous catecholamines or moderate the effects of exogenous adrenergics. The resultant effects may be ascribed to either the blockade effect to α-adrenergic agonists or to unopposed β-adrenergic receptor activity. The effect is smooth muscle relaxation. The prominent clinical effects of α-blockers include hypotension, orthostatic hypotension, tachycardia, miosis, nasal stuffiness, diarrhea, and inhibition of ejaculation. (See page 380: Clinical Autonomic Nervous System Pharmacology.)

23. C. Nonselective β-antagonists are referred to as first-generation β-blockers. These drugs include propranolol, nadolol, sotalol, and timolol. Carvedilol is a nonselective β and α_1 blocker. Second-generation drugs are those considered selective for β_1-adrenergic blockade and include atenolol, esmolol, and metoprolol. Other selective β_1 blockers include bisoprolol. (See page 380: Clinical Autonomic Nervous System Pharmacology.)

24. E. The ANS is related to several endocrine systems that control blood pressure and homeostasis. Antidiuretic hormone (ADH) is secreted by the hypothalamus in response to changes in plasma osmolality. However, many factors, such as stress, pain, hypoxia, anesthesia, and surgery, may stimulate release of ADH. Whereas β stimulation of the pancreas increases insulin release, α stimulation decreases it. The complex renin–angiotensin system modulates blood pressure and water and electrolyte homeostasis. Renin released from the juxtaglomerular complex acts on plasma angiotensinogen II, a potent vasoconstrictor. The ANS is also closely linked to adrenocortical function; glucocorticoids modulate epinephrine synthesis. (See page 378: Autonomic Nervous System Reflexes and Interactions.)

25. E. Hydralazine relaxes smooth muscle tone directly, without interacting with adrenergic or cholinergic receptors. Undesirable side effects of hydralazine include a reflex tachycardia and a lupus-like syndrome. Milrinone is a phosphodiesterase III inhibitor, which impedes the breakdown of cyclic adenosine monophosphate (cAMP). cAMP levels increase and protein kinase is activated to promote phosphorylation. In cardiac muscle, phosphorylation increases the slow inward movement of calcium current, promoting increased intracellular calcium stores; thus, inotropism increases. In vascular smooth muscle, increased cAMP activity accounts for the vasodilation, decreased peripheral vascular resistance, and lusitropism. Nitroglycerin is a venodilator, which has minimal effects on the arterial side, but it does have effects on the arterial vasculature at very high doses. Sodium nitroprusside is not just an arterial vasodilator, it is also a venodilator. It decreases afterload as well as preload. (See page 380: Clinical Autonomic Nervous System Pharmacology.)

26. B. Clonidine is a partial α_2 agonist while dexmedetomidine is a more selective α_2 agonist. Clonidine decreases central sympathetic outflow. There is decreased plasma renin activity, as well as decreased levels of norepinephrine and epinephrine.

Vasopressin is an exogenous form of endogenous antidiuretic hormone. Vasopressin acts on cardiac myocytes, vascular smooth muscle, and renal collecting ducts. The dose for vasopressin in ACLS protocols is 40 units. While adenosine should be avoided in Wolff–Parkinson–White patients with atrial fibrillation, it may be used with caution if a Wolff–Parkinson–White patient has a narrow complex tachycardia. (See page 386: Sympathomimetic Drugs.)

27. B. Isoproterenol is an inodilator; it is a balanced β_1 and β_2 receptor agonist, which increases heart rate and contractility. It is useful for treating bradycardia in patients with denervated hearts. Clinical studies suggest that dobutamine is less likely to increase heart rate than dopamine. With dopamine use, dopamine receptors are the most sensitive, followed by β receptors, then α receptors. Dopamine and dobutamine are considered to be equipotent inotropic agents. Dobutamine, but not dopamine, vasodilates the pulmonary vasculature and is helpful in treating right heart failure and cor pulmonale. (See page 380: Clinical Autonomic Nervous System Pharmacology.)

28. E. Norepinephrine acts directly on α- and β-adrenergic receptors. It produces increased cardiac output and blood pressure when given in low doses. Higher doses reduce flow because alpha arteriolar constriction is greater than beta effects. Norepinephrine is considered the first-line agent for treating hypotension in the septic patient. Phenylephrine is a pure α agonist and increases both venous and arterial constriction. It generally does not change cardiac output. Ephedrine stimulates both α and β receptors by direct and indirect actions, though predominantly indirect. Intramuscular epinephrine is the preferred route of administration for moderate to severe croup. (See page 380: Clinical Autonomic Nervous System Pharmacology.)

29. C. Atropine, scopolamine, and glycopyrrolate are called muscarinic antagonists because they interfere with the action of acetylcholine as a transmitter. Glycopyrrolate is a quaternary amine, so it does not easily penetrate the blood–brain barrier. However, atropine and scopolamine are tertiary amines so they cross the blood–brain barrier easily. Scopolamine can cause amnesia, sedation, and euphoria. However, atropine has the opposite effect including mild CNS stimulation at premedication doses, and restlessness, disorientation, hallucinations, and delirium at higher doses. Both scopolamine and atropine can cause a paradoxical bradycardia if given in low doses. Scopolamine at doses of 0.1 to 0.2 mg usually causes more slowing than atropine. Both atropine and scopolamine can cause mydriasis and cycloplegia, and should be avoided in patients with narrow-angle glaucoma. Both atropine and scopolamine block Ach transmission to sweat glands, which are innervated by the SNS even though they are cholinergic. (See page 380: Clinical Autonomic Nervous System Pharmacology.)

30. D. The indirect-acting cholinomimetic drugs are of greater importance to anesthesiologists than are the direct-acting cholinergic drugs. These drugs produce cholinomimetic effects indirectly as a result of inhibition or inactivation of the enzyme acetylcholinesterase, which normally destroys acetylcholine by hydrolysis. They are referred to as cholinesterase inhibitors or anticholinesterases. Most of these drugs inhibit both acetylcholinesterase and pseudocholinesterase. The most prominent pharmacologic side effects of the anticholinesterase drugs are muscarinic. Their most useful actions are their nicotinic effects. Muscarinic activity is evoked by lower concentrations of acetylcholine than are necessary to produce the desired nicotinic effect. Excess accumulation of acetylcholine at the motor end plates produces a depolarizing block similar to that produced by succinylcholine or nicotine. Most of the reversible cholinesterase inhibitors are quaternary ammonium compounds which cannot cross the blood–brain barrier. Physostigmine, however, is a tertiary amine that readily crosses the blood–brain barrier and can be used to treat atropine poisoning. Echothiophate is the only irreversible cholinesterase inhibitor which has medically therapeutic usage. It is used for topical treatment of glaucoma and may be effective for 2 to 3 weeks after cessation of therapy. If succinylcholine is used in such a patient, duration of action can be prolonged since it requires pseudocholinesterase for hydrolysis. (See page 380: Clinical Autonomic Nervous System Pharmacology.)

Hemostasis and Transfusion Medicine

1. Which of the following is NOT a physiologic compensation for isovolemic hemodilution?

   A. Increased cardiac output
   B. Decreased tissue oxygen extraction
   C. Increased capillary vasodilation
   D. Increased levels of 2,3-diphosphoglycerate (DPG)
   E. Acidemia

2. Which of the following is the most common infection associated with red blood cell (RBC) transfusion?

   A. Hepatitis B
   B. Human T-cell lymphotropic virus (HTLV-1 and HTLV-2)
   C. Hepatitis C
   D. Human immunodeficiency virus (HIV)
   E. Cytomegalovirus (CMV)

3. Noninfectious risks associated with transfusion include all EXCEPT:

   A. Hypothermia
   B. Dilutional coagulopathy
   C. Increase in 2,3-diphosphoglycerate
   D. Hyperkalemia
   E. Microaggregate delivery

4. Which of the following is true regarding coagulation?

   A. Most clotting factors circulate in an active form.
   B. Most clotting factors are synthesized extrahepatically.
   C. von Willebrand factor and coagulation factor VIII combine to form factor IX.
   D. Factors V and VIII have short storage half-lives.
   E. Seven clotting factors are vitamin K dependent.

5. Which of the following is not contained in cryoprecipitate?

   A. Factor VIII
   B. Factor X
   C. von Willebrand factor (vWF)
   D. Fibrinogen
   E. Fibronectin

6. Which of the following is not a vitamin K-dependent factor?

   A. II
   B. V
   C. VII
   D. IX
   E. X

7. Which of the following is not a common cause of platelet dysfunction?

   A. Splenectomy
   B. Use of nonsteroidal anti-inflammatory drugs (NSAIDs)
   C. Chronic liver disease
   D. Disseminated intravascular coagulopathy (DIC)
   E. Cardiopulmonary bypass (CPB)

8. Regarding autologous blood conservation strategies, all of the following statements are true EXCEPT:

   A. Regarding preoperative autologous donation, 4 U is typically the maximum possible donation.
   B. Erythropoietin is often accepted by Jehovah's Witnesses.
   C. Body weight of less than 100 lb is a relative contraindication to preoperative autologous donation.
   D. Acute normovolemic hemodilution commonly reduces the amount transfused by 3 to 4 U per patient.
   E. Autologous blood donation does not eliminate the risk of bacterial contamination and transmission via transfusion.

9. Which of the following conditions does NOT represent a situation that is likely associated with a decrease in the tolerance for anemia?

   A. A tachycardic and hypotensive 70-year-old healthy male undergoing exploratory laparotomy.
   B. A 70-year-old female undergoing open cholecystectomy with a history of TIAs and starting hemoglobin of 8 g/dL.
   C. A 40-year-old male with ST elevations during laparoscopic cholecystectomy.
   D. A healthy 40-year-old female having vaginal hysterectomy with urine output 0.2 cc/kg/hr over the last 12 hours.
   E. A 60-year-old male having exploratory laparotomy with mixed venous saturation of 65%.

10. Which of the following is TRUE concerning contemporary "cell saver" devices?

    A. The salvaged blood is anticoagulated.
    B. It returns blood with a hematocrit of 80% to 90%.
    C. The red blood cells (RBCs) are separated by microfiltration.
    D. It is a type of allogeneic transfusion.
    E. May be stored at 4°C for up to 24 hours.

11. Which of the following statements regarding recombinant activated factor VII (rFVIIa) is TRUE?

    A. rFVIIa is FDA approved for the treatment of coagulopathy during cases associated with major blood loss.
    B. rFVIIa is not an effective therapy for patients with hemophilia A or B.
    C. rFVIIa therapy is contraindicated in postpartum patients.
    D. No trials have shown definitive mortality benefit with rFVIIa and only a few randomized controlled trials have shown an improved clinical outcome.
    E. rFVIIa is dosed to replace normal physiologic concentrations.

12. Which of the following regarding patients undergoing massive transfusion protocol is TRUE?

    A. It should be performed in all patients with an estimated blood loss of 20% or more.
    B. It can lead to hypercalcemia and subsequent cardiac dysrhythmias.
    C. It should be performed in all patients with a pre-existing cardiac history and an estimated blood loss of 15%.
    D. It has not been shown to be of benefit if initiated when the starting platelet level is 50,000/µL.
    E. It has not been associated with coagulopathic disorders.

13. Regarding the collection and preparation of blood products for transfusion, which of the statements below is true?

    A. By Food and Drug Administration (FDA) mandate, platelets must be refrigerated and stored to a limit of 5 days.
    B. Leukoreduction is performed to remove immunoglobulins, platelets, and bacterial antigens from donated whole blood.
    C. One bag of cryoprecipitate comprises a typical adult dose.
    D. Repeated whole blood donation can occur as frequently as once a month in the United States.
    E. Cryoprecipitate is a fibrinogen-enhanced precipitate made from thawed FFP that has undergone centrifugation.

14. Which of the following statements regarding compatibility testing is TRUE?

    A. Routine RBC compatibility testing includes only ABO and RhD typing.
    B. 20% of all patients carry some form of ABO antibodies.
    C. Rh-negative patients given Rh-positive blood always have hemolytic reactions.
    D. Incompatible ABO transfusions result in intravascular hemolysis.
    E. RBC compatibility testing takes 20 minutes.

15. Which of the following statements regarding citrate intoxication is TRUE?

    A. It occurs with multiple transfusions of packed red blood cells (RBCs) over long periods of time.
    B. It may result in electrocardiographic (ECG) changes.
    C. It may result in hypertension secondary to increased systemic vascular resistance.
    D. The citrate causes a temporary increase of ionized calcium levels.
    E. Citrate is metabolized by the kidney.

16. Immediate-type hemolytic transfusion reactions:

    A. May result from incompatibility in the Kell, Kidd, Lewis, or Duffy systems.
    B. Are a rare cause of transfusion-related mortality.
    C. Are immune mediated and occur more commonly with antibodies that directly cause cellular lysis.
    D. Cannot be confirmed via laboratory assays.
    E. Are caused by RBC transfusion and cannot be initiated with transfusion of plasma.

17. Delayed hemolytic transfusion reactions:

    A. Present 3 to 10 days after an apparently compatible transfusion.
    B. Can be confirmed by an indirect Coombs' test.
    C. Does not require previous exposure.
    D. Generally result in hemolysis and have the same symptoms as immediate hemolytic transfusion reactions.
    E. Usually require extensive hemodynamic support.

18. Transfusion reactions resulting from white blood cell antigens:

    A. Are immediate and life threatening.
    B. Risk likelihood is the same regardless of the number of transfusions.
    C. May produce transfusion-related acute lung injury as a consequence of cardiogenic pulmonary edema.
    D. Rarely result in fever.
    E. Have decreased incidence since the introduction of leukoreduction and single-donor apheresis platelets.

19. Which of the following statements regarding platelet transfusion is FALSE?

    A. Prophylactic platelet transfusion should be performed prior to major surgery or invasive procedure if platelet levels are <50,000/µL.
    B. If bleeding is out of proportion to the level of thrombocytopenia and platelet levels are normal, further transfusion of platelets should not be performed.
    C. The transfusion threshold should be based on the possibility of additional causes.
    D. The average dose of platelets is one concentrate from apheresis donation or pools of 5 to 8 concentrates from whole blood.
    E. Patients about to undergo eye or central nervous system surgery should have a starting platelet count >100,000/µL.

20. Which of the following statements regarding antithrombin III (ATIII) is CORRECT?

    A. It is inactivated by heparin.
    B. It is an enzymatic complex that results in the cleaving of thrombin, VIIIa, and Va.
    C. In the presence of heparin, it can bind activated factors IX, X, and XII to accelerate anticoagulation.
    D. It is a major player in the fibrinolytic pathway by inducing the proteases in the clotting cascade.
    E. It is nonfunctional without the heparin cofactor.

21. Which of the following statements regarding fibrinolysis is TRUE?

    A. Tissue plasminogen activator (t-PA) is produced by vascular endothelial cells.
    B. The primary fibrinolytic enzyme is t-PA.
    C. Plasminogen activation occurs through a singular pathway where factors IXa, XIIa, and kallikrein activate t-PA which in turn activates the creation of plasmin t-PA.
    D. Fibrin degradation products are produced by the action of t-PA on plasminogen.
    E. Platelets have no role in inhibiting fibrinolysis.

22. Which of the following statements regarding the laboratory evaluation of coagulation is TRUE?

    A. The prothrombin time (PT) tests the extrinsic pathway of coagulation by adding tissue factors to whole blood.
    B. The thrombin time is prolonged by low amounts of any of the factors that prolong the PT.
    C. Patients with an elevated PT or PTT and an abnormal mixing study suggest a severe factor deficiency.
    D. The reptilase test uses snake venoms to confirm abnormal INR numbers.
    E. Blood temperature does not affect the PT or PTT.

23. Which of the following statements regarding von Willebrand disease is TRUE?

    A. It is a rare hereditary bleeding disorder.
    B. The activated partial thromboplastin time (aPTT) is commonly prolonged because of the diminished half-life of factor VIII in von Willebrand disease.
    C. Desmopressin (DDAVP) helps patients with all types of von Willebrand disease to some extent.
    D. Patients frequently are unaware that they have von Willebrand disease.
    E. von Willebrand factor is a small protein that circulates with factor VI.

24. Which of the following statements regarding hemophilia is TRUE?

    A. Hemophilia A is caused by a deficiency of factor IX activity.
    B. Hemophilia B is an autosomal recessive disorder that occurs almost exclusively in Ashkenazi Jews.
    C. Christmas disease is an inherited disorder following an autosomal dominant pattern.
    D. Patients with hemophilia A usually have an abnormal prothrombin time (PT) and bleeding time (BT).
    E. Hemophilia A may be treated with desmopressin (DDAVP).

25. Which of the following statements regarding disseminated intravascular coagulation (DIC) is FALSE?

    A. DIC is a disorder of plasminogen causing excessive activation of fibrinolysis.
    B. It is triggered by the appearance of excessive procoagulant material (tissue factor or equivalent) in the circulation.
    C. Prothrombin time (PT) and activated partial thromboplastin time (aPTT) may remain normal.
    D. Activated protein C should be considered in any sustained episode of DIC.
    E. Heparin has been advocated in situations in which thrombosis is clinically problematic.

26. Which of the following statements regarding low–molecular-weight heparins (LMWHs) is TRUE?

    A. Protamine successfully neutralizes LMWH.
    B. They are associated with a lower incidence of heparin-induced thrombocytopenia.
    C. Their half-life is the same as standard heparin.
    D. They cause more platelet inhibition than standard heparin.
    E. They cause PTT and PT prolongation.

27. Which of the following statements regarding thromboelastography is FALSE?

    A. It measures the rate and strength of clot formation as well as fibrinolysis.
    B. Increasing resistance to sensor oscillation creates a graphic depiction of clot formation.
    C. Can be used to help differentiate between which appropriate patient therapy is needed.
    D. The patterns produced are capable of implicating abnormal fibrinolysis.
    E. Testing cannot be performed in heparin anticoagulated patients.

ANSWERS

1. **B.** Anemia causes the oxygen dissociation curve for oxyhemoglobin to shift to the right secondary to increased levels of 2,3-diphosphoglycerate (DPG) and acidemia. This adaptive process is particularly influential for the physiologic compensation of chronic anemia and often the only mechanism necessary to maintain oxygen delivery via INCREASED tissue oxygen extraction. There are several compensatory mechanisms for anemia; most notably: (1) Increased cardiac output; (2) altered microcirculatory blood flow; and (3) improved tissue oxygen extraction from hemoglobin. Heart rate increases secondary to a sympathetic surge and higher stroke volume results from increased preload and decreased systemic vascular resistance and afterload. The decrease in blood viscosity associated with isovolemic hemodilution and chronic anemia improves blood flow especially through the microcirculation where lower shear force rates cause a pronounced vasodilation of capillary beds. (See page 419: Physiologic Compensation for Anemia.)

2. **E.** Cytomegalovirus (CMV) is the most common transfusion transmitted disease with an incidence of 1% to 3%. In immune competent recipients, the infection is often asymptomatic or mild and self-limited. However in immunocompromised patients (e.g., neonates, patients with HIV, and transplant recipients), the disease can be associated with severe multiorgan failure involving the liver, lungs, kidneys, hematologic, gastrointestinal tract, and central nervous system. The CMV is carried by white blood cells and transmitted via CMV-seropositive cellular components. Leukoreduction drastically decreases the infectivity of CMV-positive donor products, but has not completely eradicated the transfusion transmission of CMV. The rate of viral infectivity has decreased dramatically in the past 2 decades. In particular, the advent of universal (in the United States) nucleic acid testing (NAT) for HIV and the hepatitis C virus (HCV) has reduced the frequency of transmission of those agents to very low levels (one in 2 million). (See page 423: Infectious Risks of Blood Product Administration.)

3. **C.** Noninfectious risks associated with transfusion include hypothermia, dilutional coagulopathy, hyperkalemia, and microaggregate delivery. Several studies including a recent prospective randomized trial found mild hypothermia to be associated with increased blood loss, postoperative infections, cardiopulmonary morbidities, and longer hospitalization. Administration of large volumes of fluid deficient in platelets and clotting factors results in coagulopathy as a consequence of dilution. Hazard exists if large volumes of stored blood are administered rapidly. Although there is only 20 to 60 mL of plasma in a unit of packed red blood cells, contemporary infusion devices allow blood to be transfused at rates of 500 to 1,000 mL/min. The metabolic derangements that occur as a consequence of transfusion are usually not evident unless patients received a large volume transfusion or rapid infusion rates; but these often include hyperkalemia, citrate toxicity, and hypothermia. As storage time for blood products increases, the cellular components leak potassium and metabolize glucose into lactate which can result in hyperkalemia and/or acidemia in the recipient especially with rapid transfusion. During storage, blood products collect microaggregates of cellular debris, platelets, fibrin composition, and even erythrocytes and WBCs. (See page 428: Nonimmune-mediated Transfusion Reactions.)

4. **D.** The plasma half-life of most clotting factors is around 1.5 to 3 days, but those of the initiating factor VII (6 hours) and the cofactors V and VIII (8–12 hours) are much shorter. Clotting factors in the plasma are activated at sites of endothelial injury and assemble in enzymatic complexes to activate thrombin. All of these clotting factors are primarily produced in the liver, except for VIII, which also is released by endothelial cells and is well maintained in liver disease. Four critical enzyme factors—VII in the extrinsic tenase, IX in the intrinsic tenase, X in the prothrombinase, and prothrombin (II)—must be carboxylated at multiple glutamic-acid residues after translation, in order to interact with phospholipid and Ca^{++}. Vitamin K in its reduced form is the cofactor for the glutamyl–carboxylase enzyme, and thus these factors are vitamin K dependent. (See page 411: Secondary Hemostasis.)

5. **B.** Factor X is not contained in cryoprecipitate. Cryoprecipitate contains factor VIII, vWF, fibrinogen, fibronectin, and factor XIII. (See page 419: Blood Products and Transfusion Thresholds: Cryoprecipitate.)

6. **B.** Most of the coagulation proteins are synthesized by the liver. Four of the clotting factors (II, VII, IX, and X) require vitamin K for proper synthesis. (See page 409: Hemostasis and Coagulation: Secondary Hemostasis.)

7. **A.** Patients' status postsplenectomy are not commonly thrombocytopenic. Qualitative dysfunction is often associated with systemic diseases such as uremia, liver failure, and disseminated intravascular coagulopathy. It also occurs after cardiopulmonary bypass, extracorporeal circulation such as dialysis or plasmapheresis, and as a result of medication side effects. Medications that decrease platelets include NSAIDS, β-lactam antibiotics, antidepressants, GPII/IIa antagonists, phenothiazines, fish oil, garlic, and ginkgo biloba. (See page 419: Blood Products and Transfusion Thresholds: Platelets and Table 16.5: Causes of Acquired Platelet Dysfunction.)

8. **D.** A recent meta-analysis reported that acute normovolemic hemodilution does not achieve complete avoidance of allogeneic blood but that when transfusion is necessary, the amount transfused is reduced by 1 to 2 U per patient. Preoperative autologous blood donation eliminates the risk of viral infection and alloimmunization; however, it still requires blood collection and storage, which carry risks of clerical error, cardiovascular overload, bacterial infection, and transfusion-related immunomodulation.

Erythropoietin, a recombinant product, is often accepted by Jehovah's Witnesses, and its efficacy in that patient population has been demonstrated. Severe aortic stenosis, significant coronary disease or myocardial dysfunction, and low initial hematocrit and blood volume (body weight <110 lb) are relative contraindications to preoperative autologous donation. If the patient's hemoglobin level, cardiac status, and general condition permit, up to 4 U of blood can be donated at weekly intervals before surgery. (See page 429: Blood Conservation Strategies: Autologous Donations.)

9. **E.** Ultimately, the decision to transfuse RBCs should be made based on the clinical judgment that the oxygen-carrying capacity of the blood must be increased to prevent oxygen consumption from outstripping oxygen delivery. Conditions that may decrease the tolerance for anemia and influence the RBC transfusion threshold include factors that increase oxygen demand, limit the ability to increase cardiac output, cause a left shift of the oxyhemoglobin dissociation curve, and impair oxygenation to tissues. Clinical indications of tissue hypoxia include (but not limited to) tachycardia, hypotension, mixed venous O_2 saturations <50%, lactic acidosis, EKG or echocardiographic indications of myocardial infarction, and oliguria <0.5 cc/kg/hr over 6 hours. Evidence indicates that a hemoglobin level less than 9 g/dL is independently predictive of poor outcome especially in patient with cerebrovascular injury. (See page 419: Red Blood Cells and page 420: Table 16.3: Clinical Indications of Tissue Hypoxia.)

10. **A.** Contemporary "intraoperative blood salvage" devices return blood with a hematocrit of 60% to 70%. These devices anticoagulate the salvaged blood with heparin as it leaves the surgical field or postoperative drain. Suctioned blood is then collected in a reservoir, filtered to remove large debris, and centrifuged resulting in red cell concentrates. The final step of washing clears the product of residual contaminants such as plasma, platelets, free hemoglobin, cellular fragments, WBCs, and the remaining heparin or citrate. The resultant red cells are resuspended in saline and ready for reinfusion. The RBCs may be stored at 4°C for up to 6 hours with careful patient and product identification. (See page 429: Blood Conservation Strategies: Perioperative Blood Salvage.)

11. **D.** There are few randomized control trials showing improved clinical outcomes and no trials that report definitive mortality benefits of recombinant activated factor seven (rFVIIa). In fact, a recent meta-analysis published by Levi et al. demonstrated an increased risk of arterial thromboembolism especially in elderly patients receiving high doses of rFVIIa. rFVIIa was originally FDA approved for prophylaxis and treatment of patients with hemophilia A or B complicated by inhibitors to factor VIII and IX concentrates. It is now also indicated for the treatment of acquired hemophilia and factor VII deficiency. However, the majority of its use is "off-label" for the prevention and treatment of coagulopathy and major blood loss in patients with postpartum hemorrhage, trauma, reversal of various anticoagulants, and high-risk cardiothoracic, spinal, transplant, or vascular surgery. The hemostatic mechanism for rFVIIa remains unclear but likely involves more than the

physiologic role of factor VII in secondary hemostasis. The clinical dosing of rFVIIa typically exceeds normal concentrations by 1,000 fold; at these doses, rFVIIa directly activates factor X and platelets generating a thrombin burst for procoagulant activity. (See page 440: Recombinant Activated Factor Seven.)

12. **C.** Recent recommendations for intraoperative transfusion during massive bleeding focus on the patients with class II hemorrhage (blood loss of 15%–30% estimated blood volume) with pre-existing anemia or cardiovascular disease, and all patients with class III to IV hemorrhagic shock (blood loss of 30%–40% estimated blood volume). Patients undergoing massive transfusion for hemorrhage with estimated blood loss of more than two blood volumes and ongoing bleeding should have a platelet transfusion threshold of at least 75,000/μL to ensure the level does not fall below 50,000/μL. Massive transfusion patient populations are among the highest risk for Transfusion-related acute lung injury (TRALI). Citrate is a common anticoagulant used in stored blood products, and is generally metabolized by the liver and quickly eliminated. However, with rapid infusion rates, massive transfusion, or in patients with liver dysfunction, citrate accumulates in the plasma and chelates calcium resulting in hypocalcemia. Severe hypocalcemia leads to muscle weakness, tetany, arrhythmias, myocardial dysfunction, and acquired coagulopathy. Hypothermia is commonly associated with massive transfusion and can result in platelet and coagulation factor dysfunction. (See page 419: Physiologic Compensation for Anemia and page 428: Metabolic Derangements.)

13. **E.** Platelet storage is limited 5 days by FDA mandate because of the time-related risk of bacterial growth. Platelets must be stored at room temperature to preserve clotting function, but this increases the risk of bacterial growth in contaminated units, compared to other blood components. Accordingly, bacterial detection has become routine testing in many countries. Cryoprecipitate is made from barely thawed FFP, which has a precipitate enriched in fibrinogen; the precipitate is isolated by centrifugation and refrozen. Five bags of cryoprecipitate comprise a typical adult dose. In the United States, donors are deferred for 8 weeks after a whole-blood donation to avoid iron deficiency. (See page 421: Platelets and Table 16.1: Blood Components.)

14. **D.** Routine RBC compatibility testing includes ABO and RhD typing, an antibody screen for IgG non-ABO RBC antibodies, and an RBC crossmatch. RBCs must be ABO-compatible to avoid intravascular hemolysis, and Rh D-negative patients should receive D-negative RBCs to avoid anti-D alloimmunization. If hemolytic antibodies are detected on crossmatch, RBC units negative for the incompatible antigen(s) must be found, and a serologic crossmatch of patient plasma versus donor RBCs is performed to confirm compatibility. One percent of all patients and 5% to 20% of heavily transfused patients have ABO antibodies. RBC compatibility testing takes 45 to 60 minutes, and much longer if antibodies are found. (See page 419: Compatibility Testing.)

15. **B.** Citrate is a common anticoagulant used in stored blood products and is generally metabolized by the liver

and quickly eliminated. However with rapid infusion rates, massive transfusion, or in patients with liver dysfunction, citrate accumulates in the plasma and chelates calcium resulting in hypocalcemia. Severe hypocalcemia leads to muscle weakness, tetany, arrhythmias, myocardial dysfunction, and acquired coagulopathy. (See page 428: Metabolic Derangements.)

16. **A.** Acute Hemolytic Transfusion Reactions (AHTRs) remain one of the leading causes of transfusion-related mortality. They occur with the transfusion of incompatible blood products when antibodies in recipient plasma complex with donor cellular antigens causing complement activation and subsequent hemolysis. AHTRs classically result from ABO incompatibility secondary to native anti-A or anti-B antibodies; however, growing evidence exists for the implication of other red blood cell antigens such as Kidd, Kell, and Duffy causing acute hemolytic reactions in patients with a history of transfusion exposure and alloimmunization. Rarely, the transfusion of incompatible plasma (type O FFP to a patient with type A, B, or AB blood) has resulted in AHTRs as well. The diagnosis of hemolytic reactions is confirmed with laboratory analysis of free hemoglobin levels, low haptoglobin, bilirubin increases, direct antiglobulin (Coombs) test, and evidence of hematuria. (See page 426: Acute Hemolytic Transfusion Reactions.)

17. **A.** Delayed Hemolytic Transfusion Reactions (DHTRs) result from alloantibodies to minor RBC antigens in the Rh, Kell, Kidd, Duffy, MNSs, and other blood groups. They generally present 3 to 10 days after transfusion of an apparent "compatible" blood component. Typically the recipient has IgG alloantibodies to a particular RBC antigen and will mount an anamnestic immune response. Symptoms are much milder than AHTRs and rarely result in major morbidity or mortality because the hemolysis occurs extravascularly in the liver and spleen. Patients experience mild fever, and possible rash with laboratory and clinical signs of hemolysis such as jaundice, hematuria, low haptoglobin, positive direct Coombs test, and decreasing hemoglobin levels. Symptoms are generally self-limited and treated supportively with hydration to protect the renal tubules during hemolysis and further compatible transfusions to support anemia as indicated. (See page 426: Delayed Hemolytic Transfusion Reactions.)

18. **E.** Allergic and febrile reactions are the most common types of complications of transfused blood products; however, the incidence of both has decreased with the prominence of leukoreduction and single-donor apheresis platelet units. Febrile nonhemolytic transfusion reactions (FNHTRs) classically present within 4 hours of transfusion with an increase in temperature of 1°C and may be associated with chills, rigors, anxiety, and headache. They are often self-limited but can be prevented or treated with anti-inflammatory or antipyretic medication. The pathophysiology of FNHTRs involves recipient alloimmunization to human leukocyte antigens (HLAs) from donor white blood cells and the release of leukocyte-derived cytokines during product storage. Subsequently the risk of febrile reactions increases with repetitive transfusions. (See page 417: Component Processing and Storage.)

19. **B.** The indications for platelet transfusion depend on both quantitative and qualitative measures of platelet activity as well as the clinical setting. For stable patients with severe thrombocytopenia, transfusion can be held until counts fall below 10,000 to 20,000/μL as long as they have no signs or symptoms of bleeding. Prophylactic platelet transfusion is necessary for patient with severe thrombocytopenia <50,000/μL about to undergo major surgery or an invasive procedure such as lumbar puncture, liver biopsy, neuraxial anesthesia, central venous catheterization, or endoscopy with biopsy. In preparation for surgery on the eye or the central nervous system, the platelet count should be raised to >100,000/μL. Qualitative dysfunction is often associated with systemic diseases (i.e., uremia, liver failure, and disseminated intravascular coagulopathy), after cardiopulmonary bypass, dialysis, or as a result of medication side effects. Regardless of the platelet count, if bleeding is out of proportion to the level of thrombocytopenia, qualitative deficiency should be suspected and treated. The average dose of platelets is one concentrate from apheresis donation or pools of 5 to 8 concentrates from whole blood or buffy coat collections. (See page 421: Platelets.)

20. **C.** Antithrombin III (ATIII) is a circulating serine protease inhibitor that binds to thrombin and thereby inactivates it. It can bind and inactivate each of the activated clotting factors of the classical "intrinsic" coagulation cascade—factors XIIa, XIa, IXa, and Xa AT-III inhibits proteases in all clotting pathways. Its inhibitory function is greatly increased when bound to heparin. Protein C-ase is an enzymatic complex with the same structure as the coagulation complexes that thrombin cleaves and activates protein C. Activated protein C brakes clotting by cleaving VIIIa and Va, the cofactors for the external tenase and the prothrombinase complexes. (See page 412: Inhibition of Clotting Factors.)

21. **A.** The major activator of plasminogen in the blood is tissue plasminogen activator (t-PA), which is secreted from endothelial cells. Fibrin clots must be broken down after their job is done. In the end, plasminogen is activated to plasmin, which breaks down fibrin polymers (Fig. 16-4). Plasminogen activation has a minor and a major pathway. In the minor pathway, IXa, XIIa, and kallikrein can each activate plasminogen. Plasminogen activation inhibitor-1 (PAI-1) is a serpin, which binds to t-PA and urokinase and accelerates their clearance from plasma. Activated platelets release PAI-1 from α-granules. (See page 412: Fibrinolysis.)

22. **A.** A general overview of plasma clotting factor activity is obtained by the *prothrombin time (PT)* for the intrinsic (tissue) pathway and the *activated partial thromboplastin time (aPTT)* for the extrinsic (contact) pathway. These clotting tests are performed in blood specimens collected in a chelator (3.2% citrate), which binds Ca^{++} to prevent clotting in the tube. The in vitro clotting test is activated by tissue factor in the PT or negatively charged surfaces in the aPTT, using phospholipid as a platform (substituting for platelets). Ca^{++} is then added to overcome the specimen chelation, and the time is measured until complete fibrin clotting is observed. Testing is routinely performed at 37°C, but hypothermia in the patient impairs the enzymatic reactions of clot formation. Clotting physiology is

more complicated than the traditional diagrams of separate cascade pathways for these two tests. Fibrinogen activity is also a critical parameter. Most assays measure the functional conversion of fibrinogen to fibrin, although the fibrinogen protein level also can be measured for comparison to assess fibrinogen dysfunction. To investigate unexpectedly elevated PT or aPTT values, the test should be repeated after mixing the patient's plasma with equal volumes of normal plasma. Even in severe factor deficiencies, the PT or aPTT show substantial correction toward normal in a mixing study. However, if the patient's plasma contains an inhibitor or an anticoagulant, the normal plasma will also be affected and the PT or aPTT will not correct. (See page 413: Laboratory Evaluation of Secondary Hemostasis and Coagulation.)

23. **D.**   von Willebrand disease (vWD) is the most common hereditary bleeding disorder with a prevalence of approximately 1% in the general population. Most types of vWD result from decreased levels or deficient function in primary hemostasis; they present with mucocutaneous bleeding such as epistaxis, menorrhagia, and prolonged bleeding from minor wounds and dental extractions. Frequently patients are not aware of the disorder until they undergo a bleeding questionnaire in anticipation of major surgery. von Willebrand Factor (vWF) serves a central role in hemostasis by facilitating the interaction of platelets with collagen within the subendothelium and platelet-platelet interactions. It also circulates as a complex with factor VIII providing stability to the otherwise labile clotting factor. Traditional coagulation profile tests such as PT and aPTT are often normal in patients with vWD. DDAVP promotes the cleavage of vWF from FVIII and increases the availability of both. This is beneficial for most patients with type I deficiency and some type 2 subclassifications of vWD. DDAVP is not therapeutic by itself in patients with type 3 and severely depressed levels of vWF. Often these patients require treatment with additional hemostatic medications such as antifibrinolytics and/or factor replacement with plasma-derived vWF/FVIII concentrates. (See page 413: Laboratory Evaluation of Hemostasis.)

24. **E.**   Hemophilia A accounts for about 85% of the disease and stems from deficiencies of factor VIII (FVIII). Hemophilia B or the Christmas disease occurs in 14% of hemophiliacs and involves a defect in the production of factor IX. Both hemophilia A and B are X-linked recessive disorders and found almost exclusively in male patients. Factor XI deficiency is most often seen in persons of Ashkenazi Jewish descent. Hemophilia C is very rare, occurring in only 1% of all hemophiliacs; it results from genetic mutations in factor XI and is the only form that has an autosomal recessive inheritance pattern. Confirmatory laboratory in Hemophilia A includes prolonged aPTT, low factor activity levels, and normal PT and bleeding times. Treatment for all hemophilia patients involves replacement of coagulation factor deficiencies which can be accomplished with plasma transfusion or factor concentrates. Patients with mild hemophilia A and hemophilia C often benefit from treatment with DDAVP which effectively raises the circulating availability of FVIII by increasing dissociation from vWF. (See page 433: The Hemophilias.)

25. **A.**   DIC is a disorder characterized by systemic activation of coagulation that results in an imbalance of hemostasis and is always associated with a comorbid condition such as infection, inflammation, or malignancy. DIC causes diffuse thrombosis that may lead to multiorgan system failure, or consumptive coagulopathy and bleeding. The pathophysiology of DIC depends on the causative condition, but primarily involves uncontrolled activation for thrombin generation with simultaneous inhibition of fibrinolysis. Thrombin generation in DIC is initiated by tissue factor and activated factor VII in the extrinsic pathway for coagulation. The exposure of tissue factor is facilitated by extensive vascular injury, expression on neoplastic cells, or the release of proinflammatory cytokines. The compilation of prolonged PT and aPTT, thrombocytopenia, hypofibrinogenemia, and increasing fibrin degradation products in a patient with an associated condition leads to the clinical diagnosis of DIC. The management for DIC primarily involves treatment of the causative condition and supportive measures to control progressive thrombosis and control any signs of hemorrhage. Studies of patients with DIC in sepsis proved the efficacy of heparin to halt thrombin generation, improve the coagulation profile, and reduce the risk of thrombosis. (See page 413: Laboratory Evaluation of Secondary Hemostasis and Coagulation.)

26. **B.**   Low–molecular-weight heparin (LMWH) does not affect the PT and coagulation testing is usually not needed. However, if necessary, the drugs' plasma activity levels can be assessed by the aFXa assay. Like heparin, these agents inhibit factor Xa indirectly, that is, via their enhancing effect on antithrombin. Any form of heparin therapy can initiate HIT; however, UFH is more likely than LMWH to lead to immune complexes because the fractionated form is less antigenic, protamine neutralization of LMWH is reported to be incomplete. The half-life is longer than that of standard heparin, allowing for once-per-day dosing. (See page 416: Heparin Anticoagulation Testing.)

27. **E.**   Whole-blood clotting and fibrinolysis can be assessed by viscoelastic testing in thromboelastography or rotation thromboelastometry. These tests measure the rate, strength, and lysis if any, of clot formation. Thromboelastography involves the use of whole blood in a heated cup with the addition of a sensor pin. The cup or the pin oscillates while the blood clots. The increasing resistance to oscillation is transmitted through the sensor pin and a graphic depiction of clot formation is displayed in the thromboelastogram. The patterns obtained can implicate defects in factor levels, platelet function, fibrinogen concentration, and the presence of abnormal fibrinolysis (which is difficult to measure rapidly otherwise). Testing can be performed in the presence of inhibitors of heparin or fibrinolysis to help judge whether these drugs would be effective. Thromboelastography is helpful in determining the appropriate therapy, including platelets, plasma, fibrinogen replacement or antifibrinolytics, as complex bleeding syndromes such as massive hemorrhage with consumptive or dilutional coagulopathy progress. (See page 414: The Thromboelastography.)

CHAPTER 17

Inhaled Anesthetics

1. Each of the following groups contains a list of factors which decrease MAC, EXCEPT:

   A. Hypothermia, induced hypotension, and hyponatremia
   B. Metabolic acidosis, pregnancy, and lithium
   C. Increasing age, opioids, and α_2 agonists
   D. Acute ethanol administration, hypernatremia, and hypothyroidism
   E. Anemia, hypoxia, and ketamine

2. Which of the following statements about minimum alveolar concentration (MAC) is FALSE?

   A. MAC-awake is approximately 0.15 to 0.5 MAC.
   B. Based on their MAC values, sevoflurane is less potent than isoflurane.
   C. Patients tend not to lose self-awareness and recall until >0.8 MAC.
   D. Metabolic alkalosis and hyperkalemia have no effect on MAC.
   E. MAC-BAR is approximately 1.5 times the standard MAC value.

3. Which of the following best relates the relative degree to which inhalational anesthetics decrease cerebral metabolic rate?

   A. Sevoflurane = halothane < isoflurane
   B. Isoflurane < halothane < sevoflurane
   C. Sevoflurane < isoflurane < halothane
   D. Isoflurane = sevoflurane > halothane
   E. Halothane < isoflurane = sevoflurane

4. Which of the following statements regarding the central nervous system (CNS) effects of inhalational agents is FALSE?

   A. All potent inhalational agents depress the cerebral metabolic rate (CMR) while increasing cerebral blood flow.
   B. Desflurane and sevoflurane cause a similar decrease in CMR.
   C. After an isoelectric electroencephalogram (EEG) is achieved, a further increase in isoflurane concentration will cause no further decreases in the cerebral metabolic rate of oxygen consumption ($CMRO_2$).
   D. Isoflurane abolishes EEG activity at clinically used doses that are usually hemodynamically tolerable.
   E. Regarding increase in latency and decrease in amplitude, brainstem auditory evoked potentials are more sensitive to volatile anesthetics than motor evoked potentials are.

5. True statements regarding inhalational agents include all of the following EXCEPT:

   A. For less-soluble anesthetics, the rate of rise in alveolar anesthetic concentration (F_A) to inspired anesthetic concentration (F_I) over time (F_A/F_I) is not significantly affected by minute ventilation.
   B. The two major components of the second gas effect are the concentration effect and decreased solubility.
   C. The rate of rise in alveolar anesthetic concentration (F_A) to inspired anesthetic concentration (F_I) over time (F_A/F_I) for more-soluble anesthetics can be augmented by increasing minute ventilation.
   D. During emergence, washout of high concentrations of nitrous oxide can lower alveolar concentrations of O_2 and CO_2.
   E. The rate of alveolar concentration approaching the inspired concentration is inversely related to the solubility of the agent in blood.

6. True statements regarding the effects of anesthetics on the chemical control of breathing include all of the following EXCEPT:

   A. Subanesthetic concentrations of potent inhalational agents depress the hypoxic response in humans.
   B. The ventilatory response to CO_2 is depressed by all inhalational agents.
   C. With an inhalational agent at 2 MAC in a spontaneously breathing patient, the apneic threshold is generally 5 mm Hg below the resting $PaCO_2$.
   D. Residual effects of inhalation agents may impair the ventilatory drive of patients in the recovery room.
   E. Nitrous oxide decreases $PaCO_2$ during spontaneous breathing.

7. True statements concerning the hemodynamic effects of inhalational agents include all of the following EXCEPT:

   A. Forty percent nitrous oxide increases sympathetic nervous system activity and systemic vascular resistance.
   B. During rapid increases in inspired concentration, sevoflurane and isoflurane cause similar increases in heart rate from baseline.
   C. All volatile anesthetics prolong QTc interval.
   D. All volatile anesthetics slow the sinoatrial node discharge rate, as well as prolong conduction through the His–Purkinje system and ventricular conduction pathways.
   E. Reflex tachycardia from rapid increases in inspired concentration of desflurane result from stimulation of airway receptors.

8. Which of the following statements regarding metabolism of inhaled agents is FALSE?

   A. The production of compound A is enhanced during low-flow anesthesia.
   B. The volatile anesthetic which causes the most carbon monoxide production when degraded in carbon dioxide absorbents is desflurane.
   C. Compound A production is increased by warm or very dry CO_2 absorbents.
   D. There has not been a single case report of renal injury in humans from use of sevoflurane in the last 2 decades.
   E. When degraded in carbon dioxide absorbents, sevoflurane produces the most compound A, with desflurane and isoflurane producing much smaller amounts.

9. Which statement is FALSE regarding fluoride-induced nephrotoxicity?

   A. The treatment of choice is vasopressin.
   B. Sevoflurane transiently increases serum fluoride concentration.
   C. Fluoride-induced nephrotoxicity presents as high-output renal insufficiency.
   D. Nephrotoxicity is related to duration of high fluoride levels as well as the peak fluoride concentration.
   E. Faster washout may contribute to the improved safety of sevoflurane regarding fluoride concentrations compared with enflurane.

10. The FALSE statement about use of inhalational agents is:

    A. Exposure limits set by the National Institute for Occupational Safety and Health (NIOSH) are 25 ppm for nitrous oxide and 10 ppm for volatile anesthetics.
    B. Nitrous oxide decreases activity of methionine synthetase and thymidylate synthetase.
    C. Xenon and nitrous oxide are considered safe in patients susceptible to malignant hyperthermia.
    D. A brief, high concentration of volatile anesthetic may be helpful in the removal of a retained placenta.
    E. Except for nitrous oxide, inhaled anesthetics potentiate the action of neuromuscular blocking agents.

11. Each of the following statements regarding the effects of inhaled anesthetics are true EXCEPT:

    A. Seventy-five percent nitrous oxide can double the size of a pneumothorax in 10 minutes.
    B. Sevoflurane provides a stable heart rate.
    C. Desflurane slows sinoatrial (SA) node discharge.
    D. Isoflurane is associated with an increase in heart rate.
    E. Xenon does not trigger malignant hyperthermia and does not have intrinsic analgesic properties.

12. Each statement regarding inhaled anesthetics is true EXCEPT:

    A. The partial pressure of a gas in a closed container is proportional to its fractional mass.
    B. A less-soluble agent has a faster rate of rise in the ratio of alveolar anesthetic concentration (F_A) to inspired anesthetic concentration (F_I) over time (F_A/F_I).
    C. Dalton's law states that the sum of the partial pressures of each gas in a mixture of gases equals the total pressure of the entire mixture.
    D. The concentration of an inhaled anesthetic in solution depends not only on its solubility in blood, but also on the partial pressure in the gas phase at equilibrium with blood.
    E. Boiling point is the temperature at which a liquid's vapor pressure equals atmospheric pressure in an open container.

ANSWERS

1. D. All of the factors listed in the answer choices decrease MAC except for hypothyroidism. Thyroid function, whether hypothyroid or hyperthyroid, does not affect MAC. (See page 459: Table 17-5.)

2. C. MAC-awake is the dose at which 50% of patients respond to the command "open your eyes," and varies from 0.15 to 0.5 MAC. MAC values can be used to compare potency, such that the higher the MAC, the less potent the agent. Sevoflurane has a higher MAC than isoflurane and thus is less potent. Patients tend to lose self-awareness and recall at 0.4 to 0.5 MAC. Metabolic alkalosis and hyperkalemia are among a number of factors which do not affect MAC values, although metabolic acidosis decreases MAC. MAC-BAR is the alveolar concentration required to block the adrenergic response to noxious stimuli in 50% of patients; this value is approximately 1.5 times the standard MAC value. (See page 458: Neuropharmacology of inhaled anesthetics.)

3. D. Each of the potent inhaled anesthetics decreases cerebral metabolic oxygen consumption ($CMRO_2$), with the order of effect from greatest to least being Isoflurane = Sevoflurane = Desflurane > Halothane. (See page 458: Neuropharmacology of inhaled anesthetics.)

4. E. In a phenomenon called "uncoupling," all of the potent volatile agents increase cerebral blood flow in a dose-dependent manner, despite causing decreases in cerebral metabolic rate of oxygen consumption. It has been shown that, after an isoelectric EEG is achieved with isoflurane, further increases in isoflurane's concentration do not lead to further decreases in CMR. Isoflurane abolishes EEG activity at clinically used doses that are usually hemodynamically tolerated. Neuromonitoring tests vary in their sensitivity to volatile anesthetics, which can cause increases in latency and decreases in amplitude. Motor evoked potentials are extremely sensitive to depression by volatile anesthetics, while the effect of volatile anesthetics on brain stem auditory evoked potentials is negligible. (See page 458: Neuropharmacology of inhaled anesthetics.)

5. B. The rate at which the alveolar concentration approaches the inspired concentration is inversely related to the blood solubility of the anesthetic. Administration of high concentrations of one gas (e.g., nitrous oxide) facilitates the increase in alveolar concentration of another gas (e.g., halothane); this phenomenon is called the *second gas effect*. The two components of the second gas effect (increased ventilation [increased tracheal inflow] and the concentration effect) are operative at the alveolar level. Although a second gas effect exists for nearly all combinations of inhaled drugs given simultaneously, it is most pronounced when nitrous oxide is used with a more-soluble drug, such as halothane (the second gas). For more-soluble anesthetics, increasing the minute ventilation increases the rate of increase in F_A/F_I. For inhaled anesthetics with very low tissue solubility, there is an extremely rapid rise in F_A/F_I with induction; this is not significantly affected by increases or decreases in minute ventilation. Emergence from anesthesia is more rapid with low blood or tissue anesthetic solubility, increased ventilation, and replacement of nitrous oxide with nitrogen. During washout of high concentrations of nitrous oxide, alveolar concentrations of O_2 and CO_2 can be lowered. This phenomenon is called diffusion hypoxia. (See page 448: Pharmacokinetic principles.)

6. E. The ventilatory response to CO_2 is depressed more or less proportionately by all anesthetic agents. Apnea results if the anesthetic dose is high enough. If apnea occurs, the apneic threshold is approximately 4 to 5 mm Hg below the $PaCO_2$ maintained during spontaneous breathing, regardless of the type of anesthesia. It should be anticipated that the $PaCO_2$ will be 50 to 55 mm Hg at surgical planes of anesthesia when potent inhaled anesthetics are used. Surgical stimuli decrease this level by 4 to 5 mm Hg at an equivalent level of anesthesia. Nitrous oxide maintains (or may slightly increase) the $PaCO_2$ during spontaneous breathing. Subanesthetic concentrations of halothane, enflurane, and isoflurane depress the hypoxic response in humans. Residual effects of inhalational agents may impair the ventilatory drive of patients in the recovery room. (See page 468: Response to Carbon Dioxide and Hypoxemia.)

7. B. Nitrous oxide has unique cardiovascular effects; it causes an increase in sympathetic nervous system activity and vascular resistance when given in a 40% concentration. In volunteers, sevoflurane up to 1 MAC does not change heart rate, but isoflurane and desflurane cause a 5% to 10% increase in heart rate from baseline, particularly during rapid increases in inspired concentration. All volatile anesthetics can prolong QTc interval and may, in theory, increase the risk for ventricular tachycardia in patients who already have a baseline prolongation in myocardial repolarization. All volatile anesthetics slow the sinoatrial node discharge rate, as well as prolong conduction through the His–Purkinje system and ventricular conduction pathways. Desflurane has a pungency which is thought to activate upper and lower airway receptors, leading to a transient surge of sympathetic outflow characterized by hypertension and tachycardia. (See page 462: The Circulatory System.)

8. E. Sevoflurane is the only volatile anesthetic which is degraded by CO_2 absorbents to produce compound A. Sevoflurane metabolism to compound A is enhanced in low-flow or closed-circuit breathing systems and by warm or very dry CO_2 absorbents. Despite the safety concerns about sevoflurane and compound A from early rat studies, there has not been a single case report of human renal injury directly attributable to sevoflurane use in the last 2 decades. CO_2 absorbents which have been extensively desiccated (i.e., when fresh gas flows have been left on for over 24 hours) degrade sevoflurane, isoflurane, and desflurane into carbon monoxide. Desflurane produces the most carbon monoxide. (See page 471: Anesthetic Degradation by Carbon Dioxide Absorbers.)

9. A. Fluoride-induced nephrotoxicity, which is caused by inorganic fluoride, presents as high-output renal insufficiency that is unresponsive to vasopressin and is characterized by dilute polyuria, dehydration, serum hypernatremia, and hyperosmolality with elevated levels of blood urea nitrogen and creatinine. Sevoflurane undergoes 5% metabolism that transiently increases serum fluoride concentrations. The safety of sevoflurane regarding fluoride concentrations may be caused by a rapid decline in plasma fluoride concentrations because of less availability of the anesthetic for metabolism from a faster washout compared with enflurane. The "fluoride hypothesis" stated that both the duration of the high systemic fluoride concentrations (area under the fluoride–time curve) and the peak fluoride concentration (peaks above 50 μM appear to represent the toxic threshold) were related to nephrotoxicity. (See page 472: Fluoride-induced Nephrotoxicity.)

10. A. The National Institute for Occupational Safety and Health has set exposure limits of 25 ppm for N_2O and 2 ppm for volatile anesthetics. Nitrous oxide decreases the activity of vitamin B_{12}-dependent enzymes, methionine synthetase (MS), and thymidylate synthetase. The mechanism appears to be an irreversible oxidation of the cobalt atom of vitamin B_{12} by N_2O. This has led to concerns about teratogenic effects on a developing embryo/fetus. All of the potent volatile anesthetics are considered triggers for malignant hyperthermia, but xenon and nitrous oxide are considered safe in patients susceptible to malignant hyperthermia. Volatile anesthetic concentrations greater than 1 MAC may cause uterine relaxation and atony. This may be desirable in procedures such as removal of a retained placenta. With the exception of nitrous oxide, volatile anesthetics cause a direct relaxation of skeletal muscle and potentiate the effects of neuromuscular blocking agents. (See page 470: Neuromuscular System and Malignant Hyperthermia, and page 470: Genetic Effects, Obstetric Use, and Effects on Fetal Development.)

11. E. There are several concerns about nitrous oxide's potential side effects. Most of these concerns remain controversial, except for the ability of nitrous oxide to expand air-filled spaces, which appears valid and clinically relevant. Nitrous oxide will diffuse from the bloodstream into these closed gas spaces. Nitrogen in these air-filled spaces is less soluble in blood compared to nitrous oxide, and will not be readily removed via the bloodstream. Therefore, compliant spaces will continue to expand until enough pressure opposes further entry of nitrous oxide. Seventy-five percent nitrous oxide can double the size of a pneumothorax in 10 minutes, and triple the size in 30 minutes. Sevoflurane provides a stable heart rate. Desflurane, sevoflurane, and isoflurane are known to maintain cardiac output. Enflurane and isoflurane are associated with an increase in heart rate of 10% to 20% at 1 MAC. The SA node discharge rate is slowed by the volatile anesthetics. Xenon occurs naturally in air, has a MAC of 71%, does not trigger malignant hyperthermia, and provides some degree of analgesia. (See page 462: The Circulatory System.)

12. E. Within a mixture of gases in a closed container, each gas exerts a *partial pressure*: A pressure proportional to its fractional mass. Dalton's law states that the sum of each gas's partial pressure equals the total pressure of the entire mixture. Furthermore, the concentration of a gas in a mixture of gases in solution depends upon two factors: Its *partial pressure* in the gas phase during equilibrium with the solution, and its *solubility* within that solution. The most important factor in rate of rise of FA/FI is uptake of anesthetic from the alveoli into the bloodstream. Uptake is proportional to tissue solubility. Therefore, the less soluble an anesthetic (i.e., desflurane), the less uptake occurs, and the faster it reaches equilibrium with the CNS. The boiling point of a liquid, such as an anesthetic gas, is the temperature at which its vapor pressure *exceeds* atmospheric pressure in an open container. Thus, desflurane would boil at typical room temperatures if exposed to air because its boiling point is 23.5°C. (See page 448: Pharmacokinetic Principles.)

Intravenous Anesthetics

1. The rapid onset of central nervous system (CNS) effects of most intravenous (IV) anesthetics is best explained by their:

    A. Low hepatic extraction ratio
    B. Small volume of distribution
    C. High lipid solubility
    D. Large ratio of ionized to unionized drug
    E. Slow elimination half-life

2. Ketamine interacts with all of the following receptors EXCEPT:

    A. *N*-Methyl-D-aspartate (NMDA)
    B. Opioid receptors
    C. γ-Aminobutyric acid (GABA)
    D. Muscarinic receptors
    E. Monoaminergic receptors

3. Which of the following intravenous anesthetic agents has the highest degree of plasma protein binding?

    A. Thiopental
    B. Propofol
    C. Ketamine
    D. Methohexital
    E. Etomidate

4. Which of the following has the lowest hepatic extraction ratio?

    A. Ketamine
    B. Propofol
    C. Thiopental
    D. Midazolam
    E. Etomidate

5. Recovery of cognitive function after general anesthesia is slowest when which of the following agents is used for induction?

    A. Thiopental
    B. Propofol
    C. Midazolam
    D. Etomidate
    E. Ketamine

6. Concerning the antiemetic effect of propofol, all of the following hypotheses have been postulated EXCEPT:

    A. It has antidopaminergic activity.
    B. It has a depressant effect on the chemoreceptor trigger zone.
    C. It increases the release of glutamate and aspartate in the olfactory cortex.
    D. It decreases the concentration of serotonin in the area postrema.
    E. It has a depressant effect on the vagal nucleus.

7. Context-sensitive half-time describes:

    A. The time necessary for the drug concentration at the effect-compartment (effect site) to decrease by 50% after discontinuation of an infusion.
    B. The time necessary for the drug concentration in the bloodstream to decrease by 50% after discontinuation of an infusion.
    C. The time necessary for the drug concentration in the body to decrease by 50% after discontinuation of an infusion.
    D. The time necessary for the drug concentration in its volume of distribution to decrease by 50% after discontinuation of an infusion.
    E. The time necessary for the drug concentration in the liver to decrease by 50% after discontinuation of an infusion.

8. Involuntary myoclonus or myoclonus-like activity is seen with all of the following IV anesthetic drugs EXCEPT:

    A. Etomidate
    B. Propofol
    C. Methohexital
    D. Ketamine
    E. Dexmedetomidine

9. Rank the following induction agents in order of their degree of cardiovascular depression.

    A. Propofol > etomidate > thiopental
    B. Thiopental > propofol > etomidate
    C. Propofol > thiopental > etomidate
    D. Etomidate > thiopental > propofol
    E. Thiopental > etomidate > propofol

10. Which of the following statements concerning the mechanisms of action of intravenous induction agents is NOT true?

    A. Barbiturates appear to increase the duration of γ-aminobutyric acid (GABA)-activated opening of chloride ion channels.
    B. Benzodiazepines appear to increase the efficiency of coupling between GABA receptors and chloride ion channels.
    C. Ketamine produces dissociative amnesia through interaction with *N*-Methyl-D-aspartic acid (NMDA) receptors.
    D. Thiopental appears to act as a competitive inhibitor at central nicotinic acetylcholine (Ach) receptors.
    E. Propofol appears to have a mechanism of action most similar to that of the benzodiazepines.

11. Which of the following is NOT a typical induction regimen for a healthy adult patient?

    A. Etomidate, 0.2 to 0.3 mg/kg
    B. Ketamine, 0.5 to 1 mg/kg
    C. Thiopental, 1.5 mg/kg
    D. Midazolam, 0.1 to 0.2 mg/kg
    E. Propofol, 1.5 to 2.5 mg/kg

12. Ketamine is associated with all of the following physiologic effects EXCEPT:

    A. Bronchodilation
    B. Maintenance of consciousness and protective reflexes
    C. Increased oral secretions
    D. Unchanged peripheral arteriolar resistance
    E. Increased pulmonary artery pressure

13. Which of the following induction agents may facilitate the interpretation of somatosensory evoked potentials (SSEPs)?

    A. Ketamine
    B. Propofol
    C. Methohexital
    D. Midazolam
    E. Etomidate

14. For which of the following patients would ketamine be LEAST appropriate as an induction agent?

    A. A 39-year-old woman with acute asthma exacerbation who is undergoing emergency appendectomy.
    B. A 70-year-old woman with cardiac tamponade who is undergoing emergency thoracotomy.
    C. A 50-year-old woman with glaucoma who is scheduled for elective cataract resection.
    D. A 55-year-old man with mild renal insufficiency who is undergoing sigmoid resection for diverticulitis.
    E. A 7-year-old child without intravenous access who is scheduled for elective tonsillectomy.

15. Which of the following intravenous (IV) induction agents produces dissociative anesthesia?

    A. Propofol
    B. Etomidate
    C. Thiopental
    D. Ketamine
    E. Midazolam

16. Which of the following intravenous induction agents has metabolites that are pharmacologically inactive?

    A. Diazepam
    B. Ketamine
    C. Propofol
    D. Thiopental
    E. Midazolam

17. Which of the following statements about flumazenil is FALSE?

    A. It is structurally similar to benzodiazepines except that it lacks a phenyl group and has a carbonyl group instead.
    B. Its elimination half-time is approximately 1 hour.
    C. It behaves as a noncompetitive antagonist in the presence of benzodiazepine agonist compounds.
    D. A dose of 1 to 3 mg will usually antagonize a benzodiazepine for 45 to 90 minutes.
    E. Despite antagonizing benzodiazepines, flumazenil does not completely reverse respiratory depression.

18. Which of the following intravenous (IV) induction agents is associated with least respiratory depression?

    A. Ketamine
    B. Propofol
    C. Thiopental
    D. Etomidate
    E. Lorazepam

19. In terms of propensity to cause allergic reactions, which of the following intravenous (IV) anesthetics is considered to be the most immunologically "safe"?

    A. Ketamine
    B. Etomidate
    C. Propofol
    D. Midazolam
    E. Methohexital

20. Which of the following intravenous (IV) induction agents is contraindicated in patients who are predisposed to acute intermittent porphyria?

    A. Lorazepam
    B. Ketamine
    C. Etomidate
    D. Thiopental
    E. Propofol

21. Which of the following intravenous (IV) induction agents may produce adverse effects when administered in the presence of tricyclic antidepressants (TCAs)?

    A. Etomidate
    B. Midazolam
    C. Thiopental
    D. Ketamine
    E. Lorazepam

22. All of the following statements about midazolam are true EXCEPT:

    A. An induction dose in a premedicated patient is 0.1 to 0.2 mg/kg.
    B. At high doses it can cause a burst-suppressive (isoelectric) pattern on EEG.
    C. It can reduce preload and afterload, the effects of which are more marked in hypovolemic patients.
    D. It is a water-soluble compound with an acidic pH, and becomes lipid soluble upon administration into the human body at physiologic pH.
    E. It can reduce cerebral perfusion pressure, cerebral blood flow, and cerebral metabolic requirements for oxygen.

23. Which of the following statements about propofol infusion syndrome (PRIS) is FALSE?

    A. The patient can develop metabolic acidosis, cardiac dysfunction, and renal failure.
    B. The patient can develop rhabdomyolysis.
    C. It is associated with hypertriglyceridemia, hepatomegaly, and hypokalemia.
    D. It is more commonly seen in critically ill children, and critically ill patients receiving glucocorticoids and catecholamines.
    E. It is associated with propofol infusion doses greater than 4 mg/kg/hr for more than 24 hours.

24. Which of the following statements about propofol is FALSE?

    A. Initial distribution half-life is 2 to 4 minutes.
    B. The elimination half-life is 1 to 3 hours.
    C. The context-sensitive half-life for propofol infusions that have been administered for 6 to 8 hours is approximately 1 hour.
    D. Induction and maintenance doses in obese patients should be based on lean body weight.
    E. Administration of propofol may reduce cerebral blood flow, intracranial pressure, cerebral perfusion pressure, and cerebral metabolic requirements for oxygen.

25. Intravenous anesthetics in the elderly are affected by all of the following physiologic changes EXCEPT:

    A. Redistribution from vessel-rich tissue compartments is slower.
    B. The steady-state volume of distribution is reduced.
    C. The rate of hepatic clearance is reduced.
    D. The volume of the central compartment is reduced.
    E. Prolongation of β half-life.

26. All of the following statements concerning methohexital are true EXCEPT:

    A. It is preferable to thiopental or propofol for electroconvulsive therapy because it produces less depression of EEG activity.
    B. It is associated with a more profound degree of hypotension, tachycardia, and increased coronary vascular resistance compared with an equipotent dose of thiopental.
    C. It can cause hiccoughing and myoclonic-like activity.
    D. It is more than twice as potent as thiopental.
    E. Its use leads to a decrease in cardiac output and peripheral vascular resistance.

27. Accidental intra-arterial injection of barbiturates is commonly treated with any or all of the following EXCEPT:

    A. Intra-arterial administration of papaverine
    B. Intra-arterial administration of lidocaine
    C. Heparinization
    D. Tourniquet application to the affected limb
    E. Brachial plexus block

28. Each of the following statements about propofol is true EXCEPT:

    A. It causes an increase in β waves on an EEG.
    B. It can be used safely in patients with a history of acute intermittent porphyria.
    C. It can be used to decrease pruritus associated with administration of intrathecal opioids.
    D. Its effects are usually prolonged in patients with pre-existing hepatic disease.
    E. It can cause bronchodilation.

29. All of the following statements concerning etomidate are true EXCEPT:

    A. It does not stimulate histamine release.
    B. It induces involuntary myoclonic movements, which can be attenuated by prior administration of opioid analgesics.
    C. It is associated with a high incidence of postoperative nausea and vomiting.
    D. A single induction dose does not cause any measurable adrenal suppression.
    E. Its elimination half-life is increased in patients with severe hepatic dysfunction.

30. Which of the following statements concerning the cardiovascular effects of propofol is FALSE?

    A. It causes arterial dilation.
    B. It increases peripheral venous pooling.
    C. It impairs the baroreceptor reflex response.
    D. It is not a direct myocardial depressant.
    E. It decreases systemic arterial pressure.

31. Which of the following intravenous agents does NOT have intrinsic analgesic properties?

    A. Ketamine
    B. Dexmedetomidine
    C. Clonidine
    D. Thiopental

32. Which of the following statements regarding pharmacokinetics of IV anesthetics is FALSE?

   A. Elimination of a drug via first-order kinetics occurs when hepatic enzyme systems are not saturated, and the rate of drug elimination will decrease as an exponential function of the drug's plasma concentration.

   B. The diffusion rate into the CNS will be higher for IV anesthetics with a greater degree of plasma protein binding.

   C. The induction effects of IV anesthetics are terminated by redistribution from central compartments into peripheral compartments.

   D. Elimination of a drug via zero-order kinetics occurs after prolonged infusions and high steady-state plasma concentrations. The rate of elimination becomes independent of drug concentration.

   E. When a drug infusion is administered without a loading dose, it may require at least three times the elimination half-life ($t_{1/2}\beta$) to achieve a steady-state plasma concentration.

33. Which of the following statements about dexmedetomidine is FALSE?

   A. It has a slower onset and offset compared to propofol.

   B. It has amnestic and analgesic effects.

   C. It is approved by the FDA for sedation not to exceed 1 week's duration in mechanically ventilated patients in the ICU.

   D. A typical infusion rate for sedation ranges from 0.2 to 0.6 mcg/kg/hr.

   E. It is an α agonist.

ANSWERS

1. **C.** The rapid onset of IV anesthetics is primarily attributable to their high lipid solubility and the relatively high proportion of cardiac output that perfuses the brain. Only the unionized fraction of a drug can cross the blood–brain barrier, so onset is also affected by the pKa of the drug relative to the pH of body fluids; onset is also more rapid when the ratio of unionized to ionized drug is high. Although the volume of distribution, elimination half-life, and hepatic extraction ratio contribute to drug pharmacokinetics, these factors are not primarily responsible for the rapid onset of anesthetic effects. (See page 481: Pharmacokinetics and Metabolism.)

2. **C.** Ketamine interacts with NMDA and opioid, muscarinic, and monoaminergic receptors, but it does not interact with GABA receptors. This is in contrast to most intravenous anesthetics, which exert their primary effect through GABA receptors. (See page 480: General Pharmacology of Intravenous Anesthetics.)

3. **B.** Whereas about 98% of propofol is protein bound, about 85% of the barbiturates methohexital and thiopental bind to protein, and 75% of etomidate is protein bound. In contrast, only about 12% of ketamine is protein bound. (See page 481: Pharmacokinetics and Metabolism.)

4. **C.** The hepatic extraction ratio is a measure of the rate at which anesthetics are cleared from the systemic circulation by the liver. The hepatic clearance of intravenous anesthetics may be categorized into three groups: High, intermediate, and low. Thiopental, diazepam, and lorazepam have low hepatic extraction ratios, and propofol, etomidate, and ketamine have high hepatic extraction ratios. Methohexital and midazolam have hepatic extraction ratios that are intermediate between these two groups. (See page 481: Pharmacokinetics and Metabolism.)

5. **C.** In general, benzodiazepines such as midazolam are associated with a relatively prolonged time to the recovery of cognitive function compared with other intravenous anesthetics. In contrast, recovery from propofol is usually quite rapid, making it an ideal induction agent for outpatient procedures. Recovery from ketamine, etomidate, and thiopental is intermediate between the benzodiazepines and propofol. (See page 496: Sedation in the Operating Room and Intensive Care Unit.)

6. **C.** Propofol has antidopaminergic activity and depresses the chemoreceptor trigger zone and vagal nucleus. It also decreases the release of glutamate and aspartate in the olfactory cortex and reduces serotonin levels in the area postrema. All of these mechanisms are believed to contribute to propofol's antiemetic properties. (See page 486: Propofol.)

7. **A.** Context-sensitive half-time is defined as the time necessary for the effect-compartment concentration of drug to decrease by 50% after discontinuation of continuous infusion. (See page 481: Pharmacokinetics and Metabolism.)

8. **E.** Most sedative-hypnotic drugs have been reported to cause occasional EEG seizure-like myoclonic activity. Myoclonic activity is generally considered to be the result of an imbalance between excitatory and inhibitory subcortical centers, produced by an unequal degree of suppression of these brain centers by low concentrations of hypnotic drugs. Dexmedetomidine is not associated with myoclonus. (See page 483: Pharmacodynamic Effects.)

9. **C.** The cardiovascular effects of propofol are more profound than those of thiopental or etomidate. Etomidate is the induction agent considered to have the least impact on the cardiovascular system. (See page 485: Comparative Physicochemical and Clinical Pharmacologic Properties of Intravenous Agents.)

10. **E.** Propofol appears to increase the duration of GABA-mediating chloride channel opening. Therefore, its mechanism of action is most similar to that of the barbiturates, not the benzodiazepines. However, benzodiazepines also act via the GABA receptor, increasing the efficiency of coupling between the GABA receptor and chloride ion channels. Whereas thiopental is believed to exert its effect via competitive inhibition of nicotinic Ach receptors in the central nervous system, ketamine acts via NMDA receptors. (See page 480: General Pharmacology of Intravenous Anesthetics.)

11. **C.** The typical induction dose of thiopental is 3 to 5 mg/kg intravenously. All of the other choices represent typical induction drug dosages. (See page 480: General Pharmacology of Intravenous Anesthetics.)

12. **D.** Ketamine is a sympathetic stimulant that increases peripheral arteriolar resistance, arterial blood pressure, heart rate, and pulmonary artery pressure. It also possesses bronchodilatory activity. Ketamine causes a so-called dissociative anesthetic state characterized by profound analgesia and amnesia, even though patients may be conscious and maintain protective reflexes. Ketamine also increases oral secretions. Therefore, pretreatment with an antisialagogue is sometimes useful. (See page 489: Ketamine.)

13. **E.** Etomidate increases the amplitude of SSEPs and can be useful in the interpretation of SSEPs when signal quality is poor. (See page 489: Etomidate.)

14. **C.** Ketamine increases intraocular pressure and is therefore not an appropriate induction agent in patients with glaucoma. Ketamine is a sympathetic stimulant that has bronchodilatory effects. These properties make it a useful agent in a carefully defined subset of patients, such as those with acute bronchospasm, hypovolemic shock, right-to-left intracardiac shunts, and cardiac tamponade. However, its sympathomimetic effects may be ineffective in the

context of maximal sympathetic output. Ketamine may be delivered intramuscularly in patients without intravenous access. (See page 489: Ketamine.)

15. **D.**   Ketamine produces dose-dependent central nervous system depression leading to a so-called dissociative anesthetic state characterized by profound analgesia and amnesia, even though patients may be conscious and maintain protective reflexes. The proposed mechanism for this cataleptic state includes electrophysiologic inhibition of thalamocortical pathways and stimulation of the limbic system. None of the other IV anesthetic agents produce a dissociative anesthetic state. (See page 489: Ketamine.)

16. **C.**   Propofol is rapidly and extensively metabolized to inactive, water-soluble sulphate and glucuronic acid metabolites, which are eliminated by the kidneys. Midazolam undergoes extensive oxidation by hepatic enzymes to form water-soluble hydroxylated metabolites, which are excreted in the urine. However, the primary metabolite, 1-hydroxymethylmidazolam, has mild central nervous system (CNS) depressant activity. Diazepam is metabolized to active metabolites (desmethyldiazepam, 3-hydroxydiazepam), which can prolong diazepam's residual sedative effects because of their long $t_{1/2} \beta$ values. Thiopental is metabolized in the liver to hydroxythiopental and the carboxylic acid derivative, which are more water soluble and have little CNS activity. When high doses of thiopental are administered, a desulfuration reaction may occur with the production of pentobarbital, which has long-lasting CNS depressant activity. Ketamine is metabolized into norketamine, which is also pharmacologically active. (See page 483: Pharmacodynamic Effects.)

17. **C.**   Flumazenil, a 1,4-imidazobenzodiazepine derivative has a molecular structure similar to other benzodiazepines except for the absence of a phenyl group, which is replaced by a carbonyl group. Flumazenil acts as a competitive antagonist in the presence of benzodiazepine agonist compounds. Flumazenil is short acting, with an elimination half-life of approximately 1 hour. Recurrence of the central effects of benzodiazepines (resedation) may occur after a single dose of flumazenil because of the more slowly eliminated agonist drug. If sustained antagonism is desired, it may be necessary to administer flumazenil as repeated doses or by a continuous infusion. In general, 45 to 90 minutes of antagonism can be expected after 1 to 3 mg of flumazenil IV. However, the respiratory depression produced by benzodiazepines is not completely reversed by flumazenil. (See page 487: Benzodiazepines.)

18. **A.**   With the exception of ketamine (and to a lesser extent, etomidate), IV anesthetics produce dose-dependent respiratory depression, which is enhanced in patients with chronic obstructive pulmonary disease. Ketamine causes minimal respiratory depression in clinically relevant doses and can facilitate the transition from mechanical to spontaneous ventilation after anesthesia. In contrast to the other IV anesthetics, protective airway reflexes are more likely to be preserved with ketamine. The respiratory depression is characterized by a decrease in tidal volume

and minute ventilation, as well as a transient rightward shift in the CO_2 response curve. After the rapid injection of a large bolus dose of an IV anesthetic, transient apnea lasting 30 to 90 seconds is usually produced. (See page 489: Ketamine.)

19. **B.**   Severe anaphylactic reactions to IV anesthetics are extremely uncommon; however, profound hypotension attributed to nonimmunologically mediated histamine release has been reported with thiopental use. Although anaphylactic reactions to etomidate have been reported, it does not appear to release histamine and is considered to be the most "immunologically safe" IV anesthetic. Although propofol does not normally trigger histamine release, life-threatening anaphylactoid reactions have been reported in patients with a previous history of multiple drug allergies. With the exception of etomidate, all IV induction agents have been alleged to cause some histamine release. (See page 484: Hypersensitivity Reactions.)

20. **D.**   Barbiturates can precipitate episodes of acute intermittent porphyria, so their use is contraindicated in patients who are predisposed to acute intermittent porphyria. Although the benzodiazepines, ketamine, and etomidate are reported to be safe in humans, these drugs have been shown to be porphyrogenic in animal models. Propofol is not contraindicated in patients who are predisposed to acute intermittent porphyria. (See page 483: Pharmacodynamic Effects.)

21. **D.**   Ketamine can produce adverse effects when administered in the presence of TCAs because both drugs inhibit norepinephrine reuptake and may produce severe hypotension, heart failure, or myocardial ischemia. None of the other IV induction agents produces these effects when given in the presence of TCAs. (See page 489: Ketamine.)

22. **B.**   An induction dose of midazolam in a premedicated patient is usually 0.1 to 0.2 mg/kg. Benzodiazepines decrease both $CMRO_2$ and CBF analogous to the barbiturates and propofol. However, in contrast to these compounds, midazolam is unable to produce a complete burst-suppressive (isoelectric) pattern on the EEG. Accordingly, there is a "ceiling" effect with respect to the decrease in $CMRO_2$ produced by increasing doses of midazolam. Midazolam produces a decrease in systemic vascular resistance and blood pressure when large doses are administered for induction of anesthesia. The decrease in preload and afterload may be more marked in hypovolemic patients. Midazolam is a water-soluble benzodiazepine that is available in an acidified (pH 3.5) aqueous formulation. At physiologic pH, an intramolecular rearrangement occurs that changes the physicochemical properties of midazolam such that it becomes more lipid soluble. (See page 487: Benzodiazepines.)

23. **C.**   In critically ill children and adults receiving high-dose infusions of propofol, some patients have been reported to experience so-called propofol infusion syndrome [PRIS], which is characterized by cardiac failure, rhabdomyolysis, metabolic acidosis and renal failure, and is often fatal.

Hyperkalemia, hypertriglyceridemia, and hepatomegaly are also key features. It is associated with high doses and long-term use of propofol (>4 mg/kg/hr for >24 hours). It occurs more commonly in children, and critically ill patients receiving catecholamines and glucocorticoids. (See page 486: Propofol.)

24. **C.** In studies using a two-compartment kinetic model, the initial distribution half-life of propofol is 2 to 4 minutes and the elimination half-life is 1 to 3 hours. Propofol is rapidly cleared from the central compartment by hepatic metabolism and the context-sensitive half-life for propofol infusions up to 8 hours is <40 minutes. The induction dose of propofol in healthy adults is 1.5 to 2.5 mg/kg, but in the morbidly obese patient, the propofol induction and maintenance dosages should be calculated based on the patient's lean body weight. Propofol decreases $CMRO_2$ and CBF, as well as ICP. When larger doses are administered, the marked depressant effect on systemic arterial pressure can significantly decrease CPP. (See page 486: Propofol.)

25. **B.** Elderly patients have increased steady-state volume of distribution for most IV anesthetics and decreased hepatic clearance, leading to prolongation of their β half-life values. They also have decreased volume of the central compartment and slower redistribution from vessel-rich tissue to intermediate compartments. As a result, the dose of anesthetic required to elicit effect is lower and the time to recovery is longer in elderly patients than in younger patients. (See page 481: Pharmacokinetics and Metabolism.)

26. **B.** Methohexital is two to three times more potent than thiopental. Compared with thiopental, it produces a relatively more robust tachycardic response, leading to a lesser degree of hypotension. It decreases coronary vascular resistance. Therefore, if blood pressure remains stable, the myocardial oxygen supply/demand ratio will remain normal despite the increase in heart rate. Methohexital also causes myoclonic-like muscle tremors and other signs of excitatory activity (e.g., hiccoughing). (See page 485: Barbiturates.)

27. **D.** Treatments for accidental intra-arterial injection of thiobarbiturates include intra-arterial administration of papaverine and/or lidocaine, heparinization, and/or regional anesthesia-induced sympathectomy such as a brachial plexus block. Isolation of regional blood flow via tourniquet application is not appropriate. (See page 485: Barbiturates.)

28. **D.** Propofol can be used safely in patients with acute intermittent porphyria. Propofol also decreases pruritus associated with intrathecal opioid use and cholestatic liver disease. Even though propofol is metabolized by the liver, its effects are generally not prolonged in patients with pre-existing hepatic disease. Sedative doses of propofol increase β-wave activity on the EEG, analogous to benzodiazepines. (See page 486: Propofol.)

29. **D.** Etomidate sometimes induces nonepileptogenic involuntary myoclonus during induction that can be attenuated by the preinduction use of an opioid analgesic. In addition, it is associated with a high incidence of postoperative nausea and vomiting and has been shown to depress adrenocortical function for several hours after a single induction dose. Etomidate does not induce histamine release and can be safely used in patients with reactive airway disease. The high clearance rate of etomidate is a result of extensive ester hydrolysis in the liver. Severe hepatic disease causes a prolongation of the elimination half-life secondary to an increased volume of distribution and a decreased plasma clearance rate. (See page 489: Etomidate.)

30. **D.** Propofol causes arterial and venous dilatation as well as impairment of the baroreceptor reflex, all of which contribute to a decrease in systemic arterial pressure. In addition, propofol has myocardial depressant effects. All of these factors contribute to the decrease in systemic arterial pressure commonly observed after propofol induction. These cardiovascular effects are more profound than those associated with thiopental or etomidate. (See page 486: Propofol.)

31. **D.** Ketamine, dexmedetomidine, and the α_2-agonist clonidine appear to possess analgesic properties. In contrast, thiopental appears to have a mild antianalgesic effect. (See page 483: Pharmacodynamic Effects.)

32. **B.** The diffusion rate into the central nervous system will be more limited for IV anesthetics with a high degree of plasma protein binding because only the "free" unbound drug can diffuse across membranes and exert central effects. For most drugs, the hepatic enzyme systems are not saturated at clinically relevant drug concentrations, and the rate of drug elimination will decrease as an exponential function of the drug's plasma concentration (first-order kinetics). However, when high steady-state plasma concentrations are achieved with prolonged infusions, hepatic enzyme systems can become saturated and the elimination rate becomes independent of the drug concentration (zero-order kinetics). When a drug infusion is administered without a loading dose, at least three times the $t_{1/2}\beta$ value may be required to achieve a true "steady-state" plasma concentration. The initial pharmacologic effects of an IV anesthetic are related to the activity of the drug in the central compartment. The primary mechanism for terminating the central effects of IV anesthetics administered for induction of anesthesia is redistribution from the central highly perfused to the larger, but less well-perfused "peripheral" compartments. (See page 481: Pharmacokinetics and Metabolism.)

33. **C.** Dexmedetomidine is an α_2-adrenoceptor agonist. It provides comparable sedation to midazolam but has a slower onset and offset of sedation than propofol. It has been approved by the FDA for the short-term (<24 hours) sedation of mechanically ventilated patients in the ICU setting, as well as for sedation in procedures under MAC. A low-dose infusion rate of 0.2 to 0.6 mcg/kg/hr has been shown to have sedative, amnestic, and analgesic effects. (See page 491: Dexmedetomidine.)

Opioids

1. All of the following statements regarding opioid-receptor interactions are true EXCEPT:

   A. The analgesic effects of opioids are thought to result primarily from the activation of μ receptors in the brain and spinal cord.

   B. Opioid-receptor activation in peripheral tissues may play a role in the modulation of painful stimuli.

   C. Naloxone is highly specific for the μ subtype of opioid receptors.

   D. Most clinically used opioids are highly selective for the μ-subtype opioid receptor.

   E. Opioid receptors are coupled to G proteins that regulate the activity of adenylate cyclase.

2. The ability of an opioid to cross the blood–brain barrier depends on all of the following properties EXCEPT:

   A. Lipid solubility

   B. Ionization

   C. Protein binding

   D. μ affinity

   E. Molecular size

3. Which of the following is TRUE regarding context-sensitive half-time for opioids ($CSt_{1/2}$)?

   A. It is the time needed for a drug's steady-state plasma concentration to decrease to one-third upon stopping its continuous infusion.

   B. For fentanyl the $CSt_{1/2}$ is independent of the duration of the infusion.

   C. The extremely short $CSt_{1/2}$ of remifentanil is due to its rapid clearance from the plasma.

   D. The time to the loss of analgesia after an opioid infusion is solely dependent on the $CSt_{1/2}$.

4. Which of the following opioids exert their analgesic effect via both opioid and nonopioid receptors?

   A. Tramadol

   B. Tapentadol

   C. Methadone

   D. All of the above

5. Which of the following statements regarding opioid-induced muscle rigidity is TRUE?

   A. Muscle rigidity does not occur with morphine doses below 0.2 mg/kg.

   B. The phenomenon is witnessed only on induction of anesthesia without the use of neuromuscular blocking agents.

   C. Muscle rigidity may be reduced by the addition of nitrous oxide.

   D. The effects may be eliminated by naloxone.

   E. Opioid-induced muscle rigidity is mediated via σ receptors.

6. Which of the following routes of opioid administration reliably reduces the incidence of opioid-induced nausea?

   A. Intramuscular

   B. Intrathecal

   C. Subcutaneous

   D. Transdermal

   E. None of the above

7. A 46-year-old man with a history of multiple uneventful general anesthetics is undergoing a multilevel spinal fusion procedure during which 1 mg/kg of morphine is administered over 15 minutes. Shortly thereafter, the patient exhibits modest hypotension with a concomitant decrease in systemic vascular resistance, as well as an increase in pulmonary vascular resistance as measured by a pulmonary artery catheter. These findings are unaffected by the administration of 0.2 mg of naloxone. The most likely cause of this critical incident is:

   A. Morphine-induced histamine release

   B. A previously undiagnosed anaphylaxis

   C. An opioid-mediated increase in vascular permeability

   D. The central vagotonic effects of morphine

   E. Direct myocardial depression by morphine

8. The occurrence of myoclonic activity and seizures observed after repeated or prolonged administration of meperidine is most likely the result of:

   A. Direct central nervous system (CNS) effects resulting from the inherent local anesthetic actions of meperidine.
   B. Direct CNS excitation by meperidine.
   C. Neurotoxic effects of normeperidine, an active metabolite of meperidine.
   D. Insidious hypoxemia as a consequence of the prolonged clinical half-life of meperidine.
   E. Selective activation of spinal κ receptors with increasing serum levels of meperidine.

9. Which physical characteristic of fentanyl best accounts for its rapid onset of clinical effect as well as its brief duration of action?

   A. High lipid solubility
   B. High degree of ionization
   C. Relatively small molecular weight
   D. Negligible protein binding
   E. Low hepatic clearance

10. Regarding methadone, which of the statements below is FALSE?

    A. Methadone is primarily a μ agonist.
    B. After parenteral administration, the onset of analgesia is within 20 minutes.
    C. Methadone is not well absorbed orally, with only 10% bioavailability.
    D. Methadone reaches peak plasma concentration four hours after oral administration.
    E. Methadone is nearly 90% protein bound.

11. All of the following statements regarding clinical characteristics of alfentanil are true EXCEPT:

    A. On a milligram basis, the clinical potency of alfentanil is roughly ten times that of morphine and one-tenth that of fentanyl.
    B. Alfentanil displays a significantly faster onset of action than fentanyl and sufentanil.
    C. Alfentanil has a longer terminal half-life than fentanyl and sufentanil.
    D. The incidence of nausea and vomiting associated with alfentanil is no higher than that with either fentanyl or sufentanil.
    E. Similar to fentanyl and sufentanil, alfentanil may produce profound muscle rigidity when given in high doses.

12. Remifentanil exhibits a markedly shorter clinical duration of action compared with other commonly used opioids because of:

    A. Rapid redistribution resulting from high lipid solubility
    B. A lesser degree of opioid-receptor affinity
    C. A high protein-bound (α_1-acid glycoprotein) fraction
    D. A relatively high volume of distribution
    E. Metabolism of an ester side chain by blood and tissue esterases

13. Which of the following statements regarding sufentanil is TRUE?

    A. It has a clinical potency 100 to 200 times that of morphine.
    B. Bradycardia is usually not seen when pancuronium is used during anesthesia with sufentanil.
    C. Sufentanil has a higher volume of distribution than fentanyl because of its decreased plasma protein binding.
    D. Approximately 60% of an intravenous (IV) bolus dose of sufentanil is cleared from the plasma in 90 minutes.
    E. Sufentanil is extremely hydrophilic.

14. Which of the following properties regarding remifentanil is FALSE?

    A. Remifentanil is about 40 times more potent than alfentanil.
    B. Remifentanil is devoid of muscle rigidity side effects because of its rapid metabolism.
    C. Remifentanil has less depressant effect on motor evoked potentials than other opioids.
    D. Remifentanil is associated with poor postoperative pain control if it is used intraoperatively because of its rapid metabolism.
    E. Shivering is more common with remifentanil than with alfentanil.

15. All are true regarding the use of remifentanil for obstetric analgesia EXCEPT:

    A. Oxygen saturations may fall below 95% SpO_2.
    B. It can be administered as intermittent boluses or as a constant infusion.
    C. A plasma concentration between 2 and 4 ng/mL is sufficient for adequate analgesia.
    D. Remifentanil provides superior analgesia than epidural analgesia despite a poor satisfaction scoring.

16. Which of the following statements regarding opioid-induced nausea and vomiting is TRUE?

    A. Equipotent doses of opioids cause an equal incidence of nausea and vomiting.
    B. Morphine has no direct effect on the chemoreceptor trigger zone.
    C. Subcutaneous administration of opioids is associated with a lower incidence of nausea and vomiting compared with intravenous (IV) administration.
    D. Vestibular stimulation such as ambulation attenuates the nausea caused by morphine.
    E. All of the above.

17. Which of the following statements regarding morphine-induced pupillary constriction (miosis) in humans is FALSE?

    A. The presence of miosis somewhat correlates with opioid-induced respiratory depression.
    B. The effect is thought to be mediated via the nucleus of the tenth cranial nerve.
    C. A near-maximal degree of miosis is seen with as little as 0.5 mg/kg of morphine.
    D. Except if there is severe hypoxemia, the absence of miosis virtually eliminates opioids as a cause of respiratory depression.

18. The chemoreceptor trigger zone (CTZ) in the area prostema of the medulla is rich in all of the following receptors EXCEPT:

    A. Muscarinic
    B. Dopamine
    C. Histamine
    D. Nicotinic
    E. Serotonin

19. The clinical effects of meperidine that differ from those observed with other commonly used opioids include:

    A. Absence of histamine release from tissue mast cells
    B. Increase in cardiac index after high doses
    C. Less nausea and vomiting at equianalgesic doses
    D. Direct local anesthetic effects

20. Common potential disadvantages of a high-dose opioid anesthetic technique using fentanyl as the sole agent for anesthesia include all of the following EXCEPT:

    A. Hemodynamic instability and cardiac depression
    B. Impaired ventilation resulting from intense chest wall muscle rigidity
    C. Prolonged anterograde amnesia
    D. Apnea lasting for the duration of anesthetic

21. Which of the following is true regarding opioid-induced respiratory depression?

    A. Suppression of the central ventilatory drive is the sole mechanism leading to respiratory depression.
    B. Frequent hypoxemic episodes invariably do not occur after the first post operative day.
    C. Utility function curves can be used to estimate analgesic and respiratory depressant effects for different opioids.
    D. Naloxone causes a leftward shift of the dose response curve of most clinically used opioids.

22. Which of the following is true regarding the use of remifentanil?

    A. Prolonged respiratory depression with infusion techniques resulting from accumulation of active metabolites
    B. It should be administered as a constant infusion for labor analgesia
    C. Increased incidence of postoperative pain and hyperalgesia
    D. High incidence of intraoperative muscle rigidity with high doses.

23. Potential hazard in the use of naloxone to reverse opioid-induced respiratory depression include all EXCEPT:

    A. Sudden, severe pain in the postoperative period
    B. Precipitation of withdrawal syndromes in patients who are physically dependent on opioids
    C. Acute respiratory depression
    D. Acute pulmonary edema

24. Which of the following drug responses is NOT an example of pharmacogenetic variation?

    A. Variation in fentanyl-induced respiratory depression
    B. Variation in the analgesic efficacy of codeine
    C. Variation in the reversal of opioid overdose by naloxone
    D. Variation in the μ-opioid analgesic effects

ANSWERS

1. C. Most observed opioid effects involve interactions with receptor systems at spinal and supraspinal sites, although clinical studies suggest that morphine can produce analgesia by peripheral mechanisms, especially when inflammation is present. Whereas the intrinsic activity, or efficacy, of an opioid is described by the dose–response curve resulting from drug–receptor interaction, *affinity* describes the ability of a drug to bind a receptor to produce a stable complex. Most opioids used in current clinical practice are highly selective for μ receptors, but naloxone, the most commonly used opioid antagonist, is not selective for opioid-receptor type. For this reason, identification of an opioid-receptor–mediated drug effect requires demonstration of naloxone reversibility. (See page 503: The Endogenous Opioid System: Opioid Receptors.)

2. D. Physicochemical properties of the opioids influence both pharmacokinetics and pharmacodynamics. To reach its effector sites in the central nervous system (CNS), an opioid must cross biologic membranes from the blood to receptors on neuronal cell membranes. The ability of opioids to cross this blood–brain barrier depends on such properties as molecular size, ionization, lipid solubility, and protein binding (see Table 19-2). Of these characteristics, lipid solubility and ionization assume major importance in determining the rate of penetration to the CNS. (See page 507: Routes of Administration, Pharmacokinetics and Pharmacodynamics.)

3. C. Context-sensitive half-time ($CSt_{1/2}$) is defined as the time needed for the drug's plasma concentration to decrease by half from a steady-state plasma concentration after the drug infusion has stopped. The term context implies that the half time is being referred to in *context* to *the duration of the infusion* of the drug. For fentanyl the context-sensitive half-time increases with the duration of the infusion. Remifentanil has a rapid clearance from the plasma by nonspecific esterases, which is why it has a low context-sensitive half-time (2 minutes) that is independent of the duration of the infusion. In fact about 75% of remifentanil is cleared in 8 minutes after any duration of infusion. In clinical practice, besides context-sensitive half-time, "time to the loss of analgesia" after administering any given opioid depends on the dose given, the neuronal and receptor kinetic processes, and the transport of the opioids from brain to plasma. (See page 508: Pharmacokinetics and Pharmacodynamics and Figure 6.)

4. D. Tramadol has both opioidergic and monoaminergic activity thus simultaneously affecting serotonin and norepinephrine reuptake along with μ agonism. Tapentadol produces potent analgesia that is particularly useful in acute pain because of synergism between μ-receptor agonism and norepinephrine reuptake inhibition. Methadone displays an NMDA antagonism along with μ-receptor affinity which may be clinically useful in reducing opioid

tolerance and opioid-induced hyperalgesia. (See Page 505: Opioids Acting at Opioid and Nonopioid Receptors.)

5. D. Large doses of opioids may produce profound muscle rigidity, an effect that appears to be mediated by μ receptors at supraspinal sites, most notably the nucleus raphe pontis and sites lateral to it in the hindbrain. Such muscle rigidity is most often witnessed on induction with large doses of opioids, although postoperative occurrences have been observed, as have feelings of muscle tension after small doses (10–15 mg) of morphine. Opioid-induced muscle rigidity is drastically increased by the addition of 70% nitrous oxide, but it is reduced or eliminated by naloxone, drugs that facilitate γ-aminobutyric acid agonist activity, and muscle relaxants. (See page 518: Opioid-related Side Effects: Skeletal Muscle Effects.)

6. E. Opioid-induced nausea is thought to be a result of input to the vomiting center from stimulation of the chemotactic trigger zone in the area postrema of the medulla, which is rich in opioid receptors. Not only does the incidence of opioid-induced nausea appear to be irrespective of the route of administration, but clinical studies also reveal no differences among opioid species, including morphine, meperidine, fentanyl, sufentanil, and alfentanil. (See page 518: Opioid-related Side Effects: Nausea and Vomiting.)

7. A. Opioids stimulate the release of histamine from mast cells and basophils in a dose-dependent manner, an effect seen commonly after high doses of morphine. Decreases in peripheral vascular resistance and corresponding increases in pulmonary vascular resistance after morphine administration have been shown to correlate well with elevated plasma histamine concentrations. Opioid-induced histamine release is not prevented by pretreatment with naloxone, a finding suggesting a mechanism independent of opioid-receptor activation. In clinically relevant doses, morphine does not depress myocardial contractility. It does, however, produce dose-dependent bradycardia, probably by both sympatholytic and parasympathomimetic mechanisms. (See page 518: Opioid-related Side Effects: Histamine Release.)

8. C. Meperidine is metabolized primarily in the liver by N-methylation to form normeperidine, an active metabolite, and to a lesser extent by hydrolysis to form meperidinic acid. In humans, CNS effects such as restlessness, agitation, tremors, myoclonus, and seizures have been associated with increased serum levels of normeperidine. Normeperidine, which has a considerably longer elimination half-life than its parent compound, is more apt to accumulate with repeated or prolonged administration of meperidine or in patients with renal dysfunction. (See page 508: Pharmacokinetics and Pharmacodynamics: Metabolism: Meperidine.)

9. **A.** Fentanyl's high degree of lipid solubility enables it to cross biologic membranes very rapidly and to permeate highly perfused tissue groups, such as the brain, heart, and lung. This same characteristic accounts for the relatively brief clinical duration of effect seen with fentanyl because redistribution of the drug to other tissues, including muscle and fat, also results from high lipid solubility. Similarly, accumulation of fentanyl in such tissue compartments can be extensive with prolonged administration, thus creating "reservoirs" of drug. (See page 508: Pharmacokinetics and Pharmacodynamics: Piperidines, Pharmacodynamics: Fentanyl.)

10. **C.** Methadone, a synthetic opioid introduced in the 1940s, is primarily a μ agonist with pharmacologic properties that are similar to morphine. Although its chemical structure is very different from that of morphine, steric factors force the molecule to simulate the pseudopiperidine ring conformation that appears to be required for opioid activity. Methadone is well absorbed after an oral dose, with bioavailability approximately 90%, and reaches peak plasma concentration at 4 hours after oral administration. Because of its long elimination half-life, methadone is often used for long-term pain management and for treatment of opioid abstinence syndromes. After parenteral administration, the onset of analgesia is within 10 to 20 minutes. After a single dose up to 10 mg, the duration of analgesia is similar to morphine, but with large or repeated parenteral doses, prolonged analgesia can be obtained. It is nearly 90% bound to plasma proteins. (See page 508: Pharmacokinetics and Pharmacodynamics: Methadone.)

11. **C.** Alfentanil is a synthetic tetrazole derivative of fentanyl with a clinical potency nearly ten times that of morphine and one-fourth to one-tenth that of fentanyl. Alfentanil is a weaker base than other opioids, with a pKa of 6.8. As such, nearly 90% of unbound plasma alfentanil is nonionized at physiologic pH. This property, in addition to its moderately high lipid solubility, allows alfentanil to cross the blood–brain barrier rapidly and accounts for its rapid onset of action. Alfentanil has a terminal elimination half-life of 84 to 90 minutes, considerably shorter than that of fentanyl or sufentanil, mainly because of its relatively small volume of distribution. The incidences of clinical side effects with alfentanil have been shown to be similar to those with fentanyl and sufentanil when compared at equianalgesic doses. Early reports of a higher incidence of nausea and vomiting with alfentanil have not been substantiated. (See page 508: Pharmacokinetics and Pharmacodynamics: Piperidines.)

12. **E.** Remifentanil is a recently synthesized 4-anilidopiperidine opioid with a methyl ester side chain that is susceptible to metabolism by blood and tissue esterases. A unique property of remifentanil compared with other clinically useful opioids is its lack of accumulation with repeated dosing or prolonged infusion. This is because its ultrashort duration of action is the result of metabolism to a substantially less-active compound, rather than simply redistribution of an unchanged opioid. (See page 508: Pharmacokinetics and Pharmacodynamics: Piperidines, Remifentanil.)

13. **B.** Sufentanil has a clinical potency ratio 2,000 to 4,000 times that of morphine. It is extremely lipophilic. Combining vecuronium and sufentanil may cause a decrease in mean arterial pressure during induction, and significant bradycardia and sinus arrest have been reported. Bradycardia is not seen when pancuronium is used during anesthesia with sufentanil. Because of a smaller degree of ionization at physiologic pH and higher degree of plasma protein binding, its volume of distribution is somewhat smaller and its elimination half-life is shorter than those of fentanyl. Plasma sufentanil concentration decreases very rapidly after an IV bolus dose, and 98% of the drug is cleared from plasma within 30 minutes. (See page 508: Pharmacokinetics: Piperidines, Opioid-related Side Effects: Cardiovascular Effects.)

14. **B.** Remifentanil is about 40 times as potent as alfentanil. A high incidence of muscle rigidity and purposeless movement has been seen with remifentanil. Although all opioids and propofol depress motor evoked potentials in a dose-dependent fashion, remifentanil exerts less suppression than other opioids and propofol. One drawback of remifentanil use for general anesthesia is that patients require analgesics soon after an infusion is stopped. Shivering is less common with alfentanil than with remifentanil. (See page 508: Pharmacodynamics: Remifentanil.)

15. **D.** There is a paucity of data on the occurrence of hypoxia and apneic events after the use of remifentanil for obstetric analgesia but most clinical studies do not seem to mention a drop below 94% SpO$_2$. There are two approaches for the use of remifentanil for maternal analgesia, one is intermittent boluses with doses between 20 and 40 μg, and the other to provide the same dose range over 3-minute intervals. This infusion scheme provides plasma concentrations between 2 and 4 ng/mL sufficient to provide adequate maternal analgesia in most patients. Current data suggest that, even though patient satisfaction is high with remifentanil, epidurals remain superior to either PCA remifentanil or parenteral meperidine. (See Page 519: Remifentanil for Obstetric Labor Pain.)

16. **A.** The incidence of opioid-induced nausea appears to be similar irrespective of the route of administration (including oral, IV, intramuscular, subcutaneous, transmucosal, transdermal, intrathecal, and epidural). Laboratory and clinical studies comparing the incidence and severity of nausea and vomiting have found no differences among opioids (including morphine, hydromorphone, meperidine, fentanyl, sufentanil, alfentanil, and remifentanil) in equianalgesic doses. (See page 518: Opioid-related Side Effects: Nausea and Vomiting.)

17. **B.** Morphine produces dose-dependent miosis in humans, an effect that is believed to be mediated by the Edinger–Westphal nucleus of the third cranial nerve. Although significant differences exist between opioid species and their effects on pupillary size, morphine produces a near-maximal degree of constriction with 0.5 mg/kg. (See page 518: Opioid-related Side Effects: Pupil Effects.)

18. **D.** The CTZ is rich in opioid, dopamine, serotonin, histamine, and muscarinic (but not nicotinic) acetylcholine

receptors. It receives input from the vestibular portion of the eighth cranial nerve. Morphine and related opioids induce nausea by direct stimulation of the CTZ and can also produce increased vestibular sensitivity. (See page 518: Opioid-related Side Effects: Nausea and Vomiting.)

19. **D.** Meperidine is a synthetic opioid with an analgesic potency about one-tenth that of morphine. Although the analgesic effects are primarily mediated via μ-receptor activation, meperidine has demonstrated local anesthetic properties, which has led to its increasing popularity for epidural and subarachnoid administration. This local anesthetic effect is thought to be responsible for decreases in cardiac contractility contributing to a lower cardiac index observed with high plasma concentrations of meperidine, a finding not consistent with other clinically used opioids. Meperidine administration does result in histamine release, an effect that may contribute to the hemodynamic instability often encountered when high doses are used in the clinical setting. At equianalgesic doses, the respiratory depression caused by meperidine is no different from that induced by morphine, hydromorphone, meperidine, fentanyl, sufentanil, alfentanil, or remifentanil. (See page 518: Other Opioid-related Side Efects.)

20. **C.** High-dose opioid-based anesthetic techniques, particularly those using synthetic opioids (e.g., fentanyl), initially gained popularity because of the reliable hemodynamic stability that is achieved with minimal cardiovascular depression. In addition, hormonal responses to surgical stimuli are significantly blunted with such a regimen. Notable disadvantages include prolonged respiratory depression that may extend beyond the duration of anesthetic, a high incidence of clinically significant muscle rigidity on induction, and frequent reports of intraoperative awareness and recall when opioids are used as the sole anesthetic agent. (See page 508: Pharmacodynamics: Fentanyl.)

21. **C.** Opioids may cause respiratory depression by at least two mechanisms: (a) Suppression of respiratory neurons in the brainstem and (b) occlusion of upper airways due to a decrease in muscle tone. Depression of chemo and arousal reflexes by opioids may lead to a delayed upper airway obstruction responsible for recurrent periods of hypoxemia, commonly seen after the first few postoperative nights. Current data suggest that apneic events resulting in recurrent hypoxemia may occur up to the fifth postoperative night. Safety or Utility Function (UFos) curves are used to compare various opioids by assessing their side effect potential relative to their analgesic properties. Utility Functions are also useful in choosing the right opioid for specific patients. Naloxone, the drug of choice for opioid-induced respiratory depression causes a parallel rightward shift of the dose–response curve of the opioid responsible for respiratory depression. (See page 515: Opioid-induced Respiratory Depression, Figure 15.)

22. **D.** Remifentanil is rapidly metabolized by blood and tissue esterases to a substantially less-active compound. The duration of the respiratory depression seen with remifentanil has been shown to parallel the duration of its analgesic effects. The side effects of remifentanil, including a high incidence of muscle rigidity with high doses, are similar to those of other commonly used opioids at equianalgesic doses. When used for labor analgesia, remifentanil can be used either as intermittent boluses in a dose range between 20 and 40 μg with a 3-minute time interval, or as a constant infusion, based on the provider's clinical judgment. Although an ultrashort duration of action makes remifentanil an appealing agent for opioid infusion techniques and ease of titration, this characteristic poses a potential disadvantage because patients may require additional analgesics very soon after remifentanil is discontinued. Loss of consciousness is not reliably achieved with remifentanil alone. (See page 508: Pharmacodynamics: Remifentanil, Remifentanil for Obstetric Labor Pain.)

23. **C.** Naloxone is a pure opioid antagonist at μ-, κ-, and δ-opioid receptors that is used most often in clinical practice to antagonize opioid-induced respiratory depression and sedation. Since naloxone antagonizes all opioid-receptor interactions, it interrupts μ- and κ-receptor–mediated analgesia and may lead to severe pain. In some instances, acute, and sometimes fatal, pulmonary edema may ensue, an effect that is believed to result from a centrally mediated catecholamine release causing acute pulmonary hypertension. Since the duration of clinical effect seen with naloxone ranges from 1 to 4 hours, it is possible for renarcotization to occur when pre-existing opioids reactivate receptors after the effects of naloxone have subsided. (See page 510: Naloxone, Opioid-induced Respiratory Depression.)

24. **C.** Pharmacogenetics is defined as the effect of genetic variations on drug response. Variations in the gene coding for P-glycoprotein, a protein involved in the efflux of xenobiotic molecules, results in lesser efficacy of the variant protein to transport *Fentanyl* out of the brain resulting in greater respiratory depression. In patients with an inactive gene which codes for CYP2D6, this results in inability to convert the prodrug *Codeine,* into morphine-–its active component thus providing minimal or none analgesia from codeine. The antagonism of opioid induces toxic effects by *Naloxone* has not been shown to exhibit a pharmacogenetic variation. Specific genetic mutations in certain red-head individuals could lead to an increase in μ-opioid analgesia. Such phenotypes have also been shown to be resistant to the effects of midazolam and inhalation agents. (See page 515: Pharmacogenetics.)

Neuromuscular Blocking Agents

1. All of the following statements regarding a peripheral nerve are true EXCEPT:

   A. It is made up of a large number of axons of different threshold potentials.
   B. Each axon responds in an all-or-none fashion to a given stimulus.
   C. When a stimulating current reaches a high enough level, all axons are activated, and the amplitude of the action potential reaches a maximum level.
   D. There is a linear relationship between the amplitude of the muscle contraction and the current applied.
   E. Sodium channels in the nerve axon are activated in response to electrical stimulation.

2. The duration of the current delivered by a nerve stimulator should be approximately:

   A. 0.2 seconds
   B. 0.02 seconds
   C. 0.2 milliseconds
   D. 0.02 milliseconds
   E. 2 milliseconds

3. Which of the following statements regarding acetylcholine (Ach) is FALSE?

   A. The amount of Ach released with repetitive stimulation decreases.
   B. Calcium is required for vesicle binding to docking proteins and subsequent release of Ach.
   C. The action of magnesium augments the release of Ach from vesicle stores.
   D. Ach is released in quanta, each of which contains 5,000 to 10,000 molecules.
   E. In the absence of stimulation, a small amount of Ach is released at random.

4. With regard to the Acetylcholine receptors, which of the following is INCORRECT?

   A. Adult type Ach receptors at the neuromuscular junction have the conformation $(\alpha,\alpha,\beta,\varepsilon,\sigma)$.
   B. Immature or fetal Ach receptors at the neuromuscular junction have the conformation $(\alpha,\alpha,\beta,\gamma,\sigma)$.
   C. Acetylcholine receptors at the neuromuscular junction are classified as muscarinic.
   D. Depolarization requires acetylcholine to bind to both α receptors.

   E. Maintenance of adult type receptors at the neuromuscular junction is dependent upon continued nerve supply.

5. Which of the following statements regarding neuromuscular blocking drugs (NMBDs) is FALSE?

   A. The ED_{50} is the median dose corresponding to a 50% depression in twitch.
   B. The ED_{95} corresponds to the dose required to achieve neuromuscular blockade in 95% of patients.
   C. The ED_{95} of vecuronium is approximately 0.05 mg/kg.
   D. The time to maximal neuromuscular blockade can be shortened if the dose of NMBD is increased.
   E. The recovery index is the time interval between 25% and 75% of twitch height recovery.

6. Which of the following statements regarding the depolarizing blockade produced by succinylcholine is FALSE?

   A. During phase I block, fade in response to train-of-four (TOF) stimulus is not observed.
   B. Cholinesterase inhibitors do not antagonize phase II block.
   C. After administration of a 7 to 10 mg/kg dose of succinylcholine, TOF and tetanic fade typically become apparent.
   D. The prevalence of fasciculations after injection of succinylcholine is greater than 50%.
   E. Sinus bradycardia in response to succinylcholine is more common in children than in adults.

7. Regarding the clinical use of succinylcholine, all of the following statements are true EXCEPT:

   A. Infants and children are relatively resistant to succinylcholine compared with adults.
   B. The duration of neuromuscular blockade produced by succinylcholine is significantly increased in patients homozygous for an atypical form of plasma cholinesterase.
   C. Increases in serum potassium levels after succinylcholine injection can be mitigated by precurarization.
   D. Precurarization may be effective at blocking the increase in intragastric pressure observed after succinylcholine administration.
   E. At a dose of 1 mg/kg, the duration of action of succinylcholine is approximately 5 to 6 minutes.

8. All of the following statements regarding the pharmacokinetics of nondepolarizing neuromuscular blocking drugs (NMBDs) are true EXCEPT:

   A. Termination of the clinical effects of vecuronium depends primarily on redistribution rather than elimination.
   B. Termination of the clinical effects of cisatracurium depends primarily on elimination.
   C. The volume of distribution of most nondepolarizing NMBDs is approximately equal to extracellular fluid (ECF) volume.
   D. More potent drugs have a faster onset of action than less potent agents.
   E. The onset and duration of action are determined by the concentration of drug at its site of action.

9. Which of the following muscle groups demonstrates the earliest recovery from neuromuscular blockade after administration of an anticholinesterase agent?

   A. Adductor pollicis
   B. Diaphragm
   C. Geniohyoid
   D. Pharyngeal
   E. Flexor hallucis

10. Which of the following is an acetylcholinesterase inhibitor with an onset of action most similar to atropine?

    A. Glycopyrrolate
    B. Edrophonium
    C. Neostigmine
    D. Pyridostigmine
    E. Physostigmine

11. All of the following are side effects associated with anticholinesterase drugs EXCEPT:

    A. Increased salivation
    B. Increased peristalsis
    C. Bradycardia
    D. Bronchodilation
    E. Increased bladder motility

12. All of the following statements about Sugammadex are true EXCEPT:

    A. Sugammadex has no effect on succinylcholine.
    B. Concerns of hypersensitivity reactions are associated with sugammadex administration.
    C. Sugammadex acts on neuromuscular blocking agents that do not contain a steroid nucleus.
    D. In larger doses, sugammadex is an effective agent when neuromuscular blockade is deep.
    E. Sugammadex has no known major cardiovascular side effects.

13. The following statements about the nondepolarizing neuromuscular blocking drugs (NMDBs) are true EXCEPT:

    A. Laudanosine is a metabolite of cisatracurium.
    B. Pancuronium is associated with histamine release.
    C. Mivacurium is metabolized by plasma cholinesterase.
    D. *d*-tubocurarine causes histamine induced hypotension.
    E. Atracurium is metabolized by plasma cholinesterase.

14. Which of the following statements identifies an INCORRECT interaction with neuromuscular blockers?

    A. Volatile agents augment nondepolarizing drugs.
    B. Magnesium augments the effects of nondepolarizing agents.
    C. Pancuronium inhibits succinylcholine.
    D. Aminoglycosides prolong actions of neuromuscular blockers.
    E. Metoclopramide prolongs the action of succinylcholine and mivacurium.

15. The following statements regarding myasthenia gravis are true EXCEPT:

    A. They often demonstrate resistance to depolarizing neuromuscular blocking drugs.
    B. They often demonstrate resistance to nondepolarizing NMBDs.
    C. Anticholinesterase drugs are often part of the treatment.
    D. They demonstrate a voltage decrement in response to repeated stimulation at 2 to 5 Hz.
    E. Myasthenia gravis is an autoimmune disease in which the number of functional postsynaptic acetylcholine receptors is decreased.

16. The following scenarios represent patients at increased risk of hyperkalemia in response to succinylcholine administration EXCEPT:

    A. A 57-year-old woman who sustained extensive burns 1 week ago.
    B. A 20-year-old patient with T12 paralysis after a motor vehicle collision 1 month ago.
    C. A 70-year-old man 1 month following a debilitating stroke.
    D. A 40-year-old woman diagnosed with myasthenia gravis 1 year ago.
    E. A 40-year-old male with myotonic dystrophy.

17. Which of the following statements regarding train-of-four (TOF) response monitoring of the degree of nondepolarizing neuromuscular blockade is FALSE?

    A. The second twitch reappears when approximately 80% to 90% of receptors remain blocked.
    B. The third twitch reappears when approximately 70% to 80% of receptors remain blocked.
    C. All four twitches are visible when 65% to 75% of receptors are blocked.
    D. The single-twitch height has recovered to about 100% when the TOF ratio is approximately 70%.
    E. After a TOF, 10 minutes must elapse until another TOF can be attempted.

18. Regarding the differential impact of neuromuscular blocking drugs on specific muscle groups, which of the following statements is FALSE?

    A. The adductor pollicis is relatively resistant to NDMRs compared with the diaphragm.
    B. Facial nerve stimulation with monitoring of response in the eyebrow may be performed with currents of 20 to 30 mA.
    C. Recovery occurs more slowly in the adductor pollicis than in the diaphragm.
    D. The diaphragm and laryngeal muscles are relatively resistant to nondepolarizing agents.
    E. Stimulation of the posterior tibial nerve and observed contraction of the flexor hallucis muscle can be performed with results similar to that of the adductor pollicis muscle.

19. Which of the following acetylcholinesterase inhibitors can cross the blood–brain barrier?

    A. Edrophonium
    B. Pyridostigmine
    C. Neostigmine
    D. Physostigmine
    E. Atropine

ANSWERS

1. D. A peripheral nerve is made up of a large number of axons of different thresholds and sizes. Each axon responds in an all-or-none fashion, but not all axons may respond to a given stimulus. The relationship between the amplitude of the muscle contraction and the current applied is sigmoid, not linear. At low currents, an insufficient number of axons are depolarized. As the current increases, increasingly more axons are depolarized to threshold, and the strength of the muscle contraction increases up to a maximum level. The mechanism of action of nerve cell activation is via the opening of sodium channels. (See page 525: Physiology and Pharmacology: Structure.)

2. C. The duration of the current delivered by a nerve stimulator should be 0.1 to 0.2 milliseconds. At low currents, depolarization is insufficient in all axons. At a certain current threshold, recruitment of axons occurs until all axons are depolarized, propagating an action potential and muscle contraction. Additional current beyond this point is considered supramaximal as no additional muscle contraction can be achieved. (See page 525: Physiology and Pharmacology: Nerve Stimulation.)

3. C. Ach is packaged into 45-nm vesicles, each of which contains 5,000 to 10,000 molecules of Ach. Ach is spontaneously released in small quantities called quanta, producing miniature end plate potentials. When an action potential reaches the nerve terminal, about 200 to 400 quanta are released simultaneously, causing a rapid increase in the concentration of Ach at the motor end plate. Calcium enters the nerve terminals through channels that open in response to depolarization and is responsible for release of Ach from vesicles. Magnesium antagonizes the action of calcium and causes inhibition of Ach release. A few of the 75,000 to 100,000 Ach vesicles are available for immediate release. With repetitive stimulation, stored Ach vesicles are released. However, with continued stimulation, the amount of Ach released decreases rapidly. (See page 525: Physiology and Pharmacology: Release of Acetylcholine.)

4. C. Acetylcholine receptors are classified as nicotinic and have two basic conformations. The adult type has a conformation of $(\alpha,\alpha,\beta,\varepsilon,\sigma)$ and an immature of fetal type has a $(\alpha,\alpha,\beta,\gamma,\sigma)$ conformation. Adult type receptors are confined to the neuromuscular junction while immature receptors are found at the neuromuscular junction and along the whole length of the muscle fiber. In humans, the switch from immature or fetal type receptors to adult receptors occurs during the third trimester. Maintenance of the Ach receptors requires an intact nerve supply. Acetylcholine must bind to both α receptors for the receptor to function. After Ach binds to both α receptors, the inner channel opens allowing influx of sodium ions. At a critical point of sodium ion concentration, an action potential occurs along the muscle fibers entire length and a muscle contraction is obtained. Additional stimulation before relaxation from the previous contraction results in a fusion of contraction and tetanus. (See page 525: Physiology and Pharmacology: Postsynaptic Events.)

5. B. The ED_{50} and ED_{95} are two measures of NMBD potency. The ED_{50} is the median dose corresponding to a 50% depression in twitch. The ED_{95}, a more clinically relevant measure of potency, is defined as the amount of drug that produces a 95% block of a single twitch in 50% of patients. For example, the ED_{95} of vecuronium is approximately 0.05 mg/kg. The time needed to reach maximal neuromuscular blockade and duration of block are both affected by amount of drug administered. The duration of action is the time from injection to the return of 25% of a single twitch. Increasing the dose can prolong this time. The recovery index is the time from 25% to 75% twitch height, which is relatively constant. The ED_{95}, onset time, duration of action, and recovery index vary by muscle group monitored. (See page 529: Neuromuscular Blocking Agents: Pharmacologic Characteristics of Neuromuscular Blocking Agents.)

6. B. Administration of a usual intubating dose of succinylcholine produces a phase I block marked by a decrease in single-twitch height, but sustained response to high-frequency stimulation and minimal, if any, TOF or tetanic fade. Inhibitors of acetylcholinesterase potentiate phase I blockade. After administration of larger doses of succinylcholine (7–10 mg/kg) or within 30 to 60 minutes after initiating infusion, TOF and tetanic fade typically become apparent. This is referred to as phase II blockade. In contrast to phase I block, acetylcholinesterase inhibitors can antagonize phase II block. Succinylcholine produces a number of characteristic side effects. Fasciculations in response to succinylcholine injection occur in 60% to 90% of patients and can often be reduced with the prior administration of a small dose of a nondepolarizing neuromuscular blocking drug such as rocuronium. Sinus bradycardia with nodal or ventricular escape beats is a relatively common cardiovascular side effect, more so in children than adults. (See page 530: Depolarizing Drugs: Characteristics of Depolarizing Blockade.)

7. C. Succinylcholine is the only depolarizing neuromuscular blocking drug (DMR) regularly used in clinical practice. It has an onset of action of approximately 30 to 60 seconds and a duration of action of 5 to 6 minutes, making it a useful agent for rapid sequence intubations and for patients in whom prolonged muscle relaxation is not desired. Side effects commonly observed after administration of a neuromuscular blocking drug include muscle fasciculations and an elevation of intragastric, intraocular, and intracranial pressures. The risk of aspiration by an increase in intragastric pressure is offset by a stronger increase in the lower esophageal tone, provided competence of the sphincter. Succinylcholine increases intraocular pressure by 5 to 15 mm Hg and should be used with caution in open globe injuries. Intracranial pressure may be increased to some degree. These reactions can be inconsistently blocked by the prior administration of a small dose of NDMR (precurarization). Succinylcholine also increases serum potassium levels by approximately 0.5 mEq/L. This effect is not prevented by precurarization. Therefore, succinylcholine should be used with caution in patients at risk of developing clinically significant hyperkalemia. Succinylcholine is metabolized by plasma cholinesterase. Patients with atypical versions of this enzyme experience prolongation of neuromuscular blockade caused by succinylcholine. The prolongation is clinically significant in patients who are homozygous for atypical cholinesterase. (See page 530: Depolarizing Drugs: Succinylcholine.)

8. D. The duration of action of NMBDs is a function of either their elimination from the body or redistribution away from the site of effect. Cisatracurium is an intermediate-duration drug whose effects are terminated as a result of elimination. By contrast, vecuronium has a long elimination half-life but an intermediate effect duration as a result of redistribution away from the motor end plate. The volume of distribution of nondepolarizing NMBDs is about equal to the volume of the ECF compartment. The onset and duration of action of most NMBDs are determined by the time required for drug concentrations to reach a critical level at their site of action. Drug concentration at the effect site approximately parallels plasma concentration, but drug onset lags slightly behind peak plasma concentration. More potent drugs actually have slower onsets of action than less potent ones because there are fewer molecules of the more potent agent than of an equivalent dose of a less potent agent. (See page 533: Nondepolarizing Drugs: Pharmacokinetics and page 507: Onset and Duration of Action.)

9. B. The diaphragm exhibits the most rapid recovery from neuromuscular blockade. Recovery of upper airway and pharyngeal muscles (e.g., geniohyoid) and the flexor hallucis muscle generally parallels that of the adductor pollicis. (See page 543: Monitoring Neuromuscular Blockade: Choice of Muscle.)

10. B. Anticholinergic agents such as atropine and glycopyrrolate are frequently administered with neuromuscular reversal agents to blunt the cardiovascular effects of vagal stimulation produced by reversal agents. To achieve the best effect, agents with similar pharmacokinetics should be paired. The onset of action of atropine is rapid (~1 minute) and closely parallels that of edrophonium. The onset of action of neostigmine is about 7 to 11 minutes, and pyridostigmine's onset of action is 15 to 20 minutes. Physostigmine has an onset of about 5 minutes. It is not used as a neuromuscular reversal agent because of its central side effects. The pharmacokinetic profile of glycopyrrolate (onset, 2–3 minutes) is most similar to that of neostigmine. (See page 549: Reversal of Neuromuscular Block.)

11. D. Anticholinesterase agents produce vagal stimulation, leading to bradycardia and bradyarrhythmia. Other cholinergic effects observed with anticholinesterase drugs include

increased salivation and increased bladder and bowel motility. Anticholinesterases may also be associated with bronchoconstriction, not bronchodilation. (See page 549: Reversal of Neuromuscular Block.)

12. C. Sugammadex (previously referred to as ORG 25969) is a large γ-cyclodextrin that reverses neuromuscular blockade by binding to neuromuscular blocking agents in the plasma, which decreases the free or unbound drug in the plasma. Sugammadex selectively binds neuromuscular blocking agents containing a steroid nucleus such as rocuronium, vecuronium, and pancuronium. There are no known major cardiovascular side effects because it does not bind to any known receptors. In larger doses, sugammadex can be given immediately following large doses of steroidal NDMRs without the need for monitoring or concern for residual paralysis. If sugammadex becomes widely available, succinylcholine may become somewhat obsolete for intubation. (See page 549: Reversal of Neuromuscular Block.)

13. B. Laudanosine is a compound produced by the ester hydrolysis of atracurium and to a lesser degree by cisatracurium; it has been linked to seizure activity in animals. Similar to succinylcholine, mivacurium is metabolized by plasma cholinesterase. Several of the nondepolarizing NMBDs are associated with histamine release, which may cause transient hypotension after administration. Hypotension is frequently observed following *d*-tubocurarine administration, primarily because of histamine release; however, autonomic ganglionic blockade may be a contributor. Pancuronium does not release histamine, but it may cause a transient increase in catecholamine release, leading to a temporary increase in heart rate, blood pressure, and cardiac output. (See page 533: Nondepolarizing Drugs: Individual Nondepolarizing Agents.)

14. C. Volatile agents potentiate the effect of the neuromuscular blocking drugs and decrease the maintenance dose of NDMR. Most intravenous agents do not have an appreciable effect on neuromuscular blocking drugs. Aminoglycosides (neomycin and streptomycin) and polymyxins also potentiate NDMR by inhibiting neuromuscular function. Erythromycin, penicillin, and metronidazole, however, do not produce this effect. Administration of small amounts of NDMR prior to succinylcholine generally decreases the potency of the succinylcholine. With pancuronium, the effect of the succinylcholine is increased as it inhibits plasma cholinesterase. Metoclopramide also inhibits plasma cholinesterase and thus prolongs the action of succinylcholine and mivacurium. Calcium is required for the release of acetylcholine. This reaction is antagonized by magnesium and results in a decreased maintenance dose of NDMR. (See page 540: Drug Interactions.)

15. B. Myasthenia gravis is an autoimmune disorder characterized by the production of antibodies to postsynaptic acetylcholine receptors. The number of acetylcholine (Ach) quanta at the neuromuscular junction is normal or increased. The characteristic electromyographic finding in patients with myasthenia gravis is a voltage decrement in response to repeated stimulation at the 2- to 5-Hz level. Patients with myasthenia gravis have unpredictable responses to NMBDs. They are often resistant to succinylcholine, partly because of the presence of higher concentrations of Ach at the motor end plate. In contrast, sensitivity and prolonged duration of action are usually observed in response to NDMR, as a result of the decreased number of functional Ach receptors present on postsynaptic membranes. (See page 541: Altered Responses to Neuromuscular Blocking Agents: Myasthenia Gravis.)

16. **D.** An exaggerated increase in serum potassium concentration after succinylcholine administration is common in children with muscular dystrophies. The risk also occurs in children with subclinical symptoms (as they are undiagnosed); however, the receptor changes may have already occurred. Hyperkalemia may also be observed as early as 24 to 48 hours after extensive burn injuries; this response usually lessens with healing. In addition, patients with upper motor neuron lesions are more susceptible to hyperkalemia induced by succinylcholine. This response is most prominent when the drug is given 1 week to 6 months after injury, although it may occur at any time. In patients with myotonia, delayed muscle relaxation following muscle contraction can result in hyperkalemia. Hyperkalemia after succinylcholine administration is not typically associated with myasthenia gravis. (See page 530: Depolarizing Drugs: Side Effects.)

17. **E.** TOF response monitoring to nondepolarizing neuromuscular blockade involves the application of four stimuli at 0.5-second intervals (2 Hz). Recovery from neuromuscular block is measured by the return of response to these stimuli. In general, the first twitch reappears if less than 90% of receptors are blocked. The second twitch appears when 80% to 90% of receptors remain blocked, and the third appears when 70% to 80% are blocked. All four responses are usually visible when there is less than 65% to 75% receptor blockade. At this time, single-twitch height has recovered to approximately 100% of pre-relaxant height, and the height of T4 increases to approximately 70% of the height of T1. TOF can be repeated every 12 to 15 seconds in contrast with a tetanus of 50 Hz for 5-second duration which requires at least 1 to 2 minutes before repeating the tetanus. (See page 543: Monitoring Neuromuscular Block: Monitoring Modalities.)

18. **A.** Muscle groups demonstrate a differential response to muscle relaxants. The adductor pollicis is relatively sensitive to NDMRs while the diaphragm and laryngeal muscles are relatively resistant. With recovery, the adductor pollicis recovery is slower that that of the laryngeal muscles and diaphragm, imparting a degree of safety. The time to maximal blockade occurs somewhat longer in the adductor pollicis compared with the more centrally located airway muscles. Facial nerve stimulation with response monitored in the eyebrow is thought to be indicative of the action of the corrugator supercilii muscle. The impact of NDMRs on this muscle approximates that of the laryngeal adductors, so response monitoring to eyebrow movement may be a reliable predictor of adequate intubating conditions. However, monitoring in the supraorbital region may pose some technical difficulties. (See page 543: Monitoring Neuromuscular Block: Choice of Muscle.)

19. **D.** Neostigmine, edrophonium, and pyridostigmine are all charged quaternary ammonium compounds that do not cross the blood–brain barrier. Physostigmine is an uncharged molecule that can cross the blood–brain barrier and is therefore not used to reverse muscle relaxation. Atropine is not an acetylcholinesterase inhibitor but can cross the blood–brain barrier. (See page 549: Reversal of Neuromuscular Block.)

CHAPTER

21

Local Anesthetics

1. Which statement regarding myelinated nerves is FALSE?

    A. They have a diameter greater than 1 μm.
    B. They are surrounded by Schwann cells, which account for more than half of the nerve's thickness.
    C. They conduct impulses more slowly than similar-sized unmyelinated nerves.
    D. They have both afferent and efferent functions.
    E. The nodes of Ranvier are covered by negatively charged glycoproteins.

2. Which statement regarding neuronal conduction is FALSE?

    A. The resting membrane potential is predominantly maintained by a potassium gradient with at least ten times greater intracellular concentration of potassium.
    B. Generation of action potentials is primarily the result of activation of voltage-gated sodium channels.
    C. Impulse generation is an all-or-nothing phenomenon.
    D. A three-state kinetic scheme conceptualizes the change in sodium channel conformation and accounts for changes in sodium conductance during depolarization and repolarization.
    E. The resting membrane potential of neural membranes averages −30 to −40 mV.

3. The rate of absorption of local anesthetic upon injection to various sites generally increases in the following order:

    A. Intercostal, caudal, epidural, brachial plexus, sciatic/femoral
    B. Caudal, intercostal, epidural, brachial plexus, sciatic/femoral
    C. Intercostal, epidural, caudal, brachial plexus, sciatic/femoral
    D. Sciatic/femoral, brachial plexus, epidural, caudal, intercostal
    E. Intercostal, brachial plexus, epidural, caudal, sciatic/femoral

4. Which of the following about local anesthetics is FALSE?

    A. They are weak bases.
    B. The charged form of local anesthetics is lipid soluble.
    C. They have substituted benzene rings.
    D. They contain either an ester or amide linkage.
    E. They exert their effects on the intracellular side of the sodium channel.

5. Which statement concerning pKa is FALSE?

    A. The pKa is the dissociation constant.
    B. When the pH equals the pKa of a compound, 50% of it is neutral and 50% of it is charged.
    C. Increasing the pKa of a local anesthetic increases the lipid-soluble form.
    D. Onset of action is slowed by increasing the pKa.
    E. Knowing the pKa of a local anesthetic allows one to predict the relative speed of its onset of action.

6. Which statement regarding the cardiovascular toxicity of bupivacaine is FALSE?

    A. Vasodilation is a prominent feature.
    B. Bupivacaine quickly dissociates from cardiac sodium channels during cardiac diastole.
    C. Cardiac myocyte release and utilization of calcium are inhibited.
    D. Mitochondrial energy metabolism is reduced.
    E. The cardiotoxicity of bupivacaine may be mediated centrally and peripherally.

7. Which statement concerning clearance and elimination of local anesthetics is FALSE?

    A. Ester local anesthetics are primarily cleared by plasma cholinesterases.
    B. Local anesthetics with higher rates of clearance have greater margins of safety.
    C. Renal disease is important in altering the pharmacokinetic parameters of local anesthetics.
    D. Protein binding of amino amide local anesthetics is important in determining the rate of clearance.
    E. Correlation of resultant systemic blood levels between the dose of local anesthetic and the patient's weight is often inconsistent.

8. Which statement concerning treatment of systemic toxicity from local anesthetics is FALSE?

    A. Signs of central nervous system (CNS) toxicity typically occur before cardiovascular events.
    B. Propofol can terminate seizures from systemic local anesthetic toxicity.
    C. Succinylcholine (Sch) may terminate seizure activity.
    D. Ventricular dysrhythmias may be difficult to treat.
    E. Amiodarone is indicated in the treatment of bupivacaine toxicity.

9. Which statement concerning transient neurologic symptoms (TNS) after spinal anesthesia is FALSE?

   A. An increased risk of TNS is associated with lidocaine.
   B. The baricity of the local anesthetic is an important factor in the development of TNS.
   C. The dose of local anesthetic is not an important factor in the development of TNS.
   D. TNS may be a manifestation of subclinical neurotoxicity.
   E. The incidence of TNS varies with patient position.

10. Which of the following statements is FALSE?

   A. Bupivacaine 0.75% is not an acceptable concentration for obstetric use.
   B. Central nervous system (CNS) toxicity is more common with epidural local anesthetic injection than with peripheral nerve blocks.
   C. Levobupivacaine is approximately equipotent to racemic bupivacaine.
   D. Both ropivacaine and levobupivacaine appear to have approximately 30% to 40% less systemic toxicity than bupivacaine on a milligram-to-milligram basis.
   E. Levobupivacaine is an isomer of bupivacaine.

11. All of the following local anesthetics are racemic mixtures EXCEPT:

   A. Lidocaine
   B. Bupivacaine
   C. Mepivacaine
   D. Tetracaine
   E. Chloroprocaine

12. Which of the following statements concerning spinal administration of opioids is TRUE?

   A. It is primarily dependent on supraspinal mechanisms.
   B. Combining a local anesthetic with opioids results in synergistic analgesia.
   C. 2-chloroprocaine increases the summative effectiveness when co-administered with opioids epidurally.
   D. Spinal administration of opioids provides analgesia primarily by attenuating the $\alpha\delta$ fiber nociception.

13. Which of the following is TRUE regarding additives used to enhance local anesthetic activity?

   A. Co-administration of clonidine results in exclusively supraspinal neuraxial synergy.
   B. Dexamethasone will prolong the duration of anesthesia after a brachial plexus block using ropivacaine.
   C. Clonidine would improve the duration of neuraxial analgesia by at least 8 hours.
   D. The largest clinical effect of adding epinephrine is an increase in the intensity of local anesthetic block.

14. Which of the following concerning local anesthetics is FALSE?

   A. pKa determines the onset of action.
   B. Lipophilicity influences potency.
   C. Protein binding influences the peak blood levels.
   D. Clinically used local anesthetics can be alkalinized beyond a pH of 9 for best possible clinical results.

15. Which one of the following regarding systemic absorption and peak blood levels of local anesthetic is FALSE?

   A. It is linearly related to the total dose of local anesthetic injected.
   B. It is reduced with the addition of epinephrine, especially for the less lipid-soluble, less potent, shorter-acting agents.
   C. It is diminished with the more potent agents with greater lipid solubility and protein binding.
   D. It is highly dependent on the anesthetic concentration.

16. Which of the following statements concerning the central nervous system (CNS) toxicity of local anesthetics is TRUE?

   A. In general, decreased local anesthetic protein binding decreases potential CNS toxicity.
   B. Low plasma concentrations usually result in CNS excitatory effects.
   C. Highly potent lipophilic agents cause CNS excitatory effects only at higher doses.
   D. Seizure threshold may be increased by the administration of benzodiazepines.

17. Which of the following statements regarding the cardiovascular toxicity of local anesthetics is FALSE?

   A. In general, much greater doses of local anesthetics are required to produce cardiovascular toxicity than neurotoxicity.
   B. Bupivacaine cardiovascular toxicity is resistant to resuscitation.
   C. All local anesthetics disturb the cardiac conduction system by a dose dependent blockade of the sodium channels.
   D. Generally, the less potent, but more water-soluble agents are more cardiotoxic.

18. Which of the following is TRUE regarding the use of intravenous lipid to treat local anesthetic toxicity?

   A. Its efficacy to hasten cardiac function is limited to only bupivacaine-induced toxicity.
   B. Current evidence only supports its use to reverse lidocaine-induced asystole.
   C. It acts by absorption of the tissue-bound local anesthetic via a plasma–tissue partition mechanism.
   D. An initial bolus of 3 mL/kg of 20% lipid emulsion is recommended.

19. Which of the following statements concerning allergic reactions to local anesthetics is FALSE?

   A. True allergic reactions to local anesthetics are rare.
   B. Allergic reactions to local anesthetics usually involve nonworrisome type I reactions.
   C. The allergenic potential of esters may result from hydrolytic metabolism to para-aminobenzoic acid.
   D. Reactions are more common with ester than with amide local anesthetics.

20. Which of the following is NOT a clinical indication for the use of a specific local anesthetic?

   A. Eutectic mixture of levobupivacaine and lidocaine for topical anesthesia.
   B. Intravenous lidocaine to blunt the hemodynamic response to tracheal intubation.
   C. Aerosolized benzocaine to blunt airway instrumentation.
   D. Viscous lidocaine to blunt airway instrumentation.

ANSWERS

1. **C.** Myelinated nerves generally conduct impulses faster than unmyelinated nerves. The presence of myelin accelerates conduction velocity by increased electrical isolation of nerve fibers and by saltatory conduction. Increased nerve diameter accelerates conduction velocity both by increased myelination and by improved electrical cable conduction properties of the nerve. Myelinated and unmyelinated nerves carry both afferent and efferent functions. All nerves with a diameter larger than 1 μm are myelinated. Myelinated nerve fibers in the peripheral nervous system are segmentally enclosed by Schwann cells forming a bilipid membrane that is wrapped several hundred times around each axon. Myelinated nerve fibers in the central nervous system are segmentally enclosed by oligodendrocytes. Thus, myelin accounts for more than half the thickness of large nerve fibers. The nodes of Ranvier are separated by the myelinated regions. The nodes are covered by interdigitations from unmyelinated Schwann cells and by negatively charged glycoproteins. (See page 561: Anatomy of Nerves.)

2. **E.** The resting potential of neural membranes averages −60 to −70 mV, with the interior being negative compared with the exterior. This resting potential is predominately maintained by a potassium gradient with a 10 times greater concentration of potassium within the cell. An active protein pump transports potassium into the cell and sodium out of the cell through voltage-gated potassium channels. Generation of an action potential is primarily the result of voltage-gated sodium channels. After activation (opening) of the sodium channel, it spontaneously closes into an inactive state and then reverts to a resting confirmation. Thus, a three-state kinetic scheme conceptualizes the changes in the sodium channel confirmation that account for shifts in sodium conductance during depolarization and repolarization. An action potential is generated when the depolarization threshold of an axon is reached. This threshold is not an absolute voltage but depends on the dynamics of the sodium and potassium channels. After an action potential is generated, propagation of the potential along nerve fibers is required for information to be transmitted. Both impulse generation and propagation are "all-or-nothing" phenomena. Unmyelinated fibers require achievement of threshold potential at the immediately adjacent membrane, but myelinated fibers require generation of threshold potential at a subsequent node of Ranvier. (See page 561: Electrophysiology of Neural Conduction and Voltage-gated Sodium Channels.)

3. **D.** In general, local anesthetics with decreased systemic absorption have a greater margin of safety in clinical use. The rate and extent of absorption depend on numerous factors; the most important factors are the site of injection, the dose of local anesthetic, the physicochemical properties of the local anesthetic, and the addition of epinephrine. The relative amount of fat and vasculature surrounding the site of injection interact with the physicochemical properties of the local anesthetic and affect the rate of systemic uptake. In general, areas with greater vascularity have more rapid and complete uptake than those with more fat, regardless of the type of local anesthetic. Hence, multiple injections near intercostal vascular bundles have a faster uptake than injections in the buttocks and groin. The greater the total dose of local anesthetic injected, the greater the systemic absorption and peak blood levels. (See page 566: Chemical Properties and Relationship to Activity and Potency.)

4. **B.** The clinically used local anesthetics consist of a lipid-soluble substituted benzene ring linked to an amine group (tertiary or quaternary, depending on the pKa and pH) via an alkyl chain containing either an amide or ester linkage. The type of linkage separates the local anesthetics into either amino amides, which are metabolized in the liver, or amino esters, which are metabolized by plasma cholinesterases. Several chemical properties of local anesthetics affect their efficacy and potency. All clinically used local anesthetics are weak bases that can exist as either the lipid-soluble (neutral) form or as the hydrophilic (charged) form. The primary site of action of local anesthetics appears to exist on the intracellular side of the sodium channel, and the charged form appears to be the predominately active form. Penetration of the lipid-soluble (neutral) form through the lipid neural membrane appears to be the primary form of access of local anesthetic molecules. Increased lipid solubility usually hastens the rate of onset of action, increases the duration of action, and increases potency. The degree of protein binding also affects activity of local anesthetics because only the unbound form is free to exert pharmacologic effect. In general, increased protein binding is associated with an increased duration of action. (See page 566: Chemical Properties and Relationship to Activity and Potency.)

5. **C.** The combination of pH of the environment and pKa, or dissociation constant, of a local anesthetic determines how much of the compound exists in each form. Decreasing the pKa for a given environmental pH increases the percentage of the lipid-soluble form and hastens penetration of neural membranes and hence the onset of action. (See page 566: Chemical Properties and Relationship to Activity and Potency.)

6. **B.** It has been demonstrated that the central and peripheral nervous systems are involved with the cardiotoxic effects of bupivacaine, which may be exacerbated by its potent direct vasodilating properties. Bupivacaine exhibits a much stronger binding affinity to resting and inactivated sodium channels than lidocaine. It dissociates from sodium channels during cardiac diastole much more slowly than lidocaine, so slowly that complete sodium channel recovery is not achieved and a bupivacaine conduction block accumulates. Bupivacaine also inhibits myocyte release and utilization of calcium and reduces

mitochondrial energy metabolism, especially during hypoxia. (See page 572: Toxicity of Local Anesthetics.)

7. **C.** Whereas clearance of ester local anesthetics is primarily dependent on plasma clearance by cholinesterase, amide local anesthetic clearance is dependent on hepatic metabolism. Thus, hepatic extraction, hepatic perfusion, hepatic metabolism, and protein binding primarily determine the rate of clearance of amide local anesthetics. In general, local anesthetics with higher rates of clearance have greater margins of safety. Renal disease has little effect on the pharmacokinetic parameters of local anesthetics. Correlation of the resulting systemic blood levels between the dose of local anesthetic and the patient's weight often is inconsistent. (See page 569: Pharmacokinetics of Local Anesthetics.)

8. **C.** Treatment of patients with systemic toxicity is primarily supportive. Injection of the local anesthetic should be stopped. Oxygenation and ventilation should be maintained because systemic toxicity of local anesthetics is enhanced by hypoxemia, hypercarbia, and acidosis. If needed, the patient's trachea should be intubated and positive-pressure ventilation instituted. Signs of CNS toxicity occur before cardiovascular events. Seizures may increase body metabolism and cause hypoxemia, hypercarbia, and acidosis (three well-known factors that further enhance the systemic toxicity of local anesthetics). Intravenous administration of thiopental, midazolam, and propofol may terminate seizures from systemic local anesthetic toxicity. Sch may terminate muscular activity from seizures and facilitate ventilation and oxygenation; however, Sch does not terminate seizure activity in the CNS, and increased cerebral metabolic demands continue unabated. Potent local anesthetics (e.g., bupivacaine) may produce profound cardiovascular depression and malignant dysrhythmias that should be treated promptly. Oxygenation and ventilation must be immediately instituted, with cardiopulmonary resuscitation used if needed. Ventricular dysrhythmias may be difficult to treat and may need sequential electrical cardioversion, and large doses of epinephrine, vasopressin, and amiodarone. (See page 575: Treatment of Systemic Toxicity from Local Anesthetics.)

9. **B.** There is a 4% to 40% incidence of TNS after lidocaine spinal anesthesia. All local anesthetics have the potential to be neurotoxic, particularly in higher concentrations, and symptoms have been reported with multiple agents. The incidence of TNS varies with the type of surgical procedure and positioning (particularly the lithotomy position). Apparently, the incidence is unaffected by the baricity or dose. Reports of cauda equina syndrome after spinal anesthesia have led several authors to label TNS as a manifestation of subclinical neural toxicity. Other potential causes of TNS include patient positioning, early mobilization, needle trauma, neural ischemia, pooling of local anesthetics, and the addition of glucose. Clearly, the cause of TNS remains undetermined, and further studies are needed to elucidate the underlying mechanism. (See page. 576: Transient Neurologic Symptoms After Spinal Anesthesia.)

10. **B.** Enhanced awareness of potential cardiovascular toxicity with long-acting local anesthetics led to withdrawal of Food and Drug Administration approval for high concentrations of bupivacaine (0.75%) for obstetric use in the United States. The incidence of CNS toxicity with epidural injection is approximately 1 in 10,000; with peripheral nerve blocks, it is 7 in 10,000. Levobupivacaine, an isomer of bupivacaine, appears to be approximately equally potent to racemic bupivacaine for epidural anesthesia. Both ropivacaine and levobupivacaine appear to have approximately 30% to 40% less toxicity than bupivacaine on a milligram-to-milligram basis in both animal and human volunteer studies. This is likely the result of reduced affinity in brain and myocardial tissue. (See page 572: Systemic Toxicity of Local Anesthetics: Central Nervous System Toxicity.)

11. **A.** All currently available local anesthetics, with the exception of lidocaine (achiral), ropivacaine, and levobupivacaine, are racemic mixtures. Stereoisomers of local anesthetics appear to have potentially different effects on anesthetic potency, pharmacokinetics, and systemic toxicity. For example, *R* isomers appear to have greater in vitro potency for blockade of both neural and cardiac sodium channels and may thus have greater therapeutic efficacy but a greater potential for systemic toxicity. (See page 566: Pharmacology and Pharmacodynamics.)

12. **B.** Opioids have multiple sites of action with both central and a peripheral mechanism of analgesic action but spinal administration of opioids provides analgesia primarily by attenuating C-fiber nociception and is independent of supraspinal mechanisms. Co-administration of opioids with most local anesthetics results in synergistic analgesia. An exception to this analgesic synergy is 2-chloroprocaine, which appears to decrease the effectiveness of epidural opioids when used for epidural anesthesia. The mechanism for this action is unclear but does not appear to involve direct anatomization of opioid receptors. (See page 567: Additives to increase Local Anesthetic activity > Opioids.)

13. **B.** Clonidine produces analgesia via supraspinal and spinal adrenergic receptors. It also has some direct inhibitory effects on peripheral nerve conduction in the A and C nerve fibers. Current literature reports the use of dexamethasone as an adjuvant to local anesthetics, which prolongs the duration of anesthesia after brachial plexus blockade, and intravenous regional anesthesia. Clonidine has been used as an adjuvant for neuraxial and peripheral administration of local anesthetics. On average, it has been reported to improve the duration of analgesia by about 2 hours when used with either intermediate or long-acting anesthetics. The main benefits of adding epinephrine is prolongation of the local anesthetic blockade; it also decreases systemic absorption of the anesthetic and increases in the intensity of the block. (See Page 567: Additives to increase Local Anesthetic Activity.)

14. **D.** pKa determines the onset of action for a local anesthetic. The pH of commercial preparations of local anesthetics ranges from 3.9 to 6.47 and is especially acidic if they are prepackaged with epinephrine. Since the pKa of

commonly used local anesthetics ranges from 7.6 to 8.9, less than 3% of the commercially prepared local anesthetic exists as the lipid-soluble neutral form. It is this neutral form that is important for the penetration into the cell and determines the onset of action. A positive co-relation exists between local anesthetic potency and its lipid solubility as determined by the degree of the alkyl group substitution on its amide group or benzene ring. The use of the more potent agents with high protein binding results in lower systemic absorption and lower peak blood levels. Clinically used local anesthetics cannot be alkalinized beyond a pH of 6.05 to 8 before precipitation occurs, and such a pH will increase the neutral form only to about 10%. (See page 569: Pharmacokinetics of Local Anesthetics and page 567: Alkalinization of Local Anesthetic Solution.)

15. **D.** The greater the total dose of local anesthetic injected, the greater the systemic absorption and peak blood levels will be, with the relationship following a linear pattern. Epinephrine may counteract the inherent vasodilating characteristics of most local anesthetics with the reduction in blood concentration most effective for the less lipid-soluble, less potent, shorter-acting agents. The rate of systemic absorption differs amongst individual local anesthetics with the more potent, lipid-soluble agents being associated with a slower rate of absorption. This dose–absorption relationship is relatively unaffected by the anesthetic concentration and speed of injection. (See page 569: Systemic Absorption and Additives to Increase Local Anesthetic Activity: Epinephrine.)

16. **D.** Decreases in local anesthetic protein binding and clearance increase potential CNS toxicity. Local anesthetics readily cross the blood–brain barrier, and generalized CNS toxicity may occur from systemic absorption or direct vascular injection. Signs of generalized CNS toxicity from local anesthetics are dependent on the plasma concentrations achieved. Low plasma concentrations cause mild disturbances in the sensory function; however as plasma concentration increases, excitatory effects predominate that may progress to generalized depression and coma. The rate of intravenous administration of local anesthetic also affects CNS toxicity where higher rates of infusion lessen the appearance of CNS depression while leaving excitation intact. Highly potent, lipid-soluble agents cause CNS toxicity at doses that are a fraction of those of less potent agents with the toxic potential being directly related to the potency of the local anesthetic. External factors such as acidosis and hypercarbia may increase CNS toxicity perhaps by increasing cerebral perfusion and decreasing protein binding of the local anesthetic. Seizure thresholds in response to local anesthetics may also be increased by co-administration of barbiturates or benzodiazepines. (See page 572: Toxicity of Local Anesthetics: Central Nervous System Toxicity and Tables 21-4 and 21-8.)

17. **D.** In general, much greater doses of local anesthetics are required to produce cardiovascular toxicity than central nervous system toxicity. Similar to CNS toxicity, the potency for cardiovascular toxicity reflects the anesthetic potency of the agent. Physiologically all local anesthetics disturb the cardiac conduction system by blocking the sodium channels in the myocardium in a dose dependent fashion. However, attention is now being focused on the apparently exceptional cardiotoxicity of the more potent, more lipid-soluble agents (bupivacaine, etidocaine). These agents appear to have a different sequence of cardiovascular toxicity than the less potent agents. For example, whereas increasing doses of lidocaine lead to hypotension, bradycardia, and hypoxia, bupivacaine often results in sudden cardiovascular collapse from ventricular dysrhythmias that are resistant to resuscitation. (See page 572: Toxicity of Local Anesthetics: Cardiovascular Toxicity of Local Anesthetics.)

18. **C.** The use of intravenous lipid emulsion (commonly referred to as Intralipid) hastens the recovery of normal cardiac function by reversing the cardiac toxicity of most of the local anesthetics, and is not limited to any one particular agent. Current evidence has clearly demonstrated that intravenous lipids are highly efficacious in reversing bupivacaine-induced asystole. The lipid emulsion, when introduced parentally, acts as a sink to absorb the local anesthetic which is bound to tissues, including cardiac tissue. This absorption and molecular transfer is based on tissue partition principles. Lipids also prove to be a rich energy source, which spares the cardiac mitochondrial machinery. Current evidence and guidelines suggest an initial bolus dose of 1.5 mL/kg of a 20% lipid emulsion. This can be followed by a continuous infusion or repeated bolusing depending on the return of cardiac function. (See Page 575: Treatment of Systemic Toxicity from Local Anesthetics and Table 21-12: Recommended Lipid Emulsion Dosing for Treatment of Local Anesthetic Cardiovascular Toxicity.)

19. **B.** True allergic reactions to local anesthetics are rare and usually involve type I (immunoglobulin E) or type IV (cellular immunity) reactions. Type I reactions are worrisome because anaphylaxis may occur which may lead to a life threatening critical incident. Such reactions are more common with ester than with amide local anesthetics. True allergy to amide agents is extremely rare. Increased allergenic potential with esters may result from hydrolytic metabolism to para-aminobenzoic acid (a documented allergen). Added preservatives, such as methylparaben and metabisulfite, may also provoke an allergic response. (See page 577: Allergic Reactions to Local Anesthetics.)

20. **A.** A eutectic mixture of Lidocaine and Prilocaine is commonly used to provide topical anesthesia to reduce the sharp, painful sensation associated with intravenous needle placement, particularly in the pediatric population. Lidocaine and bupivacaine are incompatible as a eutectic mixture. Intravenous lidocaine may be used to decrease the hemodynamic response to laryngoscopy, intubation and extubation. Aerosolized benzocaine or viscous lidocaine may be used to provide topical anesthesia of the mucosal surface and thus blunt the reflexive response during airway instrumentation in an awake patient. (See page 571: Clinical Use of Local Anesthetics.)

Preoperative Patient Assessment and Management

1. All of the following are important predictors of cardiac postoperative complications EXCEPT:

   A. Preoperative serum creatinine of 1 mg/dL
   B. History of cerebrovascular accident
   C. Preoperative treatment with insulin
   D. History of congestive heart failure
   E. Major vascular surgery

2. After an episode of asthma, airway hyperreactivity may persist up to:

   A. 24 hours
   B. 48 hours
   C. 72 hours
   D. 4 days
   E. Several weeks

3. The current recommendation of the National Blood Resource Education Committee is that a hemoglobin of _____ g/dL is acceptable in patients without systemic disease.

   A. 9
   B. 6
   C. 7
   D. 10
   E. 8

4. Which of the following tests, if done preoperatively in a patient without risk factors, can lead to more harm than benefit?

   A. Electrocardiography (ECG)
   B. Blood urea nitrogen (BUN)/creatinine
   C. Chest radiography (CXR)
   D. Urinalysis (U/A)
   E. None of the above

5. Postoperatively, functional residual capacity may take up to _____ to return to baseline.

   A. 24 hours
   B. 48 hours
   C. 3 days
   D. 7 days
   E. 14 days

6. As a general rule, oral medications should be given to the patient _____ before arrival in the operating room.

   A. 60 to 90 minutes
   B. 30 to 60 minutes
   C. 20 minutes
   D. 10 minutes
   E. 5 minutes

7. All of the following are true regarding patients with obstructive sleep apnea (OSA) EXCEPT:

   A. Chronic pulmonary hypertension and right heart failure may be present.
   B. Increased neck circumference is a risk factor.
   C. Patients with OSA are more susceptible to the respiratory depressant effects of narcotics.
   D. Initiation of continuous positive airway pressure (CPAP) preoperatively does not reduce the perioperative risk.
   E. Patients with OSA are considered to have difficult airways.

8. All of the following place a patient at documented risk for increased perioperative cardiovascular morbidity and should be considered in a preoperative evaluation EXCEPT:

   A. Peripheral arterial disease
   B. Diabetes mellitus
   C. Hypercholesterolemia
   D. Diminished exercise tolerance
   E. Critical stenosis of a single coronary artery

9. The hallmark features of Cushing syndrome include all of the following EXCEPT:

   A. Easy bruisability
   B. Truncal "obesity"
   C. Moon facies
   D. Hypotension
   E. Skin striations

10. All of the following herbal supplements can lead to bleeding abnormalities EXCEPT:

    A. Echinacea
    B. Garlic
    C. Ginkgo
    D. Chemotherapeutic agents
    E. Ginseng

11. A preoperative electrocardiogram (ECG) should be evaluated in all of the following patient populations EXCEPT:

    A. Patients with a prior myocardial infarction.
    B. Patients with a history of hypertension, diabetes mellitus, and peripheral vascular disease.
    C. Patients without cardiac risk factors who are about to undergo vascular surgery.
    D. All women older than 50 years of age.

12. Which of the following statements about cessation of smoking is TRUE?

    A. Stopping for 4 hours reduces the vast majority of carboxyhemoglobin.
    B. Cessation for 4 days is associated with increased mucociliary clearance.
    C. Cessation for 48 hours abolishes the effects of nicotine.
    D. Stopping for 1 week is sufficient to eliminate the increased incidence of postoperative pulmonary complications.

13. A resting echocardiogram provides information about all of the following EXCEPT:

    A. Coronary anatomy
    B. Regional wall motion
    C. Ventricular wall thickness
    D. Valvular function
    E. Ejection fraction

ANSWERS

1. **A.** The Revised Cardiac Risk Index identified six independent predictors of complications: High-risk type of surgery, history of ischemic heart disease, history of congestive heart failure, history of cerebrovascular disease, preoperative treatment with insulin, and preoperative serum creatinine above 2 mg/dL. (See page 588: Cardiovascular Disease.)

2. **E.** After an episode of asthma, airway hyperreactivity may persist for several weeks. (See page 595: Asthma.)

3. **C.** The current recommendation of the National Blood Resource Education Committee is that a hemoglobin of 7 g/dL is acceptable in patients without systemic disease. (See page 599: Complete Blood Count and Hemoglobin Concentration.)

4. **C.** A preoperative CXR can identify abnormalities that may lead to either a delay or a cancellation of the planned surgical procedure or modification of perioperative care. However, routine testing in the population without risk factors can lead to more harm than benefit. The American College of Physicians suggests that a CXR is indicated in the presence of active chest disease and before intrathoracic procedures but not solely on the basis of advanced age. (See page 594: Pulmonary Disease.)

5. **E.** Functional residual capacity may take up to 2 weeks to return to baseline. (See page 594: Pulmonary Disease.)

6. **A.** As a general rule, oral medications should be given to the patient 60 to 90 minutes before arrival in the operating room. It is acceptable to administer oral drugs with up to 150 mL of water. Intravenous agents produce effects after a few circulation times, but for full effect, intramuscular medications should be given at least 20 minutes and preferably 30 to 60 minutes before the patient's arrival in the operating room. (See page 603: Pharmacologic Preparation.)

7. **D.** Patients with OSA have chronic sleep deprivation, with daytime hypersomnolence and even behavioral changes in children. Depending on the frequency and severity of events, OSA may lead to changes such as chronic pulmonary hypertension and right heart failure. Increased neck circumference, body mass index above 35 kg/m^2, severe tonsillar hypertrophy, and anatomic abnormalities of the upper airway are factors commonly associated with OSA. These patients are especially susceptible to the respiratory depressant and airway effects of sedatives, narcotics, and inhaled anesthetics. Preoperative initiation of CPAP reduces the perioperative risk, and the difficult airway algorithm should be followed, with emergency airway equipment readily available. (See page 595: Obstructive Sleep Apnea.)

8. **C.** Peripheral arterial disease has been shown to be associated with coronary artery disease in multiple studies; at least 60% of the patients scheduled for major vascular surgery exhibit at least one coronary vessel with critical stenosis. Although a critical coronary stenosis delineates an area of risk for developing myocardial ischemia, this area may or may not be the underlying cause for a perioperative myocardial infarction that occurs. In the ambulatory population, many infarctions are the result of acute thrombosis of a noncritical stenosis. Several other factors associated with atherosclerosis have been used to suggest an increased probability of CAD. This includes hypercholesterolemia. Although hypercholesterolemia increases the probability of developing CAD, it has not been shown to increase perioperative cardiac risk. Diabetes mellitus is common in elderly individuals, represents a disease that affects multiple organ systems, is associated with coronary artery disease, and increases the chance of silent myocardial ischemia and infarction. If patients experience dyspnea associated with chest pain during minimal exertion, the probability of extensive coronary artery disease is high; this has been associated with greater perioperative risk. (See page 588: Cardiovascular Disease.)

9. **D.** The prolonged use of glucocorticoids may lead to Cushing syndrome. Truncal obesity, moon facies, skin striations, easy bruisability, and hypertension are hallmark signs of Cushing syndrome. Preoperative preparations include correction of fluid and electrolyte abnormalities (e.g., hypokalemia, hyperglycemia). In patients with long-term corticosteroid use, perioperative steroid supplementation is indicated to cover the stress of anesthesia and surgery. (See page 595: Endocrine Disease.)

10. **A.** Echinacea is associated with perioperative allergic reactions, decreased effectiveness of immunosuppressants, and immunosuppression with long-term use. Both garlic and gingko have the potential to increase the risk of bleeding, especially when combined with other medications that inhibit platelet aggregation. Ginseng has the potential to increase the risk of bleeding, and can potentially decrease the anticoagulant effect of warfarin. Hematologic effects of chemotherapy include decreased platelets. (See page 584: Approach to the Healthy Patient.)

11. **D.** The preoperative 12-lead ECG can provide important information on the status of the patient's myocardium and coronary circulation. Abnormal Q-waves in high-risk patients are highly suggestive of a past myocardial infarction. Patients with Q-wave infarctions are known to be at increased risk of perioperative cardiac events and have worse long-term prognoses. Patients who exhibit left ventricular hypertrophy or ST segment changes on a preoperative ECG are also at an increased risk of perioperative cardiac events. Reasonable recommendations for a preoperative ECG include patients with systemic cardiovascular disease, diabetes mellitus, men older than 60 years of age, women older than 70 years of age, and patients with no clinical risk factors about to undergo vascular surgical procedures. (See page 591: Electrocardiogram.)

12. **C.** Cessation of smoking for 2 days may decrease carboxyhemoglobin levels, abolish the effects of nicotine, and improve mucous clearance. Between 2 days and 6 weeks, there is no real improvement, because mucociliary clearance does not improve during this time. A prospective study showed that smoking cessation for at least 8 weeks was necessary to reduce the rate of postoperative pulmonary complications. (See page 595: Tobacco.)

13. **A.** A resting echocardiogram can determine the presence of ventricular dysfunction, regional wall abnormalities, ventricular wall thickness, and valvular function. Pulsed-wave Doppler can be used to obtain the velocity–time integral. Ejection fraction then can be calculated by determining the cross-sectional area of the ventricle. Coronary angiography is currently the best method for defining coronary anatomy. Echocardiography cannot demonstrate coronary anatomy. (See page 592: Assessment of Ventricular and Valvular Function.)

CHAPTER 23

Rare and Coexisting Diseases

1. Which of the following statements about Duchenne muscular dystrophy is TRUE?

   A. The underlying defect is the lack of the muscle protein dystrophin, a major component of the muscle membrane.
   B. Cardiac muscle is spared from the disease process.
   C. Painful degeneration and atrophy of skeletal muscle is a hallmark of the disease.
   D. It is a genetic dominant trait.
   E. Death rarely occurs.

2. Anesthetic management of patients with muscular dystrophy involves attention to all of the following EXCEPT:

   A. Myocardial depressant sensitivity to inhalational agents
   B. Avoidance of succinylcholine (Sch) secondary to massive release of potassium
   C. Increased susceptibility to malignant hyperthermia
   D. Use of low doses of nondepolarizing muscle relaxants (NDMRs) because of sensitivity to these drugs
   E. Use of aspiration precautions

3. All of the following statements about myotonia are true EXCEPT:

   A. Myotonia results in delayed skeletal muscle relaxation.
   B. Myotonia diseases are similar to muscular dystrophy in that the underlying defect is a membrane-stabilizing protein.
   C. Reversal with neostigmine may provoke a myotonic contracture.
   D. Pulmonary function studies demonstrate a restrictive type of lung disease pattern.
   E. There are two types of myotonic dystrophy that are caused by abnormalities in two distinct gene loci.

4. What is an important consideration in the anesthetic management of patients with familial periodic paralysis?

   A. Maintenance of hypokalemia in all forms of myotonia.
   B. Use of succinylcholine (Sch) is acceptable in the presence of normokalemia.
   C. Maintaining mild hypothermia.
   D. No change in dosing of nondepolarizing muscle relaxants (NDMRs).
   E. Avoidance of large carbohydrate loads.

5. All of the following statements about myasthenia gravis are true EXCEPT:

   A. It is a disease of the neuromuscular junction involving the muscarinic acetylcholine (Ach) receptors.
   B. It is an autoimmune disorder with the production of antibodies against Ach receptors.
   C. The mainstay of medical therapy involves the cholinesterase inhibitor pyridostigmine, corticosteroids, immunosuppressive agents, and intravenous immunoglobulin.
   D. The hallmark of myasthenia gravis is skeletal muscle weakness.
   E. The process most likely originates in the thymus gland.

6. Intraoperative management of myasthenia gravis may include all of the following EXCEPT:

   A. Consideration of increased sensitivity to nondepolarizing muscle relaxants (NDMRs)
   B. Use of a defasciculating dose of NDMR to facilitate intubation
   C. Use of a short-acting NDMR with neuromuscular monitoring
   D. Consideration of resistance to succinylcholine (Sch)
   E. Use of an anesthetic technique that avoids the use of muscle relaxants

7. All of the following statements about Lambert–Eaton syndrome are true EXCEPT:

   A. It is a disorder of neuromuscular transmission associated with carcinomas.
   B. Antibodies against the acetylcholine (Ach) receptor are produced.
   C. Treatment involves treating the underlying malignancy.
   D. 3,4-Diaminopyridine may be used in the treatment to increase release of Ach.
   E. A typical patient is a man older than 40 years of age with proximal extremity weakness.

8. Which of the following statements about Guillain–Barré syndrome (polyradiculoneuritis) is TRUE?

   A. It is an autoimmune disorder triggered by a bacterial or viral infection.
   B. The autoimmune response is against myocytes of skeletal muscle.
   C. Ventilatory support is rarely needed.
   D. Eighty-five percent of patients do not recover.
   E. Administration of succinylcholine (Sch) is not associated with hyperkalemia.

9. Multiple sclerosis may have all of the following anesthetic considerations EXCEPT:

   A. Patients with multiple sclerosis should be advised that an exacerbation of their neurologic symptoms may occur during the perioperative period.
   B. It is speculated that demyelinated areas of the spinal cord are more sensitive to the neurotoxicity of local anesthetics.
   C. A thorough neurologic examination before surgery or anesthesia is helpful.
   D. Autonomic dysfunction is not a concern in patients with multiple sclerosis.
   E. Multiple sites of demyelination of the brain and spinal cord are the hallmarks of the disease.

10. All of the following statements concerning epilepsy are true EXCEPT:

   A. Many different types of central nervous system (CNS) disorders may cause excessive discharge of neurons to synchronously depolarize and thereby generate seizures.
   B. Grand mal seizures are characterized by tonic–clonic motor activity that may result in respiratory arrest and hypoxemia.
   C. In status epilepticus, skeletal muscle activity diminishes over time, and seizure activity can only be detected on electroencephalography (EEG).
   D. Use of ketamine for induction is a reasonable choice.
   E. Maintenance of chronic antiseizure medication is critical throughout the perioperative period.

11. Anesthetic management of patients with a medically treated seizure disorder involves which of the following considerations?

   A. Sevoflurane may be epileptogenic and is absolutely contraindicated.
   B. Patients receiving phenytoin exhibit sensitivity to nondepolarizing muscle relaxants.
   C. Potent opioids may produce myoclonic activity or chest wall rigidity, which can be confused with seizure activity.
   D. Use of ketamine for induction is indicated.
   E. Patients receiving carbamazepine exhibit sensitivity to nondepolarizing muscle relaxants.

12. Which of the following statements regarding Parkinson's disease is TRUE?

   A. It is a disease of the central nervous system characterized by destruction of dopamine-containing nerve cells in the substantia nigra of the basal ganglion.
   B. Parkinson's disease is commonly caused by a virus.
   C. Carbidopa is converted to dopamine and is the most effective drug for Parkinson's disease.
   D. Decreasing dopamine levels in the brainstem result in resolution of symptoms.
   E. It is associated with decreased levels of GABA.

13. All of the following statements are true regarding the management of anesthesia in patients with Parkinson's disease EXCEPT:

   A. Use of phenothiazines and butyrophenones is contraindicated.
   B. Gastrointestinal dysfunction is manifested by salivation, dysphagia, and esophageal dysfunction.
   C. Autonomic dysfunction is a common manifestation.
   D. Drug therapy should be discontinued before induction of anesthesia.
   E. It is associated with increased risk of aspiration.

14. All of the following statements regarding Huntington's chorea are true EXCEPT:

   A. Disordered movement and dementia are clinical hallmarks of the disease.
   B. Mental depression and suicide are common.
   C. Specific therapy is directed at control of the movement disorder.
   D. Duration of disease averages 17 months from the time of diagnosis to death.
   E. It is autosomal dominant.

15. Amyotrophic lateral sclerosis is manifested by which of the following?

   A. It is a degenerative disease involving sensory cells of the central nervous system (CNS).
   B. Although the cause is unknown, glutamate excitotoxicity and oxidant stress secondary to exposure to metal toxicity or environmental toxins are hypothesized factors.
   C. There is a decreased sensitivity to nondepolarizing muscle relaxants (NDMRs).
   D. There is sparing of pulmonary function.
   E. An increased dose of succinylcholine is indicated.

16. Which of the following factors should be considered when anesthetizing a patient with anemia?

    A. Healthy individuals do not develop symptoms until hemoglobin (Hgb) levels decrease to below 10 g/dL.
    B. Physiologic compensation includes increased cardiac output, and increased 2,3-diphosphoglycerate (2,3-DPG) levels.
    C. Symptoms are highly variable and are rarely influenced by concurrent disease processes and the speed of developing anemia.
    D. Transfusion should be administered at hemoglobin of 10 g/dL.
    E. Physiologic compensation includes decreased plasma volume.

17. Which of the following fact is TRUE regarding nutritional deficiency anemias?

    A. All deficiency anemias result in microcytic hypochromic red blood cells (RBCs).
    B. Vitamin B_{12} deficiency cannot manifest as CNS dysfunction.
    C. The use of nitrous oxide (N_2O) is contraindicated in patients with iron deficiency anemia.
    D. Causes of folic acid deficiency include alcoholism, pregnancy, and malabsorption syndromes.
    E. Ferritin levels are helpful in detecting folic acid deficiency.

18. Which of the following statements regarding spherocytosis and G6PD deficiency is TRUE?

    A. Spherocytosis is a disorder of the hemoglobin-carrying capacity of the red blood cell (RBC).
    B. Elliptocytosis is far more common than spherocytosis.
    C. The life span of an RBC in a patient with hereditary spherocytosis is 120 days.
    D. Splenectomy may be indicated in patients with hereditary spherocytosis.
    E. G6PD deficiency is characterized by elevated NAPDH.

19. Anesthetic management of a patient with sickle cell disease (SCD) involves which of the following?

    A. Avoiding the use of extremity tourniquets if at all possible.
    B. Maintenance of the hematocrit between 40% and 42%.
    C. Maintenance of mild hypothermia for all types of surgery.
    D. Maintaining mild hypercapnia throughout emergence.
    E. Maintaining moderate acidosis.

20. All of the following statements concerning rheumatoid arthritis are true EXCEPT:

    A. It is characterized by chronic inflammation of multiple organ systems.
    B. Polyarthropathy is the hallmark of the disease.
    C. Rheumatoid arthritis is a multisystem disease that spares the cardiac and pulmonary systems.
    D. Rheumatoid arthritis may affect the joints of the larynx with generalized edema and limitation of vocal cord movement.
    E. It may be associated with Felty syndrome.

ANSWERS

1. A. Duchenne muscular dystrophy is a sex-linked recessive disorder that is evident in boys and young men. In Duchenne muscular dystrophy, the underlying defect is a lack of the muscle protein dystrophin. Progressive painless muscle degeneration with atrophy of skeletal muscle occurs. Cardiac muscle and smooth muscle are not spared. Pneumonia and congestive heart failure are common causes of death, which may occur between 15 and 25 years of age. (See page 613: Duchenne Muscular Dystrophy.)

2. C. Patients with muscular dystrophy have increased susceptibility to the myocardial depressant effects of inhalation anesthetics. Use of NDMRs should be modified because of increased sensitivity to these drugs from preexisting muscle weakness. Use of succinylcholine may result in increased potassium secondary to membrane instability. It is doubtful that muscular dystrophy patients are more prone to malignant hyperthermia. Smooth muscle involvement causes intestinal hypomobility, delayed gastric emptying, and gastroparesis. (See page 613: Muscular Dystrophy: Management of Anesthesia.)

3. B. The myotonias are a group of illnesses characterized by delayed relaxation of skeletal muscle. There are two types of myotonic dystrophies that are caused by abnormalities in two different gene loci. Myotonic dystrophy is the most common form. The underlying defect is secondary to defects in sodium channels that alter ion channel function. Reversal with neostigmine may provoke a myotonic contracture. Pulmonary function studies demonstrate a restrictive type of lung disease pattern, mild arterial hypoxia, and diminished ventilatory response to hypoxia and hypercapnia. (See page 614: Myotonias.)

4. E. Familial periodic paralysis includes a subgroup of skeletal muscle channelopathies. This group includes hyperkalemic, hypokalemic, paramyotonic congenital, normokalemic periodic paralysis, and potassium-aggravated myotonia. All have persistent sodium inward current depolarization causing membrane inexcitability and subsequent muscle weakness. Anesthetic management consists of maintenance of a normal potassium level and avoiding precipitating weakness. During episodes of weakness, patients are more sensitive to NDMRs. Succinylcholine should be avoided to prevent changes in serum potassium levels. Serial potassium measurements during the perioperative period are recommended. Avoidance of hypothermia and of large carbohydrate loads is also recommended. (See page 615: Familial Periodic Paralysis: Management of Anesthesia.)

5. A. Myasthenia gravis is a disease of the neuromuscular junction in which antibodies are formed against the nicotinic Ach receptors; T-helper cells assist in this antibody production. The hallmark of myasthenia gravis is skeletal muscle weakness. The disease probably originates in the thymus gland; 90% of patients have histologic abnormalities such as thymoma, thymic hyperplasia, or thymic atrophy. Thymectomy may help in controlling the symptoms. The mainstay therapy is medical treatment with the cholinesterase inhibitor pyridostigmine. Other treatment modalities may include corticosteroids, immunosuppressants, plasmapheresis, and thymectomy. (See page 616: Myasthenia Gravis.)

6. B. Patients with myasthenia gravis are exquisitely sensitive to NDMRs, so a defasciculating dose of an NDMR may result in excessive muscle relaxation. Use of a short-acting NDMR is recommended to avoid prolonged postoperative paralysis. Response to succinylcholine includes greater resistance and prolonged duration of action (which may partially be attributable to use of pyridostigmine in the treatment of the disease). Use of regional anesthesia may avoid respiratory depression associated with opioids. Use of an anesthetic technique that avoids use of muscle relaxants may be useful. (See page 616: Myasthenia Gravis: Management of Anesthesia.)

7. B. Lambert–Eaton syndrome is a disorder of neuromuscular transmission associated with carcinomas, especially small cell carcinoma of the lung. A typical patient is a man older than 40 years of age with proximal extremity weakness. The onset may precede detection of carcinoma by years. Immunoglobulin G antibodies are produced against presynaptic calcium channels; this inhibits the proper release of Ach. Autonomic dysfunction may also occur. Patients are sensitive to both depolarizing muscle relaxants and nondepolarizing muscle relaxants. In addition to treating the underlying malignancy, the most effective symptomatic therapy includes 3,4-diaminopyridine, which improves synaptic transmission by opening voltage-gated potassium channels and increasing release of Ach. Pyridostigmine may also be used to treat symptoms of weakness. Treatment may also include immunoglobulin and plasmapheresis. (See page 618: Myasthenic Syndrome [Lambert–Eaton Syndrome].)

8. A. Guillain–Barré syndrome is an autoimmune disorder triggered by bacterial or viral infections. Antibodies are produced against myelin, which results in demyelination of nerve tissue. Symptoms include subacute or acute skeletal muscle weakness, which may result in respiratory compromise. Prognosis is good, with 85% of patients achieving full recovery. Treatment consists of plasmapheresis or high-dose immunoglobulin. Patients are exquisitely sensitive to succinylcholine, so this drug should be avoided. This response may persist after symptoms have resolved. (See page 618: Guillain–Barré Syndrome.)

9. D. Multiple sclerosis is an acquired disease of the central nervous system (CNS) that results in demyelination of the brain and spinal cord. The cause is multifactorial, and the disease occurs in genetically susceptible individuals. A viral cause has been suspected but not proven. Symptoms of multiple sclerosis are related to the site of demyelination. It is speculated that demyelinated areas of the spinal cord are sensitive to the neurotoxicity of local anesthetics. The course of the disease process is characterized by waxing and waning of symptoms. Therapy for patients with multiple sclerosis is directed at modulating the immunologic and inflammatory responses that damage the CNS. Corticosteroids are used to control acute exacerbations of symptoms but have no influence on long-term outcome. Corticosteroids have diverse effects that suppress cellular immune responses and inflammatory edema. Other treatments include interferon, glatiramer, mitoxantrone, and symptomatic treatment with baclofen and carbamazepine. Interferon alters the inflammatory response, augments natural disease suppression, and has been shown to reduce the relapse rate. Mitoxantrone, which may be cardiotoxic, can be used to treat patients with aggressive multiple sclerosis. Patient response to immunosuppressants has been variable. Patients with multiple sclerosis should be advised that an exacerbation of their neurologic symptoms might occur during the perioperative period. A thorough neurologic examination before surgery or anesthesia is helpful. Hyperthermia and metabolic and hormonal changes induced by surgery or anesthesia may exacerbate symptoms. Autonomic dysfunction caused by multiple sclerosis may exaggerate the hypotensive effects of volatile anesthetics. (See page 619: Multiple Sclerosis.)

10. **D.** Seizures may be the manifestation of many disorders of the CNS. Seizures result from excessive discharge of neurons that synchronously depolarize. Symptoms are related to the area of neuronal activity. There are more than 40 different types of epilepsy based on the clinical features. Grand mal seizures are characterized by tonic–clonic motor activity that results in respiratory arrest and arterial hypoxemia. Patients with status epilepticus have recurrent grand mal seizures with loss of consciousness lasting more than 30 minutes; mortality is high unless the condition is treated effectively. In status epilepticus, skeletal muscle activity diminishes over time, and seizure activity can only be seen on EEG. Lack of muscular activity may confuse and prevent proper diagnosis as a seizure progresses. During the perioperative period, anti-seizure medication should be continued. In the event of seizure activity, benzodiazepines are the drug of choice for treatment. Use of muscle relaxants abolishes muscular activity; however, CNS neuronal activity continues. Ketamine and methohexital may produce seizure activity in patients with known seizure disorders. (See page 619: Epilepsy.)

11. **C.** Most inhaled anesthetics, including nitrous oxide, have been reported to produce seizure activity, but it is rare with isoflurane and desflurane. Sevoflurane may be epileptogenic, but the clinical significance is uncertain. There is a potential for significant drug interaction for the same reason. Potent opioids may produce myoclonic activity or chest wall rigidity, which may be confused with seizure activity. Use of ketamine may produce seizure-like activity, so this drug is relatively contraindicated in these patients because better alternative medicines exist. Patients receiving phenytoin or carbamazepine exhibit resistance to nondepolarizing muscle relaxants. (See page 619: Epilepsy: Management of Anesthesia.)

12. **A.** Parkinson's disease is a disabling neurologic disease that primarily affects adults older than 65 years of age. It is characterized by the destruction of dopamine-containing nerve cells in the substantia nigra of the basal ganglia of the brain. Deficiency of dopamine results in increases in activity of GABA. This acid results in inhibition of brainstem nuclei, which suppress cortical motor function. This causes the characteristic features of the disease, such as resting tremor, akinesia, and postural abnormalities. Treatment of the disease is directed at increasing dopamine levels in the brain with minimal peripheral side effects. Levodopa is the single most effective drug for patients with PD. Carbidopa is a peripheral decarboxylase inhibitor and entacapone is a catechol-O-methyltransferase inhibitor that increases the bioavailability of levodopa. The etiology of Parkinson's disease is multifactorial, with genetic and environmental factors. It may also develop after encephalitis. There is little evidence for a viral cause. (See page 621: Parkinson's Disease.)

13. **D.** In Parkinson's disease, use of butyrophenones (droperidol) and phenothiazines is contraindicated because of their effects on dopamine levels in the central nervous system. Autonomic dysfunction is common; symptoms include orthostatic hypotension, gastrointestinal dysfunction, and an exaggerated response to inhalational agents. Drug therapy should not be discontinued because muscular rigidity may interfere with the ability to extubate a patient. Gastrointestinal manifestations include dysphagia, esophageal dysfunction, and salivation. Patients with Parkinson's disease should be considered at risk of aspiration pneumonitis. (See page 621: Parkinson's Disease.)

14. **D.** Huntington's disease is a neurodegenerative disease of the corpus striatum and cerebral cortex. It is an inherited disorder that is autosomal dominant. Clinical symptoms include disordered movement, dementia, clinical depression, athetosis, and dystonia. Mental depression and suicide are common. The duration of the disease averages approximately 17 years from diagnosis to death. There is no specific therapy; treatment is directed at both depression and control of movement disorders. (See page 621: Huntington's Disease.)

15. **B.** Amyotrophic lateral sclerosis is a degenerative disease of the anterior horn cell (motor cells) throughout the CNS. It is believed to be viral in origin and bears similarity to poliomyelitis. Glutamate excitotoxicity and oxidant stress secondary to exposure to toxic metals or other environmental toxins have been implicated. It is a rapidly progressive disorder in which death results within 3 to 5 years of diagnosis. Pulmonary function is severely affected, with all patients eventually requiring mechanical ventilation. Neuromuscular transmission is altered, and patients have increased sensitivity to NDMRs. These patients may also exhibit a hyperkalemic response to succinylcholine because of the emergence of extrajunctional acetylcholine receptors. (See page 622: Amyotrophic Lateral Sclerosis.)

16. **B.** There are numerous causes of anemia. Compensations include an increase in plasma volume, cardiac output, and 2,3-DPG levels as well as decreased viscosity. Symptoms depend on concurrent disease processes, and most healthy individuals can tolerate an Hgb level of 7 g/dL without significant symptoms. No specific Hgb level exists below which a transfusion should be administered. Concurrent disease and the need for increased oxygen-carrying capacity influence the need for transfusion. (See page 628 Anemias.)

17. **D.** Nutritional deficiency anemias are categorized into three subtypes: Iron, vitamin B_{12}, and folic acid deficiency. Only iron deficiency anemia produces RBCs that are microcytic and hypochromic. This anemia may be from poor iron intake or from rapid turnover of RBCs. Hemoglobin and ferritin levels are good clinical tests for iron deficiency. In vitamin B_{12} and folate deficiency, the RBCs are enlarged. Causes of folic acid deficiency include alcoholism, pregnancy, and malabsorption syndromes. N_2O is not contraindicated in iron deficiency anemia. The clinical significance of an N_2O effect on vitamin B_{12} metabolism is controversial. (See page 628: Nutritional Deficiency Anemia.)

18. **D.** Hereditary spherocytosis is a disorder of the proteins that comprise the skeleton of the RBC membrane and renders the membrane unstable; this predisposes the patient to chronic hemolysis. Spherocytosis is the most common of the RBC membrane defects. G6PD deficiency is a hemolytic disorder in which nicotinamide adenine dinucleotide phosphate (NADPH) is not produced. This results in an increased sensitivity to oxidation. G6PD deficiency also results in a reduced level of glutathione. The cells become rigid, which accelerates clearance by the spleen. Numerous drugs induce hemolysis. Patients with G6PD deficiency are unable to reduce methemoglobin, sodium nitroprusside and prilocaine should not be administered. Treatment of patients with hereditary spherocytosis consists of a splenectomy; however, splenectomy is rarely indicated before 6 years of age because of the high incidence of pneumococcal infection. The life span of a normal RBC is 120 days. Since the RBC membrane in hereditary spherocytosis is altered, the life span of the RBC is shortened. (See page 629: Hemolytic Anemias.)

19. **A.** SCD is a hereditary disorder associated with the formation of abnormal hemoglobin (Hgb). This Hgb has the tendency to sickle under specific environmental conditions (e.g., hypoxia, hypothermia, and acidosis). Individuals who are homozygous have a greater tendency to develop sickling because of the greater proportion of abnormal Hgb. Arterial tourniquets have been used safely in patients with SCD; however, these devices should be used only when they are critical to the surgical procedure because of the possibility of local hypoxia and acidosis. The incidence of complication with tourniquet use in SCD patients is 12%. Most commonly used anesthetic medications do not have an effect on the sickling process. Maintenance of a hematocrit between 30% and 35% is desired. (See page 631: Sickle Cell Disease.)

20. **C.** Rheumatoid arthritis is a chronic inflammatory disease with symmetric polyarthropathy and involvement of other systemic organs. It often causes subclinical cardiac and pulmonary dysfunction. Polyarthropathy initially occurs in the hands and wrists but may involve the joints of the lower extremities, atlantoaxial joints, temporomandibular joint, cervical spine, and joints of the larynx. Involvement of the larynx may result in generalized edema and limitation of vocal cord movement. Other potential systemic manifestations include pericarditis, aortitis, pulmonary nodules, interstitial lung disease, renal failure, and anemia. Felty syndrome is the clinical triad of rheumatoid arthritis, leukopenia, and hepatosplenomegaly. (See page 633: Rheumatoid Arthritis.)

The Anesthesia Workstation and Delivery Systems for Inhaled Anesthetics

1. The anesthesia machine, as defined by the American Society for Testing and Materials (ASTM), is the:

   A. Anesthesia pump system
   B. Anesthesia supply station
   C. Anesthesia workstation
   D. Anesthesia sleep station

2. To comply with current American Society for Testing Materials (ASTM) standards, anesthesia workstations must measure all of the following parameters EXCEPT:

   A. Exhaled tidal volume
   B. Continuous breathing system pressure
   C. Ventilatory CO_2 concentration
   D. Exhaled O_2 concentration

3. Which of the following does NOT apply to cylinders as a gas supply source?

   A. Cylinder hanger yoke assemblies are equipped with a pin index safety system.
   B. As oxygen supply pressure falls, the supply of nitrous oxide automatically decreases regardless of the supply source.
   C. If cylinders are left open to the anesthesia machine and pressures are low enough, they might inadvertently fill backward from an open pipeline source.
   D. In a two-cylinder system, exchange can be completed while gas is flowing from another cylinder into the machine.

4. Cylinder supply valves should be turned off after the pre-operative machine checkout for the following reasons EXCEPT:

   A. Cylinder depletion can occur if the pipeline supply pressures fall below 45 psig.
   B. The amount of time that a machine can operate from cylinder supply alone is not predictable.
   C. Depressing the oxygen flush valve may deplete the cylinder.
   D. The use of a pneumatically driven ventilator, particularly at high inspiratory flow rates may deplete the cylinder.

5. If there is a suspected central pipeline crossover, what action should the anesthesia provider take?

   A. Nothing, since the oxygen E-cylinder will automatically provide an appropriate oxygen source.
   B. Open the backup E-cylinder oxygen source but leave the pipeline gas sources connected.
   C. Open the backup E-cylinder source and disconnect the pipeline gas sources until the gases being piped in are identified.
   D. Should not administer general anesthesia.

6. The flow meter assembly includes all of the following EXCEPT:

   A. A physically distinguishable O_2 flow control knob
   B. A high-flow alarm to prevent turbulent flow
   C. A series arrangement when two flow tubes are present for a single gas
   D. Float stops at the top and bottom of the flow tubes

7. Which of the following statements about the Oxygen flush valve is INACCURATE?

   A. Excessive intraoperative use may lead to patient awareness.
   B. Barotrauma is not possible in fresh gas decoupled systems.
   C. The flush valve can be used to evaluate the low-pressure circuit for leaks.
   D. Flow from the flush valve enters the low-pressure circuit downstream from the vaporizer.

8. Most modern anesthetic agent–specific vaporizers have all of the following features EXCEPT:

   A. Out-of-circuit
   B. Temperature compensation
   C. Variable bypass
   D. Pressure compensation

9. Vaporizer output concentration is most likely to remain constant despite wide variations in which of the following parameters?

   A. Fresh gas flow rates
   B. Temperature
   C. Fresh gas mixture composition
   D. Back pressure

10. Which of the following statements about the Datex-Ohmeda Tec 6 vaporizer and desflurane is NOT accurate?

    A. The MAC value for desflurane set on the Tec 6 vaporizer is 10%.
    B. Desflurane has a low blood gas coefficient, making recovery from anesthesia more rapid.
    C. The Tec 6 output is affected by carrier gas composition.
    D. The Tec 6 is electrically heated and pressurized.

11. Which of the following situations is most likely to result in an anesthetic overdose?

    A. Sevoflurane vaporizer in a low-fill state used under conditions of high fresh gas flow rates (>7.5 L/min) and a high dial setting.
    B. Sevoflurane vaporizer erroneously filled with isoflurane with the dial set to 6%.
    C. Isoflurane vaporizer erroneously filled with sevoflurane with the dial set to 2%.
    D. Poorly fit O-ring junction between vaporizer and manifold.

12. With modern agent-specific vaporizers, altitude has the most impact on anesthetic depth with which of the following agents?

    A. Sevoflurane
    B. Desflurane
    C. Isoflurane
    D. Equal for all agents

13. Which of the following features is NOT consistent with a circle breathing system?

    A. Prevention of rebreathing of CO_2.
    B. Prevention of rebreathing of Nitrous oxide.
    C. Adjustment of fresh gas flow based on the minute ventilation
    D. Numerous variations of the circle arrangement are possible.

14. All of the following factors can lead to increased production of compound A from the interaction of sevoflurane and CO_2 absorbent EXCEPT:

    A. Low fresh gas flow
    B. High absorbent temperature
    C. Old absorbent
    D. Dehydration of the Baralyme absorbent

15. Factors that appear to increase the production of carbon monoxide include all of the following EXCEPT:

    A. The use of sevoflurane rather than desflurane
    B. Dryness of the CO_2 absorbent
    C. Low fresh gas flow rates
    D. High absorbent temperatures

16. The scavenging interface is the most important part of the scavenging system because:

    A. Positive-pressure and negative-pressure reliefs are provided for an active system.
    B. Positive-pressure and negative-pressure relief are provided for a passive system.
    C. Negative-pressure relief but not positive-pressure relief is provided for an active system.
    D. Negative-pressure relief is provided for a passive system.

17. Which of the following statements regarding O_2 and N_2O supply sources are not TRUE?

    A. Cylinder supply does not require regulation versus pipeline supply that does.
    B. The pipeline system supplies gases at a higher pressure than the cylinders.
    C. The fail-safe system proportionately lowers N_2O flow when O_2 flow is lowered.
    D. The second-stage O_2 regulator in the Ohmeda machine supplies a constant pressure to the O_2 flow control valve regardless of the fluctuating pipeline pressure.

18. Which of the following statements regarding flow meters is INACCURATE?

    A. The space between the float and the wall of the flow tube varies with different flow rates.
    B. The flow meters are referred to as constant pressure because the pressure across the float does not change with changing flow rates.
    C. They are made up of tapered tubes and a mobile indicator float.
    D. Flow through the annular space can only be laminar.

19. Which of the following configuration(s) for the flow meter sequence is safe?

    A. $N_2O \rightarrow Air \rightarrow O_2 \rightarrow Outlet$
    B. $O_2 \rightarrow N_2O \rightarrow Air \rightarrow Outlet$
    C. $Air \rightarrow O_2 \rightarrow N_2O \rightarrow Outlet$
    D. $O_2 \rightarrow Air \rightarrow N_2O \rightarrow Outlet$

20. When compared with traditional circle systems, fresh gas decoupled systems have the following features EXCEPT:

    A. Accurate delivery of set tidal volume
    B. Decreased risk of barotrauma
    C. Decreased risk of volutrauma
    D. Reduced risk of intraoperative awareness

21. Saturated vapor pressure for inhaled anesthetic agents:

    A. Is independent of temperature
    B. Is dependent on atmospheric pressure
    C. Is the same for all inhalation agents
    D. Is equal to atmospheric pressure at the boiling point

22. Intermittent back pressure associated with O_2 flushing ("pumping") is decreased with which of the following?

    A. Higher flow rates
    B. Rapid respiratory rates
    C. Low levels of liquid anesthetic in the vapor chamber
    D. High peak inspiratory pressure

23. Which of the following vaporizer hazards are correctly matched with their safety features?

    A. Misfilling—Keyed filling devices
    B. Tipping—Interlock system
    C. Underfilling—Filler port location
    D. Simultaneous inhaled anesthetic administration—Fail-safe system

24. Which of the following is NOT a feature of the Bain circuit?

    A. Fresh gas inflow rate 2.5 times the minute ventilation to prevent rebreathing
    B. Requirement for ventilator-assisted breathing
    C. Hazard of kinking or disconnection of the inner fresh gas hose
    D. Fresh gas entry near the patient

25. Clinical signs that the CO_2 absorbent is exhausted DO NOT include:

    A. Increased surgical bleeding
    B. Color change of Ethyl violet
    C. Increased end-expiratory level of exhaled CO_2
    D. Signs of parasympathetic activation

26. Problems associated with ventilator bellows assembly include all EXCEPT:

    A. Leaks in the bellows may lead to a change in the delivered FiO_2.
    B. Hypoventilation may occur if the ventilator relief valve is incompetent.
    C. Leaks in the bellows may cause barotrauma if ventilators use a high-pressure driving gas.
    D. Hypoventilation may occur if the ventilator relief valve is stuck in the closed position.

27. Operating room contamination with inhaled anesthetics increases with all EXCEPT:

    A. Failure to turn off gas flow at the end of an anesthetic
    B. Filling of vaporizers
    C. Use of cuffed endotracheal tubes
    D. Flushing the circuit

28. The low-pressure circuit leak test can test all of the following EXCEPT:

    A. Loose filler caps
    B. The portion of the machine that is downstream from all safety devices, except the O_2 analyzer
    C. The integrity of the machine from the flow control valves to the common gas outlet
    D. Oxygen analyzer

ANSWERS

1. C. Modern anesthesia systems administer inhaled anesthetics by incorporating a gas supply system, ventilator, built-in monitors, and protection devices. This integration of technologies is termed the "anesthesia workstation" by the American Society for Testing and Materials (ASTM). Although the unit is a variation of a pump and it does supply anesthetics, these two labels are incomplete. (See page 642: Introduction.)

2. D. To comply with 2005 ASTM standards, newly manufactured workstations must measure the following parameters: Continuous breathing system pressure, exhaled tidal volume, ventilatory CO_2 concentration, anesthetic vapor concentration, inspired O_2 concentration, O_2 supply pressure, arterial hemoglobin oxygen saturation, arterial blood pressure, and continuous electrocardiogram. The anesthesia workstation must also have a prioritized alarm system that groups alarms into three categories: High, medium, and low priority. (See page 644: Standards for Anesthesia Machines and Workstations.)

3. C. The anesthesia machines hold reserve E-cylinders if a pipeline supply source is not available or if the pipeline fails. Each hanger yoke is equipped with the pin index safety system, which is a safeguard that eliminates cylinder interchanging and the possibility of accidentally placing the incorrect gas on a yoke designed to accommodate another gas. A check valve is located downstream from each cylinder. It minimizes gas transfer from a cylinder at high pressure to one with low pressure and also from the pipeline to a cylinder source. It also allows an empty cylinder to be exchanged for a full one while gas continues to flow from another cylinder. The cylinder should be turned off except during the preoperative machine checking period or when a pipeline source is unavailable. (See page 651: Cylinder Supply Source.)

4. B. Medical gases supplied in E-cylinders are attached to the anesthesia machine via the hanger yoke assembly that orients and supports the cylinder, provides a gas-tight seal, and ensures a unidirectional flow of gases into the machine. The gas supply cylinder valves should be turned off when not in use, except during the preoperative machine pre-use checkout. If the cylinder supply valves are left open, the reserve cylinder supply can be silently depleted whenever the pressure inside the machine decreases to a value lower than the regulated cylinder pressure. For example, oxygen pressure within the machine can decrease below 45 psig with oxygen flushing or possibly even during the use of a pneumatically driven ventilator, particularly at high inspiratory flow rates. Additionally, the pipeline supply pressures of all gases can fall to less than 45 psig if problems exist in the central piping system. If the cylinders are left open when this occurs, they will eventually become depleted and no reserve supply may be available if a complete central pipeline failure were to occur. The amount of time that an anesthesia machine can operate from the E-cylinder supply is important knowledge. Oxygen can exist only in gaseous form at room temperature, and it obeys Boyle's law, which states that for a fixed mass of gas at constant temperature, the product of pressure multiplied by volume is constant. The volume of oxygen available from the cylinder is proportional to the cylinder pressure. (See page 651: Cylinder Supply Source.)

5. C. This situation is a good example of why understanding the underlying details of anesthesia equipment design and function is essential in caring for anesthetized patients. Intuitively, the correct action is to have the backup E-cylinder in the "on" position at all times to provide an automatic source of 100% oxygen; however, this would lead to an undetected exhausted oxygen backup supply. The second intuitive answer is to switch on the backup supply when a gas pipeline crossover event is suspected; however, this would ignore that the pressure difference between pipeline (50 psi) and E-cylinder (45 psi) regulators ensures a preferential supply from the compromised pipeline. (See page 650: Pipeline Supply Source.)

6. B. Contemporary flow control valve assemblies have numerous safety features. The O_2 flow control knob is physically distinguishable from other gas knobs. It is distinctively fluted, projects beyond the control knobs of the other gases, and is larger in diameter than all the other flow control knobs. If a single gas has two flow tubes, the tubes are arranged in series and are controlled by a single control valve. Flow tubes are equipped with float stops at the top and bottom of the tube. The upper stop prevents the float from ascending to the top of the tube and plugging the outlet. It also ensures that the float will be visible at maximum flows (instead of being hidden in the manifold). The bottom float provides a central foundation for the indicator when the flow control valve is turned off. There is no high-flow alarm to prevent turbulent flow. (See page 655: Flowmeter Assemblies.)

7. C. The O_2 flush valve is associated with several hazards. Improper use of a normally functional O_2 valve may also result in problems. Overzealous intraoperative flushing may dilute inhaled anesthetics and lead to patient awareness. O_2 flushing during the inspiratory phase of positive-pressure ventilation may cause barotrauma in systems that are not fresh gas decoupled. Anesthesia systems (Dräger Narkomed 6000 series, Julian, Fabius GS, and Datascope Anestar) with fresh gas decoupling are inherently safer from the standpoint of minimizing the chance of producing barotrauma from inappropriate oxygen flush valve use. Flow from the O_2 flush valve enters the low-pressure circuit downstream from the vaporizers and downstream from the Ohmeda machine check valve. Inappropriate preoperative use of the O_2 flush valve to evaluate the low-pressure circuit for leaks may be misleading, particularly on the Ohmeda machine, which has the check valve at the common outlet. Back pressure from the breathing circuit closes the check valve airtight, and large low-pressure circuit leaks may go undetected. Some machines, including the Ohmeda Modulus 2+, do not have check valves; thus, O_2 may flow in retrograde fashion through an internal relief valve located upstream from the O_2 flush valve. The O_2 flush valve may provide a high-pressure O_2 source suitable for jet ventilation. (See page 660: Oxygen Flush Valve.)

8. D. Most modern vaporizers, including the Ohmeda Tec 4, Tec 5, and Tec 7 along with the North American DraGer Vapor 19.n and 20.n, are variable bypass, flow-over, temperature-compensated, agent-specific, out-of-circuit vaporizers. *Variable bypass* refers to the method of regulating output concentration. As gas enters the vaporizer's inlet, the setting of the concentration control valve determines the ratio of flow that goes through the bypass chamber and through the vaporizing chamber. The gas channel to the vaporizing chamber flows over the liquid anesthetic and becomes saturated with vapor. Thus, *flow-over* refers to the method of vaporization. These vaporizers are temperature compensated because they are equipped with an automatic temperature-compensating device that maintains a constant vapor output over a wide range of temperatures. These vaporizers are also agent specific and out-of-circuit because they are designed to accommodate a single agent and to be located outside the breathing circuit. Most modern vaporizers are not pressure compensated. However, Tec 6 desflurane vaporizers are pressure compensated because desflurane has a vapor pressure that is three to four times that of other contemporary inhaled anesthetics. (See page 661: Vaporizers.)

9. B. If an ideal vaporizer existed, for a given concentration dial setting, its output would be constant regardless of changes in FGF rate, temperature, back pressure, and fresh gas mixture composition. Designing such a vaporizer is difficult because as ambient conditions change, the physical properties of gases and of the vaporizers themselves can change. With a fixed dial setting, vaporizer output varies with the rate of gas flowing through the vaporizer. This variation is particularly notable at extremes of flow rates. Because of improvements in design, the output of contemporary temperature-compensated vaporizers is almost linear over a wide range of temperatures. Automatic temperature-compensating mechanisms in the bypass chamber maintain a constant vaporizer output with varying temperatures. Intermittent back pressure that results from either positive pressure ventilation or use of the oxygen flush valve may result in higher-than-expected vaporizer output. This phenomenon, known as the pumping effect, is more pronounced at low FGF rates, low-concentration dial settings, and low levels of liquid anesthetic in the vaporizing chamber. Vaporizer output is influenced by the composition of the gas that flows through the vaporizer. (See page 664: Factors that influence Vaporizer Output.)

10. A. Desflurane has unique physical properties compared with other inhalation anesthetics. It has a minimal alveolar concentration value of 6% to 7%. Desflurane is valuable because it has a low blood gas solubility coefficient of 0.45° at 37°C and thus promotes rapid recovery from anesthesia.

The vapor pressure of desflurane is three to four times that of contemporary inhaled anesthetics. It boils at 22.8°C, which is near room temperature. To achieve controlled vaporization of desflurane, Ohmeda has introduced the Tec 6 vaporizer, which is electrically heated and pressurized. The vaporizer output approximates the dial setting when O_2 is the carrier gas because the Tec 6 vaporizer is calibrated using 100% O_2. At low flow rates when a carrier gas other than 100% O_2 is used, however, a clear trend toward reduction in vaporizer output emerges. This reduction parallels the proportional decrease in viscosity of the carrier gas. (See page 666: The Tec 6 and D-Vapor Vaporizers for Desflurane.)

11. B. A Sevoflurane vaporizer in a low-fill state and used under conditions of high fresh gas flow rates (>7.5 L/min) and high dial setting (such as seen during inhalational inductions) may abruptly decrease the vaporizer output to less than 2%. The causes of this problem are likely multifactorial. However, the combination of low vaporizer fill state (<25% full) in combination with the high vaporizing chamber flow, can result in a clinically significant and reproducible decrease in vapor output. In principle, if a vaporizer designed for an agent with a relatively low saturation vapor pressure (SVP) (e.g., sevoflurane—160 mm Hg at 20°C) is erroneously filled with an agent that has a relatively high SVP (e.g., isoflurane—240 mm Hg at 20°C) the output concentration of isoflurane (in vol%) will be greater than that set on the concentration dial of the sevoflurane vaporizer. Vaporizer leaks do occur frequently, and can potentially result in patient awareness during anesthesia or in contamination of the operating room environment. A loose filler cap is the most common source of vaporizer leaks. Leaks can occur at the O-ring junctions between the vaporizer and its manifold. (See page 686: Hazards.)

12. B. For the most part, traditional variable bypass vaporizers automatically compensate for altitude and for practical purposes the effect of barometric pressure can generally be ignored. The Tec 6 desflurane vaporizer is more accurately described as a dual gas "blender" than a vaporizer. Regardless of the ambient pressure, the Tec 6 will maintain a constant concentration of vapor output (vol%), not a constant partial pressure. This means that at high altitudes, the partial pressure of desflurane for any given dial setting will be decreased in proportion to the atmospheric pressure divided by the calibration pressure (normally 760 mm Hg). For example, at an altitude of 2,000 m (6,564 ft) where the ambient pressure is 608 mm Hg, the Tec 6 dial setting must be advanced from 10% to 12.5% to avoid underdosing that could potentially result in the patient having awareness. (See page 668: Factors That Influence Vaporizer Output.)

13. B. The circle system prevents rebreathing of CO_2 by use of CO_2 absorbents but allows partial rebreathing of other gases, including nitrous oxide. A circle system may be semi-open, semi-closed, or closed, depending on the amount of fresh gas inflow. A semi-closed system is associated with some rebreathing of exhaled gases and is the most commonly used application in the United States. Numerous variations of the circle arrangement are possible, depending on the relative positions of the components. (See page 672: Anesthesia Breathing Circuits.)

14. **C.** Sevoflurane has been shown to produce degradation products upon interaction with CO_2 absorbents. The major degradation product produced is fluoromethyl-2, 2-difluoro-1 (trifluoromethyl) vinyl ether, or compound A. During sevoflurane anesthesia, factors that apparently lead to an increase in the concentration of compound A include low-flow or closed-circuit anesthetic techniques, use of Baralyme rather than soda lime, higher concentrations of sevoflurane in the anesthetic circuit, higher absorbent temperatures, and fresh absorbent. Baralyme dehydration increases the concentration of compound A, and soda lime dehydration decreases the concentration of compound A. (See page 674: CO_2 Absorbents.)

15. **A.** Several factors appear to increase the production of carbon monoxide and resulting increased carboxyhemoglobin levels. They include (1) the inhaled anesthetic used (for a given MAC multiple, the magnitude of CO production from greatest to least is desflurane ≥ enflurane > isoflurane >> halothane = sevoflurane); (2) the absorbent dryness (completely dry absorbent produces more CO than hydrated absorbent); (3) the type of absorbent (at a given water content, Baralyme produced more CO than does soda lime); (4) the temperature (increased temperature increases CO production); (5) the anesthetic concentration (more CO is produced from higher anesthetic concentrations); (6) low fresh gas flow rates; and (7) reduced experimental animal (patient) size per 100 g of absorbent. (See page 675: Interactions of Inhaled Anesthetics with Absorbents.)

16. **A.** Positive-pressure relief is mandatory in both active and passive systems to vent excess gas in case of occlusion downstream from the scavenging interface. If the system is active, negative-pressure relief is also necessary. It protects the breathing circuit or ventilator from excessive subatmospheric pressure. Passive systems need only a single positive-pressure relief valve. In this system, transfer of the waste gas from the interface to the basal system relies on pressure of the waste gas itself because the vacuum is not used. The positive-pressure relief valve opens at a preset value, such as 5 cm H_2O, if an obstruction between the interface and disposal system occurs. (See page 684: Scavenging Interface.)

17. **A.** The hospital piping system provides gases to the machine at approximately 50 psig, which is the normal working pressure of most machines. The cylinder supplies are the source of backup if the pipeline fails. The O_2-cylinder source is regulated from 2,200 to approximately 45 psig, and the N_2O-cylinder source is regulated from 745 to approximately 45 psig. Most Ohmeda machines have a second-stage O_2 regulator located downstream from the O_2 supply source. This regulator supplies a constant pressure to the O_2 flow control valve regardless of fluctuating O_2 pipeline pressures. A safety device, traditionally

referred to as the fail-safe valve, is located downstream from the N_2O supply source. It serves as an interface between the O_2 and N_2O supply source. This valve shuts off, or proportionally decreases, the supply of N_2O and other gases if the O_2 supply pressure decreases. A proportioning system is a safety feature that links O_2 and N_2O flow control valves, either mechanically or pneumatically, so the minimum O_2 concentration at the common outlet is 25%. (See page 650: Anesthesia Workstation Pneumatics.)

18. **D.** The flow meter assembly precisely controls measured gas flow to the common gas outlet. The flow control valve regulates the amount of gas that enters the tapered transparent tube known as the flow tube. A mobile indicator located inside the flow tube indicates the amount of gas passing through the flow control valve. The flow meters are commonly referred to as *constant-pressure flow meters* because the pressure decrease across the float remains constant for all positions in the tube. The term *variable orifice* designates the type of unit because the annular space between the float and the flow tube varies with the position of the float. Flow through the constriction created by the float may be laminar or turbulent, depending on the flow rate. (See page 655: Flowmeter Assemblies.)

19. **A.** It has been demonstrated that in the presence of a flow meter leak, a hypoxic mixture is less likely to occur if the O_2 flow meter is located downstream from all other flow meters. A potentially dangerous arrangement has the nitrous oxide (N_2O) flow meter located in the downstream position. A hypoxic mixture may result because a substantial portion of O_2 flow passes through the leak, and all the N_2O is directed to the common outlet. A safer configuration has the O_2 flow meter located in the downstream position. A portion of the N_2O flow escapes through the leak, and the remainder goes toward the common outlet. A hypoxic mixture is less likely because all of the O_2 flow is advanced by the N_2O. A leak in the O_2 flow tube may produce a hypoxic mixture even when O_2 is located in the downstream position. (See page 657: Problems with Flow Meters.)

20. **D.** When a fresh gas decoupled (FGD) system is used, the fresh gas coming from the anesthesia workstation flow meters, via the fresh gas inlet during the inspiratory phase, is diverted into the reservoir bag by a decoupling valve that is located between the fresh gas source and the ventilator circuit. The reservoir (breathing) bag serves as an accumulator for fresh gas until the expiratory phase begins. During expiratory phase, the decoupling valve opens, allowing the accumulated fresh gas in the reservoir bag to be drawn into the circle system to refill the piston ventilator chamber (or descending bellows in the Datascope Anestar). The advantages of circle systems using FGD include more accurate delivery of the set tidal volume, and decreased risk of barotrauma and volutrauma. Possibly the greatest disadvantage to the new anesthesia circle systems that utilize FGD is the possibility of entraining room air into the patient gas circuit. As previously discussed, in a fresh gas decoupled system the bellows or piston refills under slight negative

pressure. If the volume of gas contained in the reservoir bag volume plus the returning volume of gas exhaled from the patient's lungs is inadequate to refill the bellows or piston, negative patient airway pressures could develop. To prevent this, a negative-pressure relief valve is placed in the breathing system (see Figure 24-33). If breathing system pressure falls below a preset value such as -2 cm H_2O, then the relief valve opens and ambient air is entrained into the patient gas circuit. If this goes undetected, the entrained atmospheric gases could lead to dilution of either the inhaled anesthetic agents or the enriched oxygen mixture (resulting in a lowering of the enriched oxygen concentration toward 21%) or both. If unnoticed, this dilution of patient gases could lead to intraoperative patient awareness or hypoxia. High-priority alarms with both audible and visual alerts should notify the user that fresh gas flow is inadequate and room air is being entrained. (See page 643: Anesthesia Workstation Standards and Pre-use Procedures.)

21. **D.** Saturated vapor pressure is the pressure created by the molecules in the vapor phase of a volatile liquid. As more molecules enter the vapor phase from the volatile liquid, the vapor pressure increases. Vapor pressure is dependent on the temperature and physical characteristics of the liquid; it is independent of the atmospheric pressure. The boiling point of a liquid is the temperature at which the vapor pressure equals atmospheric pressure. All inhalation agents have a unique saturated vapor pressure. (See page 661: Physics: Vapor Pressure.)

22. **A.** Intermittent back pressure associated with positive-pressure ventilation or O_2 flushing may cause higher vaporizer output concentration than the dial setting. This phenomenon, known as the pumping effect, is more pronounced at low flow rates, low dial settings, and low levels of liquid anesthetics in the vaporizing chamber. Additionally, the pumping effect is increased by rapid respiratory rates, high peak inspired pressures, and rapid decreases in pressure during expiration. (See page 664: Factors That Influence Vaporizer Output.)

23. **A.** Agent-specific, key-filling devices help prevent filling a vaporizer with the wrong agent. Overfilling of these vaporizers is minimized because the filler port is located at the maximum safe liquid level. Today's vaporizers are firmly secured to the vaporizer manifold, and there is little need to move them. Thus, problems associated with tipping are minimized. Some vaporizers are equipped with extensive baffles to make them even more immune to the problems associated with tipping. Administration of more than one inhaled anesthetic at a time is prevented by an interlock system that does not allow more than one vaporizer at a time to be operational. (See page 665: Safety Features.)

24. **B.** The Bain circuit is a modification of the Mapleson D circuit. It is a coaxial circuit in which the fresh gas flows through a narrow tube within the outer corrugated tubing. The central tube originates near the reservoir bag, but the fresh gas actually enters the circuit at the patient end. Exhaled gases enter the corrugated tubing and are vented through the respiratory valve near the reservoir bag. The Bain circuit may be used for both spontaneous and controlled ventilation. The fresh gas inflow rate necessary to prevent rebreathing of CO_2 is 2.5 times the minute ventilation. The main hazard of the Bain circuit is unrecognized disconnection or kinking of the inner fresh gas hose. (See page 673: Bain Circuit.)

25. **D.** Ethyl violet is the pH indicator added to soda lime to help assess the functional integrity of the absorbent. Ethyl violet changes from colorless to violet in color when the pH of the absorbent decreases as a result of CO_2 absorption. Unfortunately, in some circumstances ethyl violet may not always be a reliable indicator of the functional status of absorbent. For example, prolonged exposure of ethyl violet to fluorescent lights can produce photodeactivation of this dye. When this occurs, the absorbent appears white even though it may have a reduced pH and its absorptive capacity has been exhausted. Even in the absence of color changes, clinical signs that the CO_2 absorbent is exhausted include: Increased spontaneous respiratory rate (requires that no neuromuscular blocking drug be used); initial increase in blood pressure and heart rate, followed later by a decrease in both; increased sympathetic drive with skin flushing, sweating, tachydysrhythmia; hypermetabolic state (increased CO_2 production; must rule out malignant hyperthermia); respiratory acidosis as evidenced by arterial blood gas analysis; and increased surgical bleeding—due to both hypertension and coagulopathy. Although a diagnosis of depletion of CO_2 absorbent capability can be made by observation of clinical signs, the most sensitive indicator of this problem is capnography. If the end-expiratory level of exhaled CO_2 is increased, and the inspiratory level is greater than 0, then exhaustion of the CO_2 absorbent must be pursued as a possible cause. (See page 674: Carbon Dioxide Absorbents.)

26. **D.** Leaks can occur in the bellows assembly. A hole in the bellows can lead to alveolar hyperinflation and possibly barotrauma in some ventilators because high-pressure driving gas can enter the patient circuit. The oxygen concentration of the patient gas may increase when the driving gas is 100% oxygen, or it may decrease if the driving gas is composed of an air–oxygen mixture. The ventilator relief valve can cause problems. Hypoventilation occurs if the valve is incompetent because the anesthetic gases are delivered to the scavenging system instead of to the patient during the inspiratory phase. Gas molecules preferentially exit into the scavenging system because it represents the path of least resistance, and the pressure within the scavenging system can be subatmospheric. Ventilator relief valve incompetency can result from a disconnected pilot line, a ruptured valve, or from a damaged flapper valve. A ventilator relief valve stuck in the closed or partially closed position can produce either barotrauma or undesired PEEP. (See page 680: Bellows Assembly Problems.)

27. **C.** The two major causes of waste gas contamination in the operating room are the anesthetic technique used and the equipment used. Regarding the anesthetic technique, the following factors cause operating room contamination: Failure to turn off gas flow control valves at the

end of an anesthetic, poorly fitting mask, flushing of the circuit, filling anesthetic vaporizers, use of uncuffed endotracheal tubes, and use of breathing circuits such as the Jackson-Rees circuit, which is difficult to scavenge. (See page 682: Waste Gas Scavenging Systems.)

28. D.   The low-pressure leak test checks the integrity of the machine from the flow control valves to the common outlet. It evaluates the portion of the machine that is downstream from all safety devices except for the O_2 analyzer. The components located in this area are precisely the ones that may be subject to breakage and leaks. Loose filler caps on vaporizers are a common source of leaks, and these leaks can lead to delivery of sub-anesthetic doses of inhaled agents, causing patient awareness during general anesthesia. Leaks in the low-pressure system may cause hypoxia and patient awareness. The North American Drager uses a positive-pressure leak test, and the Ohmeda uses a negative-pressure leak test on the low-pressure circuit. It evaluates the portion of the machine that is downstream from all safety devices except the oxygen analyzer. (See page 647: Low-pressure Circuit Leak Test.)

CHAPTER

25

Commonly Used Monitoring Techniques

1. The O_2 sensor location is on which part of the anesthesia circuit?

   A. Expiratory limb
   B. Inspiratory limb
   C. Fail-safe valve
   D. Second-stage O_2 pressure regulator
   E. O_2 pipeline supply

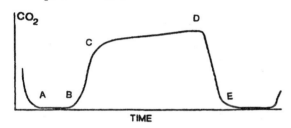

2. In the above capnograph, dead space ventilation occurs during which interval?

   A. A–B
   B. B–C
   C. C–D
   D. D–E
   E. C–E

3. In the above capnograph, the point defined as end-tidal CO_2 (ETCO$_2$) occurs at:

   A. A
   B. B
   C. C
   D. D
   E. E

4. O_2 saturation determination by a pulse oximeter is based on which physical law?

   A. Charles' law
   B. Bohr law
   C. Beer–Lambert law
   D. Boyle law
   E. Bernoulli principle

5. The correct formula for determination of mean arterial pressure (MAP) based on systolic pressure (SP) and diastolic pressure (DP) is:

   A. $DP + 1/3(SP - DP)$
   B. $SP - 1/3(SP - DP)$
   C. $DP - 1/2(SP - DP)$
   D. $(SP - DP) \times 3$
   E. $(SP + DP)/3$

6. Patients with which condition are at increased risk of developing complete heart block during insertion of a pulmonary artery catheter (PAC)?

   A. Right bundle branch block
   B. Left bundle branch block
   C. Atrial fibrillation
   D. Anterior fascicular block
   E. Posterior fascicular block

7. Which of the following monitors is the most accurate indicator of left ventricular preload?

   A. Central venous pressure (CVP) trends
   B. Pulmonary capillary wedge pressure (PCWP)
   C. Rapid infusion catheter
   D. Mixed venous saturation
   E. Urine output

8. Which of the following is NOT a method of measuring oxygen concentration?

   A. Paramagnetic analyzer
   B. Galvanic cell analyzer
   C. Polarized technograph analyzer
   D. Polarographic analyzer

9. Which of the following statements about the use of monitoring devices is FALSE?

    A. Invasive monitoring may place patients at risk for complications related to the device's application and use.
    B. Monitoring devices may measure more precisely than achievable by humans alone.
    C. Monitoring devices may make measurements at higher frequencies than is humanly possible.
    D. Monitoring devices always enhance patient safety.

10. Which of the following is NOT part of the ASA Standard II requirements?

    A. Use of an inspired oxygen analyzer with a low concentration–limit alarm during general anesthesia.
    B. When attempting a known difficult airway intubation, tracheostomy equipment should be immediately available.
    C. During all anesthetics, the means for continuously measuring the patient's temperature must be available.
    D. When using a mechanical ventilator, use of a device that is able to detect a disconnection of any part of the breathing system.
    E. Quantitative assessment of blood oxygenation during any anesthesia care.

11. End-tidal CO_2 ($ETCO_2$) values are NOT altered because of changes in which of the following?

    A. Condensation
    B. Ventilation
    C. Pulmonary blood flow
    D. Metabolic activity
    E. Cardiac output

12. The assumption that end-tidal CO_2 ($ETCO_2$) reflects $PaCO_2$ is NOT dependent on which of the following statements?

    A. Ventilation and perfusion are appropriately matched.
    B. No diffusion gradient exists for CO_2.
    C. No sampling errors occur during measurement.
    D. All alveoli empty at the same time.

13. Increasing dead space ventilation results in which change to end-tidal CO_2 ($ETCO_2$)?

    A. It increases the $ETCO_2$ value measured.
    B. It increases the baseline $ETCO_2$ value.
    C. It widens the $PaCO_2$–$ETCO_2$ gradient.
    D. It causes downsloping of the plateau phase of the capnogram.

14. The presence of a stable (three breaths) CO_2 waveform via capnography may indicate all of the following EXCEPT:

    A. An endotracheal tube (ETT) in the trachea
    B. An ETT in the pharynx
    C. An ETT in the right mainstream bronchus
    D. An ETT in the esophagus

15. Possible causes for a sudden loss of end-tidal CO_2 ($ETCO_2$) include all of the following EXCEPT:

    A. Extubation
    B. Hyperventilation
    C. Massive pulmonary embolism
    D. Disrupted sample line

16. Common clinical causes for a widened $PaCO_2$–end-tidal CO_2 ($ETCO_2$) gradient include all of the following EXCEPT:

    A. Pulmonary embolism
    B. Hypoperfusion
    C. Pulmonary shunt
    D. Chronic obstructive pulmonary disease

17. The causes of a sudden rise in nitrogen level in exhaled gases during O_2/N_2O anesthesia include which of the following?

    A. Failure of O_2 fail-safe alarm
    B. Leak in anesthesia circuit
    C. Failed inspiratory one-way valve
    D. CO_2 absorber reacting with water

18. During a laparoscopic cholecystectomy, an arterial blood gas sample is drawn because of difficulty in maintaining O_2 saturation. When reviewed, the practitioner notes a large discrepancy between $PaCO_2$ and end-tidal CO_2 ($ETCO_2$). Possible causes for this include which of the following?

    A. Air embolism
    B. Hypoxic mixture
    C. CO_2 insufflation of abdomen
    D. Pre-existing restrictive airway disease

19. Which of the following statements regarding arterial waveform devices is TRUE?

    A. They give a beat-to-beat estimation of left ventricular output.
    B. They are not accurate in patients with septic shock.
    C. All arterial waveform devices first require calibration to a reference cardiac output determined by thermodilution or lithium dilution.
    D. It is more accurate than cardiac outputs determined by thermodilution.

20. Falsely low estimations of blood pressure determined by a noninvasive cuff occur in which of the following conditions?

    A. Use of a cuff that is too small
    B. Use of a loosely applied cuff
    C. The extremity being below the level of the heart
    D. Use of excessively quick deflation of the cuff

21. The fidelity of fluid-transducing systems (i.e., arterial lines) is constrained by which of the following properties?

    A. Amplification
    B. Piezoelectric impedance
    C. Natural frequency
    D. Laminar flow

22. Which of the following is not a complication of radial arterial line placement?

    A. Median nerve injury
    B. Thrombosis of the artery
    C. Hematoma formation
    D. Ulnar nerve injury

23. Compared with the right internal jugular (IJ) vein, the left IJ vein is used less often for central venous access because of which of the following?

    A. Potential for damage to the thoracic duct
    B. Closer proximity to the carotid artery
    C. Increased risk of pneumothorax
    D. Increased risk of injury to the phrenic nerve

24. Determination of mixed venous O_2 saturation (SvO_2) allows one to assess which of the following?

    A. Adequacy of CO_2 delivery
    B. Adequacy of cerebral perfusion
    C. Determination of intracardiac and pulmonary shunts
    D. Quantity of dead space within the lungs

25. Monitoring of EEG signals via BIS or SedLine involves the translation of complex statistical models into a value of 0 to 100. Which of the following is NOT an accurate description of the number range?

    A. A BIS value of 40 to 60 is the optimal range for general anesthesia.
    B. A SedLine value of 15 to 25 is the optimal range for general anesthesia.
    C. A BIS value of 100 suggests the patient is completely awake.
    D. A SedLine value of 100 suggests the patient is completely awake.

26. Which of the following statements describes conditions in which a pulmonary artery catheter (PAC) is located in West zone 3?

    A. Pulmonary artery occlusion pressure (PAOP) > pulmonary artery end diastolic pressure (PAEDP)
    B. Inability to aspirate blood from the distal port when the PAC is wedged
    C. Nonphasic PAOP tracing
    D. Chest radiograph showing the catheter tip below the level of the left atrium

27. Pulmonary capillary occlusion pressure (PCOP) is a valid reflection of left ventricular end-diastolic pressure (LVEDP) in which of the following conditions?

    A. Ischemic left ventricle
    B. Prolonged QT interval
    C. Mitral valve stenosis
    D. Aortic regurgitation

28. The factor that DOES NOT increase the risk of mortality after a pulmonary artery catheter (PAC)-induced pulmonary artery rupture is:

    A. Hypotension
    B. Pulmonary hypertension
    C. Heparinization
    D. Coagulopathy

29. Which of the following statements is TRUE?

    A. Convection is heat loss resulting from infrared irradiation.
    B. Radiation is heat loss resulting from contact with surfaces.
    C. Evaporation is heat loss resulting from energy required for vaporization of water.
    D. Conduction is heat loss resulting from movement of air.

30. Which of the following statements about pulse oximetry is FALSE?

    A. Pulse oximetry combines the technology of plethysmography and spectrophotometry.
    B. Ambient light, nail polish, and motion may compromise the accuracy of pulse oximetry.
    C. Electrocautery can interfere with pulse oximetry.
    D. Pulse oximetry measures the fractional oxygen saturation.

ANSWERS

1. B. The O_2 monitor is located on the inspiratory limb of the anesthesia circuit. Beyond this point, the only alteration to the delivered anesthetic mixture would be the entrainment of room air, which would not produce a hypoxic mixture. The expiratory limb is downstream to the patient, providing no protection regarding what is delivered to the patient. The other possible answers are all upstream sites in the anesthesia circuit, and although they would ensure that the mixture was not hypoxic at that site, they could not ensure that downstream contamination will not occur. (See page 701: Monitoring of Inspired Oxygen Concentration.)

2. A. During the initial phase of ventilation, the gases being expired are from the conducting airways, trachea, and anesthesia circuit. These areas are not involved in gas exchange, so their composition reflects the inspired mixture. Unless the inspired mixture contains CO_2, the initial phase of expiration will be a horizontal line at 0 mm Hg of CO_2. With further exhalation, alveolar gas reaches the sampling site, and an increase in the capnograph occurs. (See page 704: Figure 25-3.)

3. D. The end-tidal CO_2 value is recorded at the end of expiration, which on the capnograph occurs just before the steep decline back to baseline. (See page 704: Figure 25-3.)

4. C. O_2 saturation detection via a pulse oximeter uses the physical principle described by the Beer–Lambert law. The Beer law states that a parallel beam of light transmitted through a clear solution with a solute dissolved within it will fall exponentially as the solute level increases. The Lambert law states that a parallel beam of light will have its intensity fall exponentially as the distance through which it must shine increases. (See page 702: Monitoring of Arterial Oxygenation by Pulse Oximetry.)

5. A. The formula for MAP is DP plus one-third the difference between the DP and SP. (See page 708: Intermittent Noninvasive Monitoring of Systemic Blood Pressure.)

6. B. Individuals who have a left bundle branch block rely on their right bundle branch to transmit the impulses from their atrioventricular node to the ventricular mass. In individuals with a left bundle branch block, passing a PAC through the right side of the heart could injure the right bundle and produce complete heart block. (See page 710: Monitoring of Central Venous and Right Heart Pressures: Complications.)

7. B. PCWP (PAOP) is accurate with the presumption that there are no complicating matters within the lungs (e.g., excessive positive end-expiratory pressure), left atrial abnormalities (e.g., mitral stenosis), or LV abnormalities (e.g., ischemia). It is assumed that during end-diastole there is cessation of forward blood flow and that a static fluid/pressure column exists between the catheter tip and the left ventricle. Urine output is also a very accurate method of detecting adequacy of left ventricular (LV) preload; however, in healthy people with inadequate LV preload, urine output may be maintained. Conversely, in numerous conditions, urine output is inadequate despite adequate LV preload. CVP measures right ventricular preload with good accuracy, however LV trends can be altered by abnormalities within the right ventricle, pulmonary circulation, and left side of the heart. Mixed venous O_2 saturation is an accurate indicator of total body O_2 balance but does not directly measure LV preload; it may be normal despite inadequate LV preload if the heart rate is increased to maintain cardiac output. Although not a selection here, the most accurate preload indicator for the left ventricle is the TEE probe because it can assess actual intracardiac chamber size and thus preload. A RIC (rapid infusion catheter) line is a large peripheral IV line placed via wire guidance over a smaller gauge catheter. (See page 710: Monitoring of Central Venous and Right-Heart Pressures.)

8. C. Oxygen is a highly reactive chemical species, providing many chemical and physical opportunities to detect its presence. Three main types of oxygen analyzer are seen in clinical practice: Paramagnetic oxygen analyzers, galvanic cell analyzers, and polarographic oxygen analyzers. The polarized technograph analyzer does not exist. (See page 701: Monitoring of Inspired Oxygen Concentration.)

9. D. Since monitors are mechanical devices, they do not become distracted. They can also make repetitive measurements more often than humans because they do not experience fatigue. Monitoring the patient's vital sign allows one to detect derangements in the patient's early stages and make interventions to prevent irreversible injury. Monitors enhance patient safety only if an appropriate intervention is undertaken to correct the perturbation in the patient's physiology. Invasive monitoring may place patients at risk for complications related to the device's application and use. (See page 700: Introduction.)

10. B. Options A, C, and D, and E are amongst the ASA standard II regulations. Option B is simply a good idea. (See page 700: Introduction.)

11. A. The production of end-tidal CO_2 is dependent on its generation (i.e., metabolic rate), transportation from the cells to the lungs (i.e., cardiac output and pulmonary blood flow), and excretion from the lung (resulting from ventilation). (See page 704: Interpretation of Inspired and Expired Carbon Dioxide Concentrations.)

12. D. Ventilation–perfusion (V/Q) mismatch results in an increase in dead space ventilation, which produces a situation in which alveolar gas is diluted by dead space gas (whose $PaCO_2$ value is 0). This increases the $PaCO_2$–$ETCO_2$ gradient. Diffusion abnormalities, such as acute respiratory distress syndrome, restrict the diffusion of CO_2

from the blood into the alveoli and thus widen the $PaCO_2$–$ETCO_2$ gradient. Sampling errors, such as excessive sampling rate in which fresh gas is entrained, or leaks in the system dilute the expired CO_2, resulting in a widened gradient. The alveolar emptying rate does not affect the gradient between $PaCO_2$ and $ETCO_2$, but it does produce the gentle upward trend of the plateau phase of the capnograph. (See page 704: Interpretation of Inspired and Expired Carbon Dioxide Concentrations.)

13. **C.** Increasing dead space ventilation results in a larger reservoir or tidal volume fraction which is not involved in respiration. During exhalation, this reservoir of nonrespiratory gas mixes with alveolar gas and dilutes its concentration of CO_2, resulting in a widening of the $PaCO_2$–$ETCO_2$ gradient. This has no effect on the baseline value seen during inspiration. Downsloping of the capnograph plateau phase can be seen when the sampling rate exceeds the exhaled volume. (See page 704: Interpretation of Inspired and Expired Carbon Dioxide Concentrations.)

14. **D.** Three stable CO_2 waveforms on a capnograph indicate that the ETT is in such a position as to be exposed to expired pulmonary gas. Thus, the ETT could be anywhere from the nose to the alveoli. Sampling gases from an ETT within the stomach may result in detection of CO_2; however, the quantity measured will decrease rapidly with subsequent breaths. (See page 704: Interpretation of Inspired and Expired Carbon Dioxide Concentrations.)

15. **B.** For $ETCO_2$ to be detected, there must be adequate pulmonary blood flow to deliver the CO_2 to the lungs for excretion, ventilation of the lungs, and an intact sampling system. The presence of a massive pulmonary embolism will cease pulmonary blood flow. Extubation in a mechanically ventilated patient would result in cessation of ventilation. A disrupted sampling line in a sidestream sampling system would result in a sudden loss of CO_2 waveform. Hyperventilation would result in a gradual lowering of $ETCO_2$, not a sudden decrease. (See page 704: Interpretation of Inspired and Expired Carbon Dioxide Concentrations.)

16. **C.** The common clinical causes associated with a widened $PaCO_2$–$ETCO_2$ gradient include embolic phenomena (thrombus, fat, air, amniotic fluid), hypoperfusion states with reduced pulmonary blood flow, and chronic obstructive pulmonary disease. In contrast, conditions that increase pulmonary shunt (perfusion in the absence of ventilation) result in minimal changes in the $PaCO_2$–$ETCO_2$ gradient. (See page 704: Interpretation of Inspired and Expired Carbon Dioxide Concentrations.)

17. **B.** During O_2/N_2O anesthesia, no nitrogen should be detected in the system. Any nitrogen in the circuit must be coming from the air surrounding the patient or the anesthesia circuit. Thus, the possible causes include venous air embolism and leaks in the anesthesia or sampling circuit. Failure of the O_2 fail-safe alarm will prevent one from detecting a loss in sufficient pipeline O_2 pressure. A failure in the inspiratory one-way valve will result in the patient's

rebreathing expired gases that, if the system is closed, will not contain nitrogen. (See page 704: Interpretation of Inspired and Expired Carbon Dioxide Concentrations: Common Problems and Limitations.)

18. **A.** The gradient between $PaCO_2$ and $ETCO_2$ is dependent on the degree of dead space ventilation. The common clinical causes associated with a widened $PaCO_2$–$ETCO_2$ gradient include embolic phenomena (thrombus, fat, air, amniotic fluid), hypoperfusion states with reduced pulmonary blood flow, and chronic obstructive pulmonary disease. Hypoxic mixture and restrictive pulmonary disease do not affect the $ETCO_2$–$PaCO_2$ gradient. CO_2 insufflation of the belly will cause increased dissolved CO_2 in the bloodstream; however, this should not cause a discrepancy in the $ETCO_2$–$PaCO_2$ gradient. (See page 704: Interpretation of Inspired and Expired Carbon Dioxide Concentrations.)

19. **A.** Analysis of the arterial waveform allows one to estimate left ventricular output. The PiCCO device makes use of an external calibration reading, whereas the FloTrac and LiDCOrapid devices use an uncalibrated, biophysical model approach. Numerous clinical studies have demonstrated that the precision and accuracy of arterial waveform analysis are acceptable when compared with thermodilution cardiac output measurements obtained by pulmonary artery catheters. (See page 713: Monitoring of Cardiac Output by Arterial Waveform Analysis.)

20. **D.** For a noninvasive blood pressure cuff to give accurate blood pressure readings, the cuff must be appropriately sized, with the width of the cuff bladder being 40% of the arm's circumference. The bladder length should be sufficient to encircle at least 80% of the extremity. Use of excessively large or small cuffs results in falsely low and falsely high pressures, respectively. The cuff must be applied appropriately tight because use of a loose cuff results in an artificially high reading. Deflation of the cuff must be slow enough to detect the Korotkoff sounds and the resultant changes with deflation. Use of excessively quick deflation results in falsely low blood pressure readings. (See page 708: Intermittent Noninvasive Monitoring of Systemic Blood Pressure.)

21. **C.** Natural frequency and damping are the two primary conditions that influence reproduction of the arterial wave measured by a fluid-filled transducer system. The natural frequency of the monitoring systems must be higher than the frequency within the arterial waveform. If the frequency within the arterial pulse wave approaches the natural frequency of the fluid-filled transducer, resonance will occur. This will be seen as overshoot or ringing. This produces amplification of the original signal by the monitoring device. Systolic pressure will be overestimated in such situations. Damping within the system impedes the transducer from detecting the changes of the pressure within the arterial waveform. This impedance results in a loss of the fine details contained within the arterial waveform. An overdampened arterial waveform results in blunting of the pulse pressure, little change in mean arterial pressure, and

loss of the dicrotic notch. Underdampened systems produce an overshoot of the systolic pressure and the development of artifacts produced not by the waveform but rather secondary to the monitoring system. (See page 706: Invasive Monitoring of Systemic Blood Pressure.)

22. **D.**   The radial artery may be damaged during catheter placement. Hematoma formation and thrombosis of the artery may occur during placement, while in situ, or during removal. The median nerve lies approximately 1 cm medial to the radial artery, sufficiently close as to risk possible injury. The ulnar nerve lies on the opposite side of the wrist along with the ulnar artery. (See page 706: Invasive Monitoring of Systemic Blood Pressure.)

23. **A.**   The right IJ vein is the jugular vein of choice for a number of reasons. It tends to be larger than the left IJ vein, and it travels in a more direct line path into the superior vena cava. The left IJ vein's more tortuous route and the presence of the thoracic duct at the left IJ vein–subclavian junction (which predisposes to thoracic duct injury) make it a less-desirable site. Both the right and left IJ veins are in similarly close approximation with the ipsilateral carotid artery and the phrenic nerve. (See page 710: Monitoring of Central Venous and Right Heart Pressures.)

24. **C.** SvO_2 allows for assessment of the total body O_2 balance. SvO_2 is dependent on cardiac output, O_2 saturation, and hemoglobin concentration. A patient can have a normal SvO_2 despite inadequate blood flow to an area of the body because a small regional area of hypoperfusion does not significantly alter SvO_2. Intracardiac or intrapulmonary shunts produce elevations of SvO_2 beyond normal (70%). The point at which the increase in the SvO_2 occurs may determine the anatomic site of the shunt. Cellular poisons and sepsis are other examples of situations in which an elevation in SvO_2 beyond normal may occur. (See page 712: Monitoring of Cardiac Output by Pulmonary Arterial Catheter.)

25. **B.**   Both the BIS and SedLine devices display a unitless number in the range of 0 to 100, which is derived from the measured EEG data by the device's proprietary algorithms. A value of 0 corresponds to an absence of any discernable electrical activity. A value of 100 corresponds to the EEG activity seen in a fully awake and alert individual. The algorithms used in the devices specify a differing "optimal range" for general anesthesia: For the BIS it is defined as between 40 and 60, for the SedLine it is 25 to 50. (See page 717: Monitoring of Processed EEG Signals.)

26. **D.**   To use a PAC to estimate left ventricular end-diastolic pressure (LVEDP) through the measurement of PAOP, the PAC must be positioned in the lungs at a site where a continuous column of blood will be present from the tip of the catheter to the left atrium when the balloon is inflated. This condition occurs in West zone 3. A PAC positioned in West zone 2 will measure airway pressure during the respiratory cycle because the alveolar pressure exceeds the capillary pressure at peak inspiration. Conditions that increase West zones 2 and 1 (e.g., hypovolemia, positive end-expiratory pressure) may convert a properly placed PAC into an improperly placed one, rendering the PAC useless for pulmonary capillary wedge pressure monitoring. A PAC in West zone 4 will be compressed by interstitial pressure, which is greater than left atrial pressure and thus gives falsely elevated PAOP values. The following characteristics suggest that a PAC is not in West zone 3: PAOP > PAEDP (if no pulmonary hypertension is present), nonphasic PAOP tracing, and an inability to withdraw blood when wedged. The location of a PAC may be confirmed by lateral chest radiography to ascertain that the catheter tip is below the level of the left atrium. (See page 710: Monitoring of Central Venous and Right Heart Pressures.)

27. **B.**   PCOP as an accurate estimation of LVEDP is predicated on normal LV compliance, the absence of aortic or mitral valve disease (aortic regurgitation, mitral stenosis, or mitral regurgitation), normal pulmonary airway pressures, normal size of pulmonary vascular bed, and normal pulmonary vascular resistance. Altering these assumptions results in the inability to predict LV loading conditions with PCOP values. (See page 710: Monitoring of Central Venous and Right Heart Pressures.)

28. **A.**   Pulmonary artery rupture is a rare but serious and possibly fatal complication of a PAC. The risk of rupture is increased in patients with pulmonary hypertension. Mortality after the rupture is aggravated further in patients who are heparinized or coagulopathic. (See page 712: Monitoring of Cardiac Output by Pulmonary Arterial Catheter.)

29. **C.**   Convection is the change in heat content resulting from the movement of air over the surface of the object. Conduction is the change in heat content resulting from the object's contact with another surface. Radiation is the change in heat content resulting from absorption or emission of photons. Evaporation is heat loss resulting from the vaporization of water. (See page 716: Monitoring of Body Temperature.)

30. **D.**   Pulse oximetry combines the technology of plethysmography and spectrophotometry. Ambient light, nail polish, and motion may compromise the accuracy of pulse oximetry. Electrocautery may interfere with pulse oximetry. Whereas pulse oximetry measures the functional oxygen saturation, co-oximetry measures the fractional oxygen saturation. (See page 702: Monitoring of Arterial Oxygenation by Pulse Oximetry.)

CHAPTER 26

Echocardiography

1. Which of the following statements regarding echocardiographic instrumentation and optimization of image quality is TRUE?

   A. Resolution increases with long wavelength sound waves.
   B. The greatest axial resolution is offered by long pulses of high-frequency ultrasound.
   C. Broadening beam size improves the lateral and elevational resolution.
   D. High frame rates and high pulse repetition frequencies (PRF) enhance resolution.

2. Which of the following parameters is the MOST important in determining potential for tissue damage with ultrasonography?

   A. Frequency
   B. Wavelength
   C. Propagation velocity
   D. Amplitude

3. Which of the following statements regarding M-mode (motion-mode) imaging is FALSE?

   A. M-mode imaging displays a series of sequentially collected brightness-mode (B-mode) images.
   B. M-mode imaging remains the best technique for examining the timing of cardiac events.
   C. M-mode imaging provides a one-dimensional, single-beam view through the heart.
   D. M-mode imaging can display shape and lateral motion information about cardiac anatomy.

4. Lateral resolution will be BEST enhanced with:

   A. Increasing sector width
   B. Increasing sector depth
   C. Decreasing the frame rate
   D. Increasing pulse repetition frequency

5. Which of the following would NOT preclude placement of a transesophageal echocardiography (TEE) probe?

   A. History of esophageal stricture, rings, or webs
   B. Recently bleeding esophageal varices
   C. Gastroesophageal reflux disease
   D. Recent gastric bypass surgery

6. The mid-esophageal ascending aorta short-axis view (ME AA SAX) is NOT useful for evaluating:

   A. The ascending aorta for the presence of dissection flaps
   B. The presence of a thrombus in the left pulmonary artery
   C. Blood flow in the main PA
   D. The presence of a wire in the SVC

7. Which of the following is the MOST accurate method for assessment of left ventricular preload?

   A. Central venous pressure (CVP) trends
   B. Pulmonary capillary wedge pressure (PCWP)
   C. Transesophageal echocardiography (TEE)
   D. Urine output

8. Which of the following is the MOST sensitive indicator of myocardial ischemia?

   A. Increased central venous pressure (CVP)
   B. Increased pulmonary artery catheter (PAC)
   C. Wall motion abnormality on transesophageal echocardiography (TEE)
   D. ST-segment change on the electrocardiographic (ECG) tracing in leads II and V_5

9. The transgastric mid-papillary short-axis (TG mid-SAX) view does NOT:

   A. Allow for the immediate diagnosis of a hypovolemic state or pump failure.
   B. Visualize the left ventricle (LV) as "doughnut shaped" in cross-section with both papillary muscles being seen.
   C. Visualize the LV walls perfused by each of the three major coronary arteries.
   D. Accurately assess blood flow velocities with Doppler.

10. Doppler assessment of blood flow CANNOT or DOES NOT:

    A. Determine the speed, direction, and timing of blood flow
    B. Require near parallel orientation to blood flow
    C. Overestimate blood flow velocity when the beam-to-flow angle divergence is greater than 30 degrees
    D. Use two techniques to evaluate blood flow

11. Pulsed-wave Doppler (PWD) DOES NOT:

    A. Offer the ability to sample only signals associated with a specific location, referred to as the sample volume.
    B. Collect data intermittently.
    C. Show aliasing (appearing on the spectral display as a signal on the other side of the baseline).
    D. Show any limitations due to the Nyquist limit being applicable to Continuous-wave Doppler (CWD) only.

12. Which of the following calculations is CORRECT given the following measurements: Left ventricular outflow tract (LVOT) time velocity integral (VTI) is 7, the LVOT diameter is 2 cm, the aortic valve (AoV) VTI is 22, and the heart rate is 100 bpm?

    A. The cardiac output is above 3 L/min.
    B. The aortic valve area is 1 cm^2.
    C. The LVOT area is about 4 cm^2.
    D. The stroke volume (SV) is about 40 cc.

13. Estimate the pulmonary artery (PA) systolic pressure, given that the central venous pressure (CVP) is 4 mm Hg. The maximum velocity of the regurgitant tricuspid jet (TR jet) is 3 cm/sec and that there is no evidence of a stenotic pulmonary valve.

    A. 40 mm Hg
    B. 36 mm Hg
    C. 32 mm Hg
    D. More data are needed.

14. Echocardiographic evaluation of left ventricular (LV) systolic function is NOT consistent with which one of the following statements?

    A. Global LV systolic function is influenced by load and contractility alterations.
    B. Wall motion is the most reliable marker of regional systolic function.
    C. The most frequently used technique to evaluate global LV function is visual estimation of the fractional area change (FAC).
    D. Ejection fraction (EF) and stroke volume are not always indicators of intrinsic systolic function.

15. Color-flow Doppler imaging (CFD) differs from conventional pulsed-wave Doppler in all the following ways EXCEPT:

    A. CFD performs multiple sample volume recordings along each scan line as the beam is swept through the sector.
    B. CFD velocity data are color-coded.
    C. CFD velocity data are superimposed on top of the gray scale 2-D image.
    D. Aliasing artifact during CFD interferes with the determination of severity of mitral valve disease.

16. Doppler echocardiography's ability to quantitatively measure blood velocity provides support for the following assessments EXCEPT:

    A. Increasing pressure half-time implies more regurgitation.
    B. Increasing velocity of flow through a narrowing implies greater stenosis.
    C. Increased area under the velocity–time curve implies greater stroke distance.
    D. Pressure gradients determine velocities of jets between chambers.

17. MOST accurate evaluation of left ventricular (LV) diastolic function implies:

    A. Estimation of left atrial (LA) pressure
    B. Finding a high E wave, low A wave, and shortened deceleration time (DT) during the impaired relaxation phase
    C. Tissue Doppler imaging, which directly measures myocardial velocities, providing load-independent diastolic function assessment.
    D. Finding higher systolic/diastolic (S/D) ratios with the pulmonary vein flow during the "pseudonormal" stage

18. Echocardiographic evaluation of aortic regurgitation DOES NOT include:

    A. Looking for associated findings including dilated aortic root, endocarditis lesions, dilated ascending aorta, calcified aortic valve, or aortic dissection
    B. Evaluation of the vena contracta usually appreciated in the mid-esophagus long-axis (ME AV LAX) view
    C. Evaluation for retrograde diastolic flow in the descending and abdominal aorta
    D. Finding a prolonged pressure half-time (PHT) (≥220 milliseconds)

19. Echocardiography is NOT useful for the placement of:

    A. Peripherally inserted central venous catheters
    B. Intra-aortic balloon pumps (IABPs)
    C. Percutaneous coronary sinus cannula
    D. Guidewires for percutaneous venous cannulae

20. Which of the following is NOT TRUE regarding epicardial and epiaortic echocardiography?

    A. Epiaortic scanning for atheroma is performed using a small-footprint transducer.
    B. High-frequency transducers are used that do not require a standoff device.
    C. It is particularly valuable when transesophageal echocardiography (TEE) probe cannot be placed or is contraindicated.
    D. Views are similar to the ones obtained via transthoracic echocardiography (TTE).

ANSWERS

1. **D.** The pulse repetition frequency (PRF) is the rate at which ultrasonic pulses are triggered. The greater the PRF, the greater the number of scan lines that are emitted in a given period. This enhances the motion display. Short pulses of high-frequency ultrasound offer the greatest axial resolution but have a decreased tissue penetration. Since resolution is highest along the axial plane, echocardiographic measurements are most precise when taken parallel to the beam's axis. The frame rate is the frequency at which the sector is rescanned. A high frame rate improves the capture of movement. Increases in sector size and depth come at the cost of a decreased frame rate and decreased PRF, respectively, producing poor motion imaging. High-frequency, short-wavelength ultrasound is more easily focused and directed to a specific target location. Image resolution increases with short-wavelength sound waves, so ultrasonic frequencies of 2 to 10 MHz are preferred in clinical echocardiography. The shorter the length of the sound pulses, the better the axial resolution of the system. The beam size determines the lateral and elevational resolution. Whereas broad beams produce a "smeared" image of two nearby objects, narrow beams can identify each object individually. (See page 724: Principles and Technology of Echocardiography.)

2. **D.** The amplitude of a sound wave represents its peak pressure and is appreciated as loudness. The level of sound energy in an area of tissue is referred to as intensity. The intensity of the sound signal is proportional to the square of the amplitude and is an important factor regarding the potential for tissue damage with ultrasound. The Food and Drug Administration limits the intensity output of cardiac ultrasonography systems to be less than 720 W/cm^2 because of concerns of potential tissue injury. Sound waves are also characterized by their frequency (f), or pitch, expressed in cycles per second or hertz (Hz), and by their wavelength (λ). These attributes significantly impact the depth of penetration of a sound wave in tissue and the image resolution of the ultrasound system. The propagation velocity of sound (v) is determined solely by the medium through which it passes. In soft tissue, the speed of sound is approximately 1540 m/sec. (See page 724: Principles and Technology of Echocardiography.)

3. **D.** Ultrasonic imaging is based on the amplitude and time delay of the reflected signals. By timing the interval between transmission and return of the reflections, the echocardiography system can precisely calculate the distance of a structure from the transducer. Current imaging is based on B-mode technology. With B-mode imaging, the amplitude of the returning echoes from a single pulse determines the display brightness of the representative pixels. M-mode imaging adds temporal information to B-mode imaging by displaying a series of sequentially collected B-mode images. M-mode echocardiography provides a one-dimensional, single-beam view through the heart but updates the B-mode images at a very high rate, providing dynamic real-time imaging. M-mode imaging remains the best technique for examining the timing of cardiac events. Two-dimensional (2-D) echocardiography is a modification of B-mode echocardiography and is the mainstay of the echocardiographic examination. Instead of repeatedly firing ultrasound pulses in a single direction, the transducer in 2-D echocardiography sequentially directs the ultrasound pulses across a sector of the cardiac anatomy. In this way, 2-D imaging displays a tomographic section of the cardiac anatomy, and unlike M-mode, reveals shape and lateral motion. (See page 726: Image Display.)

4. **D.** The pulse repetition frequency is the rate at which sound pulses are triggered. The greater the pulse repetition frequency, the greater the number of scan lines that are emitted in a given period of time. This enhances motion display. Unfortunately, sector depth must be reduced because pulse repetition frequency is inversely related to the sector depth as a longer period of time is required for the ultrasound to travel the increased distances. The frame rate is the frequency at which the sector is rescanned. A high frame rate improves the capture of movement. Typically, frame rates >30/sec are desired. The frame rate is critically dependent on the sector depth, which determines the time required for each scan line to be received, and the sector width, which increases the number of scan lines that must be transmitted. Consequently, increases in sector size and depth come at the cost of a decreased frame rate and poor motion imaging. The number of scan lines per degree of the sector (scan line density) greatly affects the image resolution. Doubling the scan lines essentially doubles the lateral resolution. However, the cost is a decrease in the frame rate and motion imaging. (See page 726: Image Display.)

5. **C.** To maintain the safety profile of TEE, each patient should be evaluated before the procedure for signs, symptoms, and history of esophageal pathology. The most feared complication of TEE is esophageal or gastric perforation. For skilled practitioners, this complication is extremely rare. Patients with extensive esophageal and gastric disease are at highest risk of perforation. Contraindications to TEE probe placement include esophageal stricture, rings, or webs; esophageal masses (especially malignant tumors); recent bleeding of esophageal varices; Zenker's diverticulum; recent radiation to the neck; and recent gastric bypass surgery. In the rare case in which TEE is essential and is the only alternative, placement of the TEE probe can be performed under direct visualization with a combined gastroscopic and echocardiographic examination. (See page 728: Transesophageal Echocardiography Safety.)

6. **B.** The ME AA SAX view is obtained by advancing the probe slightly from the upper esophagus until the ascending aorta (AA) is seen and then rotating the multiplane

angle from 0 to 45 degrees to obtain a true short axis. This "great vessel view" images the AA in short axis and the main PA with its bifurcation and right pulmonary artery in long axis. The main uses of the ME AA SAX view are to evaluate the AA for dimensions and presence of dissection flaps, evaluate the PA (position of catheter or rule out thrombus), and assess PA blood flow (by aligning the Doppler beam parallel to the blood flow in the main PA). (See page 729: Goals of the Two-Dimensional Examination.)

7. C. The most accurate method for evaluating left ventricular preload is the TEE image because it can assess actual intracardiac chamber size. Urine output is not a very accurate method of detecting adequacy of left ventricular (LV) preload. For instance, in healthy people with inadequate LV preload, urine output may be maintained. Conversely, in numerous conditions, urine output is inadequate despite adequate LV preload. CVP trends can be altered by abnormalities within the right ventricle, pulmonary circulation, and left side of the heart. PCWP is inaccurate for preload assessment as there are complicating matters within the lungs (excessive positive end-expiratory pressure), left atrial abnormalities (mitral stenosis), and LV abnormalities (ischemia). (See page 744: Left Ventricular Cavity.)

8. C. TEE-based and ST segment analysis of the ECG are the most accurate of the monitors for detecting myocardial ischemia. The most sensitive and specific method is TEE-based, specifically the regional wall motion abnormalities that occur during ischemia are readily detected by TEE. Abnormal wall thickening and inward motion of the ischemic segment occurs within seconds of the segment's becoming ischemic. However, not all wall motion abnormalities are caused by ischemia (e.g., pacing or bundle branch blocks produce nonischemic wall motion abnormalities). When comparing the TEE with ECG ST segment analysis, TEE picks up more ischemic episodes. ST analysis is very sensitive for ischemia. Increasing its sensitivity and specificity can be accomplished by placing the leads in the areas most likely to become ischemic. CVP, PAC readings, and cardiac output become abnormal with ischemia; however, they become abnormal late and are not very specific for ischemia. (See page 729: Goals of the Two-dimensional Examination.)

9. D. The TG mid-SAX view is obtained by advancing the TEE probe from the mid-esophageal position into the stomach and anteflexing until contact is made with the gastric wall. The LV is visualized as a doughnut shape in cross-section, and both papillary muscles should be seen. Advancement of the probe allows visualization of the LV apex in cross-section. The TG mid-SAX view is unique in that it visualizes all the LV walls perfused by each of the three major coronary arteries. The view is considered to be the most useful one in situations of intraoperative hemodynamic instability because it allows immediate diagnosis of hypovolemic state, pump failure, and coronary ischemia. The primary uses of the TG mid-SAX include assessment of the LV size (enlargement, hypertrophy) and cavity volume and global ventricular systolic function and regional wall motion. Two-dimensional echocardiography captures high-fidelity motion images of cardiac structures but not blood flow. Blood flow indices such as blood velocities, stroke volume, and pressure gradients are the domain of Doppler echocardiography. The direction of blood flow needs to parallel the direction of the Doppler beam for accurate estimation of velocities. (See page 729: Goals of Two-Dimensional and Three-Dimensional Examination.)

10. C. Unlike 2-D imaging, which relies on the time delay and amplitude of reflected ultrasound, Doppler technologies are based on the change in frequency that occurs when ultrasound interacts with moving objects. Reflections from RBCs are used to determine the blood flow velocity and calculate the hemodynamic parameters. The requirement of near-parallel orientation to blood flow for Doppler examinations contrasts with the near-perpendicular orientation required for 2-D imaging of cardiac structures. The *Doppler equation* $\Delta f = v \times \cos \theta \times 2\, f_t/c$ describes the relationship between the alteration in ultrasound frequency and blood flow velocity. Conceptually, the equation is simplified by observing that the change in ultrasound frequency is related to just two variables: Blood flow velocity and $\cos \theta$, where θ is the angle between the direction of flow and the direction of the Doppler beam. When the beam angle divergence is greater than 30 degrees, the value of $\cos \theta$ decreases rapidly, and the Doppler system markedly *underestimates* blood velocity. The Doppler signal is shifted only by the component of the blood velocity that is in the direction of the beam path (i.e., $v \cos \theta$). PWD and CWD are commonly used to evaluate blood flow. (See page 738: Doppler Echocardiography.)

11. D. PWD offers the echocardiographer the ability to sample blood flow from a particular location. The PWD system transmits a short burst of ultrasound toward the target and then switches to receive mode to interpret the returning echoes. Since the speed of sound (c) in tissue is constant, the time delay for a signal to reach its target and return to the transducer depends solely on the distance (d) to the target. By time gating, the electronic circuitry of the PW transducer interprets returning echoes only after a predetermined time delay after the transmission of an ultrasound pulse. In this way, only signals associated with a location, referred to as the sample volume, are selected for evaluation. Doppler data are frequently presented as a velocity–time plot known as the spectral display. Since the PWD data are collected intermittently, the maximal frequency and blood flow velocity that can be accurately measured by PWD are limited. The maximal frequency, which equals 50% of the pulse repetition frequency, is known as the Nyquist limit. At blood velocities above the Nyquist limit, analysis of the returning signal becomes ambiguous, with the velocities appearing to be in the opposite direction. The ambiguous signal from frequencies above the Nyquist limit, known as aliasing, appears on the spectral display as a signal on the other side of the baseline, hence the term *wraparound*. With continuous reception of the Doppler signal, the Nyquist limit is not applicable, and blood flows with very high velocities are recorded accurately. (See page 738: Doppler Echocardiography.)

12. **B.** Volumetric parameters are calculated using the principle that volumetric flow (Q) equals the blood flow velocity (v) times the cross-sectional area (CSA) of the conduit, that is, Q = v × CSA. In effect, the VTI (in centimeters, traced from the spectral Doppler display) represents the distance blood traveled during systole (i.e., stroke distance). By multiplying the VTI by the CSA (cm^2) of the conduit through which the blood traveled, the SV (in cm^3) is obtained: SV = VTI × CSA. The principle of conservation of mass is the basis of the continuity equation, which is commonly used to measure the AoV area. The continuity equation simply states that the volume of blood passing through one site in the heart (e.g., the LVOT) is equal to the mass or volume of blood passing through another site (e.g., the AoV).

$$\text{Volumetric flow}_1 = \text{Volumetric flow}_2$$

$$\text{Therefore, } CSA_1 \times VTI_1 = CSA_2 \times VTI_2 \text{ and } CSA_1 = CSA_2 \times VTI_2 / VTI_1$$

Based on the given data, because the LVOT diameter is 2 cm, the radius is 1 cm. The LVOT cross-sectional area or LVOT CSA is × $(\text{Radius})^2$ or approximately $22/7 \times 1$ cm^2. The SV is LVOT VTI × LVOT CSA. This equals 22 cc for the given data. Cardiac output is SV × Heart rate. This equals 2,200 cc/min or 2.2 L/min for the given data. Aortic valve area = LVOT CSA × LVOT VTI/AV VTI. Based on the given data, this works out to exactly 1 cm^2. (See page 740: Hemodynamic Assessments.)

13. **A.** Pressure gradients (PGs) are used to estimate intracavitary pressures and to assess conditions such as valvular disease (e.g., aortic stenosis), septal defects, outflow tract obstruction, and major vessel pathology (e.g., coarctation). As blood flows across a narrowed or stenotic orifice, the blood flow velocity increases. The increase in velocities relates to the degree of narrowing. In the clinical situation, the simplified Bernoulli equation describes the relation between the increases in blood flow velocity and the pressure gradient across the narrowed orifice $\Delta P = 4V^2$ where ΔP in mm Hg is the pressure gradient across the narrowed orifice and V in meters per second is the maximum velocity across that orifice measured by Doppler. Based on the given data, the pressure gradient across the tricuspid valve should equal $4 \times 3^2 = 36$ mm Hg. Since the CVP (approximating the right atrial pressure) is 4 mm Hg, the right ventricular systolic pressure should equal 40 mm Hg (36 + 4). Given no stenosis across the pulmonic orifice, a reasonable estimate of the PA systolic pressure is 40 mm Hg. (See page 741: Pressure Assessment.)

14. **B.** *Abnormal myocardial wall thickening* is a sensitive marker of myocardial ischemia that appears earlier than electrocardiographic and hemodynamic changes. The evaluation of segmental wall motion to detect ischemia is not error free. In addition to being a subjective assessment, wall motion may be affected by tethering, regional loading conditions, and stunning. Epicardial pacing of the free wall of the right ventricle (as in post-bypass period) produces a left bundle block and induces septal wall motion abnormalities. Interobserver reproducibility is better for normally contracting segments than for dysfunctional segments. Because of these issues, *wall thickening is a more reliable marker of regional function*. EF is the most frequently used estimate of LV systolic function. The evaluation of EF provides prognostic information about mortality and morbidity. EF and stroke volume are affected by factors such as preload, afterload, and heart rate and thus are not always indicators of intrinsic systolic function. Typical clinical scenarios in which EF does not represent LV systolic function include the hypercontractile LV in mitral regurgitation (in which more than half of ED volume may regurgitate inside the left atrium) or the hypocontractile LV in aortic stenosis (in which LV systolic performance is poor despite preserved contractility). The most frequently used technique to evaluate global LV function as well as preload is visual estimation of fractional area change (FAC), often referred to as "eyeball" EF. Although highly subjective, it is practiced widely and is accurate when determined by experienced echocardiographers, especially in patients with normally contracting ventricles. (See page 743: Echocardiographic Evaluation of Systolic Function.)

15. **D.** CFD provides a dramatic display of both blood flow and cardiac anatomy by combining 2-D echocardiography and PWD methods. The PWD used for CFD performs multiple sample volume recordings along each scan line as the beam is swept through the sector. This approach provides flow data at each location in the sector, which can be overlaid on the structural data obtained by 2-D imaging. The Doppler velocity data from each sample volume are color coded and superimposed on top of the grayscale 2-D image. In the most widely accepted color code, red hues indicate flow toward the transducer, and blue hues indicate flow away from the transducer. An important caveat to CFD use in the clinical setting is that CFD is susceptible to alias artifacts. *Aliasing in the color-flow map can be useful in calculating blood flow in mitral valve disease using the proximal isovelocity surface area (PISA) method.* (See page 739: Color-flow Doppler.)

16. **A.** To calculate stroke volume the instantaneous velocities during systole are traced from the spectral display and the echocardiographic system's internal software package calculates the time velocity integral (VTI, in centimeters). In effect, the VTI represents the distance (v × t = d) blood traveled during systole (i.e., stroke distance). Pressure gradients are used to estimate intracavitary pressures and to assess conditions such as valvular disease (e.g., aortic stenosis), septal defects, outflow tract obstruction, and major vessel pathology (e.g., coarctation). As blood flows across a narrowed or stenotic orifice, blood flow velocity increases. The increase in velocities relates to the degree of narrowing. The rate of decline in the pressure gradient across the valve is related to the severity of disease. This pressure half-time is the time required for the peak transvalvular pressure gradient to decrease by 50%. Typically, a larger orifice will have a shorter pressure half-time as pressures equalize faster. Intracavitary and pulmonary arterial pressures are estimated from the pressure gradient across two adjacent chambers. The pressure gradient is defined as the

difference in pressure from the "driving" chamber to the "receiving" chamber. (See page 740: Hemodynamic Assessments.)

17. C.   Diastolic dysfunction is defined as the inability of the LV to fill at normal LA pressures and is characterized by a decrease in relaxation, LV compliance, or both. The early manifestation of diastolic dysfunction is characterized by impaired relaxation, implying that the rate and duration of decrease in LV pressure after systolic contraction are prolonged, resulting in an inability of the LV to fill adequately during the rapid-filling phase. A compensatory increase in filling occurs with atrial contraction. This stage of disease is known as grade I diastolic dysfunction. In more advanced stages of disease (grades II and III of diastolic dysfunction), a decrease in LV compliance ensues. The transmitral flow Doppler (TMF) curve of an individual with abnormal relaxation is represented by a low E, high A, and prolonged DT. Progression of diastolic disease is marked by decreases in LV compliance. LA pressure increases as a compensatory mechanism to normalize the pressure gradient across the MV. In this scenario, the TMF velocities resemble the normal curve; thus, this stage is known as "pseudonormal." Because of the high LA pressure, there is less flow from the pulmonary veins during ventricular systole; this generates a lower S wave on the pulmonary vein flow (PVF) curves and thus a lower S/D ratio. One of the important caveats to assessing diastolic function using pulsed-wave Doppler is that the flow patterns depend on pressure gradients and therefore are affected by both preload and afterload. In settings in which the load conditions vary at a fast pace, such as the operating room, changes in TMF or PVF velocities may be difficult to interpret. Tissue Doppler imaging, which directly measures myocardial velocities, provides a more load-independent methodology of diastolic function assessment. (See page 746: Evaluation of Left Ventricular Diastolic Function.)

18. D.   Findings associated with aortic valve incompetence include a dilated aortic root (Marfan's syndrome), endocarditis lesions, dilated ascending aorta, calcified aortic valve, aortic dissection (may be associated with acute AI), fluttering of the anterior mitral leaflet and restricted diastolic opening of the MV from the AI jet, or a dilated LV in chronic AI. In either of the ME or the transgastric views of AV, a color-flow Doppler (CFD) sector over the AV and the left ventricular outflow tract (LVOT) demonstrate the presence or absence of the AI regurgitant jet. Vena contracta, the narrowest "neck" of the AI jet as it traverses the AV plane, is usually best appreciated in the ME AV LAX view. The largest diameter of the vena contracta in diastole is selected. The size of the vena contracta is relatively load independent and provides a reliable way to quantitate AI intraoperatively in the presence of fluctuating hemodynamics. The pressure half-time (PHT) of the AI jet is recorded in the TG LAX or deep TG LAX views. PHT expresses the pressure equilibration of the diastolic blood pressure ("driving" pressure) and the diastolic left ventricular pressure ("resistance" pressure). A short PHT (<200 milliseconds) is associated with severe AI. Retrograde

diastolic flow in the descending and abdominal aorta is sensitive and specific for severe AI. This is imaged with pulsed-wave Doppler in the ME LAX view of the distal descending aorta. (See page 749: Evaluation of Valvular Heart Disease.)

19. A.   In addition to its role in diagnostics, echocardiography is also used to assist various procedures such as placement of central venous catheter, IABPs, coronary sinus cannula, and guidewires for other venous or arterial cannulas. For patient safety reasons, the National Institute for Clinical Excellence has recommended that central lines be placed under guidance of two-dimensional ultrasound imaging. A linear-array handheld transducer with high frequencies (7.5–12 MHz) is preferred for ultrasound-guided central line placement. The technique relies on placing the transducer over the traditional anatomic landmarks and identifying the internal jugular vein (IJ) and carotid artery (CA) in the short-axis view and their anatomical relationship. Peripherally inserted central venous catheters (PICC "lines") are typically placed with fluoroscopy. Use of transesophageal echocardiography (TEE) during IABP placement allows positioning of the catheter to the preferred location, which is distal to the left subclavian artery. TEE is helpful in guiding placement of the cannula and in checking for proper position. Improper insertion of a coronary sinus cannula may result in injury to the interatrial septum or to the crux of the heart, the fragile area joining the atria and ventricles. View of the CS is obtained from the midesophagus four-chamber view by retroflexing the probe. TEE is useful in verifying the position of various other cannulas. For example, when femoral artery–femoral vein bypass is instituted, the venous cannula can be visualized as it advances in the inferior vena cava up to the level of the right atrium. Proper positioning of the guidewires used for aortic cannulation can be confirmed with TEE. (See page 758: Echocardiography-assisted Procedures.)

20. B.   During surgeries performed via sternotomy or thoracotomy, epicardial echocardiography can be performed and is particularly valuable in cases in which the TEE probe cannot be placed or is contraindicated. The epicardial views are similar to the ones obtained via TTE. In collaboration with the Society of Cardiovascular Anesthesiologists, the American Society of Echocardiography has recently issued guidelines for the performance of epicardial echocardiography. The epicardial probe uses high-frequency transducers (5–12 MHz) that may require a standoff device or saline in the mediastinum for best imaging. Epicardial imaging offers superior image quality as well as a better window to the anterior cardiac structures (aorta, aortic valve, pulmonary artery, and pulmonary vein). Because of interposition of the left bronchus, the distal ascending aorta and proximal aortic arch cannot be visualized with TEE. The ascending aorta and proximal aortic arch are of particular interest during cardiac surgeries because they represent sites for aortic cannulation. Epiaortic scanning for atheroma is performed using a small-footprint, linear-array transducer. (See page 759: Epicardial and Epiaortic Echocardiography.)

Airway Management

1. Which of the following drugs is NOT being used appropriately for pharmacologic preparation of an adult during awake intubation?

   A. 0.2 to 0.4 mg of glycopyrrolate intramuscularly (IM) or intravenously (IV)
   B. 400 to 800 mg of lidocaine administered by a nebulizer
   C. 1 μg/kg of IV dexmedetomidine over 10 minutes and then a maintenance infusion at 0.5 μg/kg/hr
   D. 2 to 24 drops of oxymetazoline instilled in each nostril
   E. Four percent cocaine topical solution with a total dose of 100 mg

2. Awake airway management may NOT be appropriate in which of the following circumstances?

   A. Patients with unstable cervical spine pathology
   B. Patients with an acute myocardial infarction
   C. Intoxicated adults
   D. Patients with increased intraocular pressure
   E. Patients with sleep-disordered breathing (obstructive sleep apnea)

3. Which of the following statements regarding the laryngeal mask airway (LMA) as a supraglottic airway tool is TRUE?

   A. In patients with asthma, the peri-induction period represents the highest risk period for wheezing.
   B. The LMA cannot be used together with an endotracheal tube (ETT).
   C. The incidence of sore throat is higher than with an endotracheal tube.
   D. It should always be removed either when the patient is deeply anesthetized or after the protective airway reflexes have returned.
   E. The LMA should always be deflated before removal.

4. Which of the following statements regarding face mask ventilation is TRUE?

   A. The sniffing position causes the tongue to be more anterior.
   B. It is made more difficult when prosthetics (dentures) are left in place.
   C. It should not be used for the duration of the anesthetic.
   D. In the presence of normal lung compliance and an open airway, face mask ventilation should require as much as 40 cm H_2O positive pressure.
   E. The sniffing position causes the esophagus to be more posterior.

5. Which of the following statements regarding airway anatomy is FALSE?

   A. The right principal bronchus is larger in diameter than the left.
   B. Cartilaginous rings support only the first two generations of the bronchi.
   C. The larynx is innervated bilaterally by two branches of each vagus nerve.
   D. The laryngeal "skeleton" consists of nine cartilages.
   E. The trachea measures approximately 15 cm in adults.

6. With regard to preoxygenation, all of the following are true EXCEPT:

   A. Preoxygenation with a fraction of inspired oxygen (FiO_2) of 1 may increase the apneic oxygenation reserve fivefold compared with room air.
   B. In emergencies, preoxygenation may be performed with eight vital capacity breaths over 60 seconds.
   C. In obese patients, preoxygenation is improved by bilevel positive airway pressure (BiPAP).
   D. The mask does not need to be tight fitting to ensure optimal preoxygenation.
   E. Without preoxygenation, nitrogen may occupy more than 60% of the functional residual capacity (FRC).

7. The maximum recommended intracuff pressure for a no. 4 laryngeal mask airway (LMA) is:

   A. 20 cm H_2O
   B. 40 cm H_2O
   C. 60 cm H_2O
   D. 80 cm H_2O
   E. none; a volume of air (30 mL) is inserted regardless of pressure

8. All of the following statements regarding endotracheal intubation in children are true EXCEPT:

   A. Elevation of the head on a pillow is not usually necessary.
   B. Cricoid pressure may be needed to displace an anterior-appearing larynx into view.
   C. A Macintosh blade is generally more useful because of a larger tongue-to-mouth ratio in children.
   D. The cricoid cartilage is the narrowest part of the child's airway.
   E. Hyperextension at the atlanto-occipital joint may cause airway obstruction.

9. Which of the following statements regarding innervation of the airway is TRUE?

   A. The oropharynx is innervated by branches of the facial, glossopharyngeal, and vagus nerves.
   B. The oropharynx is innervated by branches of the vagus, glossopharyngeal, and hypoglossal nerves.
   C. The hypoglossal nerve provides for sensation over the posterior third of the tongue, vallecula, and epiglottis.
   D. The internal branch of the superior laryngeal nerve provides all sensory innervation below the vocal cords.
   E. The external branch of the superior laryngeal nerve provides all sensory innervation above the vocal cords.

10. Laryngospasm is commonly caused by:

   A. Saliva
   B. Hypercapnia
   C. Deep anesthesia
   D. Hypoxemia
   E. Pulmonary edema

11. Which of the following statements regarding use of a laryngeal mask airway (LMA) and gastroesophageal reflux is TRUE?

   A. The LMA fits in the esophageal inlet but does not reliably seal it.
   B. There is a high incidence of aspiration when an LMA is used in the presence of a "full stomach."
   C. Aspiration is more common when an LMA is used for cardiopulmonary resuscitation than when a bag-valve-mask device is used.
   D. If regurgitation is noted when an LMA is in place, it should be removed immediately.
   E. There is a high incidence of aspiration with emergency LMA use.

12. Which of the following statements regarding the laryngeal mask airway (LMA) is TRUE?

   A. Positive-pressure ventilation is generally not useful.
   B. Gastric inflation is much more likely when positive-pressure ventilation with a pressure of 10 cm H_2O is used with an LMA than with an endotracheal tube (ETT).
   C. An LMA cannot be used in the lateral position.
   D. Tidal volumes of up to 8 mL/kg and airway pressure below 20 cm H_2O can be used in positive-pressure ventilation with an LMA.
   E. The intracuff pressure in an LMA should always be less than 20 cm H_2O.

13. Which of the following statements regarding the Sellick's maneuver is FALSE?

   A. It can obliterate the esophageal lumen while maintaining the tracheal opening.
   B. It is contraindicated when there is active vomiting.
   C. It can be used in conjunction with gentle positive-pressure ventilation.
   D. It should be used for rapid sequence induction in patients with laryngeal fractures who have full stomachs.
   E. Lateral displacement of the esophagus with the Sellick's maneuver is common.

14. Which of the following statements regarding laryngo-spasm is TRUE?

   A. It cannot be triggered by abdominal visceral stimulation.
   B. It cannot be triggered by pain.
   C. It accounts for approximately 73% of all critical post-operative respiratory events in adults.
   D. It is a possible cause of pulmonary edema.
   E. It should always be treated with muscle relaxants.

15. Which of the following statements regarding the local anesthetic cocaine is TRUE?

   A. It may be especially useful in blunting the exaggerated blood pressure response to intubation often seen in hypertensive patients.
   B. It is an excellent topical anesthetic as well as a potent vasodilator.
   C. It is poorly absorbed from the tracheal mucosa and must be given in larger doses to be effective (10% solution).
   D. It is metabolized by pseudocholinesterase and should not be given to patients with this enzyme deficiency.
   E. The total dose should be limited to 600 mg.

16. Which technique is frequently not appropriate for endo-tracheal intubation when a patient has gross blood in the airway?

   A. Retrograde wire intubation
   B. Intubating laryngeal mask airway (LMA)
   C. Esophageal–tracheal Combitube
   D. Fiberoptic bronchoscopy
   E. Cricothyroidotomy

17. Which of the following statements regarding airway management is TRUE?

   A. The backward–upward–rightward pressure (BURP) maneuver helps to expel air entrained in the stomach after bag-mask ventilation.
   B. In general, the Macintosh blade provides a better laryngeal view in patients with a smaller mandibular space.
   C. In general, the Miller blade provides a better laryngeal view in patients with a small mouth opening.
   D. The best treatment for laryngospasm is the Sellick's maneuver.
   E. Cricoid pressure (the Sellick's maneuver) can be effectively used with a laryngeal mask airway (LMA) in place.

18. Which of the following statements regarding the cricothyroid area is FALSE?

    A. The cricothyroid membrane is often crossed horizontally in its upper third by vascular structures.
    B. The cricothyroid membrane can be identified 1 to 1.5 fingerbreadths above the laryngeal prominence.
    C. The cricoid cartilage is the only circumferential cartilage in the laryngeal skeleton.
    D. Cricothyroid punctures should be made in the inferior third of the membrane and should be directed posteriorly.
    E. The cricotracheal ligament suspends the trachea superiorly from the cricoid cartilage.

19. When attempting to predict a difficult airway, it is important to acknowledge that:

    A. A small thyromental distance correlates with good descent of the larynx.
    B. Multivariate composite indices currently have the poor predictive ability for difficult laryngoscopy.
    C. A small as well as a large thyromental distance (TMD) can both predict difficult laryngoscopy.
    D. The Mallampati classification alone provides adequate information for the prediction of difficult laryngoscopy.
    E. A long descent of the larynx indicates a relatively small tongue in the hypopharynx.

20. When positioning a patient for direct laryngoscopy, it is important to remember that:

    A. Maximal mouth opening is less with atlanto-occipital extension compared with the neutral head position.
    B. Atlanto-occipital extension posteriorly displaces the tongue.
    C. Unanticipated failure of direct laryngoscopy is rarely due to improper tongue displacement.
    D. Obese patients may need the head and neck raised above the thorax with a wedge-shaped lift beginning under the scapula.
    E. Claims for laryngeal injury during direct laryngoscopy usually arise during laryngoscopies that were anticipated to be difficult.

21. Generally, when approaching a patient at risk for postextubation stridor, which of the following should NOT be considered?

    A. An endotracheal cuff leak test to rule in or rule out stridor
    B. The use of multiple-dose dexamethasone to reduce the risk of laryngeal edema
    C. Preparation of standby reintubation equipment
    D. Routine establishment of a route for reintubation and oxygenation
    E. A single dose of dexamethasone given 1 hour before extubation to reduce the likelihood of reintubation

ANSWERS

1. B. Local anesthetics are the cornerstone of awake airway control techniques. Since much of the agent used will be within the tracheal–bronchial tree and can travel to the alveoli, there is a potential for significant intravascular absorption with some techniques. In a recent study using 400 mg or 800 mg of lidocaine administered by a nebulizer, serum levels of 2.8 μg/mL and 6.5 μg/mL were measured within 10 minutes of dose completion, respectively. The toxic level of lidocaine is considered to be 4 μg/mL. Administration of antisialagogues is important to the success of awake intubation techniques; the commonly used drugs are atropine (0.5–1 mg IM or IV) and glycopyrrolate (0.2–0.4 mg IM or IV). Dexmedetomidine, a highly selective centrally acting α_2-adrenergic agonist, has been used for sedation and analgesia without respiratory depression in patients undergoing awake fiberoptic intubation. Combined with topical anesthesia, dexmedetomidine sedation provides for a smooth intubation. A loading dose of dexmedetomidine is 1 μg/kg IV over 10 minutes, and the maintenance infusion dose is 0.2 to 0.7 μg/kg/hr. Vasoconstriction of the nasal passages is required if there is to be instrumentation of this part of the airway. Oxymetazoline is a potent and long-lasting vasoconstrictor that is available over the counter. Cocaine solution 4% is a popular choice as a local anesthetic and vasoconstrictor. The total dose applied to the mucosa should not exceed 200 mg in the adult. (See page 789: Awake Airway Management.)

2. C. Patients at risk for neurologic sequelae (e.g., those with unstable cervical spine pathology) may undergo active sensory–motor testing immediately after tracheal intubation during awake airway management. In an emergent situation, there may be cautions (e.g., cardiovascular stimulation in the presence of cardiac ischemia or ischemic risk, bronchospasm, increased intraocular pressure, increased intracranial pressure) but no absolute contraindications to awake intubation. Contraindications to elective awake intubation include patient refusal or inability to cooperate (e.g., children or patients with profound mental retardation, dementia, or intoxication), or allergy to local anesthetics. Awake intubation provides many advantages over the anesthetized state, including maintenance of spontaneous ventilation in the event that the airway cannot be secured rapidly, increased size and patency of the pharynx, relative forward placement of the base of the tongue, posterior placement of the larynx, and patency of the retropalatal space. (See page 789: Awake Airway Management.)

3. D. Timing of the removal of the LMA at the end of surgery is critical. The LMA should be removed either when the patient is deeply anesthetized, or after the protective reflexes have returned and the patient is able to open the mouth on command. Removal during excitation stages of emergence can be accompanied by coughing, laryngospasm, or both. Since the halogenated inhaled anesthetics are potent bronchodilators, it is at the time of emergence, when the anesthetic is discontinued, that patients at risk for bronchospasm are most likely to wheeze. In patients managed with LMAs, there is no foreign body in the sensitive bronchorespiratory tree, and the patient can be fully emerged before removal of the device. Many clinicians remove the LMA fully inflated, so it acts as a "scoop" for secretions above the mask, bringing them out of the airway. The incidence of sore throat is approximately 10% compared with 30% with tracheal intubation, but it has been reported with a range of 0% to 70%. When tracheal intubation is mandatory (for the surgical procedure), yet concerns regarding bronchospasm exist, the Bailey maneuver should be used. In this maneuver, the deflated LMA is placed behind the in situ ETT. The ETT is removed, and the LMA is inflated. The patient is then emerged on the LMA. (See page 770: The Laryngeal Mask Airway Classic.)

4. A. In preparation for using a face mask for positive-pressure ventilation (after apnea is induced), appropriate positioning of the patient is paramount. With the patient in the supine position, the head and neck are placed in the sniffing position. This position improves mask ventilation by moving the base of the tongue and the epiglottis anteriorly, as has been demonstrated on endoscopic studies in anesthetized patients. The sniffing position moves the esophagus to a more anterior position. When a patient has presented with removable dentures, leaving the prosthetics in place can aid face mask ventilation; however, the risk of displacement should be considered. Patients with normal lung compliance should require no more than 20 to 25 cm H_2O pressure to inflate the lungs. If more pressure than this is required, the clinician should re-evaluate the adequacy of the airway, adjust the fit of the mask, seek assistance to perform two- or three-handed mask holds, or consider other devices that aid in the creation of an open passage for air flow through the upper airway. If there are no contraindications (e.g., a "full stomach" or other aspiration risk), mask ventilation can be used for the duration of anesthesia maintenance. (See page 769: The Anesthesia Face Mask.)

5. B. The laryngeal skeleton consists of nine cartilages (three paired and three unpaired) that together house the vocal folds, which extend in an anterior–posterior plane from the thyroid cartilage to the arytenoid cartilages. The larynx is innervated bilaterally by two branches of each vagus nerve: The superior laryngeal nerve and the recurrent laryngeal nerve. The trachea measures approximately 15 cm in adults and is circumferentially supported by 17 to 18 C-shaped cartilages, with a posterior membranous aspect overlying the esophagus. The right principal bronchus is larger in diameter than the left and is deviated from the plane of the trachea at a less acute angle. Cartilaginous rings support the first seven generations of the bronchi. (See page 763: Review of Airway Anatomy.)

6. D. Preoxygenation (also commonly termed denitrogenation) should be practiced in all cases when time permits. This procedure entails the replacement of the nitrogen volume of the lung (>69% of the FRC) with oxygen to provide a reservoir for diffusion into the alveolar capillary blood after the onset of apnea. Even under ideal conditions, patients breathing room air ($FIO_2 = 0.21$) will experience oxyhemoglobin desaturation to a level of less than 90% after approximately 2 minutes of apnea. Preoxygenation with 100% O_2 via a tight-fitting face mask for 5 minutes in spontaneously breathing patients can furnish up to 10 minutes of oxygen reserve after apnea (in patients without significant cardiopulmonary disease and normal oxygen consumption). A modified vital capacity technique, in which the patient is asked to take eight deep breaths in a 60-second period, shows promise in terms of prolonging the time to desaturation. In obese patients, BiPAP and the head-up position (~25 degrees) have been advocated to both reach maximal preinduction arterial oxygenation and to delay oxyhemoglobin desaturation. The most common reason for not achieving a maximum alveolar oxygen store during preoxygenation is use of a loose-fitting mask, which allows the entrainment of room air. Leaks as small as 4 mm (cross-section) may cause significant reductions in the inspired oxygen content. (See page 768: Preoxygenation.)

7. C. Before attachment of the anesthesia circuit, the LMA is inflated with the minimum amount of gas to form an effective seal. Although it is difficult to suggest a particular volume of gas to be used, the operator should be accustomed to the feel of the pilot bulb when it is inflated to 60 cm H_2O pressure, the maximum suggested seal pressure. (See page 770 : Supraglottic Airways.)

8. C. Because of the relatively larger size of the occiput in children, which produces an "anatomic sniffing position," elevation of the head (as done in adults) is not needed. On occasion, the thorax may need to be elevated instead. The relatively short neck in children gives the impression of an anterior position of the larynx. Posterior cricoid pressure is often helpful to place the laryngeal inlet into view. A straight blade is more helpful than a curved blade in displacing the stiff, omega-shaped, high epiglottis. Since the cricoid cartilage is the narrowest aspect of the airway until children are 6 to 8 years of age, one must be sensitive to resistance to advancement of the endotracheal tube that has easily passed the vocal folds. Hyperextension at the atlanto-occipital joint, as done in adults, may cause airway obstruction in children because of the relative pliability of the trachea. (See page 774: Tracheal Intubation: Use of the Direct Laryngoscope Blade.)

9. A. The oropharynx is innervated by branches of the vagus, facial, and glossopharyngeal nerves. The glossopharyngeal nerve travels anteriorly along the lateral surface of the pharynx. Its three branches supply sensory innervation to the posterior third of the tongue, the vallecula, the anterior surface of the epiglottis (lingual branch), the walls of the pharynx (pharyngeal branch), and the tonsils (tonsillar branch). The internal branch of the superior laryngeal nerve, which is a branch of the vagus nerve, provides sen-

sory innervation to the base of the tongue, epiglottis, aryepiglottic folds, and arytenoids. The remaining portion of the superior laryngeal nerve, the external branch, supplies motor innervation to the cricothyroid muscle. The hypoglossal nerve provides purely motor innervation to the tongue. (See page 789: Awake Airway Management.)

10. A. Obstruction to mask ventilation may be caused by laryngospasm, which is a reflex closure of the vocal folds. Laryngospasm may occur as a result of foreign body (oral or nasal airway), saliva, blood, or vomitus touching the glottis, or it may occur during a light plane of anesthesia. Hypoxia, as well as noncardiogenic pulmonary edema, are potential consequences of spontaneous ventilation against an obstructed airway. (See page 769: The Anesthesia Face Mask.)

11. A. Although the distal tip of the LMA's mask sits in the esophageal inlet, it does not reliably seal it. A predominant clinical perception is that the LMA does not protect the trachea from regurgitated gastric contents. During cardiopulmonary resuscitation, the incidence of gastroesophageal regurgitation is four times greater with a bag-valvemask than with an LMA. If regurgitated gastric contents are noted in the LMA, maneuvers similar to those applied when using an endotracheal tube should be instituted (i.e., the Trendelenburg position, 100% oxygen, and leaving the LMA in place and using a flexible suction device down the barrel). When populations of patients considered to have a "full stomach" are studied (in controlled trials, prospective series, or case reports), there is a very low incidence of aspiration noted with elective or emergency LMA use. (See page 770: The Laryngeal Mask Airway Classic.)

12. D. When using the LMA, tidal volumes should be limited to 8 mL/kg and airway pressure to 20 cm H_2O because this is the sealing pressure of the device under normal circumstances. Although first introduced for use with spontaneous ventilation, the LMA has shown to be useful when positive-pressure ventilation is either desired or preferred. There is no difference found in gastric inflation with positive pressures below 17 cm H_2O when comparing LMA with the ETT. Patients' airways have been managed with the LMA in the supine, prone, lateral, oblique, Trendelenburg, and lithotomy positions. The pressure within the cuff should never exceed 60 cm H_2O. (See page 770: The Laryngeal Mask Airway Classic.)

13. D. Cricoid pressure entails the downward displacement of the cricoid cartilage against the cervical vertebral bodies. In this manner, the lumen of the esophagus is ablated while the completely circular nature of the cricoid cartilage maintains the tracheal lumen. Early cadaveric studies showed that correctly applied cricoid pressure is effective in preventing gastric fluids (<100 cm H_2O pressure) from leaking into the pharynx. Cricoid pressure is contraindicated in patients with active vomiting (risk of esophageal rupture), cervical spine fracture, and laryngeal fracture. If there are difficulties in securing the airway during rapid sequence induction, gentle positive-pressure ventilation may be used while cricoid pressure is maintained. The esophagus is displaced laterally in most normal patients, questioning the utility of the Sellick's maneuver. (See page 781: NPO Status and the Rapid Sequence Induction.)

14. D. As a cause of ventilatory compromise, laryngospasm deserves special attention because of its prevalence in children and because it accounts for 23% of all critical postoperative respiratory events in adults. Laryngospasm may be triggered by respiratory secretions, vomitus, or blood in the airway; pain in any part of the body; and pelvic or abdominal visceral stimulation. The cause of airway obstruction during laryngospasm is contraction of the lateral cricoarytenoids, the thyroarytenoid, and the cricothyroid muscles. Management of patients with laryngospasm consists of immediate removal of the offending stimulus (if identifiable); administration of oxygen with continuous positive airway pressure; and if other maneuvers are unsuccessful, use of a small dose of short-acting muscle relaxant. Negative-pressure pulmonary edema may result from any airway obstruction in a patient who continues to have a voluntary respiratory effort. Negative intrathoracic pressure is transmitted to the alveoli, which are unable to expand as a result of the more proximal obstruction. (See page 784: Extubation of the Trachea.)

15. D. Among otolaryngologists, cocaine is a popular topical agent. Not only is it a highly effective local anesthetic, it is the only local anesthetic that is a potent vasoconstrictor. It is commonly available in a 4% solution. The total dose applied to the mucosa should not exceed 200 mg in adults. Cocaine should not be used in patients with known cocaine hypersensitivity, hypertension, ischemic heart disease, or preeclampsia or in those taking monoamine oxidase inhibitors. Since cocaine is metabolized by pseudocholinesterase, it is contraindicated in patients deficient in this enzyme. (See page 789: Awake Airway Management.)

16. D. Contraindications to fiberoptic bronchoscope–aided intubation are relative and revolve around the limitations of the device. Since the optical elements are small, minute amounts of airway secretions, blood, or traumatic debris can hinder visualization. Retrograde wire intubation has been described in a number of clinical situations as a primary intubation technique (elective or urgent) and after failed attempts at direct laryngoscopy, fiberoptic-aided intubation, and LMA-guided intubation. The most common indications are an inability to visualize the vocal folds because of blood, secretions, or anatomic variations; an unstable cervical spine; an upper airway malignancy; and mandibular fracture. Advantages to the esophageal–tracheal Combitube include rapid airway control, airway protection from regurgitation, ease of use for inexperienced operators, lack of requirement to visualize the larynx, and ability to maintain the patient's neck in a neutral position. This device has been shown to be useful in patients with massive upper gastrointestinal bleeding or vomiting. The LMA Fastrach is indicated for routine elective intubation and for anticipated and unanticipated difficult intubation. Since it was designed to facilitate blind tracheal intubation, the presence of airway secretions, blood, or edema does not interfere with its use. Cricothyroidotomy is predominantly

utilized in emergency situations, but may also be considered for elective procedures. (See page 797: Minimally Invasive Transtracheal Procedures.)

17. E. Treatment of laryngospasm includes removal of an offending stimulus (if it can be identified), continuous positive airway pressure, deepening of the anesthetic state, and use of a rapidly acting muscle relaxant. If a satisfactory laryngeal view is not achieved during laryngoscopy, the BURP maneuver may aid in improving the view. In this maneuver, a second operator displaces the larynx backward (B) against the cervical vertebrae, as superiorly (U) as possible and slightly lateral to the right (R), using external pressure (P) over the cricoid cartilage. As a generalization, the Macintosh blade is regarded as a better option wherever there is little room to pass an ETT (e.g., small mouth), but the Miller blade is regarded better in patients who have a small mandibular space, large incisor teeth, or a large epiglottis. The major disadvantage of the LMA in resuscitation is suboptimal mechanical protection from regurgitation and aspiration. Lower rates of regurgitation during cardiopulmonary resuscitation (3.5%) than with bag-valve-mask ventilation (12.4%) have been shown. Even in the presence of regurgitation, pulmonary aspiration is a rare event with the LMA. Unfortunately, use of the Sellick's maneuver may prevent proper seating of the LMA in a minority of instances. This may require brief removal of cricoid pressure until the LMA has been properly seated. Cricoid pressure is effective with an LMA in place. (See page 768: Clinical Management of the Airway.)

18. B. The cricothyroid membrane provides coverage to the cricothyroid space. It is located in the anterior neck between the thyroid cartilage superiorly and the cricoid cartilage inferiorly. It can be identified 1 to 1.5 fingerbreadths below the laryngeal prominence (thyroid notch) and is composed of a yellow elastic tissue that lies directly beneath the skin and a thin facial layer. It is often crossed horizontally in its upper third by the anastomoses of the left and right superior cricothyroid arteries. The membrane has a central portion known as the conus elasticus and two lateral, thinner portions. Directly beneath the membrane is the laryngeal mucosa. Because of anatomic variability in the course of veins and arteries and the membrane's proximity to the vocal folds (which may be 0.9 cm above the ligament's upper border), it is suggested that any incisions or needle punctures to the cricothyroid membrane be made in its inferior third and be directed posteriorly (posterior probing needles will strike the back side of the ring-shaped cricoid cartilage). At the base of the larynx, the signet ring–shaped cricoid cartilage is suspended by the underside of the cricothyroid membrane. The trachea is suspended from the cricoid cartilage by the cricotracheal ligament. (See page 763: Review of Airway Anatomy.)

19. C. Poor descent of the larynx results in a small TMD and may indicate a difficult direct laryngoscopy. Despite the disappointing usefulness of individual indexes for anticipating difficult direct laryngoscopy, some authors have recognized that combinations of tests may provide improved predictability. El-Ganzouri et al. designed a statistical model for stratifying risk of difficult direct laryngoscopy in a large population. This multivariate index assigned relative weights to each physical examination or historical finding based on the odds of a high-grade laryngeal view being achieved on direct laryngoscopy with an increasing examination score. Compared with the Mallampati classification alone, the multivariate composite index had improved positive predictive and specificity values at equal sensitivity. A long descent of the larynx results in a large part of the tongue being in the hypopharynx. Chou et al. also noted that the long mandibulohyoid distance can be partly caused by a shortened mandibular ramus. A short ramus results in the floor of the mouth being more rostrad and less compliant, so displacement of the tongue is more difficult. (See page 765: Limitations of Patient History and Physical Examination and page 774: Tracheal Intubation.)

20. **D.**   The extension of the atlanto-occipital joint provides wider mouth opening. Calder et al. have shown that the maximal mouth opening is 26% greater in full atlanto-occipital extension than in the neutral head position. Although atlanto-occipital extension cannot by itself allow direct laryngeal vision, it does provide anterior displacement of the mass of the tongue and brings the upper alveolar ridge into improved position relative to the tongue and larynx. Unanticipated problems with direct laryngoscopy are primarily a problem with tongue displacement. Obese patients may need further positioning to move the mass of the chest away from the plane across which the laryngoscope handle will sweep as it is manipulated in the mouth. This may require placing a wedge-shaped lift under the scapula, shoulders, and nape of neck; raising the head and neck above the thorax; and providing a grade to allow gravity to take the pandicular mass away from the airway. Domino et al.'s analysis of the American Society of Anesthesiologists' Closed Claims Database reveals that claims for laryngeal injury during direct laryngoscopy arise more often in "easy" as opposed to difficult laryngoscopies. (See page 774: Direct Laryngoscopy.)

21. **E.**   A popular test used to predict airway patency after extubation is the detection of a leak on deflation of the endotracheal cuff. Patients with a reduced cuff leak volume are at risk for postextubation stridor, although the absence of an airway leak on cuff deflation is not predictive of subsequent ventilatory failure after extubation. A randomized control trial study in 2007 revealed that multiple-dose dexamethasone effectively reduced the incidence of postextubation stridor in adult patients at high risk for postextubation laryngeal edema, but single-dose injection of dexamethasone given 1 hour before extubation did not reduce the number of patients requiring reintubation. When there is a suspicion that a patient may have difficulty with oxygenation or ventilation after tracheal extubation, the clinician may choose from a number of management strategies ranging from the preparation of standby reintubation equipment to the active establishment of a route or guide for reintubation or oxygenation. (See page 784: Extubation of the Trachea.)

Patient Positioning and Potential Injuries

1. A 67-year-old woman is scheduled for exploratory laparotomy because of a large pelvic mass. Before induction,
   she suddenly develops hypotension and tachycardia. What
   is the next most appropriate step?

   A. Increase the FIO_2 to 100%.
   B. Put the patient in the Trendelenburg position.
   C Rapidly infuse 1,000 mL of intravenous saline.
   D. Place a wedge underneath the patient's right hip.
   E. Administer 100 μg of phenylephrine.

2. All of the following statements concerning the exaggerated
   lithotomy position are true EXCEPT:

   A. It provides easy access to the perineum.
   B. The patient's pelvis is flexed ventrally on the spine.
   C. It is more easily tolerated by awake patients.
   D. This position has been associated with a high fre-
      quency of lower extremity compartment syndrome.
   E. Bulky thighs may cause abdominal compression and
      restrict ventilation.

3. All of the following statements concerning upper
   extremity injuries are true EXCEPT:

   A. The long thoracic nerve arises from nerve roots C5
      to C7.
   B. Winging of the scapula is commonly associated with
      injury of the long thoracic nerve.
   C. The long thoracic nerve is routinely involved in
      stretch injuries of the brachial plexus.
   D. Hyperabduction of the arm may push the humerus
      into the axillary neurovascular bundle.
   E. A dampened pulse oximetry tracing may be a sign of
      neurovascular compression.

4. All of the following statements concerning radial nerve
   injury are true EXCEPT:

   A. Compression at the mid-humerus level by sheets used
      to tuck the arm may cause damage to the nerve.
   B. Radial nerve injury results in wrist drop and weakness
      of thumb abduction.
   C. The most common site of injury is the olecranon
      groove.
   D. A patient with a radial nerve injury cannot extend the
      distal phalanx of the thumb.
   E. A patient with a radial nerve injury has decreased sen-
      sation in the web space between the thumb and
      index finger.

5. Which of the following statements concerning ulnar nerve
   injury is TRUE?

   A. The nerve is most susceptible to injury when the arm
      is on an arm board with the hand supinated.
   B. Elbow flexion may cause ulnar nerve damage by com-
      pression by the aponeurosis of the flexor carpi ulnaris
      muscle.
   C. The nerve is susceptible to injury as it passes in the
      ulnar groove of the lateral epicondyle.
   D. Injury causes loss of sensation in the thumb.
   E. Men have less statistical chance of postoperative ulnar
      neuropathy than women.

6. To have the pelvis retained in place on a fracture table for
   repair of a fractured femur, a vertical pole at the
   perineum should be placed:

   A. Between the genitalia and the uninjured limb
   B. Between the genitalia and the injured limb
   C. Between the limbs at the mid-thigh level
   D. Against the surface of the sacral prominence
   E. At the ankle level

7. All of the following may cause a compartment syndrome
   EXCEPT:

   A. Systemic hypotension with loss of perfusion pressure
   B. Vascular obstruction by pelvic retractors
   C. External compression by leg wrappings that are too
      tight
   D. Compression stockings
   E. Prolonged lithotomy position

8. Signs and symptoms of a compartment syndrome include
   all of the following EXCEPT:

   A. Rhabdomyolysis
   B. Hypoxic edema
   C. Renal failure
   D. Pain
   E. Deep venous thrombosis (DVT)

9. All of the following accurately describe problems resulting from the lateral decubitus position EXCEPT:

   A. Improper neck positioning may intensify pain from protrusion of a cervical disc.
   B. There is the potential for excessive ventilation of the upside lung.
   C. Respiratory compromise may be lessened if the point of flexion is at the iliac crest as opposed to the costal margin or flank.
   D. There is the potential for winging of the scapula.
   E. The saphenous nerve of the downside leg is likely to be compressed.

10. All of the following may result from the prone position EXCEPT:

   A. Conjunctival edema
   B. Breast injuries, especially if the breast is displaced laterally
   C. Distention of paravertebral vessels
   D. Increased pulmonary compliance
   E. Compression ischemia of the genitals and ventral stomas, if present

11. All of the following are complications associated with the head-elevated/sitting position EXCEPT:

   A. Paradoxical air embolus
   B. Paralysis below the fifth cervical vertebrae
   C. Stretch injury of the sciatic nerve
   D. Postural hypotension
   E. Hypertension

12. Consequences of head-down positions in an anesthetized patient include all of the following EXCEPT:

   A. Worsening of ventilation–perfusion ratio
   B. Increased intracranial pressure
   C. Compartment syndrome
   D. Decreased work of spontaneous ventilation
   E. Stretch of middle and lower divisions of the brachial plexus

13. Acute venous congestion of the optic canal is a potential etiology of ischemic optic neuropathy. All of the following help to reduce venous congestion EXCEPT:

   A. Supine positioning
   B. Short anesthetic duration
   C. Head positioned at the level of the heart
   D. Avoidance of a Wilson surgical bed frame
   E. Elevated BMI

ANSWERS

1. D. With the patient in the supine position, a mobile abdominal mass, such as a very large tumor or a pregnant uterus, may rest on the great vessels of the abdomen and compromise circulation. This is known as the aortocaval syndrome or supine hypotensive syndrome. A significant degree of perfusion may be restored if the compressive mass is rolled toward the left side of the abdomen by a mechanical device that produces leftward displacement (e.g., a wedge under the right hip). (See page 804: Variations Supine Positions.)

2. C. The exaggerated lithotomy position is rarely tolerated by awake patients. In this position, the pelvis is flexed ventrally on the spine, the thighs are flexed on the trunk, and the legs are aimed skyward. Maintenance of perfusion pressure is important because the position has been associated with a high frequency of lower extremity compartment syndrome. Controlled ventilation is usually necessary because abdominal compression by the thighs may restrict ventilation. (See page 805: Lithotomy.)

3. C. The long thoracic nerve arises from nerve roots C5 to C7 and innervates the serratus anterior muscle. Dysfunction of this nerve causes winging of the scapula. The effect of patient position is speculative because the nerve is not routinely involved in a stretch injury of the brachial plexus and because the plexus is not routinely involved when long thoracic nerve dysfunction occurs. Hyperabduction of an arm may force the head of the humerus into the axillary neurovascular bundle and may be associated with dampening of the distal pulse and the ipsilateral pulse oximeter waveform. (See page 808: Long Thoracic Nerve Dysfunction.)

4. C. The radial nerve may be injured by compression against the underlying bone as it wraps around the humerus approximately 3 cm above the lateral epicondyle. Excessive cycling of an automatic blood pressure cuff has been implicated in causing damage to the radial nerve. Compression at the mid-humerus level by sheets or towels used to tuck the arm may also result in injury. Radial nerve injury results in wrist drop, weakness of thumb abduction, inability to extend the metacarpophalangeal joints, and loss of sensation in the web space between the thumb and the index finger. (See page 808: Brachial Plexus and Upper Extremity Injuries.)

5. B. The ulnar nerve passes though the groove between the medial epicondyle and the olecranon process of the humerus. The nerve may be compressed as the arm lies abducted on a normal arm board with the hand pronated. Injury should be suspected if a pinprick on the fifth finger is not felt. Elbow flexion may cause ulnar nerve damage by several mechanisms, including compression by the aponeurosis of flexor carpi ulnaris muscle and cubital tunnel retinaculum or anterior subluxation of the ulnar nerve over the medial epicondyle of the humerus. Men are statistically more likely to have postoperative ulnar neuropathy than women. (See page 808: Brachial Plexus and Upper Extremity Injuries.)

6. A. The vertical pole on a fracture table should be well padded and placed against the pelvis between the genitalia and the uninjured limb. Damage to the genitalia and pudendal nerve and complete loss of penile sensation have been reported after improper use of the fracture table. (See page 811: Perineal Crush Injury.)

7. D. Causes of compartment syndrome that are associated with positioning include systemic hypotension with loss of perfusion pressure, vascular obstruction by intrapelvic retractors, by excessive flexion of knees or hips (as in lithotomy position), or by undue popliteal pressure from a knee crutch or by external compression by straps and wrappings that are too tight. Compression stockings and devices used to prevent deep venous thrombosis are not associated with compartment syndrome. (See page 811: Compartment Syndrome.)

8. E. Signs and symptoms of a compartment syndrome include ischemia, hypoxic edema, elevated tissue perfusion pressure within fascial compartments of the extremity, rhabdomyolysis, pain, and renal failure. A sequential compression device is used to prevent development of DVT in prolonged procedures; this is not associated with compartment syndrome. (See page 811: Compartment Syndrome.)

9. E. The lateral decubitus position may compromise ventilation and lead to injuries of the shoulder, scapula, and extremities. Damage of the peroneal nerve of the downside leg is common as it courses laterally around the neck of the fibula. The saphenous nerve courses medially and is less likely to be compressed. (See page 811: Other Supine Position Problems.)

10. D. Compression of the abdominal viscera and restricted chest expansion in the prone position decrease pulmonary compliance. Conjunctival edema is common in prone patients whose heads are at or below the level of the heart. It is usually transient, but permanent loss of vision may occur. When intra-abdominal pressure approaches or exceeds venous pressure, return of blood from the pelvis and lower extremities is reduced or obstructed, and there is distention of paravertebral vessels. Medial and cephalad displacement of the breasts is better tolerated than forced lateral displacement. Stoma that drain visceral contents through the abdominal wall are at risk in the prone position if they lie against a part of any supporting frame or pad. Compressive ischemia of the stomal orifice can cause it to slough. The same issue is present for genitals, especially the penis and scrotum of men turned prone. (See page 816: Complications of Prone Positions.)

11. **E.** Postural hypotension may occur in the sitting position because the normal protective reflexes are inhibited by drugs used during anesthesia. The sitting position predisposes patients to air embolization when venous pressure becomes subatmospheric. There is risk of peripheral nerve injury, especially stretch injuries of the sciatic nerve, as a result of marked hip flexion without bending the knees. If the neck is excessively extended, diminished cervical spinal cord perfusion pressure may cause quadriplegia. (See page 820: Complications of the Head-elevated Positions.)

12. **D.** Cephalad displacement of the diaphragm and restriction of lung expansion accompany a head-down position because of gravity-shifted abdominal viscera. Consequently, the work of spontaneous ventilation is increased for an anesthetized patient in a posture that already worsens the ventilation–perfusion ratio by gravitational accumulation of blood in the poorly ventilated lung apices. Cranial vascular congestion and increased intracranial pressure can be expected to result from head-down tilt. The use of bent knees for prevention of sliding cephalad when in steep head-down tilt can cause compressive ischemia, phlebitis or compartment syndrome. Cephalad movement, when the arms are fixated or when shoulder restraints (with either braces, tape, or "bean bag" devices) are used may result in stretch of the brachial plexus. (See page 821: Complications of Head-down Positions).

13. **E.** To prevent ischemic optic neuropathy, it is prudent to attempt to reduce venous congestion in the optic canal and to maintain optic nerve perfusion pressure. Intraoperative positioning that helps reduce intra-abdominal pressure, and therefore, venous congestion, may be useful. Prone positioning, by itself, is a risk factor and, if used, should allow the patient's head to be at level with or higher than the heart. The use of a Wilson surgical bed frame with its elevated curvature (resulting in the head being lower than the heart), obesity (with its potential elevation of intra-abdominal pressure in prone-positioned patients), and long anesthetic durations can all contribute to elevated venous congestion in the optic canal. (See page 816: Complications of Prone Positions: Blindness.)

CHAPTER 29

Monitored Anesthesia Care

1. Sedation/analgesia:

   A. Has been replaced by the term *conscious sedation* in the American Society of Anesthesiologists (ASA) practice guidelines.
   B. Describes a state in which a patient's only response is reflex withdrawal from a painful stimulus.
   C. Describes a state that allows the patient to respond purposefully to a verbal command or tactile stimulation.
   D. Is a deeper level of sedation than that provided by monitored anesthesia care (MAC).
   E. Was a term first introduced by the American Dental Association.

2. The condition in which a patient has no movement in response to a painful stimulus describes:

   A. Conscious sedation
   B. Intravenous sedation
   C. Monitored anesthesia care (MAC)
   D. Sedation/analgesia
   E. General anesthesia

3. All of the following statements regarding monitored anesthesia care (MAC) are true EXCEPT:

   A. The patient remains able to protect the airway for most of the procedure.
   B. It always involves the administration of sedative drugs.
   C. It requires performance of a preanesthesia examination and evaluation.
   D. It is reimbursed at the same level as general or regional anesthesia.
   E. It may include the administration of bronchodilators.

4. The context-sensitive half-time:

   A. Is directly related to the elimination half-time
   B. Is independent of the duration of infusion
   C. Is the half-time of equilibration between drug concentration in the blood and its effect
   D. Depends on both metabolism and distribution phenomena
   E. Is generally measured by serum assay of drug concentrations

5. Which statement about drug interactions is TRUE?

   A. Coexisting respiratory disease is not related to the frequency of respiratory depression in patients receiving opioid–benzodiazepine combinations.
   B. There is no difference in the incidence of adverse respiratory effects when midazolam is used alone or in combination with fentanyl.
   C. Most of the fatalities reported after the use of midazolam and opioids were related to adverse cardiac events.
   D. Opioids and benzodiazepines are synergistic in producing hypnosis.
   E. When an opioid is used in the analgesic dose range, there is little risk of adverse cardiorespiratory interaction.

6. When used for monitored anesthesia care (MAC), propofol:

   A. Causes greater respiratory depression than midazolam when combined with an opioid
   B. Reliably causes amnesia
   C. Possesses antiemetic effects
   D. Has excellent analgesic properties
   E. Has a context-sensitive half-time that depends markedly on the duration of the infusion

7. Advantages of midazolam over diazepam include all of the following EXCEPT:

   A. It has a lower incidence of resedation.
   B. Clearance is unaffected by cimetidine.
   C. Thrombophlebitis is rare.
   D. It is usually painless on injection.
   E. Active metabolites work synergistically with the parent drug.

8. Which statement regarding remifentanil is TRUE?

   A. Compared with other opioids, a bolus of remifentanil is associated with an increased incidence of respiratory depression.
   B. It is predominately metabolized by the P450 hepatic enzyme system.
   C. When used with midazolam, remifentanil causes less respiratory depression than other opioids.
   D. The initial infusion rate should be 1 μg/kg/min.
   E. It is supplied in a multidose vial that should be refrigerated.

9. Choose the correct order of symptoms observed with worsening local anesthetic toxicity.

   A. Muscle twitching, metallic taste, vertigo
   B. Tinnitus, numbness of the tongue, seizure
   C. Slurred speech, muscle twitching, restlessness
   D. Sedation, tinnitus, seizure
   E. Blurred vision, circumoral numbness, vertigo

10. Dexmedetomidine:

    A. Has the same half-life as clonidine
    B. Decreases cardiac vagal activity
    C. Is not associated with hypotension
    D. Is a selective α_2-receptor antagonist
    E. Is administered as an initial bolus of 0.5 to 1 $\mu g/kg$

11. Which statement regarding ketamine is TRUE?

    A. It has been shown to preserve airway reflexes when used in large doses.
    B. It is a good choice for open globe injuries.
    C. It produces a dissociative state.
    D. Doses of 0.3 mg/kg are frequently associated with significant cardiorespiratory depression.
    E. It can only be administered intramuscularly or intravenously.

12. Which of the following is TRUE regarding monitored anesthesia care (MAC)?

    A. It includes diagnosis and treatment of clinical problems that occur during a procedure.
    B. Intensive care unit nurses may provide it.
    C. Typically a longer recovery time is needed compared to general anesthesia.
    D. It does not include postprocedure anesthesia management.

13. Both monitored anesthesia care (MAC) and general anesthesia share all of the following EXCEPT:

    A. Include preoperative assessment
    B. Require continual physical presence of the anesthesiologist or nurse anesthetist
    C. Include intraoperative monitoring
    D. Always involve the administration of sedative drugs

14. All of the following describe the ideal sedation technique for monitored anesthesia care (MAC) EXCEPT:

    A. Should provide rapid and complete recovery at the end of the procedure
    B. Should have a low incidence of side effects
    C. May provide deeper sedation than that provided during sedation/analgesia
    D. Leaves the patient unable to communicate during the procedure

15. Sedation of a patient can result in all of the following EXCEPT:

    A. Loss of protective laryngeal and pharyngeal reflexes
    B. Depressed ventilatory response to hypoxia and hypercapnia
    C. Diminished swallowing reflex
    D. Decreased resting arterial partial pressure of oxygen
    E. Hypertonicity of the upper airway dilator muscles

16. Which of the following is the least likely cause of agitation during monitored anesthesia care (MAC)?

    A. Hypoxia
    B. Local anesthetic toxicity
    C. Distended bladder
    D. Cerebral hypoperfusion
    E. Laryngospasm

17. Which of the following is NOT a feature of administration of drugs by continuous infusion rather than by intermittent dosing during monitored anesthesia care (MAC)?

    A. Reduced total amount of drug administered
    B. Increased incidence of hemodynamic instability
    C. Fewer episodes of excessive sedation
    D. Fewer episodes of inadequate sedation
    E. Facilitation of a more rapid recovery

18. Which statement regarding the comparison of propofol to benzodiazepines for conscious sedation is FALSE?

    A. Immediate recovery is faster.
    B. Psychomotor function returns to baseline earlier.
    C. There is less postoperative clumsiness.
    D. The postanesthesia care unit stay is consistently markedly shorter.
    E. Propofol's context-sensitive half-time is half that of midazolam

19. Flumazenil reversal of benzodiazepine-induced sedation:

    A. Is inexpensive and should be routine
    B. Is associated with undesirable hemodynamic effects
    C. Does not reverse the amnestic effect
    D. May be associated with resedation because of its short elimination half-life
    E. The usual initial intravenous dose is 2 mg

20. Which of the following statements about the use of opioids during monitored anesthesia care (MAC) is TRUE?

    A. They are a good choice for sedation during a working spinal anesthetic.
    B. Alfentanil is a good choice for brief, intense analgesia.
    C. They are associated with reliable amnesia.
    D. They are not associated with a significant risk of nausea.
    E. Respiratory depression is not seen with remifentanil due to its short duration of action.

21. Oxygen administration during monitored anesthesia care (MAC):

    A. Can "mask" significant alveolar hypoventilation
    B. Must be administered in high concentrations to be effective
    C. Is never required in the postoperative period
    D. Is required by the American Society of Anesthesiologists (ASA) standards for basic monitoring
    E. Must always be administered via nonrebreather mask in patients with preexisting lung disease

22. Which of the following regarding Bispectral index (BIS) monitoring is FALSE?

    A. It may help avoid complications of overdosing medications.
    B. It is a processed electroencephalogram parameter.
    C. It ideally should be used as an adjunct to clinical evaluation.
    D. It increases upon deepening of sedation.
    E. It is not a replacement for clinical evaluation.

23. The American Society of Anesthesiologists (ASA) practice guidelines for sedation and analgesia by nonanesthesiologists:

    A. Suggest that the individual performing the procedure should also monitor the patient's vital signs
    B. Do not recommend routine administration of supplemental oxygen
    C. Emphasize the importance of preprocedure patient evaluations but not fasting
    D. Suggest that an individual with advanced life support skills be present during the procedure
    E. Do not recommend monitoring of patients for very minor procedures

ANSWERS

1. **C.** *Sedation/analgesia* is the term currently used by the ASA in its practice guidelines for sedation and analgesia by nonanesthesiologists. The current ASA definition of sedation/analgesia is "a state that allows patients to tolerate unpleasant procedures while maintaining adequate cardiorespiratory functions and the ability to respond purposefully to verbal command or tactile stimulation." Thus, sedation/analgesia is intended to be a lighter level of sedation than may be encountered during MAC. The term *sedation/analgesia* is used most frequently in the context of care provided by nonanesthesiologists and implies a level of vigilance that is less than that required for general anesthesia. The ASA specifically states that patients whose only response is reflex withdrawal from a painful stimulus are sedated to a greater degree than encompassed by the term *sedation/analgesia*. (See page 825: Terminology.)

2. **E.** In general anesthesia, the patient is medicated to the extent that he or she has no movement in response to a painful stimulus. (See page 825: Terminology.)

3. **B.** MAC refers to clinical situations in which the patient remains able to protect the airway during most of the procedure. Since MAC is a physician service provided to an individual patient and is based on medical necessity, it should be subject to the same level of reimbursement as general or regional anesthesia. The American Society of Anesthesiologists (ASA) states that MAC must include performance of a preanesthetic examination and evaluation. Also, the ASA states that all institutional regulations pertaining to anesthesia services shall be observed and all the usual services performed by an anesthesiologist should be provided, including administration of sedatives, tranquilizers, antiemetics, narcotics, other analgesics, β blockers, vasopressors, bronchodilators, antihypertensives, or other pharmacologic therapy as may be required in the judgment of the anesthesiologist. (See page 825: Terminology.)

4. **D.** The context-sensitive half-time is the time required for the plasma drug concentration to decline by 50% after terminating an infusion of a particular duration. The context-sensitive half-time takes into account both metabolism and distribution effects. It is highly dependent on the duration of infusion, particularly for drugs such as thiopental and fentanyl. It bears no constant relationship to the elimination half-times. Generally, it is calculated by computer simulation of multicompartmental pharmacokinetic models. (See page 827: Context-sensitive Half-time.)

5. **D.** During MAC, the maximum benefit of opioid supplementation in terms of potentiation of other administered sedatives will accrue when the opioid is used in the analgesic dose range. Within this dose range, there is great potential for an adverse cardiorespiratory interaction. Opioid–benzodiazepine combinations are frequently used to achieve the components of hypnosis, amnesia, and analgesia. The opioid–benzodiazepine combination displays marked synergism in producing hypnosis. Several fatalities have been reported after the use of midazolam, most of them related to adverse respiratory events. In many of these cases, midazolam was used in combination with an opioid. Studies have shown that midazolam usually does not produce significant respiratory effects when used alone; however, the combination of midazolam and fentanyl has a higher incidence of hypoxemia in study subjects. The respiratory depressive effects of this drug combination are likely to be even more significant in patients with coexisting respiratory or central nervous system disease or at the extremes of age. (See page 828: Drug Interactions in Monitored Anesthesia Care.)

6. **C.** Propofol has many ideal properties for use during MAC. The context-sensitive half-time remains short regardless of the length of infusion, and its rapid onset allows for easier titration. Propofol appears to have antiemetic properties but no analgesic or amnestic effects. When combined with opioids, propofol appears to result in less respiratory depression than does a benzodiazepine-opioid combination, which may cause severe respiratory depression. (See page 829: Specific Drugs Used for Monitored Anesthesia Care.)

7. **E.** The major advantages of midazolam over diazepam include the following: Midazolam is water soluble, it is usually painless upon injection, thrombophlebitis is rare, it has a short elimination half-life of 1 to 4 hours, its clearance is unaffected by histamine (H_2) antagonists, it has inactive metabolites, and resedation is unlikely. (See page 829: Specific Drugs Used for Monitored Anesthesia Care.)

8. **A.** Unlike previously available opioids, remifentanil is predominately metabolized by nonspecific esterases generating an extremely rapid clearance and offset of effect. Published data suggest that bolus administration of remifentanil is associated with an increased incidence of respiratory depression and chest wall rigidity. Since these side effects are likely to be related to high peak concentration of drug, it is recommended that remifentanil boluses be administered slowly or by using a pure infusion technique. The most logical method for the administration of remifentanil during monitored anesthesia care is by an adjustable infusion. Most investigators have used infusion rates that start at 0.1 μg/kg/min approximately 5 minutes before the first painful stimulus. This initial loading infusion is then weaned to approximately 0.05 μg/kg/min to maintain patient comfort. Remifentanil is supplied as a powder that must be reconstituted before use. (See page 829: Specific Drugs Used for Monitored Anesthesia Care.)

9. **D.** The clinically recognizable effects of local anesthetic toxicity on the central nervous system are concentration

dependent. Initial symptoms are sedation, numbness of the tongue and circumoral tissues, and a metallic taste. As concentrations increase, restlessness, vertigo, tinnitus, and difficulty focusing may occur. Higher concentrations result in slurred speech and skeletal muscle twitching, which often herald the onset of tonic–clonic seizures. (See page 839: Preparedness to Recognize and Treat Local Anesthetic Toxicity.)

10. **E.**   Similar to clonidine, dexmedetomidine is a selective α_2-receptor agonist. Stimulation of α_2 receptors produces sedation and analgesia, a reduction of sympathetic outflow, and an increase in cardiac vagal activity. The use of clonidine in the perioperative period is limited by its long half-life of 6 to 10 hours. However, dexmedetomidine has a much shorter half-life and greater α_2-receptor selectivity. Despite its α_2 selectivity, dexmedetomidine may still cause significant bradycardia and hypotension. Initial bolus doses range from 0.5 to 1 μg/kg over 10 to 20 minutes followed by a continuous infusion of 0.2 to 0.7 μg/kg/hr. (See page 829: Specific Drugs Used for Monitored Anesthesia Care.)

11. **C.**   Ketamine is a phencyclidine derivative. When used in small doses (0.25–0.5 mg/kg), its use is associated with minimal respiratory and cardiovascular depression. Ketamine produces a dissociative state in which the eyes remain open with a nystagmic gaze. Ketamine can elevate intraocular pressure and is thus relatively contraindicated in patients with open globe injuries. Increased oral secretions make laryngospasm more likely. Although it has been suggested that airway reflexes are relatively preserved with ketamine, no convincing evidence supports this notion. Ketamine can be administered by oral, intravenous, or intramuscular routes. (See page 829: Specific Drugs Used for Monitored Anesthesia Care.)

12. **A.**   MAC includes all aspects of anesthesia care, including the preoperative visit, intraoperative care, and postprocedure anesthesia management. During MAC, the anesthesiologist or a member of the anesthesia care team provides a number of specific services, including (but not limited to) monitoring of vital signs, maintenance of the patient's airway, continual evaluation of vital functions, and diagnosis and treatment of clinical problems that occur during the procedure. Conceptually, recovery from MAC should be more rapid than from general anesthesia. (See page 825: Terminology.)

13. **D.**   MAC usually is provided to conscious patients undergoing therapeutic or diagnostic procedures that would otherwise be unacceptably uncomfortable or unsafe without the attention of an anesthesiologist. As with general anesthesia, there must be a preanesthetic examination and evaluation, a prescription of anesthesia care, personal participation in or medical direction of the entire plan of care, and continuous physical presence of the anesthesia care provider. MAC always involves monitoring of a patient but does not necessarily require the administration of sedative drugs. (See page 825: Preoperative Assessment.)

14. **D.**   The ideal sedation technique involves the administration of either individual or combinations of analgesic, amnestic, and hypnotic drugs. There should be a minimal incidence of side effects such as cardiorespiratory depression, nausea and vomiting, delayed emergence, and dysphoria. Patients should be able to communicate when indicated. Recovery after the completion of the procedure should be rapid and complete. (See page 826: Techniques of Monitored Anesthesia Care.)

15. **E.**   Protective laryngeal and pharyngeal reflexes are depressed by sedation and may render the patient vulnerable to aspiration. The swallowing reflex may be depressed for a long time after the return of consciousness. Opioids depress the normal ventilatory response to hypoxia and hypercapnia. Benzodiazepines appear to have a variable effect on ventilatory response, although they clearly potentiate the respiratory depression of opioids. Hypoventilation leads to reduced oxygen saturation in the absence of supplemental inspired oxygen. Upper airway dilator muscle tone is diminished during sedation, predisposing patients to upper airway obstruction. (See page 836: Sedation and Protective Airway Reflexes.)

16. **E.**   There are many potential causes for patient agitation during MAC. Agitation can have benign causes, which are easily treated, or it may be the first sign of a potentially life-threatening development requiring timely identification and treatment. Agitation during MAC may be a result of pain or anxiety, but it is of paramount importance that hypoxia and cerebral hypoperfusion be excluded as causes. Other possible causes of agitation include local anesthetic toxicity, hypothermia, a distended bladder, nausea, an uncomfortable position and prolonged tourniquet inflation. Laryngospasm would be a very uncommon event during MAC, although assessment of the patient's airway and breathing should always occur early during diagnosis of intraoperative problems. (See page 826: Techniques of Monitored Anesthesia Care.)

17. **B.**   Continuous infusions of sedative drugs are superior to intermittent bolus dosing because they produce less fluctuation in drug concentration, thus reducing the number of episodes of inadequate or excessive sedation. The steady plasma drug concentration causes less hemodynamic instability than an intermittent bolus technique. Also, the total amount of drug may be lower, facilitating a more prompt recovery. (See page 826: Techniques of Monitored Anesthesia Care.)

18. **D.**   A study by Mackenzie showed that a group of patients receiving propofol had faster immediate recovery than the group of patients who received midazolam. Furthermore, psychomotor function was comparable to baseline values immediately after propofol sedation but did not return to baseline until 2 hours after midazolam administration. Another study by White et al. showed that propofol produced less postoperative sedation, drowsiness, confusion, and clumsiness than midazolam; however, both drugs had similar discharge times. The context-sensitive half-time of

midazolam is approximately twice that of propofol. (See page 829: Specific Drugs Used for Monitored Anesthesia Care: Propofol.)

19. D. Flumazenil is a specific benzodiazepine antagonist that reverses the sedative and anesthetic effects without adverse side effects. It has a short elimination half-time, so there is a potential for resedation after the flumazenil has been cleared. The routine use of flumazenil represents a significant cost disadvantage compared with propofol sedation. The recommended initial intravenous dose of flumazenil is 0.2 mg. This dose can be repeated every minute to achieve desired reversal of sedation. (See page 830: Benzodiazepines.)

20. B. Opioids are best used to provide the analgesic component during MAC. They are not appropriate for a sedative or anesthetic component because they cannot reliably produce sedation without significant respiratory depression, and they lack significant amnestic properties. Propofol and midazolam produce more specific sedative effects. Opioids are associated with a significant risk of nausea and vomiting in ambulatory patients. Alfentanil's pharmacokinetic profile makes it well suited for treatment of brief painful periods such as placement of a retrobulbar block. While the average duration of action of remifentanil is only 3 minutes, as a powerful opioid, it still has the potential to cause significant respiratory depression. (See page 831: Opioids.)

21. A. Even in moderate concentrations, oxygen administration is very effective for increasing a low oxygen saturation resulting from hypoventilation. However, when the patient is receiving oxygen, significant hypoventilation and hypercarbia may be present even though the oxygen saturation is normal. Oxygen administration is not required by ASA standards but should be highly considered whenever sedatives or respiratory depressants are used. Respiratory depression may persist into the recovery period; measurement of oxygen saturation on room air may be useful before discharging a patient from the post-anesthesia care unit without supplemental oxygen. The method of supplemental oxygen delivery will vary from patient to patient, and from provider to provider. Most commonly a simple nasal cannula is used, but simple face mask and even continuous positive airway pressure (CPAP) support can be provided via mask. Although patients with pre-existing pulmonary disease will likely require an increased level of supplemental oxygen compared to the healthy patient, a nonrebreather mask is usually not necessary. (See page 836: Supplemental Oxygen Administration.)

22. D. The BIS is a processed electroencephalogram parameter. Sedation monitoring is attractive because of the potential to titrate drugs more accurately and thus avoid the adverse effects of both overdosing and underdosing. An increased depth of sedation is associated with a predictable decrease in the BIS. Although the use of the BIS to monitor sedation is appealing, conventional assessment of sedation is an important mechanism whereby continuous patient contact is maintained. Ideally, BIS monitoring will be used in the future as an adjunct to clinical evaluation rather than as the primary monitor of consciousness. (See page 838: Bispectral Index Monitoring During Monitored Anesthesia Care.)

23. D. The ASA practice guidelines for sedation and analgesia by nonanesthesiologists emphasize the importance of preprocedure patient evaluation, patient preparation, and appropriate fasting periods. These guidelines also suggest that an individual other than the person performing the procedure be available to monitor the patient's comfort and physiologic status. The routine administration of supplemental oxygen is recommended, but not required. At least one person with advanced life support skills should be present during the procedure. (See page 839: Sedation and Analgesia by Nonanesthesiologists.)

CHAPTER 30

Ambulatory Anesthesia

1. Which of the following is not a candidate for outpatient surgery requiring general anesthesia?

   A. A patient with a body mass index of 35 and obstructive sleep apnea (OSA) who is having laparoscopic surgery of the upper abdomen
   B. An asymptomatic ex-premature child who is 62 weeks of postconceptional age
   C. A patient in whom a blood transfusion is anticipated
   D. Any patient in American Society of Anesthesiologists (ASA) class IV
   E. Any patient older than 80 years of age

2. Which of the following statements concerning epidural and caudal anesthesia is TRUE?

   A. Recovery from spinal anesthesia is always faster than recovery from epidural anesthesia.
   B. Bicarbonate can be added to solutions to increase the potency of epidural anesthesia.
   C. Additives for increasing duration of blockade include opioids, ketamine, clonidine, and neostigmine.
   D. Although caudal blocks result in better pain control, they do not affect discharge times.
   E. Caudal anesthesia is commonly performed on children for upper abdominal surgery.

3. Which of the following statements regarding induction with propofol is FALSE?

   A. 0.2 mg/kg of intravenous (IV) lidocaine may be used to decrease the incidence and severity of pain.
   B. Thrombophlebitis is a common problem after IV administration of this agent.
   C. 20 mL of propofol mixed with more than 20 mg of lidocaine should be avoided because it may lead to instability of the mixture.
   D. The elimination half-life of propofol is 1 to 3 hours.
   E. After induction doses of propofol, psychomotor impairment may last for up to 1 hour.

4. Which of the following statements regarding children with current or recent upper respiratory tract infections (URIs) is TRUE?

   A. URI in a child is associated with an increased risk for perioperative respiratory adverse events only when symptoms were present or had occurred within the 2 weeks before the procedure.
   B. Children with URIs are more likely to have longer lengths of hospital stays than children without URIs.
   C. The risk of adverse respiratory events is the same whether an endotracheal tube (ETT) or a laryngeal mask airway (LMA) is used.
   D. Children of parents who smoke have the same risk of adverse airway reactions as children of nonsmoking parents.
   E. Nonproductive cough carries the same risk of adverse airway reactions as does cough accompanied by copious secretions.

5. Which of the following statements regarding the current thinking on preoperative fasting and the risk of pulmonary aspiration of gastric contents in ambulatory adult patients is FALSE?

   A. There is considerable individual variation in gastric emptying times.
   B. In children who drank 7 mL/kg of clear liquids, the median half-life for gastric emptying occurred in less than 30 minutes.
   C. It is not acceptable to allow a patient to have a small solid meal the morning of a 9 am surgery.
   D. Coffee drinkers should be encouraged to drink black coffee the morning of surgery to avoid the risk of withdrawal.
   E. The new guidelines require fasting for 6 hours preoperatively only excluding the clear liquids needed to take medications.

6. Which of the following statements regarding perioperative opioids and nonsteroidal anti-inflammatory drugs is TRUE?

   A. Preoperative opioids help prevent hypotension during tracheal intubation.
   B. Morphine is helpful in controlling shivering.
   C. Preoperative celecoxib is accompanied by a reduced need for supplemental oxygen in the postanesthesia care unit.
   D. Opioids given preoperatively do not provide preoperative sedation.
   E. Opioids prevent increases in systolic blood pressure during intubation in a dose-dependent fashion.

7. Which of the following statements regarding postoperative nausea and vomiting (PONV) with ambulatory surgery is FALSE?

   A. 40 μg/kg of granisetron (a serotonin [5-HT$_3$] antagonist) is a superior antiemetic compared with 0.25 mg/kg of metoclopramide.

   B. Midazolam may possess some antiemetic properties.

   C. The ReliefBand acustimulation device is as effective as ondansetron in treating PONV in patients who are still nauseated after receiving metoclopramide and droperidol.

   D. If a dose of ondansetron is given in the operating room and the patient complains of nausea in the postanesthesia care unit (PACU), a repeat dose is often effective.

   E. Transdermal scopolamine is as effective as ondansetron or droperidol in preventing early and late PONV.

8. Which of the following statements regarding spinal anesthesia is TRUE?

   A. Chloroprocaine carries the same risk of transient neurologic symptoms (TNS) as does lidocaine.

   B. Adding fentanyl to the local anesthetic in the spinal technique does not change the tolerance for tourniquet pain.

   C. Nausea after spinal or epidural anesthesia is the same as after general anesthesia.

   D. Early ambulation after spinal anesthesia may decrease the incidence of postdural puncture headache.

   E. Headache is a common complication of lumbar puncture and needle size has no effect on the incidence of postdural puncture headache.

9. Which of the following statements regarding depth of anesthesia is FALSE?

   A. The use of bispectral index (BIS) monitoring has been shown in a meta-analysis to reduce the use of intraoperative anesthetics by up to 20%.

   B. The use of sympatholytics to treat hemodynamics is associated with faster recovery and fewer side effects than treating the hemodynamics with inhalational agents.

   C. The use of BIS monitoring may result in quicker awakening from general anesthetics.

   D. The use of BIS monitoring has significantly reduced the length of stay in the hospital.

   E. In a meta-analysis of BIS monitoring, use of BIS monitoring has a modest decrease in PACU duration.

10. Which of the following statements regarding intraoperative management of postoperative nausea and vomiting (PONV) is TRUE?

    A. Risk factors include a previous history of general anesthesia in the last 1 to 7 days.

    B. Acupuncture has not been shown to be effective in reducing the incidence of PONV.

    C. Serotonin antagonists are particularly effective in preventing PONV.

    D. Propofol increases the incidence of PONV.

    E. A risk factor for PONV is current smoking.

11. Which statement regarding the anesthetic technique and time to discharge from the ambulatory surgery unit has been shown in a recent meta-analysis?

    A. Patients receiving peripheral nerve blocks are discharged earlier than patients receiving general anesthesia or neuraxial anesthesia.

    B. Patients receiving neuraxial anesthesia are discharged earlier than patients receiving general anesthesia or peripheral nerve blocks.

    C. Patients receiving general anesthesia are discharged earlier than patients receiving peripheral nerve blocks or neuraxial anesthesia.

    D. Patients receiving neuraxial anesthesia or peripheral nerve blocks are discharged earlier than patients receiving general anesthesia.

    E. There is no difference in the time to discharge between patients receiving peripheral nerve blocks, neuraxial blocks, and general anesthesia.

ANSWERS

1. **A.** In a review of 258 morbidly obese patients who underwent outpatient surgery, they did not have a greater incidence of unplanned admissions, minor complications, or unplanned contact with health care professionals. However, morbidly obese patients have a higher incidence of OSA. The ASA has published practice guidelines for the perioperative management of patients with OSA. In the guidelines, the authors state that for patients with OSA, if local or regional anesthesia is used, the procedure can also be performed as an ambulatory procedure. Certain infants should be monitored for 12 hours after procedures because they are at risk of developing apnea. These include infants who are younger than 46 weeks of postconceptual age, infants who are younger than 60 weeks of age who also have a history of chronic lung or neurologic disease, and infants with anemia (hemoglobin <6 mmol/L). Infants without disease who are 46 to 60 weeks of age should be monitored for 6 hours after procedures. At the other extreme of life, advanced age alone is not a reason to disallow surgery in an ambulatory setting. Patients classified as ASA class III and IV should be considered for outpatient procedures provided their systemic diseases are medically controlled. The need for transfusion is also not a contraindication for ambulatory procedures. (See page 845: Places, Procedures, and Patient Selection.)

2. **C.** Epidural anesthesia takes longer to perform than spinal anesthesia. Onset with spinal anesthesia is more rapid, although recovery may be the same with either technique. In one study of patients undergoing knee arthroscopy, spinal anesthesia with small-dose lidocaine and fentanyl was compared with 3% 2-chloroprocaine administered in the epidural space. Intraoperative conditions, discharge characteristics and times, and recovery profiles were similar. Some studies suggest that bicarbonate can be added to solutions for faster onset of epidural anesthesia. Other useful (albeit controversial) additives for increasing duration of blockade include opioids, ketamine, clonidine, and neostigmine. Caudal anesthesia is a form of epidural anesthesia commonly used in children undergoing surgery below the umbilicus and to control postoperative pain. Because of better pain control after a caudal block, children can usually ambulate earlier and be discharged sooner than when a caudal block is not performed. Pain control and discharge times are no different whether the caudal block is placed before surgery or after it is completed. (See page 851: Epidural and Caudal Anesthesia.)

3. **B.** The popularity of propofol as an induction agent for outpatient surgery in part relates to its half-life: The elimination half-life of propofol is 1 to 3 hours, which is shorter than the half-lives of methohexital (6 to 8 hours) and thiopental (10 to 12 hours). Although the effect of drugs given for induction seems to be transient, they can depress psychomotor performance for several hours. Impairment after thiopental administration may be apparent for up to 5 hours; impairment after propofol administration only lasts for 1 hour. Thrombophlebitis does not appear to be a problem after IV administration of propofol, but it can be evident after thiopental administration. 0.2 mg/kg of IV lidocaine may be used to decrease the incidence and severity of pain upon propofol injection; other techniques have been tried, including 0.1 mg/kg of ketamine immediately before propofol injection or 20 mg of lidocaine plus 10 mg of metoclopramide. 20 mL of propofol mixed with more than 20 mg of lidocaine, though, should be avoided because it may lead to instability of the mixture. (See page 853: Induction.)

4. **A.** In 1-year-long survey of almost 10,000 children who underwent surgery, URI was associated with an increased risk for perioperative respiratory adverse events only when symptoms were present or had occurred within the 2 weeks before the procedure. Although a case may be cancelled because a child is symptomatic, the child may develop another URI when the procedure is rescheduled. In children, URI has not been shown to be associated with an increased length of stay in the hospital after a procedure. Independent risk factors for adverse respiratory events in children with URIs include use of an endotracheal tube (vs. use of a laryngeal mask airway [LMA] or face mask), history of prematurity, history of reactive airway disease, history of parental smoking, surgery involving the airway, presence of copious secretions, and nasal congestion. (See page 847: Upper Respiratory Tract Infection.)

5. **E.** No trial has shown that a shortened fluid fast increases the risk of aspiration. Fluids actually empty quickly from the stomach. In one study of children, 6 to 14 years who fasted overnight and then drank 7 mL/kg, median half-life for gastric emptying was 24 minutes, though there was considerable individual variation. Coffee is free of particulate matter and is accepted as a clear liquid. Coffee drinkers should be encouraged to drink coffee before their procedures because physical signs of withdrawal (e.g., headache) may easily occur. In 2011, the ASA revised practice guidelines for preoperative fasting. The guidelines allow a patient to have a light meal up to 6 hours before an elective procedure and support a fasting period for clear liquids of 2 hours for all patients. (See page 847: Restriction of Food and Liquids Before Ambulatory Surgery.)

6. **E.** Opioids can be administered preoperatively to sedate patients and decrease pain before surgery. They are useful in controlling hypertension during tracheal intubation. Opioid premedication prevents increases in systolic pressure in a dose-dependent fashion. Meperidine (but not morphine or fentanyl) is sometimes helpful in controlling shivering in the OR or the postanesthesia care unit. Preoperative administration of

nonsteroidal anti-inflammatory drugs is also useful in the early postoperative period. Celecoxib has been shown to reduce postoperative pain and need for more analgesia, but has no effect on need for oxygen postoperatively. (See page 849: Opioids and Nonsteroidal Analgesics.)

7. D. The 5-HT$_3$ antagonists seem particularly effective for PONV. For example, in one study of children who underwent strabismus surgery and were then nauseated during the first 3 hours after recovery from anesthesia, emesis-free episodes were greater after 40 μg/kg of granisetron was administered (88%) compared with 40 μg/kg of droperidol (63%) or 0.25 mg/kg of metoclopramide (58%). Midazolam and propofol, although more commonly used for sedation, have antiemetic effects that are longer in duration than their effects on sedation. When the use of a ReliefBand acustimulation device was compared with ondansetron for patients who were nauseated in the PACU after receiving metoclopramide or droperidol and who were undergoing laparoscopic surgery, nausea was most effectively treated with both the ReliefBand and ondansetron, although both therapies were equally effective individually in treating PONV. If a patient has already received ondansetron prophylaxis in the operating room and is nauseated in the PACU, another repeat dose is usually not particularly effective. In one study, premedication with transdermal scopolamine was as effective as ondansetron or droperidol in preventing early and late PONV and postdischarge nausea and vomiting, though it was associated with dry mouth. (See page 856: Nausea and Vomiting.)

8. D. Nausea is much less frequent after epidural or spinal anesthesia than after general anesthesia. Lidocaine and mepivacaine are ideal for ambulatory surgery because of their short durations of action, although lidocaine use has been problematic because of transient neurologic symptoms (TNS). Although TNS may be seen after other local anesthetics, the risk is seven times more after intrathecal lidocaine than after bupivacaine, prilocaine, or procaine administration. Likewise, lidocaine is associated with a higher rate of TNS than chloroprocaine. When fentanyl is added to spinal local anesthetic, tourniquet tolerance is improved. Bed rest does not reduce the frequency of headache. Indeed, early ambulation may decrease the incidence. Although headache is a common complication of lumbar puncture, smaller-gauge needles result in a lower incidence of postdural puncture headache. (See page 850: Spinal Anesthesia.)

9. D. BIS monitors are thought to decrease anesthetics used during general anesthesia. Since less anesthetic agent is used, titration of anesthesia with these monitors results in earlier emergence from anesthesia. In a meta-analysis of BIS monitoring for ambulatory anesthesia, BIS monitoring was shown to reduce anesthetic use by 19%, with more modest decreases in postanesthesia care unit duration (4 minutes) and PONV (6%). To be fair, not all agree that the use of depth of anesthesia monitoring decreases awareness: One group, in fact, found that when an inhalation agent was used for maintenance of anesthesia for patients with a high risk of recall that this may not be the case. They found that recall, amount of anesthesia used, and postoperative adverse outcomes were no different if BIS or end-tidal anesthesia was used to monitor depth of anesthesia. Sympatholytic drugs, instead of anesthesia, can be used to control autonomic responses to anesthesia. In fact, recovery is faster, and side effects are fewer in ambulatory patients whose blood pressure is controlled by sympatholytics instead of inhalation agents. (See page 855: Depth of Anesthesia.)

10. C. Women, especially those who are pregnant, have a higher incidence of PONV. Other risk factors include a history of motion sickness or postanesthetic emesis; surgery within 1 to 7 days of the menstrual cycle; not smoking; and procedures such as laparoscopy, lithotripsy, major breast surgery, and ear, nose, or throat surgery. The greater the number of risk factors, the greater risk for PONV. Therapies useful in controlling PONV include acupuncture, supplemental fluid therapy, clonidine (perhaps partly because it decreases anesthesia requirements), and dexamethasone. In one study, acupuncture therapy was effective in controlling both PONV and postoperative pain. Receptor antagonists, specifically selective serotonin antagonists (ondansetron, dolasetron, and granisetron), have been shown to have similar efficacy in helping to alleviate PONV. Dopamine antagonists, antihistamines, and anticholinergic drugs are useful and are generally less expensive, but they are associated with a higher incidence of side effects. Because of its ability to decrease PONV, propofol is an excellent general anesthetic for ambulatory anesthesia. (See page 853: Intraoperative Management of Postoperative Nausea and Vomiting.)

11. E. In a meta-analysis of peripheral nerve and central neuraxial blocks compared with general anesthesia, time until discharge from the ambulatory surgery unit was no different for the three groups. (See page 849: Intraoperative Management: Choice of Anesthetic Method.)

Office-Based Anesthesia

1. Approximately how many procedures were preformed in physicians' offices in 2000?

   A. 2 to 4 million
   B. 4 to 6 million
   C. 6 to 8 million
   D. 8 to 10 million
   E. 10 to 12 million

2. Which of the following statements regarding injuries during office-based anesthesia is TRUE?

   A. Intraoperative injuries are rare.
   B. The second most common incidence is in the recovery room.
   C. Less than 10% of injuries have a respiratory cause.
   D. Injuries after discharge account for about 20% of the injuries.

3. Which of the following statements regarding patient selection for office-based anesthesia is FALSE?

   A. The surgeon's office staff can arrange the surgery for patients with American Society of Anesthesiologists (ASA) status I and II.
   B. Close monitoring of oxygen saturation in an observational unit or intensive care unit (ICU) setting may be required postoperatively for patients with obstructive sleep apnea (OSA).
   C. A preoperative history and physical examination should be obtained within 90 days of the date of surgery.
   D. An anesthesiologist should contact the patient prior to an office-based procedure when possible.
   E. Preoperative anesthesia consultation should be obtained for patients with comorbid conditions.

4. All of the following statements regarding office-based anesthesia are TRUE, EXCEPT:

   A. Dantrolene should be available within 30 minutes.
   B. The ability to monitor end-tidal CO_2 is needed.
   C. The ability for continuous electrocardiographic (ECG) monitoring is needed.
   D. Monitoring of oxygen saturation is required.
   E. Continuous heart rate monitoring is required.

5. Which of the following statements is TRUE regarding the risk and management of intraoperative fires?

   A. Office-based operating rooms do not have large supplies of components required to start a fire.
   B. Office-based personnel should not be required to participate in fire drills.
   C. Flammable skin prep solutions should be quickly draped to help prevent fire.
   D. Oxygen supplies should be secured under the drapes.
   E. Facial plastic surgery creates a scenario where the risk of intraoperative fire is high.

6. Which of the following does not contribute to the mortality rate in liposuction procedures?

   A. Inadequate pain control
   B. Abdominal perforation
   C. Fat embolism
   D. Anesthetic "causes"
   E. Pulmonary embolism

7. Which of the following statements is FALSE regarding recommendations for office-based liposuction?

   A. General anesthesia can be used safely in the office setting.
   B. General anesthesia has advantages for more complex liposuction cases.
   C. Epidural and spinal anesthesia are encouraged because of the vasodilatation.
   D. Plastic surgeons should follow ASA Guidelines for Sedation and Analgesia.
   E. Moderate sedation is an effective adjunct to the anesthetic infiltrate solutions.

8. Which of the following statements regarding office-based gastrointestinal (GI) endoscopy is TRUE?

   A. Endotracheal intubation is often required for upper GI procedures.
   B. General anesthesia is usually required.
   C. Colonoscopy does not cause cardiac dysrhythmia.
   D. Hypotension may be caused by colonoscopy.
   E. The patients tend to be young patients without comorbidities.

9. All of the following ophthalmic and otorhinolaryngologic procedures are suitable for office-based anesthesia EXCEPT:

    A. Cataract extraction
    B. Ocular plastic
    C. Lacrimal duct probing
    D. Endoscopic sinus surgery
    E. Tonsillectomy

10. Which of the following statements regarding monitored anesthesia care (MAC) is FALSE?

    A. Some studies show that MAC has a higher mortality rate than general anesthesia.
    B. Complication rates for MAC are increasing.
    C. Injuries occurring during MAC procedures are less likely to be permanent than injuries sustained during general anesthesia.
    D. MAC cases are likely to lead to litigation.
    E. MAC is an appropriate office-based anesthetic.

11. Which of the following statements regarding the use of ketamine for office-based analgesia is TRUE?

    A. It is associated with nausea and vomiting.
    B. It functions as an analgesic
    C. It cannot be used as an induction agent.
    D. It increases the risk of aspiration as much as thiopental.
    E. It decreases secretions.

12. Which of the following statements regarding postoperative nausea and vomiting (PONV) in office-based anesthesia is FALSE?

    A. Use of ketorolac can result in a decreased incidence of PONV.
    B. Dexamethasone potentiates the effects of antiemetics.
    C. Routine prophylaxis using dexamethasone is more effective than symptomatic treatment.
    D. Adequate hydration may decrease PONV.
    E. 5-HT$_3$ antagonists cause less sedation than traditional first-line therapies.

ANSWERS

1. D. In the year 2000, approximately 75% of all procedures were performed on an outpatient basis; 17% in freestanding ambulatory surgical centers, and 14% to 25% (approximately 8–10 million) in physicians' offices. (See Page 861: Brief Historical Perspective of OBA.)

2. D. Injuries during office-based procedures occur throughout the perioperative period and are multifactorial in origin. Most of them occur intraoperatively. Fourteen percent occur in the postanesthesia care unit, and 21% occur after discharge. Fifty percent of injuries are respiratory and included airway obstruction, bronchospasm, inadequate oxygenation and ventilation, and unrecognized esophageal intubation. The second most common events are drug related. (See page 862: Office Safety.)

3. C. As of this writing, the patient should have a preoperative history and physical examination recorded within 30 days of the procedure, including all pertinent laboratory tests and any medically indicated specialist consultations. If the patient has an ASA status I or II, the surgeon's office can arrange the surgery as per office protocol. The anesthesiologist should have access to all of this information pre-operatively and, when possible, contact the patient prior to the scheduled procedure. However, if a patient has a significant comorbid condition, a preoperative anesthesiology consultation should be obtained before scheduling the patient for office-based surgery. Morbidly obese patients and patients with OSA present unique challenges. It has been recommended that an observational unit with close monitoring of oxygen saturation or an ICU setting be used for postoperative monitoring of patients with OSA. (See page 863: Patient Selection.)

4. A. Perioperative monitoring should adhere to the standards for basic anesthetic monitoring. These standards include continuous monitoring of heart rate and oxygen saturation, intermittent noninvasive blood pressure monitoring, end-tidal CO_2 monitoring, and the capacity for both temperature and continuous ECG monitoring. Office-based anesthesiologists should be prepared to begin the initial treatment of malignant hyperthermia, which requires having at least 12 bottles of dantrolene immediately available. (See page 865: Office Selection.)

5. E. The office must be prepared for an intraoperative fire. The ASA has recently published an advisory on the prevention and management of such an emergency. Fire requires three components known as the "fire triad": An oxidizer, an ignition source, and fuel. The modern operating room contains all three in great supply. There must be regularly scheduled fire drills that include all employees, even those with nonclinical duties. The ASA recommends that if flammable materials are used to prep the skin they should be allowed to completely dry before draping the surgical field. The field should then be draped in a manner that does not allow for oxygen to accumulate. This is important because these accumulated pockets of oxygen may flow into the surgical field where there is a source of ignition such as electrocautery. This scenario is common during facial plastic surgery. (See page 865: Office Selection and Requirements.)

6. A. Liposuction is not a benign procedure. In 2000, a census survey of the 1,200 members of the American Society of Aesthetic Plastic Surgeons (ASAPS), revealed an overall mortality rate of 19.1 per 100,000 liposuction procedures, with pulmonary embolism the diagnosis in 23.1% of deaths. Other etiologies of mortality included abdominal viscous perforation, anesthesia causes, fat embolism, infection, and hemorrhage. (See page 868: Specific Procedures: Liposuction.)

7. C. Iverson et al. developed the following considerations and recommendations regarding office-based liposuction:

1. Plastic surgeons should follow the current ASA Guidelines for Sedation and Analgesia.
2. General anesthesia can be used safely in the office setting.
3. General anesthesia has advantages for more complex liposuction procedures that include precise dosing of sedatives, controlled patient movement, and airway management.
4. Epidural and spinal anesthesia in the office setting are discouraged because of the possibility of vasodilatation, hypotension, and fluid overload.
5. Moderate sedation/analgesia augments the patient's comfort and is an effective adjunct to the anesthetic infiltrate solutions. (See page 868: Specific Procedures: Liposuction.)

8. D. The patient population for GI endoscopic procedures tends to be older, some with significant comorbid conditions. Upper GI procedures rarely require endotracheal intubation because the stomach is emptied under direct visualization. The procedure may be accomplished with sedation using midazolam and small doses of propofol. Colonoscopy is painful secondary to insertion and manipulation of the endoscope and may be associated with cardiovascular effects, including dysrhythmia, bradycardia, hypotension, hypertension, myocardial infarction, and death. (See page 869: Gastrointestinal Endoscopy.)

9. E. Ophthalmologic procedures suitable for the office include cataract extraction, lacrimal duct probing, and ocular plastics. Topical anesthesia or periorbital and retrobulbar blocks are frequently used to provide analgesia. Otolaryngology procedures acceptable for an office setting include endoscopic sinus surgery, septoplasty, and myringotomy. Tonsillectomy should not be performed in an office setting. (See page 869: Ophthalmology/Otolaryngology.)

10. C. In 1988, Cohen et al. reviewed the data from 100,000 anesthetics. They found that the group with the greatest number of mortalities had undergone procedures with sedation, whereas sedation constituted only 2% of all cases. The complication rate related to MAC anesthetics is increasing, as its use expands. In the 1990s, when injuries other than death occurred during MAC anesthetics, they were more likely to be permanent, whereas injuries occurring during GA were more frequently temporary. MAC anesthetics also tend to lead to litigation. (See page 870: Anesthetic Techniques.)

11. B. Ketamine, a phencyclidine derivative, functions as both an anesthetic and an analgesic. It does not depress respiration and increases laryngeal reflexes, thus decreasing the risk of aspiration. It is not associated with nausea and vomiting; however, ketamine may increase secretions and may cause hallucinations. (See page 871: Anesthetic Agents.)

12. C. Ketorolac decreases the incidence of PONV, and patients tolerate oral fluid and meet discharge criteria earlier than those receiving opioids. Many of the traditional first-line therapies are associated with sedation, drowsiness, and extrapyramidal side effects, and have been supplanted by 5-HT$_3$ antagonists such as ondansetron, dolasetron, and granisetron. Dexamethasone has been shown to improve the efficacy of both serotonin (5-HT$_3$) antagonists and dopamine antagonists. Routine prophylaxis use of this medication, however, has not shown any advantage over symptomatic treatment. Ensuring adequate hydration is an intervention that may be useful in the prevention of PONV. (See page 872: Post-anesthesia Care Unit (PACU).)

CHAPTER 32

Nonoperating Room Anesthesia (NORA)

1. Anesthesia equipment required in alternate sites includes which of the following?

   A. Reliable oxygen supply
   B. Invasive blood pressure monitoring setup
   C. Nitrous oxide cylinder
   D. BiPAP machine
   E. Difficult airway cart

2. The American Society of Anesthesiologists (ASA) closed claims database revealed which of the following about adverse events during nonoperating room anesthesia?

   A. Anaphylaxis to radiographic contrast dye was responsible for the majority of deaths in nonoperating room anesthesia.
   B. Nonoperating room anesthesia adverse events were associated with a low number of deaths as compared to adverse events occurring in the operating room.
   C. Half of nonoperating room anesthesia deaths were associated with monitored anesthesia care.
   D. Respiratory depression due to over-sedation was a relatively rare type of adverse event in the closed claims study.
   E. Paternal presence for pediatric cases would have decreased respiratory arrests by 50%.

3. During transfers of unstable patients between the intensive care unit or surgical suite and radiology, which of the following should be available?

   A. Central venous pressure monitor
   B. Propranolol
   C. Glidescope
   D. A manual self-inflating ventilation bag with adequate portable oxygen
   E. A method of two-way radio to the operating room desk

4. Which of the following statements regarding conscious sedation is TRUE?

   A. Cardiovascular function is often unstable.
   B. The patient should not be awake, but need to be able to maintain adequate spontaneous respirations.
   C. The patient should be able to respond to physical stimulation.
   D. Airway intervention is frequently required.
   E. Local anesthesia is rarely required for analgesia.

5. Which of the following is a method of reducing occupational exposure to ionizing radiation during nonoperating room anesthesia?

   A. Increasing distance from the source of radiation
   B. Using modern alfa-potentiometers to monitor accumulated radiation exposure
   C. Minimizing the width of walls in the room with radiation exposure
   D. Utilizing protective shielding made from titanium
   E. Avoiding dosimeters

6. Which of the following is a risk factor for intravenous contrast-induced neuropathy?

   A. Arterial hypotension
   B. Diabetes mellitus
   C. Chronic pancreatitis
   D. Melena
   E. Hypothyroidism

7. Which of the following is part of the treatment of severe hypersensitivity reactions to intravenous contrast agents?

   A. Nonsteroidal anti-inflammatory drugs
   B. Oxygen and airway protection
   C. Nonloop diuretics
   D. Bronchoconstrictors
   E. Potassium-sparing diuretic

8. Which of the following statements concerning magnetic resonance imaging (MRI) is TRUE?

   A. Cables and wires should be wound in loops in order to avoid induction-heating effects.
   B. The equipment brought into the MRI scanning room cannot be made of ferromagnetic metal.
   C. A patient with a cardiac pacemaker, an intracranial aneurysm clip, or an intravascular wire placed after January 2005 is safe for MRI.
   D. There is dangerous neutrinos radiation.
   E. Parents of pediatric patients cannot enter the MRI room.

9. Which of the following statements regarding external-beam radiation treatment is TRUE?

   A. Patients do not need to be immobile during the treatment.
   B. Sedation is preferred to general anesthesia in children.
   C. The anesthesiologist will be outside the treatment room.
   D. Patients will require a general anesthetic because of the pain associated with this procedure.
   E. A single therapy is usually all that is required.

10. Which of the following statements regarding cardioversion for atrial fibrillation is TRUE?

   A. Invasive monitoring is often required.
   B. Atrial fibrillation is associated hypertension, chronic heart failure, and valvular and ischemic heart disease.
   C. In general, patients require intubation.
   D. Propofol produces less hypotension than etomidate.
   E. A short-acting paralytic prevents patient self-injury during the procedure.

11. The physiologic response to electroconvulsive therapy (ECT) may include which of the following?

   A. Hypertrichosis
   B. Hypotension
   C. Polyuria
   D. Increase in cerebral blood flow
   E. Hyperhidrosis

12. Anesthetic considerations for electroconvulsive therapy (ECT) include which of the following?

   A. Rocuronium is associated with a longer duration of seizures.
   B. The anesthetic agent does not need to provide amnesia.
   C. Succinylcholine is most commonly used as a muscle relaxant.
   D. Propofol is contraindicated.
   E. Increased depth of anesthesia is associated with longer convulsions.

13. Which of the following statements regarding dental surgery is TRUE?

   A. Ketamine and midazolam may be given intravenously, intramuscularly, or orally.
   B. There is not an increased likelihood of postoperative laryngospasm.
   C. Tracheal intubation is often needed for airway protection.
   D. Ketamine always abolishes upper airway reflexes.
   E. Local anesthesia infiltration at the site of surgery is not beneficial during general anesthesia.

14. Which of the following is a common complication following anesthesia for dental surgery?

   A. Tracheomalacia
   B. Peripheral nerve damage
   C. Nausea and vomiting
   D. Airway obstruction from a neck hematoma
   E. Tooth injury

ANSWERS

1. A. The American Society of Anesthesiologists has developed a standard to apply to anesthesia-remote locations. Before commencing an anesthetic, it is vital to confirm the presence and proper functioning of all equipment an anesthesiologist would expect in the operating room. The location of immediately available resuscitation equipment for dealing with emergencies, including cardiopulmonary resuscitation and the management of anaphylaxis should be identified. This includes a reliable oxygen supply, full spare oxygen cylinder, adequate and reliable suction, adequate lighting, and sufficient space for personnel and equipment. (See page 877: General Principles.)

2. C. Adverse events occurring during nonoperating room anesthesia have been investigated using the ASA closed claims database. The findings demonstrated a higher number of deaths during nonoperating room anesthesia compared to anesthesia conducted in the operating room. Half of the deaths outside of the operating room were associated with monitored anesthesia care. Respiratory depression due to over-sedation was the most common adverse event in the closed claims study. (See page 877: General Principles.)

3. D. Sick, unstable patients may be transferred between the intensive care unit, the operating rooms, and nonoperating room locations for imaging or procedures. During transport the patient should be accompanied by a team member dedicated to evaluating, monitoring, and supporting the patient's medical condition. These patients are often ventilated and receiving drug infusions for both sedation and hemodynamic support. A portable oxygen source and manual self-inflating bag are essential. Infusion pumps and portable monitors should have adequate battery power for transit. Spare anesthetic and emergency drugs, equipment for re-intubation should be carried. (See page 877: General Principles.)

4. C. Conscious sedation is a state in which the patient is calm and relaxed yet able to respond to verbal or physical stimulation. The patient is able to maintain both a patent airway and protective airway reflexes during this minimally depressed level of consciousness. The patient is also responsive to verbal and physical stimuli, and their cardiovascular function is usually maintained. (See page 877: General Principles.)

5. A. Occupational exposure to ionizing radiation may come from direct exposure as well as from scattered radiation. Patients are subjected to direct exposure where the beam enters the skin. Staff working in a radiology suite are subjected to scattered radiation. Methods of limiting occupational exposure to radiation include: Limiting the time of exposure to radiation, increasing the distance from the source of radiation, using protective shielding, and using a dosimeter to limit the exposure of personnel to radiation doses. Anesthesiologists who are involved in

cases that involve exposure to ionizing radiation should wear dosimeters and be included in the institution's radiation safety program. (See page 880: Environmental Considerations for Non-operating Room Anesthesia.)

6. B. Contrast agents are eliminated by the kidneys, and contrast-induced nephropathy occurs with an incidence of 7% to 15% and is the third leading cause of hospital-acquired acute renal failure. Risk factors for CIN include: History of renal disease, prior renal surgery, proteinuria, diabetes mellitus, hypertension, gout, and use of nephrotoxic drugs. (See page 880: Environmental Considerations for Non-operating Room Anesthesia.)

7. B. Treatment of severe intravenous contrast-induced hypersensitivity reactions includes: Bronchodilation if needed, discontinuing the causative agent, and supportive therapy such as oxygen, airway protection, and cardiovascular support with fluids, vasopressors, and inotropes. (See page 880: Environmental Considerations for Non-operating Room Anesthesia.)

8. B. MRI is noninvasive and produces no ionizing radiation. There are no reports of harm from tissue contact with the magnetic field itself. Cables and wires should not be wound in loops to avoid induction-heating effects and patient burns. The equipment compatible with proximity to the MRI magnet differs in that they are made of nonferromagnetic metal such as aluminum. There have been fatalities from ferromagnetic equipment such as IV poles, gas cylinders, laryngoscopes, and pens becoming lethal projectiles if brought too close to the MRI magnet. Several types of physiologic monitors, oxygen-powered ventilators, laryngoscopic equipment, and anesthesia machines can be used within the MRI suite. Absolute or relative contraindications for MRI scanning include patients with cardiac pacemakers near the site of scanning, intracranial aneurysm clip, or intravascular wires which may all move when exposed to the magnetic field. (See page 883: Magnetic Resonance Imaging.)

9. C. Since the radiation dose is so high, all medical personnel must leave the room during external-beam radiation. Direct observation of the patient is not possible. Closed-circuit television and microphones are used. The need for patient immobility is a primary reason anesthesia is required for these procedures; it is difficult for children to keep completely still when only sedation is administered. Immobilization devices, especially those applied to the face and head, are unpleasant for the child and may cause airway concerns for the anesthesiologist. Multiple treatments usually are required. (See page 885: Radiation Therapy.)

10. B. Atrial fibrillation is associated with a number of conditions: Hypertension, chronic heart failure, and valvular and ischemic heart disease. Cardioversion is a brief but distressing procedure that is usually performed after a small bolus of intravenous induction agent. Invasive monitoring is rarely required. Propofol produces more hypotension than etomidate. In general, patients do not require intubation for cardioversion unless there is a risk of aspiration. (See page 886: Cardioversion.)

11. D.   A minimum seizure duration of 25 seconds is recommended to ensure adequate antidepressant efficacy. The cardiovascular response includes increased cerebral blood flow and intracranial pressure. Generalized autonomic nervous system stimulation results in an initial bradycardia and occasional asystole followed by a more prominent sympathetic response of hypertension and tachycardia. Occasional cardiac dysrhythmia, myocardial ischemia, infarction, or a neurologic vascular event may be precipitated. (See page 887: Electroconvulsive Therapy.)

12. C.   The anesthetic goals for a patient undergoing electroconvulsive therapy include amnesia, airway management, prevention of bodily injury from seizures, control of hemodynamic changes, and a smooth and rapid emergence. Etomidate is associated with seizures of longer duration. Propofol is an anticonvulsant and is more effective at attenuating the acute hemodynamic responses than etomi-

date. In small doses, the seizure duration is usually acceptable. Muscle relaxants are needed to prevent injury to the patient during grand mal seizures. Succinylcholine is used to prevent fractures or dislocations occurring during the seizure and is most commonly used because of its rapid onset and short duration. (See page 887: Electroconvulsive Therapy.)

13. A.   Ketamine is a useful induction agent. It may be used alone or in combination with atropine and midazolam by an intravenous, oral, intramuscular, rectal, or intranasal route. Ketamine, in standard doses, does not abolish upper airway reflexes. Tracheal intubation, often via the nasal route, is required to protect the airway, although the laryngeal mask airway has recently been used successfully in adults and children undergoing dental surgery. Laryngospasm is a postoperative concern after dental surgery and requires close observation during emergence and recovery. (See page 877: Dental Surgery.)

14. C.   After dental surgery the patient may develop postoperative complications that include bleeding, airway obstruction from retained throat packs, and laryngospasm. Later ones include and nausea and vomiting. (See page 887: Dental Surgery.)

Anesthesia for the Older Patient

1. All of the following are associated with aging EXCEPT:

    A. Free radicals and nonenzymatic glycosylation of sugars and amines are responsible for many age-related tissue changes.
    B. The cardiovascular system and lung parenchyma become stiffer with age.
    C. Mitochondrial DNA experiences more damage than nuclear DNA with aging.
    D. After elastin is damaged and removed, it is usually replaced by collagen.
    E. Many of the changes associated with aging are the result of damage to protein.

2. All of the following are associated with age-related changes in the kidney EXCEPT:

    A. Decreased ability to maintain sodium homeostasis
    B. Loss of up to 20% of glomeruli by 80 years of age
    C. Decreased renal cortical mass
    D. Reduced renal excretion of drugs
    E. Decreased glomerular filtration rate (GFR)

3. Which statement regarding drug pharmacology and aging is CORRECT?

    A. Elderly patients typically manifest a decrease in volume of distribution at steady state.
    B. Typically, the initial blood concentration of bolus drugs is lower in older patients.
    C. The most prominent pharmacokinetic effect of aging is a decrease in drug metabolism.
    D. Medications dependent on hepatic metabolism undergo increased clearance.
    E. Volume of distribution is affected by a decrease in body fat associated with aging.

4. Which of the following statements regarding aging and the cardiovascular system is FALSE?

    A. Maintenance of an adequate central blood volume becomes more critical to myocardial performance with age.
    B. There is a downregulation of β-receptors on the heart.
    C. The prevalence of atrial fibrillation increases with age.
    D. Aging diminishes or eliminates any protective effect of ischemic preconditioning.
    E. Most cases of congestive heart failure in very old individuals are attributable to diastolic dysfunction.

5. Which statement regarding postoperative mental status changes in elderly patients is FALSE?

    A. Postoperative delirium and postoperative cognitive decline are distinct clinical entities.
    B. Emergence delirium does not qualify as postoperative delirium.
    C. Low cognitive function, dementia, depression, and dehydration are risk factors for postoperative delirium.
    D. Regional anesthesia significantly reduces the incidence of postoperative delirium.
    E. Hip surgery carries a relatively high risk of postoperative delirium.

6. Which of the following statements regarding age-related changes in body composition is FALSE?

    A. The increase in body fat associated with aging is greater in women.
    B. Aging is characterized by a gradual loss of skeletal muscle.
    C. Basal metabolism is unaffected by age.
    D. Aging causes a significant decrease in plasma albumin levels.
    E. There is a reduction in total body water.

7. Which of the following statements regarding the hepatic system and aging is FALSE?

    A. Liver mass decreases with age.
    B. There is a moderate reduction in phase I drug metabolism.
    C. Liver blood flow decreases with age.
    D. Even healthy elderly patients experience markedly reduced liver reserve and markedly prolonged drug metabolism.
    E. Bile secretion decreases with age.

8. Which of the following statements regarding central nervous system changes in elderly patients is FALSE?

    A. Nearly 50% of patients older than 85 years of age have significant cognitive impairment.
    B. Changes in the function of the neurotransmitter acetylcholine (Ach) is connected to Alzheimer's disease.
    C. An 80-year-old brain has typically lost 10% of its weight.
    D. The aged brain is nearly incapable of forming new dendritic connections.
    E. Age is a major risk factor for postoperative delirium and/or cognitive decline.

9. Which of the following statements regarding the cardio-vascular system and aging is TRUE?

    A. There is increased parasympathetic activity.
    B. There is increased response to β-receptor stimulation.
    C. Veins become more compliant.
    D. Sympathetic nervous system activity decreases with age.
    E. Fibrosis of the conduction system may lead to sick sinus syndrome.

10. Which of the following statements regarding the pulmonary system in geriatric patients is TRUE?

    A. The chest wall becomes more compliant.
    B. Closing capacity typically exceeds tidal volume by 60 years of age.
    C. The diaphragm becomes more dome shaped.
    D. Lung parenchyma elasticity increases.
    E. The elderly are more likely to experience respiratory failure when required to increase minute ventilation.

11. Which of the following is not an age-associated change in the respiratory system?

    A. Aging results in less effective coughing and impaired swallowing.
    B. The majority of people older than 65 years of age have sleep-disordered breathing.
    C. There is a decreased ventilatory response to hypercapnia.
    D. Loss of muscle tone predisposes elderly individuals to upper airway obstruction.
    E. The response to hypoxia remains unchanged.

ANSWERS

1. B. A variety of deleterious processes continually attack DNA, proteins, and lipids. The primary culprits are free radicals and nonenzymatic glycosylation of sugars and amines. Whereas free radicals are a byproduct of oxidative metabolism, elevated glucose levels enhance glycosylation. Many of the changes associated with aging are the result of damage to protein. Collagen becomes stiffer from aromatic ring cleavage and by cross-linking to other collagen molecules. After elastin is damaged and removed, it is usually replaced by the stiffer collagen. In the cardiovascular system, arteries, veins, and the myocardium all stiffen with age. In contrast, lung parenchyma becomes less stiff because of loss of elastin without collagen substitution. DNA damage occurs as well, and curiously, mitochondrial DNA experiences more damage than nuclear DNA. (See page 892: The Process of Aging.)

2. B. Renal cortical mass decreases by 20% to 25% with age, but the most prominent effect of aging is the loss of up to 50% of the glomeruli by 80 years of age. The decrease in the GFR of approximately 1 mL/min/yr after 40 years of age typically reduces renal excretion of drugs to a level at which drug dosage adjustment becomes a progressively important consideration beginning at approximately 60 years of age. Nevertheless, the degree of decline in GFR is highly variable and is likely to be much less than predicted in many individuals, especially those who avoid excessive dietary protein. Aged kidneys do not eliminate excess sodium or retain sodium when necessary as effectively as kidneys of young adults. (See page 893: Changes in Body Composition and Liver and Kidney Aging.)

3. C. The most prominent pharmacokinetic effect of aging is a decrease in drug metabolism caused both by a decrease in clearance and an increase in the volume of distribution at steady state (Vdss). The increase in Vdss with age is likely attributable to the increase in body fat. When drug metabolism is via the liver, decreased liver mass and blood flow decrease clearance. (See page 894: Drug Pharmacology and Aging.)

4. B. Most cases of congestive heart failure in very old individuals are attributable to diastolic dysfunction; this occurs in the absence of clinically significant systolic dysfunction. Ventricular filling becomes more critical with age. The decreased response to β-receptor stimulation requires the ventricles to depend more on adequate end-diastolic volume to generate enough contractile strength via the length–tension (Frank–Starling) relationship. There does not appear to be a downregulation of β-receptors on the heart but rather a defect in the intracellular coupling. The diastolic dysfunction requires an increase in central blood volume and atrial pressure to maintain that end-diastolic volume. Therefore, maintenance of an adequate central blood volume becomes more critical to myocardial performance with age. (See page 897: Cardiovascular Aging.)

5. D. Postoperative cognitive decline and postoperative delirium are receiving increased attention as significant sources of debilitating morbidity. Although these two entities may yet prove to be related to each other, at present they appear to be distinct clinical syndromes. Postoperative delirium is an acute confusional state manifested by an acute onset (hours to days) and vacillating levels of attention and cognitive skill. Disorientation, perceptual disturbances (from misinterpretation of the situation to hallucinations), disorganized thinking, and problems with memory may be manifested. Emergence delirium does not qualify as postoperative delirium. The risk of postoperative delirium after major surgery in older patients is approximately 10%; however, the risk varies with the surgical procedure. The highest risk factor is associated hip surgery, with an approximate incidence of 35%. The cause of delirium is multifactorial. Patient risk factors include age, baseline low cognitive function or dementia, depression, and possibly general debility (including dehydration or visual or auditory impairment). The choice of regional versus general anesthesia does not appear to be a factor in postoperative delirium, especially if sedation is used in conjunction with the regional technique. (See page 901: Perioperative Complications.)

6. C. Changes in body composition are primarily characterized by a gradual loss of skeletal muscle and an increase in body fat, although the latter is more prominent in women. Basal metabolism declines with age, with most of the decline accounted for by the change in body composition. A reduction in total body water reflects the reduction in cellular water that is associated with a loss of muscle and an increase in adipose tissue. Aging causes a small decrease in plasma albumin levels. (See page 893: Changes in Body Composition and Liver and Kidney Aging.)

7. D. Liver mass decreases with age and accounts for most, but not all, of the 20% to 40% decrease in liver blood flow. There is also a modest reduction in phase I drug metabolism and bile secretion with age. Even in very old individuals, liver reserve should be more than adequate in the absence of disease other than for the effect of aging on drug metabolism. (See page 893: Changes in Body Composition and Liver and Kidney Aging.)

8. D. Brain mass begins to decrease slowly beginning at approximately 50 years of age and declines more rapidly later such that an 80-year-old brain has typically lost 10% of its weight. Neurotransmitter functions suffer more significantly, including levels of dopamine, serotonin, γ-aminobutyric acid, and especially the Ach system. The latter is especially important because of its connection to Alzheimer's disease. Response times increase, and learning is more difficult, but vocabulary, "wisdom," and past knowledge are better preserved. Nevertheless, of people 85 years of age and older, nearly half have significant cognitive impairment. In addition, some degree of atherosclerosis appears to be inevitable. Fortunately, and contrary to prior belief, the aged brain does make new neurons and is capable of forming new dendritic connections. Age is a major risk factor for postoperative delirium and/or cognitive decline. (See page 894: Central Nervous System Aging.)

9. **E.** Nearly all components of the cardiovascular system are affected by the aging process. The major changes include decreased response to β-receptor stimulation; stiffening of the myocardium, arteries, and veins; changes in the autonomic nervous system with increased sympathetic activity and decreased parasympathetic activity; conduction system changes; and defective ischemic preconditioning. (See page 897: Cardiovascular Aging.)

10. **E.** The most prominent effects of aging on the pulmonary system are stiffening of the chest wall and a decrease in elasticity of the lung parenchyma. Chest wall stiffening increases the work of breathing and produces a more barrel-shaped thorax that leads to flattening of the diaphragm. Closing capacity typically exceeds functional residual capacity in the mid-60s and eventually exceeds the tidal volume at some later age. The stiffened chest wall, flattened diaphragm, and the loss of muscle mass from aging all combine to make the older patient more prone to fatigue when challenged by an increase in minute ventilation, and thus more likely to experience respiratory failure. (See page 898: Pulmonary Aging.)

11. **E.** Aging leads to an approximate 50% decrease in the ventilatory response to hypercapnia and an even greater decrease in the response to hypoxia, especially at night. Generalized loss of muscle tone with age applies to the hypopharyngeal and genioglossal muscles and predisposes elderly individuals to upper airway obstruction. A high percentage of people older than 65 years of age have sleep-disordered breathing. Aging also results in less effective coughing and impaired swallowing. (See page 898: Pulmonary Aging.)

Epidural and Spinal Anesthesia

1. All of the following statements regarding epidural anesthesia are true EXCEPT:

   A. It can be used to provide postoperative analgesia.
   B. It has been shown to decrease some postoperative complications.
   C. It may improve surgical outcome.
   D. It has become absolutely indicated as the standard of care for certain procedures.
   E. It has been shown to reduce intraoperative blood loss.

2. All of the following statements are true EXCEPT:

   A. The epidural space is bounded inferiorly by the intervertebral ligament.
   B. The interspinous ligament attaches to the ligamentum flavum anteriorly.
   C. The ligamentum nuchae continues inferiorly as the supraspinous ligament.
   D. Elastin is the primary component of the ligamentum flavum.
   E. The ligamentum flavum is thickest in the midline.

3. The epidural space:

   A. Terminates cranially at C1
   B. Communicates with the intervertebral space by way of the paravertebral foramina
   C. Surrounds the vertebral canal
   D. Contains a rich network of veins posteriorly
   E. Becomes discontinuous upon injection of liquid

4. Which of the following statements regarding spinal needle insertion is TRUE?

   A. The first significant resistance encountered when advancing a needle using the paramedian approach is the interspinous ligament.
   B. If bone is repeatedly encountered at the same depth when the needle is advanced, the needle is likely walking down the inferior spinous process.
   C. The midline approach is preferred in patients with heavily calcified interspinous ligaments.
   D. Free flow of cerebrospinal fluid (CSF) after resolution of a paresthesia usually indicates that the needle is in a good position.
   E. Penetration of the dura mater is more easily detected with a beveled needle.

5. The epidural test dose:

   A. If negative, confirms that the catheter is in the epidural space
   B. Must be administered before giving a therapeutic dose
   C. May be omitted if aspiration of the catheter is negative for blood or cerebrospinal fluid (CSF)
   D. Should have an increased concentration of epinephrine if the patient is taking β-adrenergic blockers
   E. Contains epinephrine, which, if given intravenously, typically produces an immediate increase in heart rate within 10 seconds

6. Rank the following local anesthetics in order of increasing duration for spinal anesthesia.

   A. Procaine, mepivacaine, tetracaine
   B. Lidocaine, mepivacaine, procaine
   C. Lidocaine, procaine, mepivacaine
   D. Procaine, bupivacaine, mepivacaine
   E. Tetracaine, procaine, bupivacaine

7. The duration of spinal anesthesia is most prolonged when 100 μg of clonidine is added to which of the following local anesthetics?

   A. Mepivacaine
   B. Lidocaine
   C. Tetracaine
   D. Procaine
   E. Bupivacaine

8. Rank the following local anesthetics in order of increasing duration for epidural anesthesia.

   A. Ropivacaine, bupivacaine, mepivacaine
   B. Etidocaine, mepivacaine, ropivacaine
   C. Chloroprocaine, etidocaine, mepivacaine
   D. Ropivacaine, chloroprocaine, mepivacaine
   E. Chloroprocaine, mepivacaine, etidocaine

9. All of the following statements regarding complications associated with epidural and spinal anesthesia are true EXCEPT:

   A. Use of fluid instead of air for loss of resistance during epidural anesthesia reduces the risk of headache upon accidental meningeal puncture.
   B. An epidural blood patch immediately relieves postdural puncture headache (PDPH) symptoms in approximately 99% of patients.
   C. Transient reduction in hearing acuity after spinal anesthesia is more common in female than in male patients.
   D. Back pain is more common after epidural anesthesia than after spinal anesthesia.
   E. Neurologic injury occurs in about 0.03% to 0.1% of all central neuraxial blocks.

10. All of the following statements regarding spinal or epidural anesthesia and spinal hematoma are true EXCEPT:

    A. Patients taking nonsteroidal anti-inflammatory drugs (NSAIDs) and receiving mini-dose heparin are not at increased risk.
    B. Patients treated with enoxaparin are at increased risk.
    C. Patients most commonly present with numbness or lower extremity weakness.
    D. Spinal hematoma occurs at an estimated incidence of less than 1 in 150,000.
    E. The removal of an epidural or an intrathecal catheter presents nearly as great a risk for spinal hematoma as its insertion.

11. Structures traversed by a properly placed needle in the subarachnoid space via the midline approach include all the following EXCEPT:

    A. Interspinous ligament
    B. Dura mater
    C. Posterior longitudinal ligament
    D. Supraspinous ligament
    E. Ligamentum flavum

12. A patient receives a spinal anesthetic with a sensory level of T5. Which of the following is likely to occur?

    A. The small bowel will be dilated and relaxed.
    B. Glomerular filtration will be decreased by one-third.
    C. Tidal volume will be reduced by one-third.
    D. The cardioaccelerator nerves will be unaffected.
    E. Blood pressure will lower predominantly by decreasing venous return.

13. Which of the following has the lowest baricity?

    A. Lidocaine 5% in dextrose 7.5%
    B. A mixture obtained by mixing equal volumes of tetracaine 1% and water
    C. Bupivacaine 0.75% in dextrose 8.25%
    D. A mixture obtained by mixing equal volumes of tetracaine 1% and dextrose 10%
    E. Procaine 10%

14. At 37°C, the average density of cerebrospinal fluid (CSF) is _____ g/mL.

    A. 1.3
    B. 1.03
    C. 1.003
    D. 1.0003
    E. 0.03

15. Intravenous (IV) injection of a typical epidural test dose of an epinephrine-containing solution causes an average increase in heart rate of _____ bpm.

    A. 0
    B. 2
    C. 6
    D. 30
    E. 60

16. Which of the following statements concerning the addition of epinephrine to a local anesthetic solution during spinal anesthesia is TRUE?

    A. It is more effective at increasing the duration of lidocaine than tetracaine.
    B. It is important for modulating the systemic blood level of local anesthetic.
    C. It may inhibit antinociceptive afferents in the spinal cord.
    D. It is typically administered in a concentration of 10 g/mL.
    E. It is typically administered in a concentration of 1:200,000.

17. Which of the following statements concerning the choice of local anesthetic solution for epidural use is TRUE?

    A. Agents of high anesthetic potency and duration of action necessarily have slow onsets.
    B. Etidocaine is an excellent choice for obstetric use because of wide sensory/motor discrimination.
    C. Ropivacaine has a time course similar to that of lidocaine.
    D. Prilocaine has less cardiovascular toxicity than bupivacaine and lidocaine.
    E. The onset and duration of epidural anesthesia are most closely related to the volume of local anesthetic used.

18. The first function to be lost during the onset of spinal anesthesia is:

    A. Touch
    B. Motor power
    C. Temperature sensation
    D. Vibration
    E. Autonomic activity

19. Which of the following statements concerning a decrease in blood pressure of 30% during spinal anesthesia is TRUE?

    A. It is primarily the result of arteriolar dilation.
    B. It should be treated with a modest head-up position to prevent further cephalad spread of the local anesthetic.
    C. It must be treated aggressively in all patients.
    D. It may be treated effectively with a venoselective constrictor.
    E. It indicates that the patient was hypovolemic before induction of spinal anesthesia.

20. All of the following statements about postdural puncture headaches (PDPHs) are true EXCEPT:

    A. They are frequently unilateral.
    B. They are improved by recumbency.
    C. They are usually frontal or occipital.
    D. They may be accompanied by tinnitus and photophobia.
    E. They are usually self-limiting.

21. Measures to decrease the incidence of postdural puncture headache (PDPH) include all of the following EXCEPT:

    A. Use of a paramedian approach
    B. Use of small-gauge spinal needles
    C. Lowering the glucose concentration of the local anesthetic solution
    D. Maintaining the patient in the supine position for at least 12 hours after surgery
    E. Inserting the spinal needle bevel parallel to the dural fibers

22. Which of the following statements concerning high spinal anesthesia is TRUE?

    A. It is less common in parturients.
    B. It carries a high mortality rate.
    C. If it occurs, phrenic nerve paralysis is relatively short-lived.
    D. It is most likely to occur 30 minutes after the induction of spinal anesthesia.
    E. Apnea is virtually always a consequence of either ventilatory muscle paralysis or sedative medications.

23. Which of the following vertebrae has the most prominent spinous process?

    A. C5
    B. C2
    C. T1
    D. T12
    E. L5

24. Which of the following statements is TRUE?

    A. The vertebral canal is formed by two laminae anteriorly.
    B. The spinous process for C1 serves as a site for muscle and ligament attachments.
    C. Six sacral vertebrae are fused together to form the sacrum.
    D. The first cervical vertebra does not have a vertebral body.
    E. The pedicles project anteriorly from the vertebral body.

25. All of the following statements regarding vertebral anatomy are true EXCEPT:

    A. The sacral cornu are located on either side of the sacral hiatus.
    B. The twelfth thoracic rib can be helpful in identifying the twelfth thoracic vertebrae.
    C. A horizontal line at the level of the iliac crests corresponds to the L4–L5 interspace.
    D. C5 is the most prominent spinous process encountered upon palpation of the posterior neck.
    E. There are 33 spinal vertebrae.

26. All of the following statements are true EXCEPT:

    A. The subdural space lies between the dura mater and the arachnoid mater.
    B. The dura mater fuses with the filum terminale at the level of the second sacral vertebrae.
    C. The plica mediana dorsalis is usually the structure responsible for inadequate spread of epidural anesthesia.
    D. At birth, the spinal cord ends at about the level of the third lumbar vertebra.
    E. The dura mater is the outermost and thickest meningeal layer

27. Which of the following statements regarding spinal needles is FALSE?

    A. The Quincke needle has a cutting edge.
    B. The Sprotte needle requires less insertion force than the Greene needle.
    C. Use of a stylet in a spinal needle may prevent formation of dermoid tumors in the subarachnoid space.
    D. The Whitacre needle has a "pencil-point" tip.
    E. Large-gauge spinal needles are more likely to cause postdural puncture headache.

28. Combined spinal–epidural anesthesia (CSEA):

    A. Has proven to be a technique without risk or limitation
    B. Requires an epidural needle with a second lumen for the spinal needle
    C. Has recently fallen out of favor as a viable anesthetic option
    D. May result in high subarachnoid concentrations of medication administered via the epidural catheter
    E. Only local anesthetic injected into the epidural space is effective in raising the block height

29. All of the following statements regarding transient radicular irritation (TRI) are true EXCEPT:

    A. It is defined as pain or dysesthesia in the legs or buttocks after spinal anesthesia.
    B. It occurs more frequently in obese patients.
    C. It usually resolves within 72 hours.
    D. It occurs most frequently when bupivacaine is used.
    E. The risk is greater for surgery in the lithotomy position.

30. Anatomic features pertinent to the performance of neur-axial blockade include all of the following EXCEPT:

    A. In adults, the spinal cord ends at L1–L2.
    B. The angulation of the spinous processes of the thoracic vertebrae makes a paramedian approach preferable.
    C. In adults, the dural sac ends at S2.
    D. The largest interspace in the vertebral column is L2–L3.
    E. A horizontal line drawn between the iliac crests, crosses at or near the body of L4.

31. The epidural space contains all of the following EXCEPT:

    A. Cerebrospinal fluid (CSF)
    B. Blood vessels
    C. Spinal roots covered with dura
    D. Adipose tissue
    E. Connective tissue

32. Factors that may worsen hypotension during epidural anesthesia include all of the following EXCEPT:

    A. Epinephrine in the local anesthetic solution
    B. Absorption of local anesthetic from the epidural space
    C. Hypovolemia
    D. Use of chloroprocaine
    E. β_1 activation

33. Important factors that influence the distribution of local anesthetics in the subarachnoid space include the following EXCEPT:

    A. Density of the local anesthetic solution
    B. Shape of the spinal canal
    C. Position of the patient
    D. Site of injection
    E. Patient height

34. Isobaric solutions injected at the L1 level are appropriate for spinal anesthesia for:

    A. Cesarean section
    B. Femoropopliteal bypass
    C. Appendectomy
    D. Nephrectomy
    E. TURP

35. Which of the following is FALSE?

    A. The ligamentum flavum is thickest in the midline, measuring 3 to 5 mm at the L2–L3 interspace in adults.
    B. Midline insertion of an epidural needle is least likely to result in unintended meningeal puncture.
    C. In adults, the caudad tip of the spinal cord typically lies at the level of the first lumbar vertebrae.
    D. At birth, the spinal cord ends at about the level of the fifth lumbar vertebra.
    E. The arachnoid mater is avascular.

36. Spinal cord segments that contain the cell bodies of preganglionic sympathetic neurons include all of the following EXCEPT:

    A. T4
    B. C6
    C. T10
    D. L1
    E. T1

ANSWERS

1. **D.** There are no absolute indications for spinal or epidural anesthesia. Spinal and epidural anesthesia have been shown to blunt the stress response to surgery, decrease intraoperative blood loss, lower the incidence of postoperative thromboembolic events, and decrease morbidity and mortality in high-risk surgical patients. Also, both spinal and epidural techniques may be used to extend analgesia into the postoperative period and to provide analgesia to nonsurgical patients.

2. **A.** The epidural space is bounded inferiorly by the sacrococcygeal ligament covering the sacral hiatus. The interspinous ligament attaches between the spinous processes and blends anteriorly with the ligamentum flavum. Above T7, the supraspinous ligament continues as the ligamentum nuchae. The ligamentum flavum is a tough, wedge-shaped ligament composed of elastin. The ligamentum flavum is thickest in the midline, measuring 3 to 5 mm at the L2–L3 interspace in adults. (See page 907: Ligaments.)

3. **C.** The epidural space is the space that lies between the spinal meninges and the sides of the vertebral canal. The foramina magnum bounds it cranially. The epidural space is not a closed space but communicates with the paravertebral space by way of the intervertebral foramina. The epidural space is composed of a series of discontinuous compartments that become continuous when the potential space separating the compartments is opened by injection of air or liquid. A rich network of valveless veins courses through the anterior and lateral portions of the epidural space, with few, if any, veins present in the posterior epidural space. (See page 907: Epidural Space.)

4. **D.** If a paresthesia occurs upon insertion of a spinal needle, the practitioner should immediately stop advancing the needle, remove the stylet, and look for CSF at the needle hub. Obtaining CSF after resolution of a paresthesia indicates that the needle encountered a cauda equina nerve root in the subarachnoid space and the needle tip is in a good position. Of course, one should not inject local anesthetic in the presence of a persistent paresthesia. The first significant resistance encountered using the paramedian approach should be the ligamentum flavum because the interspinous ligament is bypassed. If bone is repeatedly encountered at the same depth when the needle is advanced, the needle is likely off the midline and walking along the vertebral lamina. The paramedian approach to the epidural and subarachnoid space is useful in situations in which the patient's anatomy does not favor the midline approach (e.g., the inability to flex the spine or heavily calcified intraspinous ligaments). Penetration of the dura mater produces a subtle "pop" that is most easily detected with pencil-point needles. (See page 911: Midline Approach.)

5. **B.** Because of the risk of undetected intravenous or subarachnoid migration of the catheter, a test dose must be administered before a therapeutic dose is given through the catheter. Aspiration of the catheter or needle to check for blood or CSF is helpful if positive, but the incidence of false-negative aspirations is too high to rely on this technique alone. The most common test dose is 3 mL of local anesthetic containing 5 μg/mL of epinephrine. Intravascular injection of this dose of epinephrine typically produces an average heart rate increase of 30 bpm between 20 and 40 seconds after the injection. Heart rate increases may not be as evident in some patients taking β-adrenergic blockers. In β-blocked patients, systolic blood pressure increases of 20 mm Hg or more may be a more reliable indicator of intravascular injection. (See page 914: Epidural Test Dose.)

6. **A.** The principal determinant of spinal block duration is the local anesthetic drug used. Procaine is the shortest-acting local anesthetic for subarachnoid use. Lidocaine and mepivacaine are agents of intermediate duration, and bupivacaine and tetracaine are the longest-acting drugs currently available in the United States. (See page 919: Local Anesthetic.)

7. **C.** Tetracaine is the local anesthetic that is most dramatically prolonged by addition of adrenergic agonists. Clonidine prolongs tetracaine spinal block by 50% to 70%, with a larger effect occurring at lumbar dermatomes. (See page 919: Adrenergic Agonists.)

8. **E.** Chloroprocaine is the shortest-duration local anesthetic used for epidural anesthesia. Lidocaine and mepivacaine provide blocks of intermediate duration, and bupivacaine, ropivacaine, and etidocaine produce the longest-duration epidural blocks. (See page 922: Duration.)

9. **B.** An epidural blood patch is effective in relieving symptoms within 1 to 24 hours in 85% to 95% of patients; approximately 90% of patients in whom an initial blood patch has failed do respond to a second blood patch. The use of fluid instead of air for loss of resistance during attempted epidural anesthesia does not alter the risk of accidental meningeal puncture, but it does markedly decrease the risk that the patient will subsequently develop PDPH. Compared with spinal anesthesia, back pain after epidural anesthesia is more common and lasts longer. It has been demonstrated that a 1- to 3-day transient, mild decrease in hearing acuity is common after spinal anesthesia, with an incidence of roughly 40% and a 3:1 female-to-male predominance. Multiple large studies of spinal and epidural anesthesia report that neurologic injury occurs in approximately 0.03% to 0.1% of all central neuraxial blocks, although the block was not clearly proven to be causative in most of these series. (See page 926: Complications.)

10. A. Drugs not considered putting patients at increased risk of neuraxial bleeding and spinal hematoma formation when used alone may actually increase the risk when they are combined. This may be the case when mini-dose unfractionated heparin and NSAIDs are used concurrently. Patients receiving fractionated low–molecular-weight heparin (e.g., enoxaparin) are considered to be at increased risk for spinal hematoma. Patients with spinal hematoma most commonly present with numbness or lower extremity weakness. Spinal hematoma is a rare but potentially devastating complication of spinal and epidural anesthesia, with an incidence estimated to be less than 1 in 150,000. The removal of an epidural or intrathecal catheter places the patient at nearly as great a risk of hematoma as catheter insertion. The timing of removal and anticoagulation should be coordinated. (See page 926: Complications: Spinal Hematoma.)

11. C. In the midline, the needle penetrates the skin, subcutaneous tissue, supraspinous ligament (superficial to the spinous processes), interspinous ligament (between the spinous processes), ligamentum flavum, epidural space, dura mater, and arachnoid membrane. The anterior and posterior longitudinal ligaments are anterior to the subarachnoid space, attaching to the anterior and posterior surfaces of the vertebral bodies. (See page 906: Anatomy: Ligaments.)

12. E. Spinal anesthesia to a level that affects the sympathetic nervous system (which originates from the intermediolateral cell column between T1 and L2) causes peripheral vasodilation (venodilation and arterial dilation). Blood pressure decreases as a result of decreased venous return. The cardioaccelerator nerves arise from the T1–T4 dermatomes; they are affected by spinal anesthesia to T5 because the level of sympathetic blockade can be two to six dermatomal levels higher than the sensory block. Renal blood flow and glomerular filtration rate tend to be maintained during spinal anesthesia unless the mean blood pressure decreases markedly. Spinal anesthesia causes contraction of the intestines and increased peristalsis because of unopposed vagal activity. High thoracic levels of spinal anesthesia have virtually no effect on resting ventilatory mechanics, but they compromise active exhalation. Intercostal paralysis interferes with the patient's ability to cough and clear secretions. (See page 923: Physiology: Spinal Anesthesia.)

13. B. Solutions of local anesthetic that have dextrose are hyperbaric. When an additive such as dextrose is not added, then density, and hence baricity, depend on the concentration (g%) of local anesthetic. Hence, 0.5% tetracaine has a lower baricity than 10% procaine. (See page 915: Block Height.)

14. D. The average density of CSF is 1.0003 g/mL at 37°C. (See page 915: Block Height.)

15. D. The most common test dose is 3 mL of local anesthetic containing 5 μg/mL of epinephrine (1:200,000). IV injection of this dose of epinephrine typically produces an average heart rate increase of 30 bpm between 20 and 40 seconds after injection. Heart rate increases may not be as evident in some patients taking β-blockers; systolic blood pressure increases of more than 20 mm Hg may be a more reliable indicator of intravascular injection in these patients. (See page 914: Epidural Test Dose.)

16. C. Epinephrine is frequently added to local anesthetic solutions to increase the duration of spinal anesthesia. This effect is believed to result, at least in part, from vasoconstriction of spinal cord and dural vessels. This leads to decreased vascular uptake of the local anesthetic. The fact that it is more effective for tetracaine than for lidocaine or bupivacaine may be attributed to the finding that of the three drugs, tetracaine causes the greatest (and bupivacaine the least) vasoconstriction in spinal cord blood flow. Blood concentrations of local anesthetic during spinal anesthesia are not clinically significant; hence, epinephrine is not important for modulating the systemic levels of local anesthetic. Epinephrine and related agents may cause inhibition of antinociceptive afferents, an effect that is mediated by stimulation of α_2-receptors in the spinal cord. The dose of epinephrine during spinal anesthesia usually is 0.2 to 0.3 mg (0.2–0.3 mL of 1:1,000 solution). Lesser concentrations are used during epidural anesthesia, typically 1:200,000 (1 g/200,000 mL or 5 μg/mL). (See page 919: Adrenergic Agonists.)

17. D. Bupivacaine and etidocaine are highly potent, long-duration local anesthetics. The onset of bupivacaine epidural anesthesia is relatively slow (15–20 minutes); the onset of etidocaine is more rapid. Bupivacaine has excellent sensory/motor discrimination; when used in obstetrics as a 0.125% solution, it may provide good sensory analgesia with minimal motor block. Etidocaine has relatively little sensory/motor discrimination and generally induces profound motor block. Prilocaine has less cardiovascular and central nervous system toxicities than lidocaine or bupivacaine, but it may cause methemoglobinemia when given in doses above 600 mg. Ropivacaine has a time course similar to that of bupivacaine. Within limits, the onset and duration of epidural blockade are more closely related to the mass of drug rather than to variations in volume or concentration. (See page 922: Duration.)

18. E. The onset of block is fastest at sympathetic fibers. The level of sympathetic block may extend two to six dermatomes higher than loss of pinprick sensation and four to eight dermatomes higher than motor blockade. (See page 923: Differential Nerve Block.)

19. D. Hypotension during spinal anesthesia that is below that which blocks cardioaccelerator fibers is primarily caused by venodilation leading to venous pooling and decreased cardiac output as well as decreased systemic vascular resistance resulting from arterial dilation. The amount of hypotension is related to the level of the sympathectomy. Although the cephalad spread of a hyperbaric solution may be limited by placing the patient in a head-up position, this should not be done to treat patients with existing hypotension because it will further decrease venous return. A decrease in blood pressure of 20% to 30% is usually well tolerated, but selected patients with cardiac, renal, or cerebrovascular disease may require treatment. Potential treatments may include modest head-down position, vasoconstrictors, and fluid administration. (See page 923: Spinal Anesthesia.)

20. **A.**   PDPHs are classically described as bilateral, in the occipital or frontal regions. They are worsened by the upright position, improved in the supine position, and may be accompanied by tinnitus or photophobia. Nearly all PDPHs resolve over time without invasive therapy; however, an epidural blood patch may be indicated when the symptoms are severe. (See page 926: Postdural Puncture Headache.)

21. **D.**   The incidence of PDPH is increased in young patients, women, and pregnant patients. The paramedian approach results in less CSF leakage and thus decreases the chance for development of PDPH. Small-gauge and closed-tip needles are associated with a lower incidence of PDPH. Interestingly, there appears to be a direct relationship between the glucose concentration in the local anesthetic and the incidence of PDPH. Although bed rest is indicated in the treatment of patients with PDPH, it does not decrease the likelihood of developing PDPH. (See page 926: Postdural Puncture Headache.)

22. **C.**   Excessive spread of spinal anesthesia may occur in any patient, but parturients are most susceptible. It is most likely to occur shortly after induction of spinal anesthesia, but block height may be influenced for as long as 60 minutes after injection. When recognized early and treated with pressor support and ventilation, high spinal anesthesia should be merely an inconvenience, with no mortality. If phrenic nerve paralysis occurs, it usually is short-lived. Respiratory arrest may occur as a result of respiratory muscle paralysis or dysfunction of brainstem respiratory control centers. (See page 927: Total Spinal Anesthesia.)

23. **C.**   The most prominent spinous process is T1. (See page 906: Anatomy: Vertebrae.)

24. **D.**   With the exception of C1, the cervical, thoracic, and lumbar vertebrae consist of a body anteriorly, two pedicles that project posteriorly from the body, and two laminae that connect the pedicles. The first cervical vertebra differs from this typical structure in that it does not have a body or a spinous process. The five sacral vertebrae are fused together to form the wedge-shaped sacrum. (See page 928: Vertebrae.)

25. **D.**   The sacral cornu are bony prominences on either side of the sacral hiatus and aid in identifying it. The spine of C7 is the first prominent spinous process encountered while running the hand down the back of the neck. The twelfth thoracic vertebrae can be identified by palpating the twelfth rib and tracing it back to its attachment to T12. A line drawn between the iliac crests crosses the

body of L5 or the L4–L5 interspace. (See page 906: Vertebrae.)

26. **C.**   Distally, the dura mater ends at approximately S2, where it fuses with the filum terminale. At birth, the spinal cord ends at about the level of the third lumbar vertebrae. In adults, the caudal tip of the spinal cord typically lies at the level of the first lumbar vertebrae. The inner surface of the dura mater abuts the arachnoid mater. There is a potential space between these two membranes called the subdural space. The plica mediana dorsalis is thought to be a connective tissue band running from the dura mater to the ligamentum flavum. The plica mediana dorsalis does not appear to be clinically relevant with respect to clinical epidural anesthesia. (See page 908: Dura Mater.)

27. **B.**   The Whitacre and Sprotte needles each have a pencil-point tip with a needle hole on the side of the shaft. The Greene and Quincke needles have beveled tips with cutting edges. Pencil-point needles require more force to insert than beveled-tip needles, but they provide a better tactile feel of the various tissues encountered as the needle is inserted. All spinal and epidural needles come with a tight-fitting stylet. The stylet prevents the needle from being plugged with skin or fat and dragging the skin into the epidural or subarachnoid spaces, where the skin may grow and form dermoid tumors. (See page 910: Needles.)

28. **D.**   CSEA is growing in popularity because it combines the rapid-onset, dense block of spinal anesthesia with the flexibility afforded by an epidural catheter. Special epidural needles with a separate lumen to accommodate a spinal needle are available for CSEA. However, the technique is easily performed by first placing a standard epidural needle in the epidural space and then inserting an appropriately sized spinal needle through the shaft of the epidural needle into the subarachnoid space. A potential risk of CSEA is that the meningeal hole made by the spinal needle may allow dangerously high concentrations of subsequently administered epidural drugs to reach the subarachnoid space. (See page 915: Combined Spinal–Epidural Anesthesia.)

29. **D.**   Transient radicular irritation (TRI) is defined as pain or dysesthesia in the legs or buttocks after spinal anesthesia. All local anesthetics have been shown to cause TRI, although the risk appears to be greater with lidocaine than with other local anesthetics. Additional risk factors for TRI include surgery in the lithotomy position, outpatient status, and obesity. The pain usually resolves spontaneously within 72 hours. (See page 928: Transient Neurologic Symptoms.)

30. **D.**   The largest interspace in the vertebral column is L5–S1, the site of the Taylor paramedian approach. In adults, the spinal cord ends at L1–L2, and the dural sac ends at S2. A line connecting the iliac crests most likely crosses L4 or the L4–L5 interspace. The angulation of the spinous processes of the thoracic vertebrae complicates a midline

approach, making the paramedian approach preferable in this region. (See page 906: Anatomy.)

31. A. The epidural space is a potential space that normally is filled with loose connective tissue, fatty tissue, and blood vessels. CSF is in the subarachnoid space. The spinal roots appear to traverse the epidural space, but they maintain a thin sleeve of dura around them. (See page 907: Epidural Space.)

32. E. As with spinal anesthesia, epidural anesthesia has hemodynamic effects secondary to interruption of preganglionic sympathetic vasoconstrictor fibers. In addition, the relatively large doses of local anesthetic used are absorbed rapidly and may cause hypotension because of their negative inotropic and peripheral vasodilating effects. Epinephrine absorbed from the epidural space stimulates β_2-receptors and leads to additional vasodilation and reduced diastolic blood pressure. The agents with more rapid onset, chloroprocaine and etidocaine, tend to produce greater hypotension because of rapid blockade of sympathetic fibers. Alternatively, high plasma concentrations of bupivacaine are more likely to cause myocardial depression. The hypotensive effects of epidural anesthesia are exaggerated in hypovolemic patients. (See page 923: Cardiovascular Physiology.)

33. E. Many factors are considered to influence the spread of local anesthetic in cerebrospinal fluid. The most important factors are the density of the local anesthetic solution, site of injection, shape of the spinal canal, and position of the patient (for hyperbaric and hypobaric solutions). (See page 915: Block Height.)

34. B. An isobaric solution tends to remain near the site of injection regardless of patient position (unless the solution is not truly isobaric). An isobaric injection in the lumbar region is appropriate for surgical procedures below the L1 dermatome (e.g., femoropopliteal bypass, repair of hip fracture). However, it is not appropriate for surgery at sites innervated by higher dermatomes. (See page 915: Block Height.)

35. D. The ligamentum flavum is thickest in the midline, measuring 3 to 5 mm at the L2–L3 interspace in adults. Midline insertion of an epidural needle is least likely to result in unintended meningeal puncture. In adults, the caudad tip of the spinal cord typically lies at the level of the first lumbar vertebrae. However, in 10% of individuals, the spinal cord may extend to L3. At birth, the spinal cord ends at about the level of the third lumber vertebra. (See page 906: Anatomy.)

36. B. The intermediolateral gray matter of the T1–L2 spinal cord segments contains the cell bodies of the preganglionic sympathetic neurons. (See page 909: Spinal Cord.)

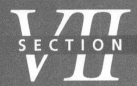

CHAPTER

35

Peripheral Nerve Blockade

1. Which of the following statements about ultrasound imaging is FALSE?

    A. It has an improved block success compared to neuro-stimulation.
    B. It has a reduced time to onset of blockade.
    C. It is associated with fewer complications.
    D. Lower frequencies offer the best spatial resolution at superficial locations.
    E. Whereas high-impedance structures appear hypere-choic, low-impedance structures appear hypoechoic.

2. The highest systemic blood concentration of local anesthesia occurs after which of the following?

    A. Epidural anesthesia with pinprick level at T6
    B. Spinal anesthesia with pinprick level at T4
    C. Bier block anesthesia to left upper extremity
    D. Bilateral intercostal blocks at T6–T12
    E. Interscalene block to the right shoulder

3. The absorption of local anesthetic drug and duration of anesthesia are related to all of the following EXCEPT:

    A. Total dose and/or concentration of local anesthetic used
    B. Addition of vasoconstrictors
    C. Site of injection
    D. Ester versus amide local anesthetic
    E. Physical properties of the local anesthetic

4. Select the correct order of anesthetic techniques with respect to systemic blood concentration from highest to lowest.

    A. Spinal anesthesia, caudal block, brachial plexus block, intercostal block
    B. Intercostal block, spinal anesthesia, brachial plexus block, caudal block
    C. Intercostal block, caudal block, epidural block, brachial plexus block
    D. Epidural block, intercostal block, caudal block, spinal block
    E. Caudal block, intercostal block, brachial plexus block, spinal block

5. All of the following concerning peripheral nerve blockade are true EXCEPT:

    A. Complaints of a "cramping" or "aching" sensation during injection may indicate intraneural injection.
    B. Use of a nerve stimulator with a variable amperage output and an insulated needle requires familiarity with anatomy.
    C. Obtaining a sensory paresthesia is an acceptable technique.
    D. Aspiration of blood or proximity of nerves to bones may make localization simpler.
    E. Ultrasound guidance to localize nerves is a simple technique to master.

6. All of the following statements concerning the trigeminal nerve are true EXCEPT:

    A. It is a sensory and motor nerve innervating the face.
    B. Its three roots arise from the medulla oblongata, separate, and exit from the skull.
    C. The mandibular nerve is the largest branch and is the only one to contain motor fibers.
    D. Most applications of trigeminal nerve block may be performed by injection of the terminal branches of the nerve.
    E. The frontal branch bifurcates into the supratrochlear and supraorbital nerves.

7. All of the following statements concerning cervical plexus blockade are true EXCEPT:

    A. The cervical plexus consists solely of nerve fibers from C1 and C2.
    B. Blockade of the cervical plexus may involve only sensory nerves because of the separation of motor and sensory fibers early in their course.
    C. Carotid endarterectomy may be performed under cervical plexus blockade.
    D. Blockade of this plexus may provide adequate anesthesia for thyroid surgery.
    E. Paresthesias are usually not necessary to perform adequate blockade of the cervical plexus.

8. Even when properly performed, cervical plexus blockade may result in all of the following EXCEPT:

   A. Intravascular injection of local anesthetic with rapid onset of seizures
   B. Phrenic nerve paralysis
   C. Recurrent laryngeal nerve blockade
   D. Epidural or subarachnoid anesthesia
   E. Ipsilateral pneumothorax

9. Interscalene blockade is typically associated with all of the following EXCEPT:

   A. Anesthesia to the shoulder and upper arm
   B. Reliable block of the ulnar border of the forearm
   C. Reliable anesthesia of the musculocutaneous nerve
   D. Reliable anesthesia to the radial and median nerves of the upper arm
   E. Possible Horner syndrome by spread to the sympathetic chain

10. The nerve-stimulation approach to interscalene brachial plexus blockade involves all of the following EXCEPT:

   A. Head positioning so that it is turned to the opposite side
   B. Palpation of the groove between the anterior and middle scalene muscle, which is located by having the patient tense the scalene muscles by raising the head slightly in the sniffing position
   C. Injection of 25 to 30 mL of local anesthetic when using a nerve-stimulation technique
   D. Introduction of the needle perpendicular to the skin in all planes so that it is directed medially, cephalad, and slightly anteriorly
   E. Locating the cricoid cartilage

11. Complications of the interscalene approach to the brachial plexus include all of the following EXCEPT:

   A. Puncture of the lung viscera and a pneumothorax
   B. Injection of local anesthesia into the epidural or subarachnoid space
   C. Intravascular injection of local anesthesia via the vertebral artery
   D. Contralateral Horner syndrome
   E. Phrenic nerve paralysis

12. All of the following statements regarding the axillary approach to the brachial plexus are false EXCEPT:

   A. It carries the greatest chance of pneumothorax.
   B. The musculocutaneous nerve is easily anesthetized.
   C. Septa within the sheath may limit the spread of local anesthetic.
   D. Injection at multiple sites in the axilla is not recommended because the axillary artery may be punctured.
   E. This block is not useful for surgery of the hand.

13. All of the following statements regarding intravenous regional anesthesia are true EXCEPT:

   A. The tourniquet should be inflated to 300 mm Hg or 2.5 times the patient's systolic blood pressure.
   B. Lidocaine, 0.5%, is an appropriate anesthetic for this procedure.
   C. If surgery is completed in 15 minutes, the tourniquet should be left inflated for the total period of time.
   D. Bupivacaine is the local anesthetic of choice in patients with lidocaine allergy.
   E. If discomfort is experienced, the distal cuff is inflated over the anesthetized area of skin, and the uncomfortable proximal cuff is released.

14. In regards to intercostal blockade of T6–T12 all of the following are true EXCEPT:

   A. It provides analgesia and motor relaxation for upper abdominal procedures.
   B. It is useful in reducing pain associated with chest tube insertion and percutaneous biliary drainage procedures.
   C. It has the potential for local anesthesia toxicity, especially if performed bilaterally.
   D. There is a high incidence of pneumothorax even when the procedure is performed by an experienced individual.
   E. It is possible to produce partial spinal or epidural anesthesia if the injection is made close to the midline.

15. All of the following statements regarding ilioinguinal/iliohypogastric nerve block are false EXCEPT:

   A. Anesthesia of the iliohypogastric nerve and ilioinguinal nerve is adequate for hernia repair.
   B. The nerve roots from T12, L1, and L2 provide fibers to these two nerves.
   C. The anteroinferior iliac spine provides the landmark for location of these two nerves.
   D. Hematoma formation is a rare complication of this nerve block.
   E. It is a technically challenging block that should not be performed without ultrasound guidance.

16. All of the following statements regarding penile nerve block are true EXCEPT:

   A. Penile blockade is used for surgical procedures of the glans and shaft of the penis.
   B. The penile branches of the pudendal nerve are targeted.
   C. The dorsal nerves lie bilaterally on the outer aspect of the dorsal arteries of the penis.
   D. A ring block is typically performed.
   E. Lidocaine with epinephrine is typically used.

17. All of the following statements regarding blocks of the terminal nerves of the lumbar plexus are true EXCEPT:

    A. When using a nerve-stimulation technique for the lateral femoral cutaneous nerve block, the primary endpoint is paresthesia over the lateral leg thigh with a current of 0.5 to 0.6 mA.
    B. An obturator nerve block may be used to prevent obturator reflex during transurethral bladder tumor resections.
    C. A lateral femoral cutaneous nerve block may be used to prevent adductor spasm in patients with multiple sclerosis.
    D. Postoperative analgesia of the knee requires both obturator and femoral nerves to be blocked.
    E. A lateral femoral cutaneous nerve block may be used as a diagnostic tool to identify cases of meralgia paresthetica.

18. Which of the following statements regarding sciatic nerve block is FALSE?

    A. When used with a saphenous nerve block, a sciatic nerve block may produce adequate anesthesia to the sole of the foot and the lower leg.
    B. The goal is to deposit local anesthetic (20–30 mL) directly within the sciatic nerve structure in the subgluteal region.
    C. The sciatic nerve is located deep within the gluteal region, making it difficult to locate.
    D. The anterior sciatic nerve block is ideal for patients who cannot be positioned laterally.
    E. In the gluteal region, the sciatic nerve is located lateral to the ischial spine and superficial to the ischial bone.

19. All of the following statements regarding an ankle block are true EXCEPT:

    A. All five nerves of the foot can be blocked at the level of the ankle.
    B. The deep peroneal nerve is located in the deep plane of the anterior tibial artery.
    C. The sural nerve is the major sensory nerve to the sole of the foot.
    D. The deep peroneal nerve may be located by palpating the tendon of the extensor hallucis longus.
    E. Epinephrine should not be added to local anesthetics used for this block in order to avoid compromising the distal circulation.

ANSWERS

1. **D.** Compared with neurostimulation, ultrasound guidance for blocks results in improved block success and completeness, prolonged duration of blocks, and reduction in complications. Whereas higher frequencies offer the best spatial resolution at superficial locations, lower frequencies offer better resolution for deeper locations. High-impedance structures result in a bright (hyperechoic) image, and low-impedance structures appear grey (hypoechoic). (See page 940: Ultrasound Imaging Basics of Technique and Equipment.)

2. **D.** The highest blood level of local anesthetic occurs after multiple intercostal nerve blocks, followed by caudal, epidural, brachial plexus, intravenous regional, and lower extremity blockade. Equivalent doses of local anesthetic may produce only 3 to 4 hours of anesthesia when placed in the epidural space, but 12 to 14 hours in the arm, and 24 to 36 hours when injected along the sciatic nerve. Of note, systemic toxicity is most often related to accidental intravascular injection, and rarely to the administration of an excessive quantity of local anesthetic to an appropriate site. The risk of systemic toxic reactions is often related to the drug used. (See page 943: Avoiding Complications: Local Anesthetic Drug Selection and Doses.)

3. **D.** The higher the dose of local anesthetic, the greater the amount of drug that is available for local effect. Epinephrine causes local vasoconstriction and therefore decreases the uptake of local anesthetic into the bloodstream. The relative absorption of local anesthetic is greatest after an intercostal nerve block. The physical properties of the local anesthetic influence the absorption of the drug and the body's ability to break down the drug and excrete it. However, there is no difference in the absorption of the drug based on the classification of the local anesthetic as an amide or ester. (See page 943: Avoiding Complications: Local Anesthetic Drug Selection and Doses.)

4. **C.** The highest blood concentration occurs after an intercostal blockade, followed by caudal blockade, epidural blockade, and brachial plexus blockade. The lowest blood concentration occurs after a spinal anesthetic. (See page 943: Avoiding Complications: Local Anesthetic Drug Selection and Doses.)

5. **E.** The traditional sign of successful localization of a nerve is eliciting a paresthesia. The patient will complain of an "electrical shock"–like sensation in the involved area. Complaints of a "cramping" or an "aching" sensation during injection is a sign of possible intraneural injection. A greater incidence of residual neuropathy is associated with this technique compared with other techniques. Use of a nerve stimulator for localization of the nerve is an alternative technique. A nerve stimulator with variable amperage allows localization of the nerve without contacting it and

may reduce the chance of nerve injury. When a low current is applied to a peripheral nerve, it will produce stimulation of the motor fibers. The closer it is in proximity to the nerve, the less amperage required to elicit the motor response. Familiarity with anatomy and technique is necessary to bring the needle in close proximity to the nerve. Transarterial localization of the brachial plexus is a technique for performing an axillary block. The axillary artery is transfixed, and the needle is passed through the artery. Local anesthetic is deposited on this side of the artery, and the needle is withdrawn until it is brought back through the proximal wall. Additional local anesthetic is deposited there as well. Ultrasound guidance to localize nerves shows promise but requires complex equipment and experience. (See page 939: Common Techniques: Nerve Stimulation and Ultrasound Imaging.)

6. **B.** The trigeminal nerve (fifth cranial nerve) is a sensory and motor nerve to the face. Its roots arise from the base of the pons, and it sends sensory branches to the large gasserian ganglion. The three major branches of this nerve are the ophthalmic, maxillary, and mandibular branches. The ophthalmic branch bifurcates to form the supratrochlear and supraorbital nerves. The maxillary branch is the middle branch and is a sensory nerve. The mandibular branch is the third and largest branch and is the only one with motor fibers. Blockade of the gasserian ganglion is used for treatment of disabling trigeminal neuralgia; however, it is very difficult to perform. Blockade of the three terminal branches is relatively simple. (See pages 945 and 955: Clinical Anatomy: Head and Neck [Trigeminal Nerve Blocks] and Specific Techniques: Head and Neck [Trigeminal Nerve Blocks].)

7. **A.** The sensory fibers of the neck and posterior neck arise from nerve roots of the C2, C3, and C4 nerves. The sensory fibers separate from the motor fibers early, so isolated sensory blockade is possible. Cervical plexus blockade can be used for surgery on the neck, such as thyroidectomy and carotid endarterectomy. Occasionally, the thyroid gland may need supplemental local anesthesia, and the carotid bifurcation will need infiltration to block reflex hemodynamic changes. Paresthesias are not required to perform this procedure. (See pages 945 and 955: Clinical Anatomy: Head and Neck [Cervical Plexus Blocks] and Specific Techniques: Head and Neck [Cervical Plexus Blocks].)

8. **E.** Complications from cervical plexus blockade may include intravascular injection into the vertebral artery, epidural or spinal anesthesia if the needle is advanced too far medially, phrenic nerve blockade, recurrent laryngeal nerve blockade, and vagal blockade. Ipsilateral pneumothorax should not occur. (See page 955: Specific Techniques: Head and Neck [Cervical Plexus Blocks].)

9. **B.**   The interscalene approach to the brachial plexus at the level of C6 provides blockade for operations on the shoulder and upper arm procedures. It frequently spares C8 and T1 fibers and therefore does not provide adequate blockade to the ulnar border of the forearm. Nerve roots for the musculocutaneous, radial, and median nerves are adequately anesthetized. However, if a tourniquet is being used, a subcutaneous ring of anesthetic is required to block the superficial intercostobrachial fibers in the axilla. Horner syndrome may occur by spread of local anesthesia to the sympathetic chain. (See page 945: Clinical Anatomy: Upper Extremity: Brachial Plexus Blockade: Interscalene Block.)

10. **D.**   For interscalene block, the patient is placed in the supine position with the head turned to the side opposite that to be blocked. The lateral border of the sternocleidomastoid muscle is identified. By tensing the scalene muscles, the groove between the anterior and middle scalene muscles may be palpated. The level of the cricoid cartilage is marked. A 22-gauge, 2.5-cm or less (≤5 cm for ultrasound guidance) needle is introduced through the skin perpendicular to all planes at the level of the cricoid cartilage so that it is directed medially, caudad, and slightly posterior. Approximately 25 to 30 mL of local anesthetic is required for adequate blockade when a nerve-stimulation technique is used. (See page 955: Specific Techniques: Upper Extremity: Brachial Plexus Blockade: Interscalene Block.)

11. **D.**   Complications from the interscalene approach to the brachial plexus are pneumothorax (if the needle is directed too inferiorly), spinal or epidural anesthesia (if the needle passes medially and enters the intervertebral foramina), intravascular injection into the vertebral artery (if the needle is too posterior because the artery passes posteriorly at the level of the sixth vertebra to lie in its canal in the transverse process), and ipsilateral Horner syndrome (because of blockade of the sympathetic chain on the anterior vertebral body). Phrenic nerve blockade may occur as well. (See page 955: Specific Techniques: Upper Extremity: Brachial Plexus Blockade: Interscalene Block.)

12. **C.**   The axillary approach to the brachial plexus carries the least chance of pneumothorax. Fascial septa within the sheath may limit the spread of local anesthetic; therefore, injection of local anesthetic at multiple sites in the axilla is recommended. The musculocutaneous nerve departs from the sheath high in the axilla and may be spared with this technique. (See page 955: Specific Techniques: Brachial Plexus: Axillary Block.)

13. **D.**   Intravenous regional anesthesia (Bier block) is a form of regional anesthesia in which local anesthetic is injected into the upper extremity distal to an occluding tourniquet. The arm is elevated and exsanguinated by an elastic bandage. The tourniquet is inflated to 300 mm Hg or 2.5 times the patient's blood pressure. The radial pulse must be tested for occlusion. This may be done by palpation or by placement of the pulse oximeter on the extremity.

Lidocaine 0.5% is the local anesthetic of choice, but it should not be used with epinephrine. Bupivacaine is not used because of its toxicity. Ideally, surgery lasting up to 1 hour may be performed by this procedure. However, the cannula may be left in place, and medication may be reinjected after 90 minutes. For surgical procedures between 20 and 40 minutes long, the tourniquet should be deflated, reinflated, and then subsequently deflated in an attempt to minimize sudden reabsorption of local anesthetic. (See page 955: Specific Techniques: Upper Extremity: Intravenous Regional Anesthesia [Bier Block].)

14. **D.**   Intercostal blockade may provide both motor and sensory anesthesia of the abdomen and chest. This technique is also useful for reducing pain from chest tube insertion and percutaneous biliary drainage. It is advantageous over spinal or epidural blockade because there is no accompanying sympathetic blockade. Intercostal blockade results in the highest blood concentration of local anesthetic and therefore has the greatest likelihood of toxicity from local anesthetic. The incidence of pneumothorax is rare in experienced hands. It is possible to produce partial spinal or epidural anesthesia if the injection is made close to the midline and the anesthetic tracks along a dural sleeve to the epidural or subarachnoid space. (See page 955: Specific Technique: Trunk Nerve Blocks: Intercostal Nerve Blockade.)

15. **D.**   Ilioinguinal/iliohypogastric nerve blockade provides sensory anesthesia to the lower portion of the abdomen and groin. It is used for anesthesia for hernia repair, but blockade of these two nerves alone is inadequate for hernia repair. Subcutaneous infiltration is needed as well. These two nerves are easily located because of their anatomic relationship to the anterosuperior iliac spine. Nerve roots from L1 and sometimes T12 provide fibers to these two nerves. Complications of this block are generally volume-related and include systemic toxicity and transient femoral nerve palsy. Hematoma formation is a rare complication of this block. This block is performed easily with blind technique, although ultrasound imaging may be used to help improve the success rate of nerve localization and deposition of local anesthetic. (See page 955: Specific Techniques: Trunk Nerve Blocks: Inguinal Nerve Block.)

16. **E.**   Penile block is used in surgical procedures involving the glans and the shaft of the penis. The dorsal nerves (terminal branches of pudendal nerve, S2–S4) lie bilaterally on the outer aspect of the dorsal arteries of the penis. From the base of the penis, they divide several times and encircle the shaft of the penis before reaching the glans. The penile branches of the pudendal nerve (S2–S4) are blocked by a circumferential infiltration of the root of the penis (ring block). To avoid compromising penile circulation, epinephrine-containing solutions should not be used. (See page 955: Specific Techniques: Penile Block.)

17. **D.**   Blockade of the lateral femoral cutaneous nerve may be used as a diagnostic tool to identify cases of meralgia

paresthetica. An obturator nerve block aids in preventing the obturator reflex during transurethral bladder tumor resections and for adductor spasms (seen in patients with multiple sclerosis). Procedures on the knee require anesthesia of the femoral and the obturator nerves, although postoperative analgesia of the knee can usually be provided by femoral nerve block alone. When using nerve-stimulation technique for blockade of the lateral femoral cutaneous nerve, the primary endpoint is paresthesia of the lateral thigh with a current of approximately 0.5 to 0.6 mA. (See page 955: Specific Techniques: Lumbar Plexus and Lower Extremity: Separate Blocks of the Terminal Nerves of the Lumbar Plexus.)

18. B.   When used with a saphenous nerve block, a sciatic nerve block may produce adequate anesthesia to the sole of the foot and the lower leg. The sciatic nerve is difficult to locate because of its deep location. With the aid of ultrasound-guided blockade, the identification of various anatomic landmarks may help identify its location. In the gluteal region, the sciatic nerve is seen on ultrasonography lateral to the ischial spine and superficial to the ischial bone. For the anterior sciatic nerve block, the patient is positioned supine with the selected leg to be blocked externally rotated, making this block ideal for patients who cannot be positioned laterally. The goal is to deposit local anesthetic (20–30 mL) next to, but not directly within, the sciatic nerve structure in the subgluteal region. A hypoechoic local anesthetic fluid collection is often seen around the hyperechoic nerve within the sheath compartment during injection. (See page 955: Specific Techniques: Lower Extremity: Sciatic Nerve Blockade using Posterior, Anterior, and Posterior Popliteal Approaches.)

19. C.   Five peripheral nerves are anesthetized for an ankle block: The posterior tibial, sural, saphenous, deep peroneal, and superficial peroneal nerves. The posterior tibial nerve is the major nerve to the sole of the foot and is located just posterior to the posterior tibial artery. The sural nerve also innervates the sole of the foot. The saphenous nerve, which is located medially, innervates the anterior surface of the foot. The deep peroneal nerve is located in the deep plane of the anterior tibial artery and may be located by identifying the anterior tibial artery or the tendon of the extensor hallucis longus. The superficial peroneal nerve is located along the skin crease between the anterior tibial artery and the lateral malleolus. Epinephrine should only be added with caution to local anesthetics used for this block in order to avoid compromising the distal circulation. (See page 955: Specific Techniques: Lower Extremity: Ankle Blockade.)

CHAPTER 36

Anesthesia for Neurosurgery

1. Considering cerebrospinal fluid (CSF), which statement is TRUE?

   A. Normal volume is 250 mL, but four times this amount is produced each day.
   B. Normal volume is 150 mL, but three times this amount is produced each day.
   C. Normal volume is 100 mL, but four times this amount is produced each day.
   D. Normal volume is 50 mL, but three times this amount is produced each day.
   E. Normal volume is 250 mL, but two times this amount is produced each day.

2. Which of the following statements regarding intracranial pressure (ICP) is TRUE?

   A. ICP fluctuates significantly in normal states.
   B. ICP is not changed with changes in cerebrospinal fluid (CSF) volume.
   C. ICP never changes quickly, always gradually reaching new states of equilibrium.
   D. ICP is dependent on the volume of intracranial blood, brain tissue, and CSF.
   E. ICP is increased with any small increase in intracranial volume.

3. Which of the following statements regarding autoregulation of cerebral blood flow (CBF) is FALSE?

   A. Autoregulation leads to constant CBF over a range of mean arterial pressures (MAPs).
   B. Autoregulation maintains constant CBF between MAPs of approximately 60 to 150 mm Hg.
   C. At the low end of the autoregulation plateau, the cerebrovascular resistance (CVR) is at a maximum.
   D. Cerebral perfusion pressure (CPP) is dependent on MAP and intracranial pressure (ICP).
   E. CBF is maintained by adjusting CVR in response to changes in CPP.

4. Which of the following statements regarding the effects of anesthetics on cerebral blood flow is TRUE?

   A. Inhalation anesthetics cause cerebral vasodilatation in a dose-dependent manner.
   B. Inhalation anesthetics have no effect on cerebral metabolic rate (CMR).
   C. Thiopental causes increased cerebral blood flow (CBF) and decreased CMR.
   D. Propofol causes vasoconstriction and increased CMR.
   E. Ketamine decreases CBF and decreases CMR.

5. Which of the following statements regarding the use of hyperventilation to provide brain relaxation is TRUE?

   A. Hyperventilation is recommended in all patients with traumatic brain injury (TBI).
   B. Hyperventilation should be continued for 48 hours.
   C. Hyperventilation is helpful for ischemia because it decreases cerebral blood flow (CBF).
   D. Hyperventilation is always contraindicated in patients with TBI.
   E. Hyperventilation should be used for brief periods to manage acute increases in intracranial pressure (ICP).

6. Which of the following statements regarding venous air embolism (VAE) is TRUE?

   A. The sitting position carries reduced risk of VAE.
   B. A multi-orifice catheter placed in the superior vena cava is optimal.
   C. The presence of a patent foramen ovale (PFO) increases the risk of paradoxical emboli.
   D. Precordial Doppler has not been shown to help detect VAE.
   E. Patients with a PFO should be placed in an upright seated position for surgery.

7. All of the following complications may occur in patients with aneurysmal subarachnoid hemorrhage EXCEPT:

   A. Cardiac dysfunction
   B. Neurogenic pulmonary edema
   C. Cardiogenic pulmonary edema
   D. Hydrocephalus
   E. Secondary hyperthyroidism

8. Which of the following statements regarding blood pressure during carotid surgery is TRUE?

   A. It should be maintained 20% below baseline throughout surgery.
   B. It should be maintained as close to baseline as possible throughout surgery.
   C. It should be maintained as close to baseline as possible except during carotid cross-clamping, when it should be increased 20%.
   D. It should be maintained 20% below baseline except during carotid cross-clamping, when it should be increased to 20% above baseline.
   E. It should be maintained 20% above baseline throughout surgery.

9. Which of the following is NOT an indication for endotracheal intubation in a patient with traumatic brain injury (TBI)?

   A. Decreased level of consciousness
   B. Hypertension
   C. Increased risk of aspiration
   D. Hypoxemia
   E. Need for sedation during diagnostic studies

10. Cushing's response to elevated intracranial pressure (ICP) includes:

    A. Hypertension and bradycardia
    B. Hypotension and tachycardia
    C. Hypertension and tachycardia
    D. Hypotension and bradycardia
    E. Vasodilation and prolonged QRS

11. Cauda equina syndrome is defined by which symptoms?

    A. Back pain extending to the lower extremities
    B. Loss of pain and temperature sensation with sparing of proprioception in the lower extremities
    C. Loss of motor and touch sensation ipsilateral to the lesion and urinary retention
    D. Perineal anesthesia, urinary retention, fecal incontinence, and lower extremity weakness
    E. Loss of motor sensation in the lower extremities with no sensory deficit

12. Which of the following statements regarding electroencephalography (EEG) is TRUE?

    A. Brain ischemia disrupts the EEG but not in a reliable pattern.
    B. Brain ischemia may lead to EEG silence.
    C. It is easy to differentiate ischemia from anesthetic effects on EEG.
    D. EEG asymmetry between the right and left sides of the brain is not a particularly useful tool during carotid endarterectomy.
    E. The goal in neurosurgery is to typically produce an isoelectric EEG.

13. Which of the following statements regarding evoked potentials is TRUE?

    A. Inhalation agents disrupt evoked potentials more than intravenous (IV) anesthetics.
    B. Certain anesthetic agents should be avoided when brainstem auditory evoked potentials (BAEPs) will be recorded.
    C. No muscular relaxation can be used during the case when monitoring of motor evoked potentials (MEPs) is planned.
    D. Total IV anesthesia is not recommended when monitoring MEPs.
    E. Opioids and benzodiazepines significantly affect evoked potentials.

14. Which of the following statements concerning intracranial pressure (ICP) monitoring is TRUE?

    A. ICP provides a direct measurement of cerebral blood flow (CBF).
    B. Ideally, ICP should be maintained below 30 mm Hg.
    C. Patient position has no affect on ICP.
    D. It is possible to drain cerebrospinal fluid (CSF) to lower ICP.
    E. ICP monitoring is not recommended for patients with severe traumatic brain injury (TBI) and a normal CT scan.

15. Which of the following statements regarding profound hypothermia is FALSE?

    A. Profound hypothermia has well-known cerebroprotective effects.
    B. Cardiopulmonary bypass is necessary when using profound hypothermia.
    C. Hypothermia-induced coagulopathy is a concern when using profound hypothermia.
    D. When core temperature is below 25°C, circulatory arrest is tolerated for 30 minutes.
    E. Profound hypothermia increases cerebral activity, but decreases the energy required for cellular housekeeping.

16. Which statement regarding the hemodynamic changes during induction of anesthesia is TRUE for patients undergoing neurosurgery?

    A. Hypertension is a desirable finding because it shows that the patient has an intact stress response.
    B. Hypertension may lead to worsening ICP and brainstem herniation.
    C. The brief period of hypertension surrounding laryngoscopy has been shown to have no effect on the bleeding from a cerebral aneurysm.
    D. TBI patients are particularly tolerant of periods of apnea.
    E. Although significant blood loss may predispose to systemic hypotension, aggressive fluid resuscitation prior to induction should be avoided.

17. The use of succinylcholine is absolutely contraindicated in all of the following situations EXCEPT in:

    A. A patient with denervation from myelopathy
    B. A patient with L4 and L5 cord transaction 5 years previously
    C. A patient with denervation from a stroke
    D. A patient with a stroke that occurred over 72 hours ago
    E. A patient with a stroke that occurred 24 hours ago

18. Which of the following is not a contraindication for immediate extubation in a neurosurgical patient?

    A. Prolonged prone surgery
    B. Facial edema and no cuff leak
    C. Rales and low oxygen saturation
    D. Massive transfusion and no cuff leak
    E. Blood pressure 138/76

19. Which of the following statements regarding endovascular treatment of cerebral aneurysms is FALSE?

    A. It is a minimally invasive surgery.
    B. It typically requires general anesthesia.
    C. It may cause hemorrhage.
    D. Cardiopulmonary bypass may be necessary.
    E. It is typically performed in an interventional radiology suite as opposed to an operating room.

20. Which of the following is a relative contraindication to an "awake" craniotomy?

    A. Tumor resection surgery
    B. Epilepsy
    C. Multiple opioid allergies
    D. Difficult airway
    E. Anemia

21. Which of the following statements regarding hypertonic saline to manage elevated intracranial pressure (ICP) is TRUE?

    A. It must be used before attempting ICP control with mannitol.
    B. It has never been compared with mannitol for efficacy in controlling ICP.
    C. It causes more significant electrolyte disturbances than mannitol does.
    D. Unlike mannitol, it does not cause a brisk diuresis.
    E. It causes significantly more brain relaxation than does mannitol.

22. Risk factors for postdecompressive hypotension include all the following EXCEPT:

    A. Low Glasgow Coma Scale (GCS) score
    B. Absence of basal cisterns on CT
    C. Bilateral dilated pupils
    D. Use of inhalation anesthetics

23. Spinal column damage may cause spinal cord ischemia through which of the following mechanisms EXCEPT:

    A. Hemorrhage
    B. Compression
    C. Vasospasm
    D. Emboli

24. Which of the following statements regarding urgent intubation of a patient with a spinal cord injury is TRUE?

    A. Never assume that a patient has a cervical spine injury until there is radiologic evidence.
    B. Intubation should wait until radiographic studies are available.
    C. Rapid sequence induction is only rarely indicated.
    D. Assessment of neck mobility is important before induction.
    E. Manual in-line stabilization is appropriate.

25. Autonomic hyperreflexia is characterized by:

    A. Tachycardia and hypotension in a patient with a spinal cord lesion above T7
    B. Bradycardia and hypertension in a patient with a spinal cord lesion above T7
    C. Tachycardia and hypertension in a patient with a spinal cord lesion above T7
    D. Bradycardia and hypertension in a patient with a spinal cord lesion below T12
    E. Bradycardia and hypotension in a patient with a spinal cord lesion below T12

26. Which of the following statements regarding postoperative visual loss is FALSE?

    A. It occurs in surgeries with long durations.
    B. It is most commonly bilateral.
    C. It has been proven to be directly correlated with levels of hypotension and hematocrit.
    D. It is commonly caused by ischemic optic neuropathy (ION).
    E. Risk factors include obesity, male gender, and use of a Wilson frame.

ANSWERS

1. **B.** Although CSF volume is approximately 150 mL, more than three times this amount is produced in a 24-hour period. (See page 997: Neurophysiology.)

2. **D.** Intracranial pressure (ICP) is low except in pathologic states. The Monro–Kellie doctrine states that in the setting of a nondistensible cranial vault, the volume of blood, CSF, and brain tissue must be in equilibrium. An increase in one of these three elements or the addition of a space-occupying lesion can be accommodated initially through displacement of CSF into the thecal sac, but only to a small extent. A further increase, as with significant cerebral edema or accumulation of an extradural hematoma, quickly leads to a marked increase in ICP because of the low intracranial compliance. (See page 997: Neurophysiology.)

3. **C.** CBF remains approximately constant despite modest swings in arterial blood pressure. The mechanism by which CBF is maintained is called autoregulation of CBF. As CPP (MAP − ICP) changes, CVR adjusts to maintain stable flow. Although this range is frequently quoted as a mean arterial pressure range of 60 to 150 mm Hg, there is significant variability between individuals, and these numbers are only approximate. At the low end of the plateau, CVR is at a minimum, and any further decrease in CPP compromises CBF. At the high end of the plateau, CVR is at a maximum, and any further increase in CPP results in hyperemia. (See page 997: Neurophysiology.)

4. **A.** Inhalation anesthetics tend to cause vasodilation in a dose-related manner. Higher doses result in dominance of the vasodilatory effect and an increase in CBF. They also decrease cerebral metabolism. Intravenous agents, including thiopental and propofol, cause vasoconstriction coupled with a reduction in metabolism. Ketamine, on the other hand, increases flow and metabolism. (See page 999: Anesthetic Influences.)

5. **E.** Hypocapnic cerebral vasoconstriction provides anesthesiologists with a powerful tool for manipulating CBF. Hyperventilation is routinely used to provide brain relaxation and optimize surgical conditions. But because hyperventilation decreases CBF, it has the theoretical potential for causing or exacerbating cerebral ischemia. Clinically, it has been associated with harm only in the early period of TBI, but it is still recommended to be avoided in all patients with TBI except when necessary for a brief period to manage acute increases in ICP. (See page 1010: Ventilation Management.)

6. **C.** For neurosurgery, the sitting position confers the greatest risk for VAE. A Doppler device should be placed on the chest, end-tidal CO_2 should be monitored, and plans should be made for treating a VAE if it occurs. A multi-orifice catheter can be placed in the right atrium to evacuate air. Its location can be confirmed either electrocardiographically

or with echocardiography. The presence of a PFO increases the risk of paradoxical embolism. Therefore, patients to be placed in the sitting position should be evaluated for a PFO, either preoperatively or intraoperatively, and an alternate position should be considered for those who have one. (See page 1012: Surgery for Tumors.)

7. **E.** Patients with aneurysmal subarachnoid hemorrhage (SAH) are at risk for numerous complications that may affect the anesthetic plan. These include cardiac dysfunction, neurogenic or cardiogenic pulmonary edema, hydrocephalus, and further hemorrhage from the aneurysm. Secondary hyperthyroidism is not a known complication of an SAH. (See page 1013: Cerebral Aneurysm Surgery and Endovascular Treatment.)

8. **B.** Blood pressure should be maintained as close to baseline as possible throughout carotid surgery. Without evidence to support it, some advocate increasing the blood pressure during carotid cross-clamping to improve flow through collateral vessels. This practice presupposes that collateralization is marginal and will be helped by the elevation in pressure. Although collateral flow may be marginal, it may also be absent or entirely adequate. In the latter two situations, elevation in blood pressure, through the use of phenylephrine, will only increase myocardial oxygen demand. (See page 1014: Carotid Surgery.)

9. **B.** If the patient's trachea is not intubated after traumatic brain injury (TBI), immediate attention should focus on assessing the airway and making preparations for intubation. Patients with TBI usually have several indications for intubation, including a decreased level of consciousness, increased risk of aspiration, and concern for hypoxemia and hypercarbia. Sometimes these patients must be tracheally intubated and sedated simply to allow further diagnostic studies. Hypertension by itself is not an indication for intubation. (See page 1016: Overview of Traumatic Brain Injury.)

10. **A.** Patients may demonstrate Cushing's response of hypertension and bradycardia, which signifies brainstem compression from increased ICP. (See page 1016: Anesthesia and Traumatic Brain Injury: Anesthetic Management: Emergent Surgery.)

11. **D.** Cauda equina syndrome is the result of injury below the level of the conus, or caudal end of the spinal cord, typically below L2. Compression of the cauda equina results in perineal anesthesia, urinary retention, fecal incontinence, and lower extremity weakness. (See page 1020: Spinal Cord Injury.)

12. **B.** A progressive reduction in cerebral blood flow produces a reliable pattern change in EEG, and the eventual progression to EEG silence. The monitor is therefore useful when surgical procedures jeopardize the perfusion of

the brain, such as during cross-clamping of the carotid artery during carotid endarterectomy. EEG is particularly useful in this setting because the spectral analysis on the at-risk side can be compared in real time with the unaffected side, facilitating detection of ischemia by the resultant asymmetry of EEG. The changes in the EEG spectrum seen with ischemia may occur as a result of other influences, however. Intravenous anesthetic agents such as propofol and thiopental, as well as inhaled agents such as isoflurane, cause a similar change in a dose-related manner, with eventual progression to a drug-induced isoelectric EEG. Typically, the goal in neurosurgery is to achieve a state called *burst suppression*. In this state, periods of isoelectric EEG are punctuated by "bursts" of EEG activity. When burst suppression is the goal, a suppression ratio can be calculated as the percentage of an epoch in which the patient's EEG is isoelectric. The suppression ratio allows one to achieve near-complete suppression (>90%) of EEG activity, while remaining certain that regular EEG activity will return in a short while with cessation of administration of the drug. In contrast, when complete isoelectric EEG is achieved, time to arousal becomes unpredictable. (See page 1000: Central Nervous System Function: Electroencephalogram.)

13. **A.** Inhalation agents, including nitrous oxide, generally have more depressant effects on evoked potential monitoring than IV agents. Whereas cortical evoked potentials with long latency involving multiple synapses are exquisitely sensitive to the influence of anesthetic, short-latency brainstem and spinal components are resistant to anesthetic influence. Thus, BAEPs can be recorded under any anesthetic technique. Monitoring of MEPs in general precludes the use of muscle relaxant, although use of a short-acting neuromuscular blocking agent for the purpose of tracheal intubation is not contraindicated if its effect wears off before monitoring and surgery begins. MEP is exquisitely sensitive to the depressant effects of inhalation anesthetics, including nitrous oxide. Although it can be recorded with low-dose agents, the signals are so severely attenuated that this practice is generally not advisable. Total IV anesthesia without nitrous oxide is the ideal anesthetic technique for MEP monitoring. Opioids and benzodiazepines have negligible effects on recording of EPs. (See page 1000: Monitoring: Central Nervous System Function: Evoked Potential Monitoring.)

14. **D.** Although monitoring ICP does not provide direct information about CBF, it allows one to calculate CPP, which must be in an appropriate range for CBF to be adequate. When ICP is high and CPP is low, interventions can target either ICP or mean arterial pressure to restore a favorable balance of the two. Ideally, ICP should be maintained below 20 mm Hg. Interventions to lower ICP include suppression of cerebral metabolic activity, positional changes to decrease cerebral venous blood volume, drainage of CSF, removal of brain water with osmotic agents such as mannitol, and if absolutely essential, mild to moderate hyperventilation to further decrease cerebral blood volume. ICP monitoring is recommended in all salvageable patients with severe TBI

(GCS ≤ 8) and an abnormal CT scan (hematomas, contusions, swelling, herniation, or compressed basal cistern), and in patients with severe TBI with a normal CT scan if two or more of the following features are noted at the admission: Age > 40 years, unilateral or bilateral motor posturing, or SBP < 90 mm Hg. (See page 1004: Intracranial Pressure Monitoring.)

15. **E.** Profound hypothermia is well known for its neuroprotective effects. When core body temperature is below 20°C, circulatory arrest of less than 30 minutes appears to be well tolerated. The practical constraints against using deep hypothermia in settings in which cerebral ischemia is anticipated are numerous. Foremost is the need for cardiopulmonary bypass during the cooling and warming portion of the procedure. Hypothermia-induced coagulopathy is another concern during surgical procedures in cold patients. Profound hypothermia both decreases cerebral activity and decreases the energy required for cellular housekeeping. (See page 1007: Hypothermia.)

16. **B.** During induction of anesthesia, hypotension, hypertension, and prolonged apnea should be avoided. Hypertension due to laryngoscopy is poorly tolerated by patients after aneurysmal subarachnoid hemorrhage because systolic hypertension is thought to be a cause of recurrent hemorrhage from the aneurysm. Additionally, hypertension may worsen elevated ICP and possibly lead to herniation of cranial contents into the foramen magnum. Apnea results in a predictable increase in $PaCO_2$, and corresponding cerebral vasodilation. Although most patients tolerate the increase in cerebral blood volume, patients with poor intracranial compliance may develop severe intracranial hypertension and decompensate from apnea, as well as suffer a decrease in cerebral perfusion. TBI patients in particular are frequently intolerant of apnea. Furthermore, these patients may have concomitant injuries with significant blood loss that may predispose to systemic hypotension. Vigorous resuscitation with isotonic fluid and/or blood should be administered prior to induction and continued until the patient is euvolemic. (See page 1009: Induction and Airway Management.)

17. **E.** Many neurosurgical and spine surgery patients have conditions in which succinylcholine is contraindicated. Muscle denervation from stroke, myelopathy, and spinal cord injury result in upregulation of acetylcholine receptor isoforms across the muscle belly. This upregulation leads to massive release of potassium with use of succinylcholine; this has the potential to lead to a cardiac arrest. However, it is generally (but not necessarily absolutely) safe to use succinylcholine in the first 24 to 72 hours after an injury. (See page 1009: Induction and Airway Management.)

18. **E.** For extensive spine surgeries in the prone position, significant dependent edema frequently occurs. Although the predictive value of an air leak from around the endotracheal tube cuff is poor in general, the combination of pronounced facial edema and an absent cuff leak after

prone surgery should make one suspicious for upper airway edema. Delaying extubation of the trachea under these circumstances is appropriate. Other factors that may delay extubation in these patients include the development of pulmonary edema and hypoxemia from fluid administration, as well as persistent hemodynamic instability. (See page 1011: Emergence.)

19. D. In contrast to aneurysm surgery, endovascular treatment of aneurysms is a minimally invasive procedure performed in the interventional radiology suite. Despite the less invasive nature of this procedure, it can have equally severe complications as surgery, including further hemorrhage, stroke, and vessel dissection. Although the procedure is not particularly stimulating, the general anesthetic needs to be performed with great care. (See page 1013: Cerebral Aneurysm Surgery and Endovascular Treatment.)

20. D. Frequently, the decision to perform a procedure "awake" has been made by the neurosurgeon before the patient meets the anesthesiologist. Typically, these surgeries are for tumors adjacent to the eloquent cortex or for resection of an epileptic focus. It is the role of the anesthesiologist to determine whether the patient is an appropriate candidate for an "awake" procedure. Although patients with difficult airways, obstructive sleep apnea, or orthopnea may present relative contraindications to an "awake" craniotomy, patients with severe anxiety, claustrophobia, or other psychiatric disorders may be particularly inappropriate for this type of procedure. (See page 1015: Epilepsy Surgery and the Awake Craniotomy.)

21. D. Both hypertonic saline (HS) and HS-Dextran have been used to manage patients with elevated ICP, primarily in the setting of intracranial hypertension refractory to mannitol therapy. Since the blood–brain barrier reflection coefficient to sodium ions is approximately 1, HS establishes a gradient that facilitates the movement of water from the brain into the intravascular space. A randomized trial showed that 3% saline and mannitol have equivalent brain relaxation effects, but with the former having less electrolyte and vascular volume sequelae. In addition to efficacy, the proposed benefit of HS is lack of severe electrolyte disturbance, which is common with mannitol. The brisk diuresis seen with mannitol is absent from HS therapy. (See pages 1016: Overview of Traumatic Brain Injury and 1012: Surgery for Tumors.)

22. D. Profound hypotension may occur after anesthesia induction or, more likely, after craniectomy when the intrinsic stimulus for blood pressure elevation dimin-

ishes. Risk factors for postdecompressive hypotension include low GCS score, absence of basal cisterns on CT, and bilateral dilated pupils. (See page 1019: Emergent Surgery: Neurosurgical.)

23. D. Damage to the spinal column may occur without injury to the spinal cord or may cause spinal cord injury through various insults, including compression, hemorrhage, and vasospasm, all of which result in spinal cord ischemia and infarction. (See page 1020: Spinal Cord Injury.)

24. E. Cervical spine injury should be presumed in any trauma patient requiring intubation before complete physical and radiographic evaluation. Intubation should proceed with little movement of the cervical spine. A rapid sequence induction with cricoid pressure and manual in-line stabilization is appropriate unless a difficult airway is anticipated. (See page 1021: Urgent Airway Management.)

25. B. Patients with chronic spinal cord lesion above T7 may develop autonomic reflexia when stimulated below the site of the lesion. This is a condition characterized by intense vasoconstriction below the site of the lesion accompanied by cutaneous vasodilation above, hypertension, and bradycardia. This is the result of reflex sympathetic stimulation below the lesion unmodulated by supraspinal influence from above. (See page 1024: Autonomic Hyperreflexia.)

26. C. The complication of postoperative visual loss is of particular concern in prone spine surgery, although it can occur in other settings. The visual loss is commonly bilateral and is caused by ischemic optic neuropathy (ION), although retinal artery occlusion and cortical blindness may also occur. These incidents of visual loss occur despite the absence of pressure on the eyes from positioning errors, which would result in central retinal artery thrombosis rather than anterior or posterior ION. Suggested risk factors for ION may include hypovolemia, hypotension, anemia, venous congestion, edema, adverse drug effects, and individual patient variation in anatomy and physiology of the optic nerve blood flow. There has been no association demonstrated with direct pressure or embolic events. A recent case-control study comparing the index cases in the POVL registry with controls suggest that the risk factors for ION include obesity, male gender, use of Wilson frame, long surgical duration, and greater estimated blood loss. Of note, there was no association with level of blood pressure or hematocrit. (See page 1024: Postoperative Visual Loss.)

Anesthesia for Thoracic Surgery

1. The leading cause of cancer mortality in the United States is:

   A. Lung cancer
   B. Colorectal cancer
   C. Breast cancer
   D. Prostate cancer
   E. None of the above

2. The leading cause of cancer death in women in the United States is:

   A. Lung cancer
   B. Colorectal cancer
   C. Breast cancer
   D. Ovarian cancer
   E. None of the above

3. During a preanesthetic interview, you elicit the history of severe exertional dyspnea from an elderly man who smokes cigarettes. This implies:

   A. He is at increased risk of high peak airway pressures on mechanical ventilation.
   B. Wet crackles will be heard at his lung bases on auscultation.
   C. Preoperative flow volume loops will demonstrate a restrictive pattern.
   D. He has a severely diminished respiratory reserve and is at high risk of postoperative ventilatory support.
   E. He will require mechanical ventilatory tidal volumes of 15 to 20 mL/kg.

4. Acute lung injury, an early form of acute respiratory distress syndrome, is sometimes seen after thoracic surgery. Risk factors for acute lung injury after chest surgery include:

   A. Alcohol abuse
   B. Planned pneumonectomy
   C. High intraoperative ventilatory pressures
   D. Excessive amounts of fluid administration
   E. All of the above

5. Which statement regarding the physical examination of a patient undergoing thoracic surgery is FALSE?

   A. Deviation of the trachea indicates potentially difficult intubation.
   B. Clubbing is often seen in patients with a left-to-right shunt.

   C. If cyanosis is present, the patient's PaO_2 level is typically below 55 mm Hg.
   D. The compliance of the pulmonary circulation is reduced in patients with chronic obstructive pulmonary disease (COPD).
   E. A narrowly split second heart sound is a sign of pulmonary hypertension.

6. Which of the following can increase pulmonary vascular resistance?

   A. Systemic acidemia
   B. Septicemia
   C. Systemic hypoxia
   D. Positive end-expiratory pressure (PEEP)
   E. All of the above

7. Which statement regarding flow–volume loops is FALSE?

   A. Small airway resistance is best displayed at expiration between 25% and 75% of vital capacity.
   B. Lung volume is displayed on the horizontal axis.
   C. Patients with restrictive lung disease have a decreased maximum midexpiratory flow rate.
   D. The flow–volume loop displays essentially the same information as the spirometer.
   E. Effort-dependent areas of the loop determine large airway patency.

8. All of the following statements regarding the treatment of wheezing are true EXCEPT:

   A. Ipratropium bromide causes bronchodilation by increasing $3'5'$-cyclic guanosine monophosphate levels.
   B. Aminophylline should be used cautiously in patients with myocardial ischemia.
   C. Cromolyn sodium is of little value in the treatment of acute wheezing episodes.
   D. Steroids decrease mucosal edema and prevent the release of bronchoconstricting substances.
   E. β-agonist aerosols cause bronchodilation by increasing $3'5'$-cyclic adenosine monophosphate levels.

9. The following are true regarding intraoperative monitoring during thoracic surgery EXCEPT:

   A. Pulmonary artery (PA) catheters often cannot be relied on to accurately assess left ventricular end-diastolic volume (LVEDV).
   B. The central venous pressure (CVP) is helpful in determining right ventricular performance.
   C. A central line placed in the external jugular vein often kinks after patient positioning.
   D. The CVP has been shown to have a poor correlation with left atrial pressure in patients with pulmonary disease.
   E. Patients with chronic obstructive pulmonary disease (COPD) presenting for lung resection usually have a left-sided heart strain pattern on the electrocardiogram (ECG).

10. Pulmonary artery (PA) catheters:

    A. Are most often directed to the left upper lobe
    B. Should lie in the nondependent lung when one-lung ventilation is used
    C. Are most reliably inserted through the right internal jugular vein
    D. Yield inaccurate data when placed in the dependent lung
    E. Provide a good approximation of left ventricular end-diastolic volume (LVEDV)

11. Which of the following is TRUE regarding the diffusing capacity for carbon monoxide (DLCO)?

    A. A preoperative DLCO less than 60% of predicted indicates high risk of mortality after lung resection.
    B. DLCO testing is of little clinical use.
    C. DLCO correlates well with forced expiratory volume in 1 second (FEV_1).
    D. It is impaired by interstitial lung disease.
    E. Predicted postoperative diffusing capacity percent is a poor predictor of mortality after lung resection.

12. With respect to the intraoperative use of transesophageal echocardiography (TEE), which of the following statements is FALSE?

    A. TEE is useful for detecting ventricular dysfunction.
    B. Peripheral and central lung tumors are equally easy to locate with TEE.
    C. TEE may be used to detect pulmonary artery compression by a mediastinal tumor.
    D. TEE can help determine whether cardiopulmonary bypass is necessary for tumor resection.
    E. Aortic dissection may be diagnosed with TEE.

13. Which of the following statements is TRUE regarding changes seen when a patient is positioned in the lateral decubitus position?

    A. Blood flow to the nondependent lung is significantly greater than it is to the dependent lung.
    B. The distribution of blood flow is turned by 180 degrees compared with the supine position.

C. An awake, spontaneously breathing patient will demonstrate poor ventilation–perfusion matching in the dependent lung.
D. Ventilation in the dependent lung is greater than in the nondependent lung.
E. The nondependent hemidiaphragm is displaced higher into the chest.

14. A patient undergoing a right thoracotomy with one-lung ventilation is given vecuronium bromide and is placed in the left lateral decubitus position. The following statements are true EXCEPT:

    A. Thirty-five percent of the cardiac output participates in gas exchange in the left lung.
    B. Hypoxic pulmonary vasoconstriction reduces blood flow to the nondependent hypoxic lung by 50%.
    C. The patient's functional residual capacity (FRC) is reduced by receiving vecuronium bromide.
    D. One-lung ventilation causes a right-to-left shunt through the nonventilated lung.
    E. Atelectasis may inhibit optimal ventilation to the dependent lung.

15. When positioning a double-lumen tube:

    A. Insertion through the vocal cords is performed with the distal curvature facing laterally.
    B. The tube should be advanced until moderate resistance is encountered.
    C. The Miller laryngoscope blade yields a much easier tube insertion than does a Macintosh laryngoscope blade.
    D. The stylet should be removed after the tube is rotated 90 degrees.
    E. A left-sided tube should be rotated 90 degrees to the right after the tip passes through the vocal cords.

16. All the following are absolute indications for one-lung ventilation EXCEPT:

    A. Pneumonectomy
    B. Massive pulmonary hemorrhage
    C. Bronchopleural fistula
    D. Unilateral abscess
    E. Bronchopulmonary lavage

17. When checking the position of the double-lumen tube, all of the following are true EXCEPT:

    A. Use of an underwater seal is a good method to verify separation before bronchopulmonary lavage.
    B. Inflation of the bronchial cuff rarely requires more than 2 mL of air.
    C. Selective capnography can be used to ensure correct placement.
    D. A pediatric bronchoscope should be passed through the tracheal lumen first.
    E. If breath sounds are not equal after the tracheal cuff is inflated, the tube should be advanced 2 to 3 cm.

18. All of the following antagonize hypoxic pulmonary vasoconstriction EXCEPT:

    A. Propofol
    B. Pulmonary hypertension secondary to pulmonary embolism
    C. Epinephrine
    D. Mitral stenosis
    E. Infection

19. All of the following are true regarding patients with mediastinal masses EXCEPT:

    A. Local anesthesia is an anesthetic option for biopsy.
    B. Airway obstruction on induction of anesthesia may be relieved with neuromuscular blocking agents.
    C. Hypotension on induction of anesthesia may be secondary to cardiac compression.
    D. Mediastinal masses may cause superior vena cava syndrome.
    E. Passage of a rigid bronchoscope beyond the obstruction may be lifesaving.

20. Mediastinoscopy:

    A. Commonly occludes the left radial pulse
    B. May be associated with right hemiparesis
    C. May cause injury to the superior laryngeal nerve
    D. Is a procedure with potential for life-threatening hemorrhage
    E. Must be performed with the patient under general anesthesia

21. Regarding lung volume reduction surgery, all of the following are true EXCEPT:

    A. This procedure may be indicated in patients with end-stage emphysema.
    B. Ventilation can usually be decreased after the chest is open.
    C. Nitrous oxide should be avoided.
    D. Pneumothorax may be difficult to diagnose.
    E. Patients have a greater amount of functional lung tissue after surgery.

22. Which of the following statements regarding bronchopulmonary lavage is TRUE?

    A. The cuff seal of an endobronchial tube should be adjusted so that no leak is present at 50 cm H_2O.
    B. Most patients require 3 days of mechanical ventilation after lavage.
    C. The patient is turned so the lavage side is uppermost.
    D. After lung separation is achieved while the patient is under general anesthesia, the patient is allowed to regain consciousness for the procedure.
    E. The onset of rales in the ventilated lung indicates heart failure.

23. Which of the following statements regarding fiberoptic bronchoscopy is FALSE?

    A. Suction through the bronchoscope leads to a decreased PaO_2.
    B. Airway obstruction after fiberoptic bronchoscopy is a rare complication.
    C. Positive end-expiratory pressure (PEEP) should be discontinued before passage of the fiberscope.
    D. The adult fiberscope can pass through a 7.5-mm endotracheal tube.
    E. Jet ventilation may be achieved by attachment to the suction channel.

24. Which of the following statements regarding choice of anesthesia for thoracic surgery is FALSE?

    A. Ketamine produces bronchodilation.
    B. Remifentanil in combination with propofol significantly blunts hypoxic pulmonary vasoconstriction.
    C. Morphine increases bronchomotor tone.
    D. Isoflurane may be beneficial because it increases the cardiac arrhythmia threshold.
    E. Morphine may cause bronchoconstriction.

For questions 25 to 39, choose A if 1, 2, and 3 are correct; B if 1 and 3 are correct; C if 2 and 4 are correct; D if 4 is correct; or E if all are correct.

25. The goals of performing pulmonary function tests (PFTs) in patients scheduled for lung resection for treatment of a malignancy are to:

    1. Establish the maximum amount of resectable lung tissue
    2. Identify patients needing postoperative ventilatory support
    3. Evaluate the benefits of bronchodilators in reversing existing airway obstruction
    4. Evaluate whether increased inspired O_2 concentration increases ventilation and therefore the work of breathing

26. Which of the following sympathomimetic drugs are β_2-selective and typically produce minimal cardiac effect from β_1-stimulation?

    1. Albuterol
    2. Terbutaline
    3. Metaproterenol
    4. Epinephrine

27. Respiratory changes that occur after lower abdominal surgery include:

    1. Total lung capacity decreases to the same extent after abdominal surgery as after extremity surgery.
    2. Tidal volume is decreased for approximately 2 weeks.
    3. Pulmonary compliance increases.
    4. Vital capacity decreases by 25% to 50%.

28. Which of the following statements regarding pulmonary evaluation for lung resectability is TRUE?

    1. It is more useful to use the percent of predicted forced expiratory volume in 1 second (FEV_1) rather than the absolute value.
    2. A patient with an abnormal vital capacity has a 33% likelihood of complications.
    3. An FEV_1 of less than 500 mL in a 70-kg patient is an absolute contraindication to lung resection.
    4. A ratio of residual volume to total lung capacity of 10% is consistent with a high risk for pulmonary resection.

29. Which of the following statements concerning smoking is TRUE?

    1. Smoking decreases forced vital capacity and maximum midexpiratory flow rate.
    2. Cessation of smoking for 48 hours before surgery shifts the oxyhemoglobin curve to the left.
    3. Most of the beneficial effects of smoking cessation do not occur before 2 to 3 months.
    4. Smoking increases mucociliary transport.

30. Which of the following statements concerning oxygenation and ventilation is TRUE?

    1. Arterial blood gases are unnecessary as long as end-tidal CO_2 is monitored.
    2. The alveolar dead space affects the arterial–alveolar CO_2 gradient.
    3. Hypercarbia is usually a greater problem than systemic hypoxia during one-lung ventilation.
    4. CO_2 readings may help indicate correct double-lumen tube placement.

31. Which of the following statements regarding bronchial blockers is TRUE?

    1. They are effective in maintaining lung isolation despite surgical manipulation.
    2. An advantage is that they are useful in patients with difficult airways.
    3. Placement of an endobronchial catheter into the bronchus should be performed blindly.
    4. A bronchial blocker may be used in a 12-year-old child.

32. During one-lung ventilation:

    1. Tidal volumes should be adjusted to 10 to 12 mL/kg.
    2. Continuous positive airway pressure (CPAP) to the nondependent lung increases arterial O_2 concentration.
    3. Hyperventilation can lead to a decreased PaO_2 level.
    4. A fraction of inspired oxygen (FiO_2) of 1 is frequently used.

33. Hypoxic pulmonary vasoconstriction:

    1. Is increased in the presence of potent inhaled anesthetics
    2. Is indirectly inhibited by hypothermia
    3. Is increased by volume overload
    4. Is activated by collapse of the nondependent lung

34. Rigid bronchoscopy is the procedure of choice for:

    1. Assessing vascular tumors of the lower airway
    2. Securing an airway in a difficult intubation
    3. Bronchoscopy in small children
    4. Evaluation of upper lobe lesions

35. Which of the following statements regarding myasthenia gravis is TRUE?

    1. Examination of pupillary size may differentiate between myasthenic and cholinergic crisis.
    2. These patients are very sensitive to depolarizing muscle relaxants and are resistant to nondepolarizing muscle relaxants.
    3. Thymectomy is considered to be the treatment of choice in many patients with generalized myasthenia gravis.
    4. This condition is associated with a markedly decreased release of acetylcholine from nerve terminals.

36. Which of the following statements regarding video-assisted thoracoscopic surgery (VATS) is TRUE?

    1. CO_2 may be insufflated into the pleural cavity.
    2. Continuous positive airway pressure (CPAP) may interfere with the surgical procedure.
    3. The need for one-lung ventilation is greater for VATS than for open thoracotomy.
    4. It may take 30 minutes for complete lung collapse.

37. Which of the following statements about central venous catheters/central venous pressure (CVP) monitoring is TRUE?

    1. It reflects right-sided heart function.
    2. One common use is for the infusion of vasoactive drugs.
    3. A CVP catheter can be placed from either the internal or external jugular vein.
    4. It reliably reflects intravascular status.

38. Which of the following statements about double-lumen endobronchial tubes (DLT) is TRUE?

    1. The depth required for insertion of the tube correlates with the patient's height.
    2. A left-sided tube is preferred for both right- and left-sided procedures.
    3. The width of the left bronchus is directly proportional to the width of the trachea.
    4. A 37-Fr double-lumen tube is the correct size for most women.

39. Which of the following statements concerning malposition of a double-lumen tube (DLT) is TRUE?

1. If the DLT is not inserted far enough, breath sounds are not audible over the contralateral side.
2. The mean distance from the carina to the right upper lobe orifice is 2 to 3 cm.
3. If the DLT is inserted too far down either bronchus, breath sounds will be heard bilaterally when ventilating through the bronchial lumen.
4. Tracheal rupture is a rare complication.

40. Which of the following statements concerning postoperative pain management of thoracic surgeries is TRUE?

1. Epidural morphine is contraindicated in thoracic surgeries.
2. Patients who receive technically perfect rib blocks frequently complain of shoulder discomfort postoperatively.
3. Ketamine infusions of 1 to 2 mg/kg/hr are commonly used as an adjunct to epidural analgesia.
4. The incidence of chronic pain following VATS procedures may be similar to the rates seen following open thoracotomies.

ANSWERS

1. A. Lung cancer has long been the most common cause of cancer mortality in the United States The most recent statistics from the American Cancer Society indicate that approximately 221,130 new cases of lung cancer would be diagnosed in 2011 (115,060 among men and 106,070 among women). The Society also estimates that there will be 156,940 deaths from lung cancer, which represents 27% of all cancer deaths. (See page 1030: Key Points.)

2. A. In 1987, lung cancer surpassed breast cancer as the leading cause of cancer death in women in the United States. (See page 1030: Key Points.)

3. D. During all preanesthetic assessments, it is important to ask about dyspnea. Dyspnea is a sensation of shortness of breath that occurs when a patient's requirement for ventilation is greater than his or her ability to respond to that demand. When the anesthesiologist quantitates the degree of physical activity required to produce the sensation of dyspnea, certain postoperative predictions can be made. If a patient complains of dyspnea produced by minimal exertion, the ventilatory reserve is implicitly significantly diminished, and the forced expiratory volume in 1 second (FEV_1) is predicted to be less than 1,500 mL; the patient does not necessarily have restrictive airway disease. It is not unusual for these patients to need postoperative ventilatory support. High peak airway pressures during mechanical ventilation can involve multiple factors, including light anesthetic and obstructive, or restrictive pulmonary disease; however, it is not the most commonly seen effect of exertional dyspnea. Wet sounds (crackles) are usually caused by excessive fluid in the airways and indicate sputum retention or edema. Mechanical ventilation volumes of 15 to 20 mL/kg are excessive except in a recruitment maneuver. (See page 1031: Preoperative Evaluation.)

4. E. Patients with a preoperative history of alcohol abuse have been identified as being at increased risk for acute lung injury after thoracic surgery. Patients who undergo pneumonectomy, who are exposed to high airway pressures on mechanical ventilation, or who receive an excessive amount of fluid relative to their needs have also been identified as being at increased risk for acute lung injury. (See page 1031: History.)

5. B. Clubbing is seen frequently in patients with congenital heart disease associated with a right-to-left shunt, in patients with chronic lung disease, and in patients with malignancies. If cyanosis is present, the arterial saturation is 80% or less, which correlates with a PaO_2 level of 50 to 52 mm Hg. Displacement of the trachea should alert the anesthesiologist to the potential for difficult intubation. Patients with COPD have reduced compliance of the pulmonary capillary bed (in other words, the capillaries have a decreased ability to distend with increasing blood flow). The second heart sound is a combination of the aortic valve and pulmonic valve closing in close succession. A narrowly split second heart sound can be a sign of pulmonary hypertension, as distinguished from the normal physiologic splitting of the second heart sound which is heard during deep inspiration. (See page 1032: Respiratory Pattern: Evaluation of the Cardiovascular System.)

6. E. Systemic acidosis, sepsis, hypoxemia, and PEEP can increase pulmonary vascular resistance, which may place the patient at risk of right ventricular failure. This paradoxical change (pulmonary vascular resistance being the opposite of systemic vascular resistance under the same circumstances) is believed to be due to the body attempting to shift blood flow to the most highly ventilated portions of the lung. The resultant risk of right ventricular failure is further increased in a patient with chronic obstructive pulmonary disease, characterized by distention of the pulmonary capillary bed with decreased compliance in response to increased pulmonary blood flow. (See page 1032: Evaluation of the Cardiovascular System.)

7. C. In patients with restrictive lung disease, the maximum midexpiratory flow rate is usually normal, but total lung capacity is reduced (the opposite trends are seen in obstructive lung disease). Lung volume is displayed on the horizontal axis of a flow–volume curve, and flow is displayed on the vertical axis. The shape and peak of flow rates during expiration at high volumes are effort dependent and indicate the patency of the larger airways. Effort-independent expiration occurs at low lung volumes and usually reflects smaller airway resistance. The best measurement for small airway disease is to measure the maximum midexpiratory flow rate at 25% to 75% of vital capacity. Obstructive disease should be suspected if the FEF 25% to 75% is less than 50% of predicted. This change usually occurs before the decrease in FEV_1/FVC ratio in this population. The flow–volume loop essentially displays the same information as the spirometer but is more convenient for measurement of specific flow rates. (See page 1033: Flow–Volume Loops.)

8. A. The balance between 3′5′-cyclic adenosine monophosphate (which produces bronchodilation, and is proportionately increased by β_2-agonists like albuterol) and 3′5′-cyclic guanosine monophosphate (which produces bronchoconstriction) determines the state of contraction of the bronchial smooth muscle. Ipratropium bromide blocks the formation of 3′5′-cyclic guanosine monophosphate and therefore has a bronchodilatory effect. Aminophylline may cause ventricular dysrhythmias, so it should be used cautiously when treating patients with cardiac disease. Steroids decrease mucosal edema and prevent the release of bronchoconstricting substances. Cromolyn sodium stabilizes the mast cells and inhibits degranulation and histamine release. It is useful in the prevention of bronchospastic attacks but is of little value in the treatment of acute exacerbations. (See page 1036: Wheezing and Bronchodilation.)

9. **E.** Patients presenting for lung surgery often have COPD owing to cigarette smoking and right-sided heart strain evident on the ECG. The right-sided strain is partially the result of the heart working to overcome increased pulmonary vascular resistance seen in this disease. A CVP catheter reflects right ventricular performance, venous tone, and can reflect the patient's blood volume (although this is no longer considered an accurate guide for fluid responsiveness). The major disadvantage of using the external jugular vein for placement of a CVP is that the catheter may kink when the patient is turned laterally. The CVP has been shown to have poor correlation with the left atrial pressure in patients with pulmonary disease. A major limitation of the PA catheter is the assumption that the pulmonary capillary wedge pressure provides a good approximation of LVEDV. This assumption is inaccurate in certain situations, such as high levels of PEEP or acute respiratory failure. The false reading occurs due to distension of the right ventricle causing septal bulging and resultant decrease in the size of the left ventricle. (See page 1036: Intraoperative Monitoring.)

10. **C.** The tip of a flow-directed PA catheter usually ends up in the right lower lobe because this is the area of highest pulmonary blood flow (although flow also depends on patient positioning to some extent). The PA catheter is most reliably inserted through the right internal jugular vein using a modified Seldinger technique. During thoracotomy with one-lung ventilation, a catheter in the dependent lung should produce accurate hemodynamic measurements. Due to lung deflation, the nondependent lung will not have sufficient blood flow for accurate interpretation of data. A major limitation of PA catheters is the assumption that the pulmonary capillary wedge pressure (PCWP) provides a good approximation of LVEDV. The use of PCWP directly to assess preload assumes a linear relationship between ventricular end-diastolic volume and ventricular end-diastolic pressure. However, alterations in ventricular compliance affect this pressure–volume relationship during surgery. Decreases in ventricular compliance may occur with myocardial ischemia, shock, right ventricular overload, or pericardial effusion. (See page 1037: Pulmonary Artery Catheterization.)

11. **D.** Gas exchange ability by the lungs can be evaluated by testing the DLCO. This parameter is impaired in disorders such as interstitial lung disease. A predicted postoperative DLCO of less than 40% after lung resection surgery is associated with an increased risk of postoperative respiratory complications and mortality. Predicted postoperative diffusing capacity percent is the strongest single predictor of risk of complications and mortality after lung resection. Little relationship exists between predicted postoperative DLCO and predicted postoperative FEV_1. (See page 1034: Diffusing Capacity for Carbon Monoxide.)

12. **B.** TEE can consistently locate central lung tumors, but peripheral lung tumors are located only 30% of the time. TEE is a useful intraoperative monitor for ventricular function, valvular function, and wall motion abnormalities. TEE may help determine when cardiopulmonary bypass is necessary for mediastinal tumor resection (e.g., if tumor is invading into the heart itself). TEE may also show mediastinal tumors compressing the pulmonary artery. In an exploratory thoracotomy for hemothorax, intraoperative TEE revealed the presence of a subacute aortic dissection, which was believed to be the cause of the hemothorax. (See page 1038: Transesophageal Echocardiography.)

13. **D.** In the spontaneously breathing patient in a lateral decubitus position, blood flow and ventilation to the dependent lung are significantly greater than to the nondependent lung. This can also be true in the mechanically ventilated patient; however, lack of diaphragmatic contraction and increased pressure on the diaphragm from the abdominal organs shift ventilation in the favor of the nondependent lung. In the lateral decubitus position, the distribution of blood flow and ventilation is similar to that in the upright position but turned by 90 degrees. Good ventilation–perfusion matching at the level of the dependent lung results in adequate oxygenation in the awake, spontaneously breathing patient. The dependent hemidiaphragm is pushed higher into the chest by the abdominal contents than is the nondependent diaphragm. (See page 1038: Physiology of One-lung Ventilation, Lateral Position, Awake, Breathing Spontaneous, Chest Closed.)

14. **A.** Before the initiation of one-lung anesthesia, the average percentage of cardiac output participating in gas exchange is 45% in the nondependent lung and 55% in the dependent lung. After the initiation of one-lung anesthesia, hypoxic pulmonary vasoconstriction reduces the blood flow to the nondependent lung by 50% (the resultant calculated total shunt during one-lung ventilation is 27.5% through the nondependent lung, and 72.5% of blood flow through the dependent lung). The FRC and the total lung volume decrease during one-lung ventilation. There are several reasons for this, including general anesthesia, paralysis, pressure from the abdominal contents, compression by the weight of mediastinal structures, and suboptimal positioning on the operating table. Atelectasis is one cause of suboptimal ventilation to the dependent lung. (See page 1038: Physiology of One-lung Ventilation, One-lung Ventilation, Anesthetized, Paralyzed, Chest Open.)

15. **B.** Advancement of a double-lumen tube should be stopped when moderate resistance to further passage is encountered, which indicates that the tube tip has been seated in the stem bronchus. (Of note, a more proximal resistance occurs when advancing the tracheal opening/offset portion of the tube through the arytenoids and vocal cords. This can be a significant difficulty, even requiring changing to a smaller diameter DLT.) A Macintosh laryngoscope blade is preferred for intubation with a double-lumen tube because it provides the largest area through which to pass the tube. The insertion of the tube between the vocal cords is performed with the distal concave curvature facing anteriorly. It is important to remove the stylet before rotating or advancing the tube farther to avoid tracheal or bronchial lacerations. After the tip of the tube passes the vocal cords, the stylet is removed. A right-sided tube then is rotated 90 degrees to the right; a

left-sided tube is rotated 90 degrees to the left. (See page 1043: Placement of Double-lumen Tubes.)

16. **A.**   In clinical practice, a double-lumen tube is commonly used for lobectomy or pneumonectomy; however, these are relative indications for lung separation. Separation of the lungs to prevent spillage of pus or blood from an infected or bleeding source is an absolute indication for one-lung ventilation. Bronchopleural or bronchocutaneous fistulae represent low-resistance escape pathways for the tidal volume delivered by positive-pressure ventilation; these are both absolute indications for one-lung ventilation. During bronchopulmonary lavage, an effective separation of the lungs is mandatory to avoid accidental spillage of fluid from the lavaged lung to the nondependent ventilated lung. (See page 1041: Absolute Indications for One-lung Ventilation and page 1042: Relative Indications for One-lung Ventilation.)

17. **E.**   If breath sounds are not equal after the tracheal cuff is inflated, the double-lumen tube is likely too far down. Withdrawing the tube by 2 or 3 cm usually restores equal breath sounds. Conversely, if breath sounds are equal with inflation of the bronchial cuff, the placement may not be distal enough. Inflation of the bronchial cuff rarely requires more than 2 mL of air. The bronchoscope usually is introduced first through the tracheal lumen. The carina is visualized, and bronchial cuff herniation should not be seen. Common methods of ensuring the correct placement of a double-lumen tube include fluoroscopy, chest radiography, selective capnography, and the use of an underwater seal. If the bronchial cuff is not inflated and positive-pressure ventilation is applied to the bronchial lumen of the double-lumen tube, gas will leak past the bronchial cuff and will return to the tracheal lumen. If the tracheal lumen is connected to an underwater seal system, gas will be seen bubbling up through the water. The bronchial cuff can then be gradually inflated until no gas bubbles are seen. (See page 1043: Placement of Double-lumen Tubes.)

18. **A.**   It is generally believed that inhaled agents inhibit hypoxic pulmonary vasoconstriction (HPV), but intravenous drugs do not have this effect. Of note, these data are mostly the result of in vitro laboratory studies; most clinical studies show an insignificant difference between inhaled and intravenous anesthetics. Factors associated with an increase in pulmonary artery pressure antagonize the effects of resistance caused by hypoxic pulmonary vasoconstriction and result in increased flow to the hypoxic region (i.e., greater shunt). Therefore, one can predict that these indirect inhibitors of hypoxic pulmonary vasoconstriction would include mitral stenosis, thromboembolism, and vasopressors such as epinephrine. Direct inhibitors of hypoxic pulmonary vasoconstriction include infection and vasodilator drugs. (See page 1055: Effects of Anesthetics and Hypoxic Pulmonary Vasoconstriction.)

19. **B.**   When a patient has a mediastinal mass and there is concern that airway obstruction may occur during anesthetic induction, an awake fiberoptic intubation is the technique of choice. Spontaneous respiration should be maintained because muscle paralysis may result in airway compression and may worsen the obstruction. Ventilatory difficulties may be relieved by passing the rigid bronchoscope beyond the obstruction under direct laryngoscopy or by changing the patient's position. Mediastinal masses may cause superior vena cava syndrome. Cardiac compression may become apparent after the induction of anesthesia. (See page 1058: Diagnostic Procedures for Mediastinal Masses.)

20. **D.**   Mediastinoscopy is a means of assessing the spread of lung carcinoma. Hemorrhage is a real risk and may be life threatening, so blood must be available. Pressure on the innominate artery by the mediastinoscope has been thought to cause transient left hemiparesis; therefore, it is recommended that blood pressure be monitored in the left arm and that the right radial pulse be monitored continuously (in order to detect compression of the innominate artery). Recurrent laryngeal nerve injury may occur either by the mediastinoscope or by tumor involvement. If both recurrent laryngeal nerves are damaged, upper airway obstruction may result. Most surgeons and anesthesiologists prefer general anesthesia using an endotracheal tube and continuous ventilation because this offers a more controlled situation and greater flexibility in terms of surgical manipulation; however, the procedure can be performed under local anesthesia with various sedation techniques. (See page 1060: Mediastinoscopy.)

21. **B.**   Extensive bullae represent end-stage emphysematous destruction of the lung. After the chest is open during lung volume reduction surgery, more of the tidal volume may enter the compliant bullae, which are no longer limited by chest wall integrity, and an increase in ventilation is needed until the bullae are resected. Nitrous oxide should be avoided because it may cause expansion of bullae. The diagnosis of pneumothorax may be made by a unilateral decrease in breath sounds, which may be difficult to distinguish in a patient with bullous disease. Other factors seen in pneumothorax include an increase in ventilatory pressure, progressive tracheal deviation, wheezing, or cardiovascular changes. Treatment of a pneumothorax involves the rapid placement of a chest tube. Unlike most cases of pulmonary resection, after bullectomy, patients are left with a greater amount of functional lung tissue than was previously available to them, and the mechanics of respiration are improved. (See page 1063: Lung Cysts and Bullae.)

22. **A.**   During bronchopulmonary lavage, the cuff seal should be checked to maintain perfect separation of lungs at a pressure of 50 cm H_2O to prevent leakage of lavage fluid. A stethoscope should be placed over the ventilated lung to check for rales that may indicate leakage of lavage fluid into this lung. After the trachea is intubated, the patient is turned so the side to be treated is lowermost (so that gravity assists in preventing lavage flow into the ventilated lung), and the double-lumen tube position and seal are checked again. After another period of ventilation, most patients can be extubated in the operating room. The whole lung lavage procedure is carried out entirely under general anesthesia, although it possible to perform

segmental lavage under local/sedation anesthetics. (See page 1064: Bronchopulmonary Lavage.)

23. **B.** During and after fiberoptic bronchoscopy, patients experience increased airway obstruction. These changes are believed to be secondary to direct mechanical activation of irritative reflexes in the airway and possibly to mucosal edema. Lidocaine topicalization appears to aid in reducing this response. The standard adult fiberoptic bronchoscope has an external diameter of 5.7 mm and a 2-mm diameter suction channel. If suction at 1 atm is applied to the fiberscope, air is removed at a rate of 14 L/min. If the fiberscope is in the airway, this causes decreases in the fraction of inspired oxygen (FiO_2), PaO_2, and functional residual capacity, leading to decreased PaO_2. Therefore, suctioning should be kept brief. The adult fiberscope can be passed through endotracheal tubes of 7 mm or greater internal diameter. Clearly, passage through an endotracheal tube decreases the cross-sectional area available for ventilating the patient, so if fiberoscopy is planned, an endotracheal tube of the largest possible diameter should be used. Insertion of the bronchoscope also causes a significant PEEP effect that may result in barotrauma in ventilated patients. If PEEP is already being used, it should be discontinued before passage of the fiberscope. Postendoscopy chest radiography is advisable to exclude the presence of mediastinal emphysema or pneumothorax. The suction channel of the adult fiberoptic bronchoscope has been used to oxygenate and ventilate the lungs of patients. (See pages 1056: Anesthesia for Diagnostic Procedures and 1058: Fiberoptic Bronchoscopy.)

24. **B.** The potent inhaled anesthetic agents all have been shown to decrease airway reactivity and reduce bronchoconstriction provoked by hypocapnia or inhaled or irritant aerosols. Their mechanism of action is probably a direct one on the airway musculature itself, and potent inhaled anesthetic agents are therefore the drugs of choice in patients with reactive airways. For an inhalation induction, halothane or sevoflurane may be preferable because they are less pungent, although after the patient is asleep, isoflurane can be used because it increases the cardiac arrhythmia threshold and provides greater cardiovascular stability than halothane. Fentanyl and Remifentanil do not appear to influence bronchomotor tone, but morphine may increase tone by a central vagotonic effect, and also by releasing histamine. In patients with reactive airways, ketamine may be the drug of choice for induction due to its potent bronchodilatory effect (it has also been successfully used in the treatment of patients with refractory asthma). Propofol infused in doses of 6 to 12 mg/kg/hr does not abolish HPV during one-lung ventilation in humans. Propofol infusion in combination with remifentanil will typically result in stable one-lung ventilation with no effect on HPV. (See page 1054: Choice of Anesthesia for Thoracic Surgery.)

25. **A.** Preoperative PFTs allow the surgeon and anesthesiologist to determine the maximum amount of resectable lung before the patient would become a pulmonary cripple. Historically, an FEV_1 of 800 cc would be a contraindication

for surgery; however, when attempting a procedure such as a pneumonectomy, it is possible to transiently occlude the pulmonary artery (in the OR) and measure PA pressures. If the pressures are elevated, the patient cannot tolerate loss of the vascular bed and further resection would be contraindicated. Obviously, if the amount of planned resection would cause significant morbidity, reconsideration of the surgical plan may be in order. PFTs also allow one to plan for postoperative ventilatory support after lung resection. Preoperative PFTs also evaluate whether the patient exhibits airway obstruction and whether that obstruction reverses completely or partly after bronchodilator therapy. PFTs do not evaluate whether increased FiO_2 increases the work of breathing. (See page 1033: Pulmonary Function Testing and Evaluation for Lung Resectability.)

26. **A.** Albuterol, terbutaline, and metaproterenol are β_2-selective sympathomimetic drugs that have little effect on β_1-receptors (cardiac receptors). They are used to increase intracellular cyclic adenosine monophosphate (cAMP) concentrations in bronchial smooth muscle and thereby produce bronchodilation (bronchoconstriction occurs with increased cGMP and is relieved by increased cAMP). Epinephrine stimulates both β_1- and β_2-receptors, as do isoproterenol, isoetharine, and ephedrine. (See page 1036: Wheezing and Bronchodilation.)

27. **C.** Tidal volume decreases by 20% within 24 hours after surgery and gradually returns to normal after 2 weeks. Vital capacity is decreased by 25% to 50% within 1 to 2 days after surgery and generally returns to normal after 1 to 2 weeks. Pulmonary compliance decreases by 33% with similar reductions in functional residual capacity. Total lung capacity decreases after abdominal surgery but not after extremity surgery. (See page 1033: Effects of Anesthesia and Surgery on Lung Volume.)

28. **A.** A patient with an abnormal vital capacity has a 33% likelihood of complications and a 10% risk of postoperative mortality from lung resection. An FEV_1 of less than 500 mL in a 70-kg patient is probably incompatible with life and is an absolute contraindication to lung resection. Historically, an FEV_1 of 800 cc would be a contraindication for surgery; however, if a surgeon still feels that the patient may have a positive prognosis, it is possible to clamp the arterial flow to the offending portion of lung and check for elevated PA pressures (which would then be an absolute contraindication). It is preferable to indicate the percentage of predicted rather than just using the absolute value. The percentage of predicted takes into account the age and size of the patient, and the same number may have a different implication in another patient. A ratio of residual volume to total lung capacity of more than 50% is generally indicative of a high-risk patient for pulmonary resection. (See page 1033: Spirometry.)

29. **B.** Most of the beneficial effects of smoking cessation, such as improvement in ciliary function, improvement in closing volume, increased maximum midexpiratory flow rate, and reduction in sputum, usually occur 2 to 3 months after smoking cessation. Smoking increases airway irritability,

decreases mucociliary transport, and increases secretions. Smoking also decreases forced vital capacity. Smoking cessation 48 hours before surgery has been shown to decrease the level of carboxyhemoglobin and to shift the oxyhemoglobin dissociation curve to the right, thus increasing O_2 availability. (See page 1035: Smoking.)

30. **C.** Normally, a small arterial–alveolar CO_2 gradient of approximately 4 to 6 mm Hg is dependent on the alveolar dead space. The capnogram waveform is helpful in diagnosing airway obstruction, incomplete relaxation, and incorrect positioning of the double-lumen tube. Adequacy of ventilation should be confirmed by monitoring arterial blood gases and $PaCO_2$, in particular. This may be estimated continuously and noninvasively by using capnography. During one-lung ventilation, systemic hypoxia is usually a greater problem than hypercarbia, making it necessary to monitor arterial oxygenation. This is because CO_2 is 20 times more diffusible than O_2; arterial CO_2 concentration is more dependent on ventilation, but arterial O_2 concentration is more dependent on perfusion. (See page 1038: Monitoring of Oxygenation and Ventilation.)

31. **C.** A Bronchial blocker or Univent (a single-lumen endotracheal tube with a movable endobronchial blocker) tube may be helpful for cases in which changing the double-lumen tube to a single-lumen tube may be difficult (e.g., after bilateral lung transplantation). The bronchial blocker may be used with a single-lumen tube to obtain lung isolation, thereby avoiding the use of a double-lumen tube in a patient with a difficult airway. The bronchial blocker technique may be useful in achieving selective ventilation in adults and may be used in children younger than 12 years old. It should be placed via bronchoscopic guidance. These tubes are not used very commonly because they are easily displaced (e.g., by surgical manipulation). Displacement of the bronchial blocker necessitates a pause in surgery while it is replaced under bronchoscopic guidance. (See page 1042: Methods of Lung Separation.)

32. **E.** During one-lung ventilation, the dependent lung should be ventilated with a tidal volume of 10 to 12 mL/kg Of note, acute lung injury occurs in 4% of patients post-pneumonectomy and 1% of patients postlobectomy. There has been suggestion that a lower tidal volume would help prevent some instances of acute lung injury. This may be a practice model change in the future. The single most effective maneuver to increase arterial O_2 concentration during one-lung ventilation is the application of CPAP to the nondependent lung. During a VATS procedure, CPAP to the nondependent lung will decrease the free space available for the surgeon in the field, and it may be necessary to transiently increase and decrease the CPAP levels based on surgical requirements, providing the patient will tolerate such manipulation. It is important not to hyperventilate the patient's lungs because hypocapnia will increase vascular resistance in the dependent lung, inhibit nondependent lung hypoxic pulmonary vasoconstriction, increase the shunt, and therefore decrease the PaO_2 concentration. An FiO_2 of 1 is usually used during one-lung ventilation. This high oxygen concentration serves to protect against hypoxemia during

the procedure. (See pages 1051: Tidal Volume and Respiratory Rate and 1052: Continuous Positive Airway Pressure to the Nondependent Lung.)

33. **C.** Normally, collapse of the nonventilated, nondependent lung results in the activation of reflex hypoxic pulmonary vasoconstriction. It is generally believed that inhaled potent anesthetics inhibit HPV. Other indirect inhibitors of HPV include mitral stenosis, volume overload, thromboembolism, hypothermia, vasoconstrictor drugs, and a large hypoxic lung segment. Direct inhibitors of HPV include infection, vasodilator drugs such as nitroglycerin and nitroprusside, hypocarbia, and metabolic alkalemia. (See page 1055: Hypoxic Pulmonary Vasoconstriction.)

34. **B.** The rigid bronchoscope is the instrument of choice for removal of foreign bodies, control of massive hemoptysis, assessment of vascular tumors, bronchoscopy in small children, and resection of endobronchial lesions. Flexible bronchoscopy is useful in evaluating upper lobe lesions and in securing an airway in difficult intubations. (See page 1057: Table 37-6. Instruments of Choice for Bronchoscopy.)

35. **B.** The distinction between a myasthenic crisis and a cholinergic crisis may be made using a Tensilon test or by examining pupillary size (which is large during a myasthenic crisis but small during a cholinergic crisis). Thymectomy is now considered the treatment of choice in many patients with myasthenia gravis. After thymectomy, approximately 75% of patients either go into remission or show some improvement. Patients with myasthenia gravis are sensitive to the nondepolarizing relaxants and are resistant to succinylcholine. (The ED_{95} is 2.6 times normal in these patients. Clinically, however, the use of succinylcholine has been without incident, with the usual clinical doses producing adequate relaxation for endotracheal intubation and a normal recovery time, despite the occasionally reported early onset of phase II block. Doses of 0.2 to 1 mg/kg have been used in a number of patients with MG, and most did not show fasciculation before becoming paralyzed.) The basic abnormality in myasthenia gravis is a decrease in the number of postsynaptic acetylcholine receptors at the end plates of the affected muscles. Myasthenia gravis is an autoimmune disorder, and most affected patients have circulating antibodies to the acetylcholine receptors, the problem is not release of acetylcholine itself. (See page 1065: Myasthenia Gravis.)

36. **E.** During VATS, CO_2 may be insufflated into the pleural cavity to help visualization by the surgeon. CPAP may interfere with the surgical procedure and should be used only as a last resort in VATS. The need for one-lung ventilation is greater with VATS than with open thoracotomy because it is not possible to retract the lung during VATS, although it is possible during open thoracotomy. It may take 30 minutes for complete lung collapse; thus the operated lung should be deflated as soon as possible after tracheal intubation and positioning of the double-lumen tube. (See page 1061: Video-assisted Thoracoscopic Surgery.)

37. A. The CVP reflects right-sided heart function, not left ventricular performance. Uses of central venous catheters or large-bore introducers include insertion of a transvenous pacemaker, infusion of vasoactive drugs, and insertion of a pulmonary artery (PA) catheter, which may subsequently be required during surgery or in the postoperative period. A recent study in healthy subjects indicated that, contrary to common belief, the CVP did not consistently reflect intravascular volume status. The CVP catheter may be placed centrally from the external or the internal jugular vein, from the subclavian veins, or from one of the arm veins. The success rate is highest using the right internal jugular vein, and a pacemaker or PA catheter may be inserted most easily from this vein. The major disadvantage of using the external jugular vein during thoracotomy is that the catheter often kinks when the patient is turned to the lateral decubitus position. (See page 1037: Central Venous Pressure Monitoring.)

38. E. Since the left main bronchus is considerably longer than the right bronchus, there is a narrower margin of safety on the right main bronchus with potentially a greater risk of upper lobe obstruction whenever a right-sided DLT is used. Hence, a left-sided DLT is preferred for both right- and left-sided procedures, with the obvious exception of upper bronchial involvement in the surgery (e.g., a bronchial sleeve resection), in which case the contralateral DLT should be placed. In patients in whom the left main bronchus cannot be directly measured, the left bronchial diameter can be accurately estimated by measuring tracheal width. The width of the left bronchus is directly proportional to the width of the trachea. The left bronchial width is estimated by multiplying the tracheal width by 0.68. Typically, most women fit a 37-Fr DLT, and most men can be adequately managed with a 39-Fr DLT. The depth required for insertion of the DLT correlates with the height of the patient. For any adult who is 170 to 180 cm tall, the average depth for a left DLT is 29 cm. For every 10-cm increase or decrease in height, the DLT is advanced or withdrawn approximately 1 cm. (See pages 1042: Methods of Lung Separation and 1042: Double-lumen Endobronchial Tubes.)

39. C. Upon insertion, the DLT may be passed too far down into either the right or the left mainstem bronchus. In this case, breath sounds are very diminished or are not audible over the contralateral side. This situation is corrected when the tube is withdrawn and until the opening of the tracheal lumen is above the carina. A right-sided DLT may occlude the right upper lobe orifice. The mean distance from the carina to the right upper lobe orifice is 2.3 ± 0.7 cm in men and 2.1 ± 0.7 cm in women. Upon insertion, the DLT may not be inserted far enough, leaving the bronchial lumen opening above the carina. In this position, good breath sounds are heard bilaterally when ventilating through the bronchial lumen even after its cuff is inflated, but no breath sounds are audible when ventilating through the tracheal lumen because the inflated bronchial cuff obstructs gas flow arising from the tracheal lumen. The cuff should be deflated and the DLT rotated and advanced into the desired mainstem bronchus. A rare complication with DLTs is tracheal rupture. Overinflation of the bronchial cuff, inappropriate positioning, and trauma owing to intraoperative dislocation that resulted in bronchial rupture have been described in association with the Robertshaw tube and the disposable DLT. (See pages 1042: Methods of Lung Separation and 1042: Double-lumen Endobronchial Tubes.)

40. C. Epidural morphine produces profound analgesia lasting from 16 to 24 hours after thoracotomy and does not cause a sympathetic block or sensory or motor loss. These are significant advantages over systemic opioids or infiltration of local anesthetics. Epidural opioids are most effective at alleviating pain when administered at the thoracic level. Epidural morphine has been shown to decrease pain and improve respiratory function in post-thoracotomy patients. Low-dose ketamine infusion at 0.05 mg/kg/hr was reported to be a useful adjunct to epidural analgesia for post-thoracotomy pain management (1–2 mg/kg/hr would be an exceedingly high dose, which would certainly be of benefit to pain management, but likely with deleterious side effects, and thus is not utilized). Rib blocks provide 6 to 24 hours of moderate pain relief, but patients still complain of diaphragmatic and shoulder discomfort caused by the chest tubes. The incidence of chronic pain after VAT may be comparable with that following thoracotomy. The pain that occurs may be related to trauma to intercostal nerves by insertion of the surgical trocars or by compression during the surgery. (See page 1068: Postoperative Pain Control).

CHAPTER 38

Anesthesia for Cardiac Surgery

1. The area of the myocardium most vulnerable to ischemia is the:

   A. Right ventricle
   B. Apex of the left ventricle
   C. Interventricular septum
   D. Portion of the right atrium containing the sinoatrial node
   E. Subendocardial region of the left ventricle

2. The principal determinants of myocardial oxygen demand are:

   A. Wall tension and contractility
   B. Systemic vascular resistance and heart rate
   C. Mean arterial blood pressure and heart rate
   D. Preload and afterload
   E. Mean arterial blood pressure and systemic vascular resistance

3. Under normal conditions, approximately what is the oxygen saturation of blood entering the coronary sinus?

   A. 10%
   B. 25%
   C. 50%
   D. 75%
   E. 90%

4. Regarding perfusion of the left ventricular subendocardium, which one of the following statements is most accurate?

   A. It occurs mostly during systole.
   B. It occurs mostly during diastole.
   C. It increases with an increase in left ventricular end-diastolic pressure.
   D. It is unaffected by heart rate.
   E. It decreases with an increase in aortic diastolic pressure.

5. The normal area of the aortic valve is:

   A. 0.2 to 0.4 mm^2
   B. 2 to 4 mm^2
   C. 0.2 to 0.4 cm^2
   D. 4 to 8 cm^2
   E. 2 to 4 cm^2

6. Which of the following conditions best describes a physiologic change associated with mitral stenosis?

   A. Left ventricular outflow obstruction
   B. Left ventricular dysfunction resulting from chronic pressure overload
   C. Left ventricular dysfunction resulting from chronic volume overload
   D. Decreased right ventricular pressure
   E. Increased left atrial pressure and concomitant right ventricular hypertrophy

7. An advantage of membrane over bubble oxygenators in cardiopulmonary bypass circuits is:

   A. The uptake of inhaled anesthetics is more predictable with membrane oxygenators.
   B. There is less trauma to blood constituents.
   C. Pulsatile flow is possible with the use of a membrane oxygenator.
   D. Membrane oxygenators offer a cost advantage over bubble oxygenators.
   E. Carbon dioxide exchange is significantly more effective.

8. The most commonly used test to evaluate the adequacy of anticoagulation for cardiopulmonary bypass is:

   A. Heparin concentration assay
   B. Antithrombin III index
   C. Activated partial thromboplastin time (APTT)
   D. Activated clotting time (ACT)
   E. Prothrombin time (PT)

9. Advantages of centrifugal versus roller pump cardiopulmonary bypass (CPB) machines include all of the following EXCEPT:

   A. Less blood trauma
   B. Less risk of air emboli
   C. Elimination of tubing wear and the risk of plastic microemboli
   D. Ability to deliver pulsatile blood flow
   E. Reduction in line pressures

10. For each degree of Celsius decrease in body temperature, metabolic rate is decreased by approximately:

    A. 1%
    B. 2%
    C. 4%
    D. 8%
    E. 10%

11. Nitric oxide dilates pulmonary vascular beds via:

    A. Production of cyclic adenosine monophosphate (cAMP)
    B. Inhibition of cAMP
    C. Production of cyclic guanosine monophosphate (cGMP)
    D. Inhibition of cGMP
    E. None of the above

12. A patient with previously normal left ventricular function is undergoing elective coronary artery bypass grafting. Immediately after separation from cardiopulmonary bypass (CPB), the following measurements are noted: A blood pressure via radial intra-arterial catheter of 78/52 mm Hg, a heart rate of 94 bpm, a pulmonary artery pressure of 28/18 mm Hg, and a cardiac index of 2.7. The most prudent initial intervention would be:

    A. Direct measurement of intra-aortic pressures to verify radial artery correlation
    B. The addition of a phenylephrine infusion to provide α-receptor–mediated vasoconstriction
    C. The addition of an epinephrine infusion to provide both inotropic support and α-receptor–mediated vasoconstriction
    D. An intra-aortic volume infusion using pulmonary capillary wedge pressures as a guide to the adequacy of left ventricular filling
    E. A trial of atrial pacing after placement of epicardial leads

13. The most frequent cause of perioperative neurologic complications after coronary artery bypass grafting is:

    A. Changes in carotid artery flow dynamics during aortic cross clamping
    B. Low-flow states in patients with pre-existing cerebrovascular disease
    C. Emboli
    D. Intraoperative hemodilution
    E. Ischemia to watershed regions of the brain during the rewarming phase of cardiopulmonary bypass

14. Of the following anesthetic techniques for cardiac surgery, the one associated with the best outcome in terms of perioperative morbidity is:

    A. A predominantly opioid-based anesthetic in conjunction with benzodiazepines
    B. A "balanced" anesthetic technique using opioid analgesics combined with potent inhalation agents titrated for varying degrees of stimulation
    C. Continuous high-dose sufentanil infusion
    D. A predominantly potent inhalation agent–based technique with epidural catheter placement for postoperative analgesia
    E. None of the above

15. In the immediate postcardiopulmonary bypass period, milrinone may be particularly useful in the treatment of right ventricular failure secondary to high pulmonary vascular resistance because:

    A. The positive chronotropic effect of milrinone results in improved cardiac output from the noncompliant right ventricle.
    B. Milrinone improves right ventricular contractility while decreasing pulmonary vascular resistance.
    C. Milrinone decreases preload to the right ventricle by decreasing resistance in venous capacitance vessels.
    D. The improvement in left ventricular performance afforded by milrinone in turn decreases right ventricular afterload.
    E. All of the above.

16. The most common cause of persistent bleeding after heparin reversal in cardiac surgical patients is:

    A. Heparin rebound
    B. Hypothermia
    C. Reduced platelet count or function
    D. Diminished capillary integrity
    E. Inactivation of antithrombin III

17. Compared with volatile anesthetics, which of the following statements about propofol is FALSE?

    A. Propofol is associated with more favorable cardiac function.
    B. Propofol is associated with higher need for inotropic support.
    C. Propofol is associated with elevated plasma troponins after cardiac surgery in elderly patients.
    D. Propofol is associated with a predictable and fairly rapid awakening after discontinuation.
    E. Propofol may be continued postoperatively in the intensive care unit (ICU).

18. Which of the following statements regarding magnesium is FALSE?

    A. It has coronary vasodilating properties.
    B. It reduces the size of myocardial infarction in the setting of acute ischemia.
    C. It acts as an antiarrhythmic agent.
    D. It decreases mortality associated with infarction.
    E. It increases myocardial reperfusion injury.

19. Which of the following statements regarding hypertrophic cardiomyopathy (HOCM) is FALSE?

    A. HOCM is a dynamic obstruction.
    B. The obstruction is attenuated by any intervention that reduces ventricular size.
    C. HOCM is a genetically determined disease.
    D. Angina during exercise occurs even in the absence of epicardial coronary artery disease.
    E. Hypotension is managed with volume replacement and vasoconstrictors.

20. What is the average prime volume for a cardiopulmonary bypass machine for adults?

    A. 500 to 1,000 cc
    B. 1,500 to 2,500 cc
    C. 3,000 to 4,000 cc
    D. 4,000 to 4,500 cc
    E. 5,500 to 6,500 cc

21. Which of the following statements regarding heparin is FALSE?

    A. Intravenous heparin's peak onset of action is less than 5 minutes.
    B. Heparin is a polyionic mucopolysaccharide.
    C. Heparin's half-life is approximately 90 minutes after intravenous (IV) injection.
    D. Hypothermia decreases the half-life of heparin.
    E. Heparin's anticoagulant effect is because of its ability to potentiate the antithrombin III activity.

22. The critical factors influencing coronary blood flow include all of the following EXCEPT:

    A. Perfusion pressure
    B. Vascular tone
    C. Perfusion time (heart rate)
    D. Severity/degree of intra-luminal obstructions
    E. Absence of collateral circulation

23. The following hemodynamic goals for patients with coronary artery disease are matched correctly EXCEPT:

    A. Preload—normal to small
    B. Afterload—normal to high
    C. Contractility—normal to high
    D. Rate—normal to slow
    E. Rhythm—sinus

24. With respect to sodium nitroprusside, which of the following is INCORRECT?

    A. It should be shielded from light to prevent deterioration.
    B. Toxicity may result from doses exceeding 8 to 10 μg/kg/min.
    C. Possible methemoglobinemia accumulation leading to toxicity may occur at high infusion rates.
    D. The triad of toxicity included: Elevated mixed venous O_2, increasing dose requirement (tachyphylaxis), and metabolic acidosis.
    E. Treatment of toxicity may include modalities such as: 100% O_2 administration, amyl nitrate inhaler, intravenous sodium nitrite, and intravenous thiosulfate.

25. The following hemodynamic goals for patients with aortic stenosis are matched correctly EXCEPT:

    A. Preload—normal to high
    B. Afterload—normal to high
    C. Contractility—normal to high
    D. Rate—normal to slow
    E. Rhythm—sinus

26. The following hemodynamic goals for patients with hypertrophic cardiomyopathy are matched correctly EXCEPT:

    A. Preload—low to normal
    B. Afterload—normal to high
    C. Contractility—low to normal
    D. Rate—normal
    E. Rhythm—sinus

27. The following hemodynamic goals for patients with aortic insufficiency are matched correctly EXCEPT:

    A. Preload—normal slightly elevated
    B. Afterload—normal to high
    C. Contractility—normal
    D. Rate—normal to high
    E. Rhythm—sinus

28. The following hemodynamic goals for patients with mitral stenosis are matched correctly EXCEPT:

    A. Preload—normal avoid hypovolemia
    B. Afterload—normal avoid pulmonary vasoconstriction
    C. Contractility—normal
    D. Rate—normal
    E. Rhythm—usually not a problem

29. The following hemodynamic goals for patients with mitral regurgitation are matched correctly EXCEPT:

    A. Preload—normal to slightly increased
    B. Afterload—normal to high
    C. Contractility—normal to slightly depressed
    D. Rate—slightly increased
    E. Rhythm—controlled ventricular rate

30. The following hemodynamic goals for patients with acute aortic dissection are matched correctly EXCEPT:

    A. Preload—normal to slightly increased
    B. Afterload—depressed
    C. Contractility—normal to slightly depressed
    D. Rate—normal
    E. Rhythm—controlled ventricular rate

31. In regard to patients with heparin allergies/sensitivity/resistance, which of the following is INCORRECT?

    A. Patients with congenital AT-III deficiency require higher doses of heparin to achieve adequate anticoagulation.
    B. Fresh frozen plasma (FFP) is a means of providing AT-III to deficient patients.
    C. Type-II heparin induced thrombocytopenia is characterized by antibody production.
    D. Type-I heparin induced thrombocytopenia is characterized by a transient decrease in platelet count.
    E. Hirudin and bivalirudin are useful anti-coagulants in patients with AT-III deficiency as they bind to and increase the potency of the native AT-III.

32. Which of the following statements regarding protamine is INCORRECT?

    A. Protamine is a polycationic protein derived from salmon sperm.
    B. True anaphylaxis or anaphylactoid reactions may occur following protamine administration.
    C. Protamine reactions are mediated by thromboxane and C5a anaphylatoxin.
    D. Reaction can be characterized by skin flushing, increased airway pressures, hypotension, and decreased pulmonary vascular resistance.
    E. Patients can become sensitized to protamine, which increases incidence of reactions.

33. The following statements regarding the use of nitroglycerin in the treatment of myocardial ischemia are correct EXCEPT:

    A. Is a coronary arterial vasodilator
    B. Is predominantly a venodilator
    C. May reverse acute coronary vasospasm
    D. Reflex tachycardia may result via baroreceptor mechanisms
    E. Improves venous return

34. Physiologic effects of nitroglycerin include all of the following aside from:

    A. Systemic venodilation
    B. Reflex tachycardia
    C. Coronary artery dilation
    D. Cyanide production
    E. Decreased afterload

35. Pharmacologic agents with coronary artery dilator properties include all of the following EXCEPT:

    A. Nifedipine
    B. Nitroglycerin
    C. Diltiazem
    D. Magnesium
    E. Esmolol

36. The following statements about cardiac tamponade are true EXCEPT:

    A. Clinical signs and symptoms include paradoxical pulse, tachycardia, and hypotension.
    B. Stroke volume decreases.
    C. Cardiac output becomes rate dependent.
    D. Compression of the right atrium is usually the most severe.
    E. A vasodilator should be administered to relieve LV pressure.

37. Which of the following statements regarding the normal function of an intra-aortic balloon pump (IABP) is FALSE?

    A. It is designed to reduce afterload.
    B. It is designed to increase diastolic blood pressure.
    C. A properly inserted IABP should have its distal tip just below the subclavian artery.
    D. The balloon is designed to deflate during diastole.
    E. The balloon should be above the renal arteries.

38. Techniques commonly used for perioperative blood conservation during cardiac surgery include all of the following EXCEPT:

    A. Red blood cell scavenging
    B. Perioperative administration of antifibrinolytic agents
    C. Intraoperative autologous hemodilution
    D. Use of membrane oxygenators
    E. Return of platelets via the blood-salvaging device

39. True statements regarding intraoperative electrocardiographic monitoring include all of the following EXCEPT:

    A. Lead II may be monitored to detect ischemia in the inferior wall of the left ventricle, as well as to assist in the detection of cardiac arrhythmias.
    B. Lead V_5 aids in the detection of ischemia to the posterior wall of the left ventricle.
    C. Lead V_5 is monitored to detect ischemia in regions of the myocardium supplied by the left anterior descending coronary artery.
    D. Ischemia of the lateral wall of the left ventricle is detected by monitoring leads I and aVL.
    E. Lead V_5 aids in the detection of ischemia to the anterior wall of the left ventricle.

40. Relatively strong indications for the perioperative placement of a pulmonary artery catheter in a patient undergoing cardiac surgery include:

    A. Procedures in which continuous retrograde cardioplegia is to be used during cardiopulmonary bypass
    B. Pulmonary hypertension
    C. Access to central circulation for the infusion of vasoactive drugs
    D. Assistance in the management of a patient with normal left ventricular function
    E. Coronary artery bypass grafting

41. Examples of congenital cardiac lesions in which cyanosis develops as a result of obstruction to pulmonary flow include:

    A. Patent ductus arteriosus
    B. Ventricular septal defect
    C. Coarctation of the aorta
    D. Tetralogy of Fallot
    E. Atrial septal defect

42. Which of the following statements regarding amrinone and milrinone is FALSE?

    A. They are phosphodiesterase inhibitors.
    B. They increase myocardial contractility.
    C. They decrease pulmonary vascular resistance.
    D. They increase systemic vascular resistance.
    E. They decrease myocardial contractility.

ANSWERS

1. **E.**   Although zones of ischemic myocardium may result from inadequate coronary blood flow through the vessels supplying each region, the area of myocardium most vulnerable to ischemia is the subendocardial region of the left ventricle. This is not only because of a greater metabolic requirement in the presence of greater systolic shortening, but also because subendocardial blood flow is restricted during systole. (See page 1077: Coronary Blood Flow.)

2. **A.**   Wall tension and contractility are the principal determinants of myocardial oxygen demand. Wall tension, in turn, is directly proportional to intracavitary pressure and ventricular radius and is inversely proportional to the thickness of the ventricular wall. Wall Stress = Pressure × Radius/2 × Wall thickness, and is based on preload and afterload. Other key determinants of myocardial oxygen demand are heart rate and contractility. Myocardial oxygen demand may be reduced by interventions that prevent or treat ventricular distention and reduce contractility. (See page 1077: Coronary Artery Disease: Myocardial Oxygen Demand.)

3. **C.**   Oxygen extraction in the coronary circulation is extremely efficient; blood entering the coronary sinus is typically about 50% saturated. Although extraction may be increased somewhat in response to stress, the principal mechanism by which oxygen supply is increased in response to increased oxygen demand is through an increase in coronary blood flow. (See page 1077: Coronary Artery Disease: Myocardial Oxygen Supply.)

4. **B.**   The left ventricular subendocardium is one of the areas of the heart that is most vulnerable to ischemia because of its high metabolic requirements. Perfusion of the subendocardial tissue of the left ventricle takes place mostly during diastole; this is in contrast to perfusion of the right ventricle, which occurs principally during systole. Perfusion pressure is defined as the difference between aortic diastolic pressure and left ventricular end-diastolic pressure. Whereas an increase in aortic diastolic pressure increases perfusion, an increase in left ventricular end-diastolic pressure decreases perfusion. Insofar as changes in heart rate affect diastolic time, changes in heart rate do cause changes in perfusion. (See page 1077: Coronary Artery Disease: Coronary Blood Flow.)

5. **E.**   The normal aortic valve diameter is 1.9 to 2.3 cm, and the normal aortic valve area is 2 to 4 cm². Aortic stenosis is classified based on the degree of narrowing of the aortic valve area. Aortic stenosis is considered critical when the area of the aortic valve is below 0.8 cm². Patients with this degree of aortic stenosis are almost always symptomatic, and surgical correction is indicated. Classic symptoms include, dyspnea (50%), angina (35%), and syncope (15%) resulting in predicted mortality of 2, 5, and 3 years respectively if not corrected. Clinical risk factors associated with the development of aortic stenosis include: Older age, male gender, smoking, hypertension, and hyperlipidemia. Patients with mechanical stresses from a bicuspid valve, those with mineral metabolism abnormalities such as Paget disease or renal failure, and patients with autoimmune factors such as in rheumatic heart disease are also at increased risk. (See page 1081: Valvular Heart Disease: Aortic Stenosis.)

6. **E.**   In mitral stenosis, left atrial pressure elevation is a consequence of a narrowed mitral orifice. This increased pressure is transmitted back through the pulmonary circulation, leading to right ventricular hypertrophy. Conversely, the left ventricle is not subject to pressure or volume overload, and normal function is generally preserved. (See page 1086: Mitral Stenosis.)

7. **B.**   Oxygenators serve two main purposes: Oxygenate venous blood and remove carbon dioxide. The two types of oxygenators are bubble and membrane. Bubble oxygenators are efficient and work on the principle of direct gas–blood contact. A large interface surface is created with bubble production allowing the more insoluble oxygen to diffuse on the bubbles' surfaces. The gas–blood interface has destructive forces and is responsible for hemolysis, platelet destruction, and microemboli with CPB time exceeding 90 minutes. Membrane oxygenators eliminate the large gas–blood interface by allowing blood to pass through microporous membranes. In these membranes blood comes in close contact with gas molecules allowing diffusion of oxygen and carbon dioxide and avoiding the degree of hemolysis, platelet destruction, and microemboli posed by bubble oxygenators. (See page 1090: Cardiopulmonary Bypass: Oxygenators.)

8. **D.**   The ACT indicates the time required for thrombus formation after a sample of whole blood is mixed with a clotting accelerator. A value of more than 400 seconds is generally believed to reflect a degree of anticoagulation that is adequate for cardiopulmonary bypass. (See page 1090: Cardiopulmonary Bypass: Anticoagulation.)

9. **D.**   Centrifugal CPB machines operate by a magnetically controlled impeller and an electric motor and are rapidly replacing the older roller pump systems. Advantages of the centrifugal system include less trauma to blood entering the system, lower line pressures, reduced risk of air emboli, and elimination of tubing wear and plastic emboli resulting from tubing compression (spallation). Neither roller pumps nor centrifugal pumps may deliver physiologically significant pulsatile blood flow. (See page 1090: Cardiopulmonary Bypass: Pumps.)

10. **D.**   For each degree of Celsius decrease in body temperature, there is a reduction of 8% in the metabolic rate. (See page 1090: Cardiopulmonary Bypass: Heat Exchanger.)

11. C. Nitric oxide exerts most of its effects by stimulating the guanylyl cyclase enzyme, leading to increased production of cGMP. In turn, cGMP stimulates phosphodiesterases, which relax vascular smooth muscles, promoting vasodilation. (See page 1090: Cardiopulmonary Bypass.)

12. A. Although frequently accurate, radial artery pressure may be as much as 30 mm Hg lower than central aortic pressure after CPB. Peripheral vasodilation during rewarming is thought to be the cause of the discrepancy, which may be readily detected by direct transduction of intra-aortic pressure via the operative field. This aortic–radial pressure gradient usually dissipates within 45 minutes of separation from bypass. (See page 1094: Arterial Blood Pressure.)

13. C. Although the incidence of stroke after coronary artery bypass grafting is approximately 3%, the incidence of subtle cognitive deficits elicited by postoperative neuropsychiatric testing is much higher (60%–70%). The origin of perioperative neurologic insults is believed to be primarily embolic. Macroemboli, such as atheroma and particulate matter, account for most overt perioperative strokes. Microemboli (air, platelet aggregates) are likely responsible for the subtle cognitive changes seen after coronary artery bypass grafting. Most neuropsychiatric deficits improve over the initial 2 to 6 months after cardiac surgery, although significant numbers of patients (13%–39%) exhibit residual impairment. Risk factors for neurologic complications include: Advanced age (>70), preexisting cerebrovascular disease (carotid stenosis > 80%), history of prior stroke, peripheral vascular disease, ascending aorta atheroma, and diabetes. Operative risk factors include: Duration of CPB, intra-cardiac procedures, excessive warming during or post CPB, and possibly perfusion pressure during CPB. (See page 1095: Central Nervous System Function and Complications.)

14. E. Two large outcome studies by Tuman et al. and Slogoff and Keats reinforced the premise that the choice of anesthetic per se has no effect on outcome in patients undergoing cardiac surgery. More important is the ability of the anesthesiologist to preserve compensatory cardiovascular mechanisms while preventing perioperative episodes of myocardial ischemia. Since no data exist to document the superiority of any one anesthetic technique for cardiac surgery, it becomes apparent that the proper management of the anesthetic is more important than the technique used. (See page 1095: Selection of Anesthetic Drugs.)

15. B. A phosphodiesterase III inhibitor, milrinone, acts via a non–β-receptor pathway to effect a decrease in pulmonary vascular resistance while improving left and right heart contractility. Such interventions are the treatments of choice in conditions of right ventricular failure secondary to high pulmonary vascular resistance; overdistention of the ventricle is carefully avoided. (See page 1099: Discontinuation of Cardiopulmonary Bypass.)

16. C. The usual causes of persistent oozing after heparin neutralization include inadequate surgical hemostasis and reduced platelet count or function, although insufficient doses of protamine, dilution of clotting factors, and (rarely) "heparin rebound" may be contributing factors. Thrombocytopenia and diminished platelet function are frequent consequences of extracorporeal circulation, resulting from platelet activation and destruction when in contact with the bypass circuit. (See page 1104: Postbypass Bleeding.)

17. A. Compared with volatile anesthetics, propofol is associated with less favorable cardiac function, a higher need for inotropic support, and elevated plasma troponins after cardiac surgery in elderly patients. It may be continued postoperatively in the ICU, and it affords a predictable and fairly rapid awakening after discontinuation. (See page 1080: Intravenous Sedatives and Hypnotics.)

18. E. Magnesium has use in the treatment of myocardial ischemia. It has coronary artery vasodilating properties, reduces the size of myocardial infarction in the setting of acute ischemia, and decreases mortality associated with infarction. In addition, it is an antiarrhythmic agent, and it minimizes myocardial reperfusion injury. (See page 1080: Treatment of Ischemia.)

19. B. Hypertrophic cardiomyopathy is a genetically determined disease. In patients with HOCM, systolic septal bulging into the left ventricular outflow tract (LVOT), malposition of the anterior papillary muscle, drag forces, and a hyperdynamic ventricular contraction may contribute to creation of a LVOT gradient. This type of obstruction is dynamic and is accentuated by any intervention that reduces ventricular size. Therefore, increases in contractility and heart rate or decreases in either preload or afterload are harmful because they facilitate septal–leaflet contact. In patients with HOCM, myocardial oxygen balance is tenuous, and angina during exercise occurs even in the absence of epicardial coronary artery disease when the coronary microcirculation is unable to supply the hypertrophied myocardium. In patients with HOCM, angina results from the elevated left ventricular systolic pressure. Pharmacologic management of hypotension in patients with HOCM should be done with volume replacement and vasoconstrictors rather than inotropes and vasodilators. (See page 1083: Hypertrophic Cardiomyopathy.)

20. B. Many institutions use a standard volume prime for all adult patients, and others use a minimum volume based on body weight or body surface area. The average prime volume is 1,500 to 2,500 cc. The blood is generally replaced by crystalloids with the addition of albumin (to decrease postoperative edema), mannitol (to promote diuresis), electrolytes (calcium to counteract citrated transfused blood), corticosteroids (for anti-inflammatory effects), and heparin (to ensure proper anti-coagulation) when needed. The addition of crystalloid provides a dilutional anemia that is useful in offsetting increased blood viscosity due to hypothermia. (See page 1090: Cardiopulmonary Bypass: Prime.)

21. D. Heparin is a polyionic mucopolysaccharide extracted from either bovine lung or porcine intestinal mucosa. After IV injection, the peak onset of heparin is less than 5 minutes with a half-life of approximately 90 minutes in normothermic patients. In hypothermic patients, there is a progressive increase in the half-life proportional to the degree of hypothermia. The anticoagulant effect of heparin is derived from its ability to potentiate the activity of anti-thrombin III (AT-III), altering its structural configuration and increasing its AT-III-thrombin inhibitory potency by more 1,000 times. By inhibiting thrombin, AT-III prevents fibrin clot formation via both the intrinsic and extrinsic pathways in addition to inhibiting factors IX, Xa, XIa, XIIa, kallikrein, and plasmin. (See page 1090: Cardiopulmonary Bypass: Anticoagulation.)

22. E. In patients with diseased native coronary vessels, the development of collateral vessels maintains supply to the distal muscle. Perfusion pressure is defined as the difference between aortic diastolic pressure and left ventricular end diastolic pressure (AoDP – LVEDP). The presence of significant intra-luminal obstruction or increase in coronary vascular tone results in a decrease in perfusion pressure and thus a drop in coronary blood flow. Normal coronary vasculature may dilate, thereby increasing flow to 3 to 5 times that of baseline. As coronary stenosis progresses, the vasculature reaches a critical point in which no further dilatation can occur, supply to demand is not matched, and ischemia results. Due to the relatively high left ventricular intra-luminal pressure, the LV subendocardium is perfused almost entirely in diastole. Increase in heart rate result in less LV perfusion time. Tachycardia has therefore been shown to be the most important trigger of intraoperative and perioperative ischemia. (See page 1077: Coronary Artery Disease: Coronary blood flow.)

23. C. The goal in preventing ischemia is to match coronary blood supply and demand. In patients with coronary artery disease, the goals are as follows. Preload should be low to normal to minimize wall tension and LVEDP. Afterload should be maintained with hypertension better than hypotension. Contractility and heart rate should be normal to low, decreasing myocardial oxygen demand. (See Table 38-1: Coronary Artery Disease—Hemodynamic Goals.)

24. C. Sodium nitroprusside decreases peripheral vascular resistance by metabolic or spontaneous reduction to nitric oxide and improves ventricular compliance in the ischemic myocardium. The dose ranges from 0.5 to 3 μg/kg/min. At doses exceeding 8 to 10 μg/kg/min, toxicity due to cyanide and thiocyanate may develop. Adverse effects of SNP include rebound hypertension, intracranial hypertension, blood coagulation abnormalities, increased pulmonary shunting, and hypothyroidism. The triad of tachyphylaxis, metabolic acidosis, and increase mixed venous O$_2$ indicates toxicity. Patients may also appear flushed. Treatment of toxicity includes modalities such as: 100% O$_2$ administration, amyl nitrate inhaler, intravenous sodium nitrite, and intravenous thiosulfate. The SNP solution must be shielded from light and should not be infused with other drugs. Toxicity from nitroglycerin, not SNP,

involves methemoglobinemia production. (See page 1080: Treatment of Ischemia.)

25. D. The goal in aortic stenosis is to balance cardiac perfusion with cardiac activity. In the hypertrophied and thick ventricle, diastolic filling will be lessened. Heart rate control in AS patients is critical. Significant tachycardia results in less diastolic filling and cardiac ischemia. The left ventricle with its narrow valve has a low and relatively fixed stroke volume such that the cardiac output is determined by heart rate. Bradycardia will lead to a decreased cardiac output and low systemic blood pressure. Afterload should be relatively maintained to enable adequate coronary perfusion pressure. Aortic stenosis patients often rely on their atrial kick to account for 30% to 40% of LVEDV and this maintenance of sinus rhythm becomes crucial. (See Table 38-3: Aortic Stenosis—Hemodynamic Goals.)

26. A. The goal in patients with hypertrophic cardiomyopathy is to maintain forward flow. In the hypertrophied and thick ventricle, preload is crucial as is sinus rhythm for adequate cardiac output. Aggressive fluid resuscitation should be maintained and every attempt to ensure sinus rhythm as these patients often rely of the atrial kick. Transcutaneous pacing or pacing via a pulmonary artery catheter should be considered. Heart rate control in hypertrophic cardiomyopathy should be normal. Contractility is these patients should be kept low and may be accomplished using volatile anesthetics. (See Table 38-4: Hypertrophic Cardiomyopathy—Hemodynamic Goals.)

27. B. The goal in patients with aortic insufficiency is to avoid increased LV wall stress. The ventricle has undergone eccentric hypertrophy, constantly struggling to pump the additional regurgitant volume. The ventricle may benefit from afterload reduction, promoting forward flow; however, this may require augmenting preload. The most appropriate rate is controversial. Tachycardia will prevent diastolic runoff time and reduce ventricular wall distension, but also will increase the myocardial oxygen demand. Bradycardia should be avoided as it results in ventricular distension, elevations in left atrial pressures, and pulmonary congestion. Contractility and rhythm are not usually a problem. (See Table 38-5: Aortic Insufficiency—Hemodynamic Goals.)

28. E. In patients with mitral stenosis, increased cardiac output or decreased diastolic filling time results in significant increases in left atrial pressures. This explains why pregnancy, thyrotoxicosis, infection, and atrial fibrillation may lead to decompensated pulmonary edema in patients with MS. The atrial kick is not the concerning feature as in AS but rather it is the extremely fast rate at which the atria contract that lead to a decompensation in MS patients. Therefore, in patients with MS, ventricular rate should be controlled and tachycardia avoided. Preload should be maintained with careful titration of vasoconstrictors as needed. Afterload should be maintained with avoidance of hypoxia, hypercarbia, and acidosis as they increase pulmonary vascular resistance and may precipitate right heart failure. Contractility is usually intact, however, the right ventricle is of concern especially if significant pulmonary hypertension is present. This may present a problem when separating from cardio-pulmonary bypass. (See Table 38-6: Mitral Stenosis—Hemodynamic Goals.)

29. B. In patients with mitral regurgitation, the left atrium receives a larger volume of blood during the cardiac cycle. In turn, the LV received a larger preload causing both left-sided chambers to dilate. The regurgitant volume is related to the orifice size, therefore, increase in heart rate and decrease in preload reduce the LV size and lessen the regurgitant volume. Vasodilation decreases afterload and thereby reduces the LV to LA systolic gradient, promoting forward flow. Following valve replacement, the newly competent valve increases afterload, which may present a problem following cardio-pulmonary bypass and necessitate inotropic support. Mitral regurgitation results from mechanical issues such as: Leaf prolapse, restrictive leaf motion (rheumatic disease), and leaf perforation (endocarditis). Mitral regurgitation may occur following LV structural or functional changes (ischemic MR). (See Table 38-8: Mitral Regurgitation—Hemodynamic Goals.)

30. D. In patients with acute aortic dissection, the goal is emergent surgical resection with adequate intravenous access, invasive hemodynamic monitoring, and slow and careful titration of drugs. Preload should be adequate or increased in cases of acute aortic insufficiency or tamponade. Afterload should be decreased with careful titration using combinations of drugs to a blood pressure of <120/60. Contractility should be depressed. The heart rate should be brought to <60 bpm; myocardial oxygen consumption may be an issue if the dissection extends to involve the coronary vessels. Cardio-pulmonary bypass may require alternate site cannulation and deep hypothermic circulatory arrest if cerebral vessels are involved. (See Table 38-9: Acute Aortic Dissection—Hemodynamic Goals.)

31. E. Both patients receiving pre-operative heparin and those with congenital AT-III deficiencies may require a higher dose of heparin to achieve acceptable anti-coagulation for CPB. Heparin resistance is defined by activated clotting time (ACT) <380 seconds after 400 U/kg of intravenous heparin. Exogenous AT-III can be administered by transfusing FFP or by a commercial human AT-III concentrate (Thrombate III). Heparin allergies are classified as Type-I and Type-II heparin induced thrombocytopenia (HIT). Type-I HIT, is a generally mild decrease in platelet count. Type-II HIT is an autoimmune-mediated formation of antigenic heparin compounds which causes platelet clumping and microvascular thrombosis. Heparin alternatives such as hirudin and bivalirudin should be used in these patients. Hirudin and bivalirudin are direct thrombin inhibitors. Their action is independent of AT-III. (See page 1090: Cardiopulmonary Bypass: Anticoagulation.)

32. D. Protamine is a polycationic protein derived from salmon sperm and neutralizes heparin. Idiosyncratic reactions may be true anaphylaxis or anaphylactoid and characterized by increased airway pressures, decreased systemic vascular resistance and hypotension, increased pulmonary vascular resistance, and skin flushing. Patients may become sensitized to protamine after exposure in cardiac catheterization, hemodialysis, cardiac surgery, exposure to neutral protamine Hagedorn insulin. Reactions are mediated by thromboxane and C5a anaphylatoxin. Protamine should be infused slowly preferable into a peripheral venous site. (See page 1104: Reversal of Anticoagulation.)

33. E. Nitroglycerin is a modest coronary arterial dilator and as such is the drug of choice for the acute treatment of coronary artery vasospasm. The reduction in venous return afforded by the venodilatory effect of nitroglycerin leads to a lessening in myocardial wall tension and thus to a reduction in myocardial oxygen demand. The use of nitroglycerin may result in reflex tachycardia caused by a sudden decrease in venous return. (See page 1080: Nitrates.)

34. D. Nitroglycerin is a systemic venodilator. In addition, at higher doses, nitroglycerin dilates systemic arterial beds. Therefore, it both reduces preload (by decreasing venous return) and reduces afterload (by decreasing systemic arterial pressure). Nitroglycerin is the drug of choice in the treatment of patients with coronary vasospasm because it is also an effective dilator of the coronary arterial bed, including stenosed arteries and collateral beds. However, nitroglycerin may also cause methemoglobinemia, especially in patients with deficiencies of methemoglobin reductase. Sodium nitroprusside, not nitroglycerin, may produce cyanide and thiocyanate upon metabolism, posing the risk of toxicity during prolonged infusions or after administration of relatively large quantities over short time periods. (See page 1077: Coronary Artery Disease: Treatment of Ischemia.)

35. E. Nifedipine and diltiazem are calcium channel blockers that dilate coronary arteries and are used as antianginal agents in the prevention of coronary vasospasm. Nitroglycerin also has coronary artery dilating properties associated with the production of nitric oxide. Magnesium is another coronary artery vasodilator that has been used to reduce infarct size and minimize reperfusion injury in the setting of acute ischemia. Esmolol is an ultra-short acting β1-selective blocker, with a half-life of 9.5 minutes. Its usefulness stems from its ability to transiently decrease heart rate and this myocardial oxygen demand. No specific direct coronary effects are noted. (See page 1077: Coronary Artery Disease: Treatment of Ischemia.)

36. E. Cardiac tamponade involves an elevation in intrapericardial pressure, which impairs venous return and may cause cardiac chamber collapse. Under this circumstance, the chambers with the lowest intracardiac pressures (atria and right ventricle during diastole) are most at risk of collapse, especially during diastole. Stroke volume in cardiac tamponade is relatively fixed, so cardiac output becomes dependent on heart rate. Prompt surgical intervention is vital. Drugs with arteriolar or venous dilatory effects and those causing myocardial depression should be avoided in patients with hemodynamic compromise. (See page 1106: Postoperative Considerations, Tamponade.)

37. D.   The IABP uses a synchronized counterpulsation method to improve myocardial function by decreasing myocardial oxygen demand and increasing myocardial oxygen supply. The device is most commonly inserted into the femoral artery and advanced so the distal tip lies just below the subclavian artery and the proximal end is above the renal arteries. The balloon inflates during diastole, increasing aortic diastolic pressure and improving coronary perfusion as well as facilitating forward flow. During the subsequent systole, the balloon deflates, reducing systemic afterload and facilitating left ventricular ejection. (See page 1093: Preoperative and Intraoperative Management: Intra-aortic Balloon Pump.)

38. E.   Antifibrinolytic agents such as tranexamic acid, epsilon-aminocaproic acid, and aprotinin have been shown to decrease blood loss in high-risk patients undergoing cardiac surgery. Such agents act to inhibit the fibrinolytic cascade triggered by the effects of extracorporeal circulation. Intraoperative hemodilution achieved by the removal of autologous blood provides a safe source of whole blood for reinfusion while being spared the damaging effects of the bypass circuit. The returned blood has a hematocrit of approximately 70%; however, platelets and coagulation factors are washed out. After re-infusion of conserved blood dilutional effects may further decrease platelet and coagulation factor count. (See page 1092: Blood Conservation in Cardiac Surgery.)

39. B.   Simultaneous monitoring of multiple electrocardiographic leads improves the sensitivity of ischemia detection while aiding in its localization. Leads II, III, and aVF are the most sensitive to ischemic changes in the inferior ventricular wall, typically supplied by the right coronary artery. Lead V$_5$ is commonly used to monitor the anterior wall of the left ventricle (left anterior descending artery), and leads I and aVL provide the greatest information concerning the lateral left ventricular wall (left circumflex artery). (See page 1108: Monitoring.)

40. B.   Although indications for the placement of a pulmonary catheter vary among institutions, conditions in which left ventricular filling pressures cannot be reliably predicted by transduced right atrial pressures generally predicate pulmonary artery catheter placement. These conditions include pulmonary hypertension, left ventricular dysfunction or decreased compliance, and valvular dysfunction. Other indications include operations requiring prolonged operative time or combined procedures (valve replacement plus coronary grafting). (See page 1108: Monitoring.)

41. D.   In patients with tetralogy of Fallot, the right ventricular outflow obstruction may lead to cyanosis as a result of decreased pulmonary flow. The presence of a ventricular septal defect complicates the problem by providing a path of preferential flow in the setting of decreased systemic vascular resistance. Whereas ventricular septal defects and patent ductus arteriosus result in increased pulmonary blood flow from volume overload, coarctation of the aorta results in left ventricular pressure overload. (See page 1107: Table 38-21.)

42. E.   Amrinone and milrinone are two drugs in a class of phosphodiesterase III inhibitors. These agents are very effective at decreasing pulmonary vascular resistance and increasing myocardial contractility. They are also systematic arterial vasodilators and therefore reduce left ventricular afterload, reducing myocardial work. (See page 1106: Preoperative Evaluation: Discontinuation of Cardiopulmonary Bypass.)

CHAPTER 39

Anesthesia for Vascular Surgery

1. The most effective medical therapy for atherosclerotic peripheral vascular disease is:

   A. Dipyridamole
   B. Urokinase
   C. Warfarin (Coumadin)
   D. Aspirin
   E. Smoking cessation

2. In patients presenting for vascular surgery, the incidence of significant coronary artery disease (stenosis > 70%) detected by angiography in patients without any clinical symptoms of coronary stenosis is approximately:

   A. <1%
   B. 11%
   C. 37%
   D. 78%
   E. >90%

3. Most neurologic deficits after carotid endarterectomy are thought to result from:

   A. Concomitant contralateral carotid stenosis
   B. Prolonged carotid artery cross-clamp in the absence of shunt use
   C. Thromboembolism
   D. Perioperative vasospasm
   E. Inadequate intraoperative carotid artery perfusion pressure

4. Each of the following is a potential postoperative complication specific to carotid endarterectomy EXCEPT:

   A. Hypertension
   B. Bradycardia
   C. Neurologic deficits
   D. Respiratory insufficiency
   E. Renal insufficiency

5. Distal ischemia as a consequence of aortic surgery generally results from:

   A. Prolonged aortic occlusion
   B. Inadequate distal runoff
   C. Thrombosis resulting from inadequate anticoagulation
   D. Postperfusion vasospasm
   E. Atheroemboli

6. The most important factor shown to be of clinical importance in preserving renal function during aortic cross-clamping is:

   A. Lisinopril
   B. Fenoldopam
   C. Dopamine
   D. Intravascular volume status
   E. Mannitol

7. Strategies that have been shown to reduce the incidence of myocardial ischemia in patients undergoing vascular surgery include all of the following EXCEPT:

   A. Treatment of tachycardia with β-adrenergic blocking agents
   B. Prevention of hypothermia
   C. Correction of anemia
   D. Prophylactic infusions of nitroglycerin
   E. Continuation of Statin therapy

8. Which of the following statements regarding carotid artery occlusive disease is TRUE?

   A. It is rarely bilateral.
   B. Plaques most often develop proximal to the carotid bifurcation.
   C. Patients who present with transient ischemic attacks have a 40% risk of stroke during the subsequent year.
   D. The most common cause is atherosclerosis.
   E. Stroke in these patients is usually due to carotid artery obstruction.

9. All of the following are methods that have been used to determine the need for shunt placement during carotid endarterectomy EXCEPT:

   A. Intraoperative electroencephalography evaluation
   B. Measurement of cerebral spinal fluid pressure via a lumbar drain
   C. Transcranial Doppler techniques
   D. Somatosensory evoked potential (SSEP) monitoring
   E. Xenon-gated measurements of cerebral blood flow

10. Factors that may contribute to systemic hypotension or organ dysfunction after aortic occlusion and subsequent reperfusion include all of the following EXCEPT:

    A. Metabolic acidosis
    B. Activated complement
    C. Oxygen-derived free radicals
    D. Endotoxemia
    E. More distal cross-clamp position

11. Which of the following statements regarding the artery of Adamkiewicz is TRUE?

    A. It is responsible for more than 85% of the spinal cord blood supply.
    B. It originates between L3 and S1 in 10% of patients.
    C. It is the sole source of arterial flow to the posterior portions of the spinal cord.
    D. It originates between T8 and T12 in 75% of patients.
    E. The posterior spinal arteries account for 50% of the spinal blood flow.

12. Which of the following measures have demonstrated definitive utility in the prevention of spinal cord ischemia associated with aortic occlusion during vascular procedures?

    A. Early use of sodium bicarbonate
    B. Maintenance of normal cardiac function
    C. Cerebrospinal fluid (CSF) drainage
    D. Low threshold for transfusion to maintain a hematocrit >35%
    E. Prophylactic mannitol infusion

13. In comparing surgical approaches for either occlusive or aneurysmal abdominal aortic disease, differences in outcome of a retroperitoneal over a traditional transabdominal approach include:

    A. Lower incidence of ileus and small bowel obstruction
    B. Fewer postoperative pulmonary complications
    C. Longer intensive care unit (ICU) stays
    D. Decreased long-term incisional pain
    E. Increased fluid shifts

14. Which of the following statements with respect to surgical techniques used during occlusion of the thoracic aorta to decompress the heart and allow some degree of distal perfusion is FALSE?

    A. One can decompress the heart and allow some degree of distal perfusion by placement of an aortic shunt.
    B. One can decompress the heart and allow some degree of distal perfusion by use of partial bypass.

    C. One can decompress the heart and allow some degree of distal perfusion by placement of an ex vivo axillo-femoral bypass graft.
    D. One can decompress the heart and allow some degree of distal perfusion by segmental surgical repair.
    E. Distal perfusion in the context of thoracic aortic occlusion reduces reperfusion acidosis.

15. Which of the following statements regarding renal function after aortic reconstruction procedures is TRUE?

    A. Procedures involving infrarenal aortic occlusion do not adversely affect renal function.
    B. Dopamine has been shown to be highly effective in preventing renal failure.
    C. Intraoperative urine output is a reasonable predictor of postoperative renal function.
    D. The best measures to prevent perioperative renal compromise are maintenance of adequate intravascular volume and of myocardial function.
    E. Patients with preoperative impaired renal function are at no increased risk for postoperative renal failure.

16. Potential advantages of a regional anesthetic technique over general anesthesia for lower extremity vascular bypass procedures include all of the following EXCEPT:

    A. Avoidance of hyperdynamic responses to tracheal intubation and extubation
    B. Reduced postoperative hypercoagulability
    C. Reduced incidence of postoperative respiratory complications
    D. A reduction in perioperative cardiac complications
    E. Reduced postoperative graft failure

17. During endovascular repair of an aortic aneurysm, all of the following are potential incidents or complications related to the intervention EXCEPT:

    A. Potential renal impairment secondary to intravenous dye
    B. Aneurysm rupture
    C. Graft migration
    D. Pneumothorax
    E. Retroperitoneal hematoma

ANSWERS

1. **E.** Although antiplatelet medications such as aspirin may slow the progression of atherosclerosis and may be associated with decreased cardiovascular events, cessation of smoking is by far the most effective form of medical therapy. This emphasizes the dramatic impact of tobacco abuse on the progression of atherosclerotic disease. Smoking cessation rates are approximately 25% after major surgery. Despite the low success rates, the benefits of smoking cessation are so great that such programs may be cost effective. Systemic anticoagulation and thrombolytic agents are generally reserved for cases of acute ischemia. (See page 1114: Medical Therapy for Atherosclerosis.)

2. **C.** Hertzer et al. performed coronary angiography in 1,000 consecutive patients slated to undergo vascular surgery and identified significant coronary artery stenosis (>70% occlusion) in 37% of patients who had no symptoms of coronary disease. These data indicate a high index of suspicion for coronary artery stenosis in patients presenting for vascular surgery even in the absence of a prior history of cardiac disease. (See page 1114: Coronary Artery Disease in Patients with Peripheral Vascular Disease.)

3. **C.** Although maintenance of adequate carotid artery perfusion pressure is an anesthetic goal during carotid endarterectomy, most studies indicate that as many as 65% to 95% of all neurologic deficits after carotid endarterectomy may result from thromboembolic events. These may occur during surgical manipulation of the diseased vessel or in association with shunt placement. An embolism-related stroke rate of at least 0.7% has been reported in association with shunt placement; no convincing data exist to indicate that routine shunt insertion reduces the incidence of postoperative neurologic deficits. (See page 1124: Monitoring and Preserving Neurologic Integrity.)

4. **E.** Common problems arising after carotid endarterectomy include the onset of new neurologic dysfunction, hemodynamic instability during emergence from general anesthesia, and respiratory insufficiency. Blood pressure abnormalities are common after carotid endarterectomy; hypertension is more common than hypotension. Severe hypertension seems to occur more often in patients with poorly controlled preoperative hypertension. (See page 1123: Carotid Endarterectomy.)

5. **E.** Although heparin is routinely administered before aortic occlusion to reduce the risk of thrombus formation, it is recognized that distal ischemic events after aortic surgery are generally the result of dislodgment of atheroemboli from the diseased aorta. It is believed by some that in the absence of major distal occlusive disease, systemic heparinization may be unnecessary when repairing abdominal aortic aneurysms. (See page 1128: Aortic Reconstruction.)

6. **D.** Renal protection is still a controversial topic, with no therapies proven to yield superior outcome. Many different methods of renal protection have been advocated, most of them centering on improving renal blood flow or glomerular flow. These include dopamine, fenoldopam, angiotensin-converting enzyme inhibitors, prostaglandins, vasodilators, isovolemic hemodilution, furosemide, and mannitol. Outcomes have not been shown to improve with any of these techniques. One of the most important factors for preventing postoperative renal failure remains good hydration (as the most important factor for maintaining renal blood flow) during clamping and postclamp release. (See page 1130: Monitoring and Vascular Access.)

7. **D.** In high-risk patients undergoing noncardiac surgery, there is an increased incidence of myocardial ischemia associated with anemia (hematocrit level of <28) and hypothermia (presumably resulting from increased oxygen consumption accompanying postoperative shivering). Statin therapy has been shown to decrease perioperative cardiac complications in vascular surgery patients when they are started at least 30 days preoperatively. Discontinuing statin therapy, pre- or postoperatively, increases the risk of cardiac complications. Although the perioperative treatment of tachycardia with β-adrenergic blocking agents has proven efficacious in the prevention of myocardial ischemia, the use of prophylactic infusions of intravenous nitroglycerin has not been shown to reduce the incidence of ischemic episodes in patients with known or suspected coronary artery disease who are undergoing noncardiac surgery. (See page 1118: Prevention of Myocardial Injury.)

8. **D.** The most common cause of carotid occlusive disease is atherosclerotic plaque, which usually develops at the lateral aspect of the carotid bifurcation. It is bilateral in approximately 50% of cases. The natural history of patients who present with transient ischemic attacks resulting from carotid occlusive disease is an approximate 10% risk of stroke during the ensuing year. Only 30% of strokes in patients with carotid disease are due to occlusion, the majority of strokes are embolic. (See page 1123: Carotid Endarterectomy.)

9. **B.** Surgeons who perform shunt procedures selectively use a monitor of cerebral perfusion to identify appropriate subjects for shunt insertion. Methods used include carotid SSEP monitoring, intraoperative electroencephalography, and direct monitoring of cerebral blood flow (e.g., xenon-gated flow measurements). However, none of these techniques has been shown to significantly improve neurologic outcomes in patients undergoing carotid vascular surgery. Measurement of cerebral spinal fluid pressure has no role in determining the need for shunt placement. (See page 1124: Monitoring and Preserving Neurologic Integrity.)

10. **E.** Hypoxia to tissues distal to aortic occlusion leads to anaerobic metabolism and resultant acidosis. In addition,

oxygen-derived free radicals, prostaglandins, cytokines, and other vasoactive mediators are produced, and this may result in hypotension and organ dysfunction when reperfusion occurs. Among the many factors described are renin, angiotensin, epinephrine, norepinephrine, prostacyclin, endothelin, prostaglandin F_1, thromboxane A_2 and B_2, lactate, potassium, oxygen-derived free radicals, platelet activators, cytokines, and activated complements (C3 and C4). Reactive hyperemia after reperfusion of ischemic vascular beds contributes to systemic hypotension resulting from a redistribution of blood flow. Hypoxic insult to the intestines during aortic occlusion and the associated increase in gut permeability may produce endotoxemia. An aneurysm occurring lower on the aorta allows for positioning of the aortic cross-clamp more distally. More distal aortic occlusion allows for continued perfusion of mesenteric and renal arteries. Reducing the size of the area of reperfusion reduces the magnitude of the above mediators of hypotension. (See page 1133: Aortic Cross-clamping and Unclamping.)

11. D. The blood supply to the thoracolumbar spinal cord (from T8 to the conus terminalis) is derived in large part by the major radicular artery known as the artery of Adamkiewicz. It arises from the left side in 60% of cases. In 75% of patients, it joins the anterior spinal artery between T8 and T12; it arises between L1 and L2 in 10% of patients. Although much of the blood flow in the anterior spinal artery is dependent on the artery of Adamkiewicz, the posterior portions of the spinal cord are supplied by the paired posterior spinal arteries, derived in part from the vertebral system; these arteries account for approximately 25% of spinal cord blood flow. (See page 1122: Prevention of Perioperative Spinal Cord Ischemia.)

12. B. Spinal cord ischemia with resultant paraplegia is a devastating complication of aortic occlusion and occurs in 1% to 11% of procedures involving the distal descending thoracic aorta. Although attempts to improve spinal cord perfusion pressure through CSF drainage and hyperventilation have been undertaken, the only definitive methods in the prevention of spinal cord ischemia are rapid surgery and the maintenance of normal cardiac function. (See page 1122: Prevention of Perioperative Spinal Cord Ischemia.)

13. A. In a randomized, prospective trial comparing the traditional transabdominal approach with the retroperitoneal approach for elective infrarenal aortic reconstruction, the retroperitoneal approach was associated with a lower incidence of ileus and small bowel obstruction, less fluid shift, shorter stays in the hospital and ICU, and lower hospital costs. There was no difference in postoperative pulmonary complications, however, and the retroperitoneal approach was accompanied by an increase in long-term incisional pain. (See page 1133: Surgical Approach.)

14. D. The placement of aortic (Gott) shunts, the use of temporary ex vivo axillofemoral bypass grafts, and partial bypass techniques have been used as a means to decompress the heart and provide distal perfusion in the face of thoracic aortic occlusion. These techniques attenuate the hemodynamic response to aortic unclamping, reduce reperfusion acidosis, and possibly ameliorate the hormonal and metabolic aberrations associated with aortic occlusion. Although segmental, sequential surgical repair may minimize the duration of ischemia to any given vascular bed, it does not allow for decompression or distal perfusion during periods of occlusion. (See page 1122: Prevention of Perioperative Spinal Cord Ischemia.)

15. D. The development of acute renal failure after aortic reconstruction is associated with a mortality rate of more than 30%. Although it is more common in patients requiring supraceliac aortic occlusion, infrarenal occlusion is not without risk, as evidenced by data indicating that infrarenal aortic cross-clamping decreased renal blood flow by 38%, increased renal vascular resistance by 75%, and redistributed blood flow from the renal cortex. Indeed, infrarenal aortic reconstruction may be associated with a 3% incidence of renal failure. Previous data have shown that intraoperative urine output is a poor indicator of postoperative renal function. The best predictor of postoperative renal failure is preoperative renal function. Although various strategies, including administration of mannitol, furosemide, and low-dose dopamine, have been used to increase renal blood flow and promote diuresis, none has been shown conclusively to prevent renal failure. Maintenance of adequate intravascular volume and maintenance of myocardial function are the most successful preventative measures. (See page 1120: Etiology and Epidemiology of Kidney Injury.)

16. D. It is a widely held belief that regional anesthetic techniques are associated with fewer postoperative respiratory complications than are general anesthetic techniques. Data indicate that regional techniques may reduce postoperative hypercoagulability and graft thrombosis in patients undergoing lower extremity vascular bypass procedures. A reduction in cardiac complications is often cited as a reason for avoiding general anesthesia. Although some studies have suggested a possible reduction of cardiac complications, this remains unsubstantiated. (See page 1139: Management of Elective Lower Extremity Revascularization.)

17. D. The technique for implantation of endovascular aortic grafts generally requires bilateral common femoral artery or iliac artery cutdown in the supine position. Preimplantation angiography is required to identify the vasculature. Dye loads may be considerable (100–250 mL). Major complications in endovascular stent grafting have included aneurysm rupture during the time of graft implantation, renal insufficiency secondary to contrast use, and late complications such as graft migration with late aneurysmal rupture. Retroperitoneal hematoma is a possible complication, which can cause significant morbidity and mortality. There does not appear to be an increased incidence of pneumothorax during EVAR. (See page 1130: Endovascular Abdominal Aneurysm Repair (EVAR): Other Complications.)

CHAPTER 40

Obstetrical Anesthesia

1. Plasma volume and red blood cell (RBC) volume increase by which of the following percentages in pregnancy?

   A. Plasma volume, 70%; RBC volume, 50%
   B. Plasma volume, 40%; RBC volume, 40%
   C. Plasma volume, 40%; RBC volume, 20%
   D. Plasma volume, 60%; RBC volume, 20%
   E. Plasma volume, 60%; RBC volume, 60%

2. Which of the following factors does not influence the placental transfer of drugs?

   A. Fetal osmolality
   B. The placental area
   C. Ionization of the drug
   D. Molecular weight
   E. Concentration in fetal blood

3. Which dermatomes are affected in the first stage of labor?

   A. T5 to T10
   B. S2 to S4
   C. T10 to L1
   D. T12 to L2
   E. T6 to L2

4. The most common side effect of neuraxial anesthesia for obstetrics is:

   A. Meningitis
   B. Decreased variability of fetal heart rate
   C. Nausea and vomiting
   D. Hypotension
   E. Nerve group damage

5. Considering regional anesthesia for cesarean section, which of the following is TRUE?

   A. Epidural anesthesia is by far the most common regional technique.
   B. Aspiration of the epidural catheter for blood is reliable for detection of catheter misplacement.
   C. Epidural anesthesia consistently eliminates visceral discomfort during exteriorization of the uterus.
   D. Spinal narcotics are contraindicated in parturients.
   E. Epidural anesthesia has the advantage of a slower onset than spinal.

6. When considering anesthetic complications relating to cesarean section, which of the following is TRUE?

   A. Fatality with general anesthesia is equal to that with regional anesthesia.
   B. Paresthesia and pain with spinal needle placement are common, and the procedure should proceed despite these complaints.
   C. Phenylephrine should not be used to treat hypotension in pregnant patients.
   D. Colloid is superior to crystalloid prehydration in preventing hypotension associated with neuraxial anesthesia.
   E. The risk of hypotension with regional anesthesia is increased in women in labor compared with nonlaboring women.

7. The incidence of postdural puncture headache after dural puncture with a 25- or 26-gauge spinal needle in pregnant women is approximately:

   A. 0%
   B. 1%
   C. 3%
   D. 5%
   E. 10%

8. Many of the symptoms associated with preeclampsia may result from an imbalance between the placental production of:

   A. Renin and angiotensin
   B. Endothelin and nitric oxide
   C. Prostacyclin and thromboxane
   D. Platelets and antithrombin III
   E. Progesterone and estrogen

9. The greatest change in cardiac output in pregnant patients occurs:

   A. During the second trimester
   B. After the delivery of the placenta
   C. During the third trimester
   D. During the first stage of labor
   E. During the second stage of labor

10. When considering fetal heart rate, which of the following is TRUE?

    A. The normal fetal heart rate is 80 to 120 bpm.
    B. Acceleration of fetal heart rate in response to fetal stimulation is ominous.
    C. A fetal heart rate of more than 170 bpm may be caused by intravenous narcotics.
    D. Baseline variability of fetal heart rate may be affected by ephedrine.
    E. Baseline variability of fetal heart rate is a reflection of the integrity of the sympathetic nervous system but is not affected by the parasympathetic nervous system.

11. Normal fetal oxygen saturation is:

    A. 90% to 100%
    B. 50% to 100%
    C. 50% to 80%
    D. 30% to 70%
    E. 10% to 50%

12. The average arterial blood pH of healthy, vigorous infants is:

    A. 7.04
    B. 7.14
    C. 7.24
    D. 7.34
    E. 7.44

13. The initial breath during neonatal resuscitation may entail a peak positive pressure up to _____ cm H_2O.

    A. 10 to 15
    B. 15 to 20
    C. 20 to 30
    D. 30 to 40
    E. 40 to 50

14. The studies that relate surgery and anesthesia during pregnancy to fetal outcomes have found that:

    A. Only gynecologic surgery in the third trimester is correlated with increased fetal death.
    B. Neither surgery nor anesthesia can be correlated with an increase in congenital disorders.
    C. Maternal condition at the time of surgery has no affect on fetal outcomes.
    D. Operative exposure to nitrous oxide dramatically increases the chance of congenital disorders in humans.
    E. General anesthesia is associated with a significant increase in the incidence of congenital disorders.

15. Which of the following statements concerning lung volume changes during pregnancy is TRUE?

    A. Functional residual capacity (FRC) decreases by >40%.
    B. Inspiratory reserve volume decreases.
    C. Tidal volume is unchanged.
    D. Minute ventilation increases by 50%.

16. Considering a pregnant patient's response to anesthetic, which of the following is TRUE?

    A. Progesterone levels have no effect on minimum alveolar concentration (MAC).
    B. Lower doses of local anesthetics are needed per dermatomal segment for an epidural or spinal block.
    C. A decrease in MAC is not seen until after 20 weeks of gestation.
    D. Pregnancy leads to decreased neurosensitivity to local anesthetics.

17. Which of the following is a side effect of systemic meperidine analgesia for labor?

    A. Increased variability of the fetal heart rate
    B. Fetal bradycardia
    C. Neonatal depression
    D. Prolongation of the first stage of labor

18. Considering paracervical block, which of the following statements is TRUE?

    A. Paracervical blocks are ineffective until the completion of the first stage of labor.
    B. Bupivacaine is the local anesthetic agent of choice.
    C. Paracervical block may cause fetal asphyxia.
    D. Paracervical block is performed using 5 to 10 mL of concentrated local anesthetic.

19. Which of the following would not be part of the classification of severe preeclampsia?

    A. Intrauterine growth retardation
    B. Systolic blood pressure of 170 mm Hg
    C. Oliguria (400 mL/24 hr)
    D. Intense sciatic pain

20. Which of the following statements is TRUE?

    A. Magnesium increases the duration of action of depolarizing muscle relaxants.
    B. Magnesium does not affect the duration of action of nondepolarizing muscle relaxants.
    C. Magnesium increases the amount of the acetylcholine liberated from motor nerve endings.
    D. Magnesium makes the end plate more sensitive to acetylcholine.

21. Which of the following statements concerning pregnancy and human immunodeficiency virus (HIV) is TRUE?

    A. Pregnancy accelerates the progression of HIV.
    B. There is no risk of vertical transmission through breastfeeding.
    C. Intrapartum transmission accounts for 90% of the risk of HIV transmission.
    D. Zidovudine prophylaxis decreases vertical transmission to less than 2%.

22. When considering neonatal adaptations at birth, which of the following statements is FALSE?

    A. Functional closure of the ductus arteriosus occurs within hours to days.
    B. There is a dramatic increase in pulmonary vascular resistance with increasing pulmonary arterial oxygen tension.
    C. Prompt expansion of the lungs is of primary importance.
    D. The foramen ovale functionally closes almost immediately.

23. Considering nonobstetric surgery in pregnant women, which statement is TRUE?

    A. Hyperventilation is necessary for fetal well-being.
    B. It is necessary to monitor for uterine contractions intraoperatively but not postoperatively in patients in their third trimester.
    C. Left uterine displacement is not necessary until the start of the second trimester.
    D. Chewable antacid should be given to all pregnant patients before induction of anesthesia.

24. Changes to the blood coagulation mechanisms during pregnancy include:

    A. Increased fibrinogen, decreased protein S, decreased D-dimer complex formation
    B. Decreased fibrinogen, increased protein S, decreased protein C
    C. Increased fibrinogen, decreased platelets, decreased D-dimer complex formation
    D. Decreased fibrinogen, increased protein S, decreased MAC complex formation
    E. Increased fibrinogen, decreased protein S, increased D-dimer complex formation

25. Amongst the changes in plasma protein composition during pregnancy:

    A. Plasma albumin decreases proportionally more than other serum globulins.
    B. The albumin–globulin ratio is increased because of high prealbumin.
    C. Plasma cholinesterase decreases by 50% to 60%, prolonging succinylcholine effect.
    D. The total amount of protein in the circulation decreases.
    E. Relatively less potency is seen in drugs that are fractionally plasma bound.

26. Cardiovascular changes during pregnancy do NOT include:

    A. Increases of cardiac output by 30% to 50% above that of the nonpregnant state
    B. Arterial blood pressure decreases from reduced PVR
    C. Cardiac output may reach 12 to 14 L/min during labor
    D. Maternal blood vessels increase responsiveness to angiotensin and other pressors
    E. When lying supine, cardiac output decreases in some pregnant women

27. During pregnancy, respiratory adaptations include:

    A. Increases in Mallampati scores, but with simpler direct laryngoscopies
    B. The diaphragm is displaced in the caudal direction, creating a larger thoracic cage
    C. Functional residual capacity (FRC) decreases by 50% to 75%
    D. Progesterone induces increases in minute ventilation
    E. Alveolar dead space decreases so that its ratio with tidal volume ratio is preserved

28. The metabolism of pregnant women is altered in which of the following ways?

    A. Basal oxygen consumption increases by 50% by the end of the pregnancy.
    B. Increased alveolar ventilation leads to a reduction in the partial pressure of CO_2.
    C. Maternal blood pH decreases to 7.2 to 7.3 due to increased respiration.
    D. There is an increased risk of maternal hypoglycemia in the third trimester.
    E. The partial pressure of oxygen in blood is reduced due to fetal steal.

29. Which of the following is true regarding opioid use in labor and delivery?

    A. Maternal dosing of naloxone immediately prior to delivery is the safest way to avoid neonatal respiratory depression.
    B. Nalbuphine and butorphanol are biotransformed into active metabolites.
    C. Meperidine dosing is associated with a high incidence of maternal sedation.
    D. Remifentanil for labor pain can be dosed with minimal side effects.
    E. Ketamine is associated with a high incidence of nausea and neonatal depression.

30. Regarding the use of inhaled anesthetics during labor and delivery:

    A. Self-administered nitrous oxide is the most commonly used inhalation agent for labor analgesia.
    B. For uterine relaxation, intravenous nitroglycerin is recommended to be administered in a dose of 400 to 600 μg.
    C. A gas scavenger is needed for labor analgesia utilizing potent inhalants, but not with nitrous oxide.
    D. General anesthesia is not utilized for vaginal deliveries.
    E. Nitrous oxide provides complete analgesia in most parturients.

31. Which of the following is FALSE regarding local anesthetic systemic toxicity?

    A. It can manifest as seizures and progress to cardiovascular collapse.
    B. Twenty percent lipid emulsion therapy is dosed at 5 mL/kg/min.
    C. Benzodiazepines are the initial treatment for local anesthesia–mediated seizures.
    D. Initial epinephrine dose of 10 to 100 μg of epinephrine is recommended as the initial treatment for cardiovascular collapse.
    E. Cardiopulmonary bypass should be considered if intralipid therapy fails.

32. Preeclampsia is a serious condition of pregnancy because:

    A. It involves elevated blood pressure after the 20th week, with or without proteinuria.
    B. Pulmonary edema is seen in approximately 20% of severe preeclamptic patients.
    C. Placental ischemia leads to increased circulating angiotensin, which furthers hypertension and tissue hypoxia.
    D. Elevated liver enzymes and thrombocytopenia and >5 g of proteinuria per 24 hours are the defining symptoms of the HELLP syndrome.
    E. Cerebral hemorrhage and edema account for over 80% of the deaths seen with preeclampsia–eclampsia.

33. Which of the following statements regarding treatment of preeclampsia is FALSE?

    A. Delivery of the fetus and placenta is the definitive treatment.
    B. Magnesium sulfate 4 g over 5 minutes is dosed to prevent convulsions.
    C. Hydralazine is commonly used to decrease blood pressure.
    D. The use of spinal anesthesia for C-section in patients with severe preeclampsia is absolutely contraindicated due to the resulting refractory hypotension.
    E. General anesthesia with ketamine is contraindicated.

34. Which of the following is TRUE regarding obstetric hemorrhage?

    A. Antepartum hemorrhage is associated only with abruptio placentae.
    B. Delivery of a placenta previa pregnancy carries a <1% risk of maternal mortality.
    C. The risk of placenta accreta in women with previa increases by 8% with each additional cesarean section.
    D. Postpartum hemorrhage is typically defined as blood loss greater than 2,000 mL following vaginal or cesarean section.
    E. A spinal or saddle block is the preferred anesthetic in patients with uncontrolled blood loss requiring dilation and curettage.

35. Eisenmenger's syndrome in the parturient causes:

    A. Up to a 30% mortality rate in the mother
    B. Severe pulmonary hypertension leading to left-to-right shunt
    C. Left ventricular dysfunction more frequently than right ventricular dysfunction
    D. Decreased risk of shunt with N_2O due to decreased pulmonary vascular resistance
    E. Slower arm-to-brain times with IV medications due to shunting

36. Which of the following is FALSE with regards to advanced maternal age in pregnancy?

    A. About one in seven births in the United States are in women of 35 years of age or older.
    B. Cesarean section rate for mothers >34 years of age is approximately 30% higher than mothers of 30 to 34 years of age.
    C. Studies suggest that advanced maternal age patients prefer Cesarean delivery.
    D. Cesarean delivery is safer for the majority of patients of advanced maternal age.
    E. Multiple gestations are more common in patients of advanced maternal age.

37. True statements with respect to binding of drugs in fetal serum include:

    A. Bupivacaine and lidocaine are each 50% bound in fetal serum.
    B. Lidocaine is bound 50% and bupivacaine is bound 25% in fetal serum.
    C. Lidocaine binds 25% and thiopental binds 75% in fetal serum.
    D. Fetal serum binds thiopental 25% and bupivacaine 50%.
    E. Meperidine is approximately 50% bound and bupivacaine is 25% bound.

38. During pregnancy, the gastroesophageal sphincter tone begins to decrease after __ weeks.

    A. 12
    B. 20
    C. 28
    D. 34
    E. 37

ANSWERS

1. C. Increased mineralocorticoid activity during pregnancy produces sodium retention and increased body water content. Thus, plasma volume and total blood volume begin to increase in early gestation, resulting in a final increase of 40% to 50% and 25% to 40%, respectively, at term. The relatively smaller increase in RBC blood volume (20%) accounts for the reduction in hematocrit during pregnancy. (See page 1145: Physiologic Changes of Pregnancy.)

2. A. Drugs cross biologic membranes by simple diffusion, the rate of which is determined by the Fick principle. The Fick equation is dependent on the diffusion constant of the drug, which depends on molecular size, lipid solubility, and degree of ionization. Other factors important in the Fick equation include surface area available for exchange or placental area, concentration of free drug in maternal blood, concentration of free drug in fetal blood, and thickness of the diffusion barrier. Most drugs commonly used by anesthesiologists have molecular weights below 500 and are easily transferred through the placenta. (See page 1147: Placental Transfer and Fetal Exposure to Anesthetic Drugs.)

3. C. In early labor, only the lower thoracic dermatomes T11 and T12 are affected, but with progressing cervical dilation and the transitional phase, adjacent dermatomes may be involved, and pain is referred from T10 to L1. In the second stage of labor, additional pain impulses resulting from distention of the vaginal vault and perineum are carried by the pudendal nerve, which is composed of lower sacral fibers S2 to S4. (See page 1147: Placental Transfer and Fetal Exposure to Anesthetic Drugs.)

4. D. Hypotension resulting from sympathectomy is the most frequent complication that occurs with central neuraxial blockade. Therefore, maternal blood pressure must be monitored at regular intervals, typically 2 to 5 minutes for the first 20 minutes after initiating the block. Meningitis is a rare complication of neuraxial anesthesia, as is nerve group damage. Nausea and vomiting may result from hypotension. Fetal heart rate variability is much less affected by neuraxial anesthesia than by intravenous anesthetics. (See pages 1152: Neuraxial Anesthesia and 1154: Anesthetic Complications.)

5. E. Subarachnoid or spinal block is the most commonly administered regional anesthetic technique for cesarean delivery because of its speed and reliability. Despite an adequate dermatomal level with either spinal or epidural anesthesia, women may experience varying degrees of visceral discomfort, particularly during exteriorization of the uterus and traction on abdominal viscera. Improved perioperative anesthesia and analgesia may be provided with the addition of narcotics to the neuraxial local anesthetic solution. In contrast to spinal anesthesia, epidural anesthesia is associated with a slower onset of action and more controllability. Aspiration of the epidural catheter for blood or cerebrospinal fluid is not reliable for detection of catheter misplacement, particularly with single-orifice catheters. (See page 1152: Anesthesia for Cesarean Delivery.)

6. D. A recent study of anesthesia-related death in the United States (between 1979 and 1990) revealed that the case fatality rate for general anesthesia was 16.7 times greater than that for regional anesthesia. Hypotension is a common complication of neuraxial anesthesia for cesarean section, and colloid prehydration has been shown to be superior to crystalloid solution in preventing this hypotension. The risk of hypotension after regional anesthesia is lower in women who are in labor compared with nonlaboring women. In the presence of maternal tachycardia, 25 to 50 μg of phenylephrine may be substituted for ephedrine. Pressure or trauma exerted by a needle on spinal nerve roots or the spinal cord produces immediate pain. Needle advancement should stop immediately upon patient complaint of paresthesia or pain, and if the pain does not resolve within seconds, the needle or catheter should be withdrawn and repositioned. (See page 1154: Anesthetic Complications.)

7. B. The frequency of postdural puncture headache development is related to the diameter of the puncture needle, ranging from more than 70% after the use of a 16-gauge needle to <1% with a smaller 25- or 26-gauge spinal needle. The incidence of the headache is reduced with the use of atraumatic pencil-point needles (e.g., Whitacre or Sprotte needles). (See page 1154: Anesthetic Complications—Postdural Puncture Headache.)

8. C. Many of the symptoms associated with preeclampsia, including placental ischemia, systemic vasoconstriction, and increased platelet aggregation, may result from an imbalance between the placental production of prostacyclin and thromboxane. During normal pregnancy, the placenta produces equivalent quantities of these prostaglandins. During preeclamptic pregnancy, up to seven times more thromboxane than prostacyclin may be present. (See page 1155: Management of High-risk Parturients—Preeclampsia–Eclampsia.)

9. B. During labor, cardiac output increases above antepartum levels. Between contractions, the cardiac output increases approximately 30% during the first stage and 45% during the second stage. The greatest change occurs immediately after delivery of the placenta, when cardiac output increases to an average of 80% above prepartum values. In some cases, it may increase by as much as 150%. (See page 1161: Heart Disease.)

10. D. The baseline fetal heart rate is measured between contractions and ranges from 120 to 160 bpm. An acceleration of fetal heart rate in response to fetal stimulation (e.g., during vaginal examination or fetal capillary blood sampling) is a reassuring sign that the fetus is not acidotic. Persistently elevated fetal heart rates may be associated with chronic fetal distress, maternal fever, or administration of drugs such as ephedrine or atropine. Fetal hypoxia and acidosis often lead to low fetal heart rates. The baseline fetal heart rate variability, which is normally present, reflects the beat-to-beat adjustments of parasympathetic and sympathetic nervous symptoms to various internal and external stimuli. Fetal central nervous system depression by asphyxia may decrease baseline variability. Therefore, a smooth fetal heart rate may be an ominous finding. Ephedrine may increase fetal heart rate variability. Intravenous opioids can cause a decrease in fetal heart rate variability. (See page 1166: Fetal Monitoring—Electronic Fetal Monitoring.)

11. D. Fetal oxygen saturation between 30% and 70% is considered normal. Saturation readings consistently below 30% for a prolonged period of time (i.e., 10–15 minutes) are suggestive of acidemia. Fetal blood scalp sampling or prompt obstetric intervention may be indicated. (See page 1166: Fetal Monitoring—Ancillary Tests and Fetal Pulse Oximetry.)

12. C. Uterine contractions decrease or even eliminate the blood flow through the intervillous space of the placenta. On the fetal side, cord compression occurs during the final stages of approximately one-third of vaginal deliveries. Thus, mild degrees of hypoxia and acidosis occur even during normal labor and delivery and play an important role in initiation of ventilation. On average, healthy, vigorous infants have a pH of 7.24 at birth. (See page 1169: Newborn Resuscitation in the Delivery Room—Fetal Asphyxia.)

13. D. Initial resuscitative methods include rubbing the back and slapping the neonate's feet. If the newborn is apneic or gasping, or if the heart rate is <100 bpm after initial stabilization, then positive pressure ventilation (PPV) should begin. PPV via bag and mask should be instituted at a rate of 40 to 60 breaths per minute. The initial breath may require pressures of 30 to 40 cm H_2O. Subsequent inflation pressures should be reduced to 15 to 20 cm H_2O in an infant with normal lungs. A small plastic oropharyngeal airway may help maintain patency of the upper airway. Endotracheal intubation may be required if bag–mask ventilation is ineffective or prolonged. (See page 1170: Resuscitation.)

14. B. Available evidence, stemming from two large studies, suggests that there is no correlation among surgery, anesthesia, and congenital disorders. There was an increased risk of spontaneous abortion in women who had received general anesthesia during the first or second trimesters, which was most evident after gynecologic operations. Although many commonly used anesthetics are teratogenic at high doses in animals, few, if any studies support teratogenic effects of anesthetic or sedative medications in the doses used for human anesthesia care. (See page 1173: Anesthesia for Nonobstetric Surgery in the Pregnant Woman.)

15. D. From the fifth month, the expiratory reserve volume, residual volume, and FRC decrease. The latter decreases by 20% to 30% compared with the nonpregnant state. Concomitantly, there is an increase in inspiratory reserve volume, so total lung capacity remains unchanged. Minute ventilation increases from the beginning of pregnancy to a maximum of 50% above normal at term. This is accomplished by a 30% to 50% increase in tidal volume and a small increase in respiratory rate. (See page 1146: Respiratory Changes.)

16. B. The MAC for inhaled agents is decreased by 8 to 12 weeks of gestation and may be related to an increase in the progesterone levels. Lower doses of local anesthetics are needed per dermatomal segment for epidural or spinal block; this has been attributed to an increased spread of local anesthetic within the epidural and subarachnoid spaces, which occurs as a result of epidural venous engorgement. In addition, an increased neurosensitivity to local anesthetics has been suggested (which may be mediated by progesterone). (See pages 1145: Physiologic Changes of Pregnancy—Altered Drug Responses and 1173: Anesthesia for Nonobstetric Surgery in the Pregnant Woman.)

17. C. Historically, meperidine has been the most commonly used systemic opioid during the first stage of labor; however, there has been a move away from this agent in the past decade. The major side effects include nausea and vomiting, dose-related depression of ventilation, orthostatic hypotension, and potential for neonatal depression. Meperidine may cause transient alterations of fetal heart rate, such as decreased beat-to-beat variability and tachycardia. No studies have shown that systemic opioids prolong the first stage of labor. (See page 1149: Opioids.)

18. C. Although the paracervical block effectively relieves pain during the first stage of labor, the technique has fallen out of favor because it was associated with a high incidence of fetal asphyxia and poor neonatal outcome (particularly with the use of bupivacaine). This may be related to uterine artery constriction or increased uterine tone. The technique is basically simple and involves submucosal injection of 5 to 10 mL of dilute local anesthesia at the vaginal fornix. (See page 1151: Paracervical Block.)

19. D. Preeclampsia is classified as severe if it is associated with any of the following: Systolic blood pressure above 160 mm Hg, diastolic blood pressure of 110 mm Hg, proteinuria of 5 g/24 hr, oliguria (400 mL/24 hr), cerebral or visual disturbances, pulmonary edema, epigastric pain, and intrauterine growth retardation. (See page 1155: Management of High-risk Parturients—Preeclampsia–Eclampsia.)

20. A. Magnesium potentiates the duration and intensity of action of depolarizing and nondepolarizing muscle relaxants. It seems to do this by decreasing the amount of acetylcholine liberated from the motor nerve terminals and diminishing the sensitivity of the end plate to acetylcholine. It has also been found to depress the excitability of the skeletal muscle. (See page 1155: Management of High-risk Parturients—General Management.)

21. D. Women now represent nearly half of the people worldwide living with HIV. There is no evidence that pregnancy accelerates the progression of the disease. However, there is compelling interest to prevent vertical transmission of HIV from mother to fetus. The risk of intrauterine infection of the fetus is 4.4%. Intrapartum transmission accounts for 60% of the risk of peripartum transmission; the remainder is through breastfeeding. However, when zidovudine prophylaxis is given to women with HIV perinatally and to the newborn in the first weeks of life, vertical transmission is reduced by 66% (to less than 2%). (See page 1165: HIV and AIDS.)

22. B. Many morphologic and functional changes occur in neonates. The onset of ventilation and expansion of the lungs opens the pulmonary vasculature, resulting in decreased resistance and a significant increase in pulmonary blood flow. Pulmonary vascular resistance decreases as oxygen tension increases and the carbon dioxide level decreases. As soon as the pulmonary perfusion increases, the foramen ovale (which constitutes a communication between the inferior vena cava and the left atrium) undergoes functional closure. Cessation of the umbilical circulation reduces pressure in the inferior vena cava and right atrium. The increase in pulmonary blood flow increases the pressure in the left atrium. The smooth muscle of the ductus arteriosus constricts in response to increased oxygen tension. Catecholamines also help to constrict the ductus arteriosus. However, the ductus does not constrict abruptly or completely after birth; in fact, functional closure may take hours or even days. (See page 1169: Neonatal Adaptations at Birth.)

23. C. It is generally agreed that only surgical procedures that cannot be delayed for months, including emergency surgery, should be performed during pregnancy. Beginning in the second trimester, uterine displacement must be maintained at all times during surgery. Fifteen to thirty milliliters of a nonparticulate (but not chewable) antacid should be administered within one-and-half hour before induction of anesthesia. Maternal hyperventilation should be avoided, and end-expiratory PaCO$_2$ or arterial blood gases should be monitored. Hyperventilation may decrease uterine blood flow and change fetal pH. Monitoring uterine activity should be continued after the operation to detect preterm labor. (See page 1173: Anesthesia for Nonobstetric Surgery in the Pregnant Woman.)

24. E. Several procoagulant factor levels increase during pregnancy, most notably fibrinogen, which doubles in mass. Anticoagulant activity decreases, as evidenced by decreased protein S concentrations and activated protein C resistance, and fibrinolysis is impaired. Increases in D-dimer and thrombin–antithrombin complexes indicate increased clotting and probable secondary fibrinolysis. Indeed, pregnancy has been referred to as a state of *chronic compensated disseminated intravascular coagulation*. These coagulation changes peak at the time of parturition.

25. A. Serum cholinesterase activity declines to a level of 20% below normal by term and reaches a nadir in the puerperium. However, it is doubtful that moderate succinylcholine

doses lead to prolonged apnea in otherwise normal circumstances. Although the total amount of protein in the circulation increases, plasma protein concentration declines to <6 g/dL at term because of dilution from increased plasma volume. The albumin–globulin ratio declines because of the relatively greater reduction in albumin concentration. A decrease in serum protein concentration may be clinically significant because the free fractions of protein-bound drugs can be expected to increase. (See page 1145: Hematologic Alterations.)

26. D. Systemic vascular resistance declines as maternal vessels lose their responsiveness to angiotensin and other pressors. Cardiac output increases by 30% to 50% above that of the nonpregnant state due primarily to a 20% to 50% increase in stroke volume and also to mild elevations in heart rate. Arterial blood pressure decreases slightly because the decrease in peripheral resistance exceeds the increase in cardiac output. Additional increases in cardiac output occur during labor (when cardiac output may reach 12–14 L/min) and also in the immediate postpartum period because of added blood volume from the contracted uterus. Supine hypotensive syndrome, which occurs in 10% of pregnant women, occurs because the supine position leads to vena cava occlusion and thus decreased preload to the heart, resulting in lowered cardiac output and blood pressure, tachycardia, maternal mental status changes, nausea and presyncope. (See page 1145: Cardiovascular Changes.)

27. D. Mallampati scores increase during pregnancy and laryngoscopies tend to become more difficult in the pregnant population. The diaphragm is displaced cephalad (by the enlarging uterus). FRC decreases by 20% to 30% from the fifth month onward. Progesterone induces increases in minute ventilation from the very start of pregnancy (minute ventilation can increase up to 50% above nonpregnant values at term). Alveolar dead space increases such that the dead space to tidal volume ratio remains unchanged. (See page 1146: Respiratory Changes.)

28. B. Basal oxygen consumption increases during early pregnancy, with an overall increase of 20% by term. Increased alveolar ventilation leads to a reduction in the PaCO$_2$ to 32 mm Hg and an increase in the PaO$_2$ to 106 mm Hg. The plasma buffer base decreases from 47 to 42 mEq/L and, therefore, the pH remains practically unchanged. Human placental lactogen and cortisol increase the tendency toward hyperglycemia and ketosis, which may exacerbate preexisting diabetes mellitus.

29. C. The major side effects of meperidine include a high incidence of nausea and vomiting, maternal sedation, dose-related depression of ventilation, orthostatic hypotension, and the potential for neonatal depression. As with all systemic opioids, it is unclear whether remifentanil patient-controlled analgesia can provide satisfactory analgesia without an unacceptably high incidence of maternal, fetal, and neonatal side effects. Butorphanol and nalbuphine are biotransformed into inactive metabolites and have a ceiling effect on depression of ventilation. Naloxone, a pure opioid antagonist, should not be administered to the mother shortly before delivery to prevent neonatal ventilatory depression because it reverses maternal analgesia at a time when it is most needed and, in some instances, has caused maternal pulmonary edema and even cardiac arrest. If necessary, the drug should be given directly to the newborn intramuscularly (0.1 mg/kg). In low doses (0.2–0.4 mg/kg), ketamine provides adequate analgesia without causing neonatal depression. (See page 1149: Systemic Medication.)

30. **A.**   Nitrous oxide, 50% by volume, is the most commonly used inhalation agent for analgesia during labor, and the mother is trained to intermittently self-administer the gas at the onset of a contraction. Studies are conflicting as to whether nitrous oxide provides benefit to the parturient. All inhalation anesthetics require a waste gas scavenging system. Intravenous nitroglycerin (50–250 μg) has largely replaced the need for general anesthesia for uterine relaxation. General anesthesia is rarely used for vaginal delivery, but may be required when time constraints prevent induction of regional anesthesia. (See page 1153: General Anesthesia.)

31. **B.**   Seizure activity should be treated with an intravenous benzodiazepine such as midazolam 1 to 5 mg or other sedative hypnotic. New guidelines recommend consideration of early administration of 20% lipid emulsion (1.5 mL/kg over 1 minute, followed by 0.25 mL/kg/min for at least 10 minutes after attainment of hemodynamic stability). If cardiovascular collapse occurs, it should be treated according to advanced cardiac life support protocols. Initial small boluses of epinephrine (10–100 μg) are preferred; vasopressin is not recommended. Failure to respond to lipid emulsion and vasopressor therapy should prompt consideration of cardiopulmonary bypass. (See page 1155: Local Anesthetic Systemic Toxicity.)

32. **C.**   Preeclampsia is defined by hypertension with proteinuria. Placental ischemia results in a release of uterine renin and an increase in angiotensin. Widespread arteriolar vasoconstriction occurs, causing hypertension, tissue hypoxia, and endothelial damage. The HELLP syndrome is a particular form of severe preeclampsia characterized by *h*emolysis, *e*levated *l*iver enzymes, and *l*ow *p*latelet count (thrombocytopenia). In contrast to preeclampsia, elevations in blood pressure and proteinuria may be mild. Pulmonary edema occurs in approximately 2% of severe preeclamptic patients as a result of heart failure, circulatory overload, or aspiration of gastric contents during convulsions. Cerebral hemorrhage and edema account for 50% of deaths with preeclampsia–eclampsia. (See page 1156: Preeclampsia–Eclampsia.)

33. **D.**   The definitive treatment of preeclampsia–eclampsia remains delivery of the fetus and placenta. The mainstay of anticonvulsant therapy is magnesium sulfate with a typical intravenous loading dose of 4 g in a 20% solution over 5 minutes. Therapeutic blood levels are maintained by continuous infusion of 1 to 2 g/hr. Hydralazine is the most commonly used vasodilator in preeclampsia because it increases uteroplacental and renal blood flow. In surgical delivery of preeclamptic patients, the use of ketamine and ergot alkaloids should be avoided. Studies have shown that the incidence and severity of hypotension is similar in women with severe preeclampsia having a cesarean delivery with spinal compared with epidural anesthesia. Thus, spinal anesthesia is emerging as a suitable alternative to epidural anesthesia for cesarean delivery in severely preeclamptic women. (See page 1156: Preeclampsia–Eclampsia.)

34. **B.**   Antepartum hemorrhage occurs in association with placenta previa and abruptio placentae. Placenta previa complicates approximately 0.4% of pregnancies, resulting in up to 0.9% incidence of maternal mortality. The risk of placenta accreta in women with previa increases from 3% in primary cesarean section to 61% in quaternary section. Postpartum hemorrhage is usually defined as blood loss greater than 500 mL after vaginal delivery or greater than 1,000 mL after cesarean section. General anesthesia is indicated in the presence of uncontrolled hemorrhage and/or severe coagulation abnormalities. A saddle block is an option for anesthesia when dilation and curettage for treatment of postpartum hemorrhage is indicated AND the patient is hemodynamically stable. (See page 1159: Obstetric Hemorrhage.)

35. **A.**   Eisenmenger's syndrome occurs when uncorrected left-to-right shunt results in pulmonary hypertension, which, when severe, reverses flow to a right-to-left shunt. Pregnancy is not well tolerated and mortality can approach 30%, most commonly from embolic phenomena. Arm-to-brain circulation times are rapid owing to right-to-left intracardiac shunts; drugs given intravenously have a rapid onset of action. Invasive monitoring of arterial and cardiac filling pressures is indicated as the right ventricle is at greater risk of dysfunction than the left ventricle. Nitrous oxide may increase pulmonary vascular resistance and should be avoided. (See page 1161: Congenital Heart Disease.)

36. **D.**   In 2002, almost 14% of all births in the United States occurred in women aged 35 years or older. Older women believe that their age makes their infant more vulnerable and, as such, believe a controlled cesarean delivery is safer than vaginal delivery. Other explanations for increased requests for cesarean delivery include concerns about physical stamina, protection of the pelvic floor from damage, refusal to undergo labor pain, and social convenience. Women over 34 years of age were twice as likely to request cesarean delivery compared with those aged 25 years or younger. The cesarean delivery rate for mothers of 30 to 34 years of age was 37% and for mothers >34 years of age, it was 48%. Cesarean delivery is associated with increased maternal risk compared with uncomplicated vaginal delivery; hysterectomy occurs 10 times more frequently following cesarean delivery compared with vaginal delivery, and the risk of maternal death is 16 times greater. Perinatal complications are also significant in patients with advanced maternal age; multiple gestations, both iatrogenic and naturally occurring, are more common in older gravidae. (See page 1163: Advanced Maternal Age.)

37. C. Most drugs used in anesthesia exhibit only low-to-moderate degrees of binding in the fetal serum: Approximately 50% for etidocaine and bupivacaine, 25% for lidocaine, 52% for meperidine, and 75% for thiopental. (See page 1164: Preterm Delivery.)

38. B. Gastric emptying is essentially normal in the first two trimesters, but is prolonged in the third. Gastroesophageal sphincter tone is decreased after 20 weeks, thus caution regarding the unprotected airway is essential. (See page 1173: Anesthesia for Nonobstetric Surgery in the Pregnant Woman.)

Neonatal Anesthesia

1. The neonatal period is defined as the period that begins with birth and ends at:

   A. 24 hours
   B. 14 days
   C. 30 days
   D. 6 months
   E. 1 year

2. Which of the following statements regarding the fetal circulation is FALSE?

   A. Fetal pulmonary vascular resistance is relatively high compared with the systemic vascular resistance.
   B. The ductus arteriosus allows 90% of the blood leaving the right ventricle to bypass the lungs and flow through the ascending aorta.
   C. Persistent probe patency of the foramen ovale is seen in 10% to 20% of adult patients.
   D. Pulmonary vascular resistance decreases acutely at the time of birth and reaches neonatal levels within 1 hour.
   E. The ductus arteriosus is dilated secondary to a low PaO_2 level.

3. True statements regarding the transition of the cardiopulmonary system and persistent pulmonary hypertension (PPH) include all of the following EXCEPT:

   A. The goal of therapy is to keep PaO_2 between 80 and 90 mm Hg.
   B. Pulmonary circulation is sensitive to O_2, pH, and nitric oxide.
   C. Hypoxia and acidosis are pivotal etiologic factors in PPH.
   D. Because of the elevated pulmonary vascular resistance, a right-to-left shunt develops.
   E. Patency of the ductus arteriosus beyond 4 days of age is abnormal regardless of the infant's gestational age.

4. Which of the following corresponds with the location of glottis in full-term neonates?

   A. C2
   B. C3
   C. C4
   D. C5
   E. C6

5. Which of the following statements regarding O_2 consumption in adults versus neonates is correct?

   A. 7 cc/kg/min in adults; 3 cc/kg/min in neonates
   B. 6 cc/kg/min in adults; 5 cc/kg/min in neonates
   C. 10 cc/kg/min in adults; 4 cc/kg/min in neonates
   D. 3 cc/kg/min in adults; 7 cc/kg/min in neonates
   E. 5 cc/kg/min in adults; 5 cc/kg/min in neonates

6. The ratio of minute ventilation to functional residual capacity (FRC) is approximately 1.5:1 in adults and approximately _____: 1 in neonates.

   A. 0.5
   B. 1
   C. 1.5
   D. 2
   E. 5

7. Which of the following is not a shunt present in fetal circulation?

   A. Placenta
   B. Foramen ovale
   C. Ductus arteriosus
   D. Foramen secundum
   E. Ductus venosus

8. Persistent pulmonary hypertension (PPH) may be caused by all of the following EXCEPT:

   A. Sepsis
   B. Respiratory distress
   C. Meconium aspiration
   D. Delivery of high concentrations of oxygen
   E. Congenital diaphragmatic hernia

9. Which of the following statements regarding the neonatal kidney is TRUE?

   A. The neonatal kidney is more than 90% mature by 1 week of age.
   B. Fluids should be restricted intraoperatively.
   C. The half-life of renally excreted drugs is decreased.
   D. Urine output in neonates is 1 to 2 mL/kg/hr.
   E. Glomerular filtration rate (GFR) is very high in utero and decreases after birth.

10. Which of the following statements regarding neonatal airway is FALSE?

    A. The head is flexed forward when the patient is in the supine position.
    B. Neonates are obligate nose breathers.
    C. They have a relatively large tongue.
    D. The vocal cords are the narrowest portion.
    E. The larynx is more cephalad.

11. Which of the following statements regarding the neonatal pulmonary system is TRUE?

    A. Neonates have a high closing volume.
    B. Neonates have rigid ribs.
    C. Neonates' O_2 consumption is equal to adults.
    D. Neonates have a low ratio of minute ventilation to functional residual capacity (FRC).
    E. Neonates have high lung compliance.

12. Which of the following statements regarding the neonatal cardiovascular system is FALSE?

    A. Increases in cardiac output are primarily achieved through an increase in heart rate.
    B. The parasympathetic system dominates over the sympathetic system in the heart.
    C. Cardiac output may typically be increased by no more than 40% in neonates.
    D. Neonates have immature baroreceptors.
    E. The neonatal heart is very compliant.

13. Which of the following statements about muscle relaxants in pediatrics is FALSE?

    A. The duration of action of vecuronium is twice as long in children younger than 1 year of age than it is in older children.
    B. Rocuronium currently is considered the drug of choice for intermediate action.
    C. Epinephrine may be indicated after succinylcholine-induced hyperkalemia.
    D. Succinylcholine should be used in boys younger than 8 years of age only for rapid sequence induction, difficult airway, and other emergencies.
    E. There is little difference in duration of action between a typical induction dose of rocuronium and a rapid sequence dose.

14. Which of the following statements regarding neonatal anesthetic requirement is TRUE?

    A. Neonates require as much anesthetic as older infants.
    B. In premature infants, the minimum alveolar concentration (MAC) is decreased by 30%.
    C. Premature infants have decreased endorphins.
    D. Immature infants have mature blood–brain barriers.
    E. The highest MAC occurs at 2 years of age.

15. Which of the following statements regarding regional anesthesia in neonates is FALSE?

    A. The requirement for intraoperative opioids may be eliminated.
    B. The dose of muscle relaxants can be reduced.
    C. The most common response to a high spinal anesthesia is respiratory insufficiency.
    D. The requirement for inhalation anesthetics is reduced.
    E. Brachial plexus blocks are not considered safe in neonates.

16. Which of the following statements regarding anesthetic uptake in infants versus adults is TRUE?

    A. The ratio of alveolar ventilation to FRC is greater in adults than in infants.
    B. Neonates have a lower cardiac index.
    C. Infants have higher blood–gas partition coefficient.
    D. In neonates, the brain and heart receive relatively more cardiac output.
    E. Infants have a lower respiratory rate.

17. Which of the following statements regarding congenital diaphragmatic hernia is FALSE?

    A. The occurrence of symptoms partly depends on the effect on the pulmonary circulation.
    B. Most congenital diaphragmatic hernias are left sided.
    C. After diagnosis, the patient requires immediate intubation.
    D. High-frequency ventilation has not been shown to be beneficial.
    E. Goal peak inspiratory pressure should be less than 25 cm H_2O.

18. Omphalocele is associated with:

    A. A 60% incidence of congenital heart disease
    B. Extra-abdominal contents without a sac (amnion)
    C. Beckwith–Wiedemann syndrome
    D. More fluid loss preoperatively than is associated with gastroschisis
    E. Interruption of the omphalomesenteric artery

19. Which of the following statements regarding tracheo-esophageal fistula is FALSE?

    A. Eighty-five percent of these connections consist of a fistula between the distal trachea and the esophagus, with a blind proximal esophageal pouch.
    B. Fifty percent of these patients have associated congenital anomalies.
    C. Primary repair can be done 24 to 48 hours after diagnosis.
    D. A major complication is dehydration.
    E. Infants presenting for surgical repair commonly have gastrostomy in place.

20. Which of the following statements regarding meningomyelocele is TRUE?

    A. Fifty percent to ninety percent of meningomyeloceles can be detected by maternal serum α-fetoprotein.
    B. Serum α-fetoprotein is more reliable than amniotic fluid α-fetoprotein.
    C. Meningocele contains the neural elements.
    D. Regional anesthesia is absolutely contraindicated in patients with meningocele.
    E. Twenty percent of these patients have hydrocephalus requiring shunting.

21. Which of the following statements regarding postoperative apnea is FALSE?

    A. Premature infants with congenital anomalies are at highest risk.
    B. Compared to general anesthesia, spinal anesthesia may decrease the incidence of postoperative apnea.
    C. The cause is multifactorial.
    D. A 44-week postconceptional infant undergoing a spinal anesthetic does not require prolonged postoperative monitoring.
    E. Caffeine may be an effective treatment for life-threatening apnea and bradycardia.

22. Which of the following metabolic abnormalities is classically described in a patient with pyloric stenosis?

    A. Hyponatremia, hypokalemia, hypochloremia, and metabolic acidosis
    B. Hypernatremia, hypokalemia, hypochloremia, and metabolic acidosis
    C. Hyponatremia, hypokalemia, hypochloremia, and metabolic alkalosis
    D. Hypernatremia, hyperkalemia, hyperchloremia, and metabolic alkalosis
    E. Hyponatremia, hyperkalemia, hyperchloremia, and respiratory alkalosis

23. Which of the following statements regarding pyloric stenosis is TRUE?

    A. It is a surgical emergency.
    B. Dextrose 5% in water should be used for fluid replacement.
    C. It is usually evident in the first week of life.
    D. Postoperative apnea is a concern in these patients.
    E. Potassium should not be replaced.

24. Which of the following statements regarding retinopathy of prematurity (ROP) is FALSE?

    A. The exact cause is unknown.
    B. Hypoxia may be a cause.
    C. Prolonged bright-light exposure appears to contribute to this disease.
    D. In a premature infant, a pulse oximetry reading of 96% is appropriate.
    E. The most advanced stage of the disease is characterized by complete retinal detachment.

25. Which of the following is NOT a reason that drug pharmacokinetics would differ in neonates?

    A. Increased fetal hemoglobin concentration.
    B. Immature renal and hepatic function.
    C. Decreased fat stores.
    D. Decreased protein binding.
    E. Larger volume of distribution.

26. Select the choice that correctly places the blocks in order of decreasing chance of local anesthetic toxicity.

    A. Caudal > Intercostal > Epidural > Femoral
    B. Femoral > Epidural > Caudal > Intercostal
    C. Intercostal > Caudal > Epidural > Femoral
    D. Intercostal > Epidural > Caudal > Femoral
    E. Epidural > Femoral > Caudal > Intercostal

ANSWERS

1. C. The neonatal period is defined as the first 30 days of extrauterine life and includes the newborn period. The newborn period is the first 24 hours of life. (See page 1179: Physiology of the Infant and the Transition Period.)

2. D. The pulmonary vascular bed has a high vascular resistance because the alveoli are relatively closed and filled with fluid, and the blood vessels are compressed. However, the ductus arteriosus represents a low-resistance system, which is dilated secondary to low PaO_2. Therefore, the blood that leaves the right ventricle by the pulmonary artery is shunted preferentially (90%) through the ductus arteriosus to the aorta; only 10% of the cardiac output of the right ventricle flows through the pulmonary artery into the pulmonary vascular bed. The transition of alveoli from a fluid-filled state to an air-filled state results in a reduced compression of the pulmonary alveolar capillaries and thus a reduction in pulmonary vascular resistance. It takes 3 to 4 days for the pulmonary vascular resistance to decrease to the eventual level that it will achieve during the neonatal period. Anatomic closure of the foramen ovale usually occurs in the first year of life, but may remain probe patent into adulthood in 10% to 20% of patients. (See page 1179: Fetal Circulation.)

3. A. Patency of the ductus arteriosus beyond the fourth day of life is abnormal regardless of the infant's gestational age. The major transition of circulatory system occurs over the first 24 hours of life. The pulmonary circulation is extremely sensitive to O_2, pH, and nitric oxide. Hypoxia and acidosis, along with inflammatory mediators, may cause the pulmonary artery pressure to either persist at a high level or to increase to pathologic levels; the result is PPH. The goals of therapy are to achieve a PaO_2 of between 50 and 70 mm Hg with a $PaCO_2$ of between 50 and 55 mm Hg. The elevated pulmonary vascular resistance causes both the ductus arteriosus and foramen ovale to remain open, with subsequent right-to-left (bypassing the pulmonary circulation) shunting. (See page 1182: Persistent Pulmonary Hypertension of the Newborn.)

4. C. In healthy adults, the glottis is at the level of C5 to C6. In full-term infants, the glottis is at the level of C4. In premature infants, it is at the level of C3. (See page 1185: Anatomy of the Neonatal Airway.)

5. D. The O_2 consumption of infants is 7 to 9 cc/kg/min; it is 3 cc/kg/min in adults. Therefore, varying degrees of early obstruction have more impact on O_2 delivery and reserve in neonates, infants, and children than in adults. (See page 1180: The Pulmonary System.)

6. E. Tidal ventilation for neonates is the same, in cubic centimeters per kilogram, as for adults, but neonatal O_2 consumption is three times greater; thus, the respiratory rate must be three times greater (which results in an alveolar ventilation that is three times greater). Consequently, whereas the ratio of minute ventilation to functional residual capacity is approximately 1.5:1 in adults, it is 5:1 in neonates. (See page 1180: The Pulmonary System.)

7. D. Fetal circulation is characterized by the presence of four main shunts: The placenta, foramen ovale, ductus venosus, and ductus arteriosus. The relatively low pressure in the left atrium and the high pressure in the right atrium cause the foramen ovale to be open. (See page 1179: Fetal Circulation.)

8. D. Persistent pulmonary hypertension (PPH) is a syndrome that may be primary, with no recognized origin, or it may be secondary to meconium aspiration, sepsis, pneumonia, respiratory distress, or congenital diaphragmatic hernia. Delivering a high concentration of oxygen to a neonate is generally avoided, as it predisposes to conditions such as retinopathy of the newborn. This practice does not seem to increase the incidence of PPH. (See page 1182: Persistent Pulmonary Hypertension of the Newborn.)

9. D. By the time the healthy full-term infant is 1 month of age, the kidneys are approximately 60% mature. Urine output is low in the first 24 hours, but it then increases to an expected level of at least 1 to 2 mL/kg/hr. After the first day of life, a urine output of less than 1 mL/kg/hr should be considered indicative of either hypovolemia or decreased renal function. From an anesthetic standpoint, the half-life of medications excreted by means of glomerular filtration will be prolonged. The relative inability to conserve water means that neonates, especially in the first week of life, poorly tolerate fluid restriction. The fetal kidneys receive little blood flow and have a low glomerular filtration rate (GFR). (See page 1183: The Renal System.)

10. D. Neonates are obligate nose breathers; therefore, anything that obstructs the nares will compromise a neonate's ability to breathe. The large tongue occupies relatively more space in the infant's airway and makes it difficult to perform direct laryngoscopy and intubate an infant's trachea. The neonate larynx is more cephalad and the vocal cords are angled slightly anterior. Unlike in adults, the narrowest portion of a neonate's airway is not the vocal cords but the cricoid ring. Neonates have large occiputs, so their heads flex forward onto the chest when they are lying supine and the head is in midline. (See page 1185: Anatomy of the Neonatal Airway.)

11. A. Anatomically and physiologically, the neonatal pulmonary system differs in several respects from that of adults: High O_2 consumption, high closing volumes, high ratio of minute ventilation to FRC, low lung compliance, and pliable ribs. (See page 1180: The Pulmonary System.)

12. E. Any increase in neonatal cardiac output must be accomplished by an increase in the heart rate. For this reason, infants are said to be rate dependent for their cardiac output. Especially in the first 3 months of life, the parasympathetic nervous system's influence on the heart is more mature than the sympathetic system, and the myocardium does not respond to inotropic support as well as in older children and adults. The neonatal heart can increase cardiac output by 30% to 40%. Neonates have immature baroreceptors; the baroreceptors are responsible for the reflex tachycardia that occurs in response to hypotension. The hear t of the neonate is relatively noncompliant. (See page 1179: The Cardiovascular System.)

13. **E.**   Rocuronium is the drug of choice among the intermediate-acting nondepolarizing muscle relaxants for neonates. A rapid sequence dose of rocuronium (1–1.2 mg/kg) will result in longer duration of action. In infants younger than 1 year of age, the duration of action of vecuronium is approximately twice that observed in older children (because of their immature livers). The reports of hyperkalemia with cardiac arrest in boys younger than 8 years of age (because of unrecognized muscular dystrophy) have caused some clinicians to recommend that succinylcholine should not be used routinely in this age group. However, succinylcholine is still recommended in rapid sequence situations, in patients with potential difficult airways, and if airway emergencies develop with desaturation. If the circulation is unstable with severe bradycardia, hypotension, or cardiac arrest, the first drug of choice is epinephrine. (See page 1187: Neuromuscular Blocking Agents.)

14. **B.**   Neonates and premature infants have lower anesthetic requirements than older infants and children. In premature infants, the MAC value will decrease by 20% to 30%. The reason for the lower MAC requirements is thought to be multifactorial: An immature nervous system, progesterone from the mother, elevated levels of endorphins, and an immature blood–brain barrier. The highest MAC values occur at 1 to 6 months of age. (See page 1196: Anesthetic Dose Requirements of Neonates.)

15. **E.**   Regional anesthetic techniques allow for early extubation in neonates because they may eliminate the need for intraoperative narcotics, reduce the need for muscle relaxants, and reduce the concentration of volatile agents needed. High spinal anesthesia presents as respiratory insufficiency rather than hypotension; the reason for this is the lack of sympathetic tone. Brachial plexus blocks can be safely performed on neonates and infants for upper extremity surgery. (See page 1196: Regional Anesthesia.)

16. **D.**   Various reasons for the faster uptake of anesthetic in infants have been proposed, including the ratio of alveolar ventilation to functional residual capacity is 5:1 in infants and 1.5:1 in adults; in neonates, more of the cardiac output goes to the vessel-rich group of organs, which include the heart and the brain; neonates have a greater cardiac output per kilogram of body mass and infants have lower blood–gas partition coefficients for volatile anesthetics. Infants have a higher respiratory rate than adults. (See page 1196: Uptake and Distribution of Anesthetics in Neonates.)

17. **D.**   The left side of the diaphragm closes later than the right side, resulting in a higher incidence (90%) of left-sided congenital diaphragmatic hernias (foramen of Bochdalek). The occurrence of symptoms depends on the degree of herniation and interference with pulmonary function. At times, the degree of interference is so great that the neonate's clinical condition begins to deteriorate immediately. In other situations, it may be several hours before the infant's condition is fully appreciated. Immediate supportive care includes tracheal intubation and control of the airway, along with decompression of the stomach. High-frequency ventilation has been used in place of conventional ventilation in an attempt to reduce barotrauma and has been demonstrated to be beneficial. The goal of ventilation is to maintain preductal arterial saturation above 85%, using peak inspiratory pressures below 25 cm H_2O and allowing the PCO_2 to rise to 45 to 55 mm Hg. (See page 1202: Congenital Diaphragmatic Hernia.)

18. **C.**   Failure of part or all of the intestinal content to return to the abdominal cavity results in omphalocele that is covered with a membrane called an amnion. The amnion protects the abdominal contents from infection and loss of extracellular fluid (ECF). In gastroschisis, the intestines and viscera are not covered by any membrane and are susceptible to infection and loss of ECF. Interruption of the omphalomesenteric artery results in ischemia and atrophy of the layers of the abdominal wall and formation of a gastroschisis, not an omphalocele. There is a high instance of associated congenital anomalies with omphalocele, but not with gastroschisis. Congenital heart defects are found in approximately 20% of infants with omphalocele. The Beckwith–Wiedemann syndrome consists of mental retardation, hypoglycemia, congenital heart disease, an enlarged tongue, and omphalocele. (See page 1204: Omphalocele and Gastroschisis.)

19. **E.**   Approximately 85% of tracheoesophageal fistulae consist of a fistula from the distal trachea to the esophagus and a blind proximal esophageal pouch. Fifty percent of affected infants have associated congenital anomalies, of which approximately 15% to 20% involve the cardiovascular system. The two major complications of esophageal atresia with a distal tracheal fistula are aspiration pneumonia and dehydration. If the infant is in good condition, primary repair can be performed 24 to 48 hours after diagnosis. When the degree of reflux is so severe that the pulmonary system must be protected, a gastrostomy is performed; but this is rarely required. (See page 1206: Tracheoesophageal Fistula.)

20. **A.**   Elevation of maternal serum α-fetoprotein will detect 50% to 90% of open neural tube defects, but this test has a false-positive rate of 5%. Amniotic fluid α-fetoprotein is more reliable. By definition, the lesion involves both meninges and neural components. Alternatively, a meningocele does not contain neural elements. Regional anesthesia has been reported as an alternative to general anesthesia in neonates with meningomyelocele. Hydrocephalus requiring shunting develops in approximately 80% to 90% of infants with myelomeningocele. (See page 1208: Meningomyelocele.)

21. D. The infants at highest risk for postoperative apnea are those born prematurely, those with multiple congenital anomalies, those with a history of apnea and bradycardia, and those with "chronic" lung disease. The cause of apnea is multifactorial. Spinal anesthesia without supplemental sedation decreases the incidence of postoperative apnea and bradycardia in high-risk infants. The most conservative approach is to monitor all infants younger than 60 weeks postconceptual age overnight after surgery. Infants with a history of life-threatening apnea and bradycardia may be receiving CNS stimulants such as caffeine and theophylline. (See page 1200: Postoperative Apnea.)

22. C. The classic electrolyte pattern in infants with severe vomiting consists of hyponatremia, hypokalemia, hypochloremia, and metabolic alkalosis with compensatory respiratory acidosis. (See page 1210: Pyloric Stenosis.)

23. D. Pyloric stenosis is a medical emergency, not a surgical one. These patients need fluid resuscitation (full-strength, balanced salt solution), and after the infant begins to urinate, potassium chloride should be added. Pyloric stenosis may appear as early as the second week of life. The risk of postoperative apnea in these patients is a concern. (See page 1210: Pyloric Stenosis.)

24. C. Although the exact cause of retinopathy of prematurity (ROP) is unknown, variations in arterial oxygenation (hypoxia or hyperoxia) are believed to play significant roles. At one time, there was a concern that exposure to bright ambient light could cause ROP, but this has been disproven. The risks of the development of ROP from hyperoxia have been of concern to anesthesiologists who anesthetize preterm neonates for any type of surgery. It is not known whether supplemental oxygen may start the development of ROP in preterm patients. A study demonstrated that the use of supplemental oxygen for a prolonged period of time, not just for the short duration of a general anesthetic, was not deleterious as long as the pulse oximetry readings were kept in the 96% to 99% range. The spectrum of this disease is classified into stages one through five, with completely detached retina (stage five) as the most advanced form. (See page 1200: Retinopathy of Prematurity.)

25. A. Neonates have a greater proportion of water than adults, and therefore, have a larger volume of distribution. This can increase the required dose of water-soluble medications. Neonates have decreased circulating plasma proteins for binding of drugs, resulting in a larger fraction of free drug, and creating a potential for toxicity. The fat and muscle content of the neonate is much less than that of an adult. This means drugs that redistribute to face and muscle will have higher levels in neonates. The decreased renal and hepatic functions of neonates also predispose them to increased blood levels. Fetal hemoglobin does not affect anesthetic doses or effect. (See page 1186: Anesthetic Drugs in Neonates.)

26. C. The risk of local anesthetic toxicity is generally increased in areas with increased vasculature, because this leads to increased uptake of drug into the circulation. Listed in decreasing order of potential local anesthetic toxicity with injection: Intercostal blocks, caudal space injections, epidural space injections, and peripheral nerve blocks. (See page 1189: Local Anesthetic Solutions.)

Pediatric Anesthesia

1. Studies show that parental presence at induction of anesthesia is more effective than pharmacologic alternatives at reducing anxiety in both the child and the parents.

   A. True
   B. False

2. Which of the following statements regarding pediatric patients with upper respiratory infections (URIs) is FALSE?

   A. They are at a higher risk if they live in a household with parents who smoke.
   B. At least 2, and preferably 4 weeks, should pass after a URI before any elective surgery is undertaken.
   C. They have fewer perioperative complications if a laryngeal mask anesthetic is used rather than an endotracheal tube.
   D. Children younger than 1 year of age with a URI are at a greater risk for respiratory complications than are older children undergoing anesthesia.
   E. Asthmatic children undergoing mask induction with sevoflurane will not gain any extra benefit from preoperative bronchodilator therapy.

3. Which of the following is an important consideration for children with obstructive sleep apnea (OSA)?

   A. Daytime somnolence is a common clinical feature of OSA in children.
   B. OSA occurs more commonly in boys than in girls.
   C. There is an increased opioid sensitivity in children with nocturnal desaturations >85%.
   D. Premedication including midazolam must be decreased in children with OSA.
   E. OSA in childhood can only be diagnosed via polysomnography.

4. An infant younger than 50 weeks postconceptual age undergoing general anesthesia, with a previous history of bronchopulmonary dysplasia, may be discharged after an uneventful 2-hour recovery.

   A. True
   B. False

5. Healthy children undergoing elective minor surgery require the following preoperative tests:

   A. Complete blood count
   B. Electrolytes
   C. Chest radiography
   D. Hematocrit and hemoglobin
   E. No routine tests needed

6. In younger infants who still feed frequently, formula should be given up to _____ hours preoperatively.

   A. 2
   B. 4
   C. 6
   D. 8
   E. 10

7. Which statement regarding the American Society of Anesthesiologists (ASA)'s practice guidelines for preoperative fasting is TRUE?

   A. Solids are always prohibited after midnight.
   B. Formula is not allowed within 8 hours of surgery.
   C. Breast milk is allowed until 4 hours of surgery.
   D. Flat cola is not allowed within 6 hours of surgery.
   E. Apple juice is not allowed within 4 hours of surgery.

8. Which statement regarding oral premedications is TRUE?

   A. The effect of oral midazolam lasts about 2 hours.
   B. Fifteen minutes is required to obtain adequate sedation after oral midazolam.
   C. Ketamine and midazolam should not be combined for preoperative sedation, due to enhanced side effects profile.
   D. The recommended dose of oral ketamine is 1 mg/kg.
   E. The appropriate dose of oral midazolam is 0.1 mg/kg.

9. Oral clonidine reliably causes sedation and decreased anesthetic and analgesic requirements for a duration similar to that of oral midazolam.

   A. True
   B. False

10. Dexmedetomidine is not effective for preoperative sedation in children.

    A. True
    B. False

11. Which dose range for intramuscular ketamine reliably provides for a quiet, breathing, and minimally responsive pediatric patient in approximately 5 minutes?

    A. 0.1 to 0.2 mg/kg
    B. 0.5 to 1 mg/kg
    C. 1 to 2 mg/kg
    D. 2 to 5 mg/kg
    E. 8 to 9 mg/kg

12. Emergence delirium is a phenomenon of recovery from inhaled anesthetic use in children. For this reason, intravenous anesthetic induction is recommended for most pediatric patients.

    A. True
    B. False

13. Intravenous anesthetics that act on the N-methyl-D-aspartic acid receptor or the γ-aminobutyric acid receptor have been associated with neurodegeneration in animal studies. For this reason, they should be considered relatively contraindicated in pediatric patients.

    A. True
    B. False

14. Which of the following statements regarding the use of succinylcholine in pediatric patients is TRUE?

    A. Patients with muscular dystrophy can safely receive succinylcholine without a concern for hyperkalemia.
    B. Succinylcholine is indicated for rapid airway control in cases of laryngospasm.
    C. The use of succinylcholine in all children is absolutely contraindicated.
    D. Succinylcholine is not contraindicated after a recent burn injury.
    E. Succinylcholine is not contraindicated in a patient with a family history of malignant hyperthermia.

15. Which statement regarding postoperative nausea and vomiting (PONV) in pediatric patients is TRUE?

    A. The effectiveness of ondansetron as the best rescue medication has been proven.
    B. Younger ages are associated with incidence of PONV peaking between 6 and 10 years of age.
    C. Postoperative nausea and vomiting (PONV) is common after orchiopexy, strabismus surgery, and tonsillectomy.
    D. The type of anesthetic technique has no effect on PONV.
    E. Even if the child requests it, he/she should not be given something to drink before discharge so as to avoid PONV.

16. An otherwise healthy 10-kg, 2-year-old girl presents for a 2-hour eye muscle surgery. She has been fasting since 10 PM and enters the operating room at 8 AM. Approximately, how much intravenous fluid should she receive during the first hour of anesthesia?

    A. 50 mL
    B. 100 mL
    C. 150 mL
    D. 250 mL
    E. 350 mL

17. The average hourly maintenance fluid requirement for a 22-kg child is approximately how many milliliters?

    A. 42
    B. 52
    C. 54
    D. 62
    E. 84

18. The hourly maintenance fluid requirement for a pediatric patient weighing 16 kg is:

    A. 36 mL/hr
    B. 42 mL/hr
    C. 46 mL/hr
    D. 52 mL/hr
    E. 56 mL/hr

19. What is the maximum allowable blood loss (MABL) for a 4-kg term infant with a starting hematocrit of 32% and a target hematocrit of 24%?

    A. 70 mL
    B. 80 mL
    C. 90 mL
    D. 100 mL
    E. 110 mL

20. Which of the following is the smallest size catheter capable of allowing rapid transfusion of packed red cells in small children?

    A. Peripherally inserted central catheters (PICC)
    B. # 26 gauge IV
    C. #24 gauge IV
    D. #22 gauge IV
    E. #20 gauge IV

21. In pediatric patients, the endpoint(s) of fluid and blood therapy is:

    A. Adequate blood pressure
    B. Adequate tissue perfusion
    C. Adequate urine output
    D. Correction of identifiable deficiencies in hemostasis
    E. All of the above

22. Which of the following regarding anesthesia in children with anterior mediastinal masses is FALSE?

    A. These children frequently require general anesthesia or sedation for biopsies, MRI or CT scans, or central line placements.
    B. These tumors frequently include lymphomas, teratomas, thymomas, and thyroid cancers.
    C. Local anesthetic and sedation is the preferred anesthetic choice when possible.
    D. Positive pressure ventilation is required with general anesthesia, as spontaneous ventilation in the anesthetized patient causes airway collapse.
    E. Anesthesia may need to be induced in the lateral position if the patient cannot lie flat.

23. Which of the following medications is not recommended for managing pediatric pain?

    A. Ketorolac
    B. Codeine
    C. Acetaminophen
    D. Meperidine
    E. Diclofenac

24. Which of the following is NOT impacted by the intraoperative pediatric anesthetic?

    A. Cases of emergence agitation
    B. Ensuring the child recovers from mild hypothermia
    C. Planning to manage nausea and vomiting
    D. Analgesia in the recovery phase
    E. Positioning in the "recovery position"

25. Which of the following patients may be at increased risk for developing postoperative apnea after general anesthesia?

    A. A 2-year-old child undergoing strabismus surgery
    B. A 4-month-old infant who was delivered at 35 weeks
    C. A 1-year-old child undergoing inguinal hernia surgery
    D. A 3-month-old infant undergoing tonsillectomy and adenoidectomy
    E. A 3-year-old child 2 weeks following a URI

26. Which of the following is the appropriate drug and dose amount for preoperative sedation?

    A. Midazolam orally 1.5 mg/kg
    B. Ketamine orally 2 mg/kg
    C. Clonidine orally 2 μg/kg
    D. Methohexital rectally 2.5 mg/kg
    E. Dexmedetomidine orally 20 μg/kg

27. Which statement(s) regarding mask induction of general anesthesia in pediatric patients is TRUE?

    A. A right-to-left intracardiac shunt quickens the rate of mask induction.
    B. Desflurane has an acceptable incidence of laryngospasm when used for mask induction.
    C. The incidence of bradycardia, hypotension, and cardiac arrest is highest in patients younger than 1 year of age.
    D. The minimum alveolar concentration (MAC) of sevoflurane is approximately 1.5% for young infants compared with 2% for adolescents and adults.
    E. All inhalational anesthetics impair cerebral autoregulation in children at any MAC.

28. Which statement(s) regarding airway management in pediatric patients is FALSE?

    A. With an uncuffed endotracheal tube, air should leak out at 20 to 25 cm H_2O.
    B. The narrowest portion of the pediatric airway is at the level of the cricoid cartilage.
    C. The appropriately sized endotracheal tube may be determined by comparison with the fifth digit.
    D. If a cuffed tube is used, the cuff pressure should not exceed 20 cm H_2O.
    E. The appropriate length of the tube from mid-trachea is calculated 5+ age in years.

29. Which of the following statements regarding regional anesthesia in pediatric patients is FALSE?

    A. The dural sac is at the S1 level at 1 year of age.
    B. The recommended dose of bupivacaine for a caudal anesthetic is 1 mL/kg of 0.175% solution.
    C. The sitting position facilitates free flow of cerebrospinal fluid (CSF) when placing a spinal block in neonates.
    D. A spinal anesthetic is contraindicated in preterm infants.
    E. A #20-gauge catheter is appropriate for caudal anesthesia in children over the age of 2 years.

ANSWERS

1. B. Two systematic reviews established that parental presence reduced the anxiety of parents but not the children. Children 1 to 6 years of age are those for whom parental presence may be most beneficial. Parents who are most insistent on being present at induction of anesthesia are often the most disruptive, least likely to calm their child, and actually provoke further noncompliant behavior in their child. If the parent is unable to cope with the OR environment or the child's loss of consciousness, he/she should not be present at their child's induction of anesthesia. (See page 1239: Preoperative Preparation: Anxioloysis.)

2. E. Children who have had a recent URI ideally should not undergo elective anesthesia for at least 4 weeks after the infection, to ensure resolution of the pathologic effects in the small airways. Since young children have 6 to 7 URIs per year, most clinicians proceed with anesthesia 2 to 4 weeks after the original infection. Additional factors that increase the risk of adverse airway events include cigarette smoking in the house, atopy, asthma, prematurity, young age, and secretions. In an infant (<1 year of age) presenting for surgery with a URI, there should be a low threshold for cancellation since perioperative respiratory complications in these infants are substantive. If the airway must be manipulated, a supraglottic airway is less likely to trigger airway reflex responses than a tracheal tube. Preoperative bronchodilator therapy should be administered to children with mild-to-moderate asthma even if they are not wheezing, as this reduces airway resistance by approximately 25% during sevoflurane anesthesia and tracheal intubation. If wheezing persists, the child should be referred to their pulmonologist for reassessment and the anesthetic deferred. (See page 1230: Preoperative Assessment: Medical Conditions.)

3. C. Children have obstructed airways during sleep that are associated commonly with hypercapnia and intermittent hypoxia. The gold standard for the diagnosis is a polysomnogram, although many children present for surgery with a diagnosis of OSA, but without a polysomnogram. In these cases, the diagnosis is made "clinically" by the presence of loud snoring, witnessed apneas, nocturnal enuresis, attention deficit disorder and behavioral problems, and inability to concentrate in school or poor school performance. OSA occurs equally in boys and girls. Daytime somnolence is not a feature in children with OSA. Although children with OSA may be premedicated with very small risk, those with nocturnal desaturation <85% are at increased risk for perioperative desaturation and airway events when the usual doses of opioids are administered. (See page 1230: Preoperative Assessment: Obstructive Sleep Apnea.)

4. B. Infants who were born prematurely (<37 weeks gestational age) and are <60 weeks postconceptual age require 12 to 24 hours of postanesthesia monitoring for apnea and hemoglobin oxygen saturation, irrespective of the type of surgery. Factors that increase the risk of perioperative apnea in ex-premature infants include age (<60 weeks postconceptual age), anemia (<12 g% Hb), and secondary diagnoses (e.g., intraventricular hemorrhage). Once the infant has been 12 hours apnea-free, he/she may be discharged home. In contrast to general anesthesia, regional anesthesia does not increase the risk of perioperative apnea and does not require prolonged perioperative monitoring unless the infant also received sedation, has multisystem disease, or a history of perioperative apneas. (See page 1230: Preoperative Assessment: Ex-premature Infants.)

5. E. It is currently the standard of care that healthy children undergoing elective minor surgery require no laboratory evaluation. Routine chest radiography and urinary analysis are also unnecessary. Commonly used coagulation screening tests, such as bleeding time and prothrombin time, do not reliably predict abnormal perioperative bleeding. (See page 1231: Laboratory Testing.)

6. C. Solids are prohibited within 6 to 8 hours, formula within 6 hours, breast milk within 4 hours, and clear liquids within 2 hours of surgery. Regardless of the length of fasting, a defined population of children is at an increased risk for aspiration of stomach contents: Those with delayed gastric emptying times and abdominal pathology. (See page 1230: Fasting Guidelines and Table 6.)

7. C. According to the ASA's practice guidelines for preoperative fasting, solids are prohibited within 6 to 8 hours of surgery, formula within 6 hours, breast milk within 4 hours of surgery, and clear liquids within 2 hours of surgery. Indeed, liquids such as apple or grape juice, flat cola, and sugar water may be encouraged up to 2 hours before the induction of anesthesia, because their consumption has been shown to decrease the gastric residual volume. (See page 1230: Fasting Guidelines and Table 6.)

8. B. The most common oral sedative premedication in the United States is midazolam. In a dose of 0.5 to 0.75 mg/kg, a 98% success rate of sedating children within 10 to 15 minutes occurs. Most premedications (including midazolam) do not delay recovery and/or hospital discharge for surgeries at least 30 minutes in duration. Some studies have combined oral midazolam and ketamine in a 50:50 mixture with good success. Oral ketamine as a sedative should be dosed at 5 to 6 mg/kg. (See page 1240: Pharmacologic Sedation.)

9. B. Both clonidine and dexmedetomidine take 60 to 90 minutes to affect sedation and anxiolysis. They may produce bradycardia and sedation that persist beyond the duration of the anesthetic. Compared with midazolam, the onset of action is slower and the duration is longer. (See page 1240: Pharmacologic Sedation.)

10. B. Dexmedetomidine is an α_2 agonist (as is clonidine) that has been used as on oral sedative for pediatrics. It has been effective in doses of 2 μg/kg orally. (See page 1240: Pharmacologic Sedation.)

11. D. A dose of 2 to 5 mg/kg of ketamine intramuscular yields a minimally responsive spontaneously breathing child in approximately 5 minutes. Planning for the management of oversedation, respiratory depression and increased secretions are important before the administration of ketamine. (See page 1240: Pharmacologic Sedation.)

12. B. Use of mask-inhaled anesthesia induction has several advantages over intravenous induction in children, particularly with potent, less soluble, and nonpungent agents such as sevoflurane. The agitation behaviors observed after rapid emergence from inhaled anesthetics (sevoflurane and desflurane) may be decreased using intravenous medications, including midazolam, ketorolac, fentanyl, propofol, and dexmedetomidine. The exact reason for this disturbance is not clear. (See page 1251: Emergence Agitation.)

13. B. When alcohol and NMDA receptor antagonists were noted to cause apoptosis (programmed cell death) in newborn rodents, investigators also discovered that most general anesthetics and sedatives cause apoptosis in newborn rodents and nonhuman primates. Most anesthetics, with the exception of xenon, dexmedetomidine, and opioids, cause apoptosis in newborn rodents and primates after relatively prolonged exposure (>12 hours). Brief anesthesia with ketamine (≤3 hours) or isoflurane (<2 hours) failed to induce neurocognitive dysfunction. Since most anesthetics in young children last less than 3 hours, these data may have limited external validity, at least in terms of humans. In addition, the doses of intravenous anesthetics and sedatives in rodents and primates are up to tenfold greater than in humans. Lastly, studies in humans who received anesthesia at a young age suggested that cognitive disability in those who received anesthesia before the age of 3 years may be more prevalent than in those who did not. (See page 1218: Apoptosis.)

14. B. Succinylcholine can be recommended only when ultrarapid onset and short duration of action are of paramount importance such as is laryngospasm. Its use is absolutely contraindicated in patients with muscular dystrophy, recent burn injury, spinal cord transaction or immobilization, as well as a family history of malignant hyperthermia. The need for succinylcholine has been decreased by the availability of fast-acting nondepolarizing agents such as rocuronium. (See page 1225: Neuromuscular blocking agents.)

15. C. PONV is particularly prominent after certain surgical procedures such as orchiopexy, strabismus surgery, and tonsillectomy. The type of anesthetic used for a particular surgical procedure also influences the incidence of PONV. No drug has been proven to be clearly superior for rescue. For instance, when propofol is used in place of inhaled

agents as the primary anesthetic for high-risk procedures, there is evidence that PONV is decreased. IV dexamethasone (0.0625–0.15 mg/kg; maximum 10 mg) and ondansetron (0.05–0.15 mg/kg) reduce the perioperative incidence of PONV by up to 80%. The incidence of vomiting increases with increasing age, peaking in children 10 to 16 years of age. Few children vomit in the PACU; most children who vomit, do so after ingesting their first fluids in the ward, in the car on the way home, or at home. Hence, it is appropriate to administer large volumes of IV fluids intraoperatively and in PACU (20–30 mL/kg), and recommend oral fluids only when the child requests to drink. (See page 1251: Vomiting.)

16. D. The hourly maintenance fluid requirement for a child who weighs less than 10 kg is 4 mL/kg. This child would have an hourly requirement of 40 mL (10 kg × 4 mL/kg). The fluid deficit is then calculated by multiplying the hourly fluid requirement by the time since the last oral fluid intake (40 mL × 10 hours = 400 mL). Generally, half of the total deficit (200 mL) is replaced in the first hour of the anesthetic, in addition to the scheduled fluid maintenance under anesthesia. Since the third-space and evaporative losses are minimal during eye surgery, the hourly intraoperative maintenance is approximately 4 mL/kg. Hence, approximately 240 mL should be given in the first hour. (See page 1245: Fluid Management.)

17. D. For the "first" 10 kg, the hourly fluid requirement is 4 mL/kg/hr. For the "next" 10 kg, it is 2 mL/kg/hr. For the "remaining" kilogram, it is 1 mL/kg/hr. Hence, the average hourly maintenance fluid requirement is 62 mL (40 + 20 + 2). (See page 1245: Fluid Management.)

18. D. The hourly maintenance fluid requirement for pediatric patients is 4 mL/kg for the first 10 kg plus 2 mL/kg for each kilogram between 11 and 20 kg, and 1 mL/kg for each kilogram over 20 kg. For the foregoing example with a 16-kg patient, this would be 40 mL/hr (first 10 kg) + 2 mL/hr × 6 kg = 52 mL/hr. (See page 1245: Fluid Management.)

19. C. MABL is estimated as follows:

$$MABL = \frac{EBV \times (\text{starting hematocrit} - \text{target hematocrit})}{\text{starting hematocrit}}.$$

In general, estimated blood volume (EBV) is 90 mL/kg for term infants, so the EBV = 4 kg × 90 mL/kg = 360 cc. Therefore:

$$MABL = 360 \text{ mL} \times \frac{32 - 24\%}{32\%} = 90 \text{ mL}.$$

(See page 1246: Blood Transfusion Therapy.)

20. D. For procedures that are likely to result in significant tissue trauma or blood loss, appropriate size IV access must be provided for transfusion of the blood and blood products needed for volume replacement. Packed red cells cannot be rapidly infused through either #24-gauge intravenous catheters or most peripherally inserted central catheters. A #22-gauge catheter is the smallest intravenous cannula through which blood can be infused rapidly. (See page 1246: Blood Transfusion Therapy.)

21. E.   All of the options are true regarding goal-directed fluid and blood component therapy for pediatric (and adult) patients. (See page 1245: Fluid Management.)

22. D.   Children with anterior mediastinal masses require general anesthesia and/or sedation for tissue (lymph node) biopsies, CT scan or MRI for diagnosis, or indwelling central line for chemotherapy. Children with these tumors present a significant risk for anesthesia, since cardiac arrest has been reported. Four tissues are typically found in anterior mediastinal masses in children: Lymphomas, teratomas, thymomas, and thyroid. The most rapidly growing tumor in the anterior mediastinum is the lymphoblastic T cell lymphoma, a nonHodgkins lymphoma. The decision to proceed with local, regional, or general anesthesia depends on the age and level of co-operation of the child, the extent of mediastinal organ compromise, and the accessibility of the node or tumor being biopsied. Those children who can tolerate the surgery under local anesthesia and sedation are managed in this manner. If the child cannot lie flat, anesthesia can be induced and the trachea intubated with the child positioned in the left lateral decubitus or less desirably, in the sitting position. The trachea should be intubated at induction of anesthesia to ensure a patent airway should it become necessary to turn the child prone because circulatory collapse occurs. Tracheal intubation is performed without muscle relaxation to preserve spontaneous respiration. Spontaneous respiration best preserves the negative intrathoracic pressure gradient to suspend the tumor above the mediastinal structures and avoid pressure on the pulmonary artery and right atrium as well as the tracheobronchial tree. (See page 1234: Anterior Mediastinal Mass.)

23. D.   Ketorolac is effective in the management of pediatric pain. Avoiding ketorolac in cases of underlying hemostasis disorders and nephropathies should not preclude its appropriate use in other aspects of pediatric pain management. Meperidine is no longer recommended as an analgesic because of the risk of seizures (from normeperidine) and the accumulation of normeperidine after repeated doses of meperidine. (See page 1228: Opioids.)

24. E.   The preparation for anesthesia recovery should be made before the procedure is begun. Children in the recovery phase may exhibit emergence agitation after a general anesthetic (more common after certain procedures such as strabismus surgery and a sevoflurane based anesthetic). Pediatric patients also exhibit a natural disorientation as they recover, so having a plan to soothe the child by having a parent available or adjuvant pharmacology is helpful. Nausea and vomiting should be expected after procedures associated with a higher-nausea risk, and the adjustment of anesthetic techniques used may decrease the risk. Analgesia preparations are also done by administering a customized anesthetic technique and having a recovery team that is familiar with managing pediatric patients as they recover from procedures and anesthetics. Having the child lie in the lateral decubitus position, neck extended with their mouth open is known as the "recovery position." In this position, oropharyngeal secretions, blood, or vomitus will drain onto the gurney rather than collect in the parapharyngeal region, and trigger upper airway reflex responses. The child is placed in this position after the anesthetic. (See page 1250: PACU Complications.)

25. B.   Infants who were born prematurely (<37 weeks gestational age) and are <60 weeks postconceptual, require 12 to 24 hours of postanesthesia monitoring for apnea and hemoglobin oxygen saturation, irrespective of the type of surgery. Factors that increase the risk of perioperative apnea in ex-premature infants include age (<60 weeks postconceptual age), anemia (<12 g% Hb), and secondary diagnoses (e.g., intraventricular hemorrhage). Opioids are best avoided in these infants and local anesthetic blocks are preferred. In contrast to general anesthesia, regional anesthesia does not increase the risk of perioperative apnea and does not require prolonged perioperative monitoring, unless the infant also received sedation, has multisystem disease, or a history of perioperative apneas. (See page 1232: Ex-premature Infants.)

26. C.   Midazolam is the most commonly used sedative premedication in the United States. It has rapid onset and predictable effect without causing significant cardiorespiratory depression. In an oral dose of 0.5 to 0.75 mg/kg, midazolam peaks approximately 30 minutes after administration, and its effect lasts approximately 30 minutes. Oral ketamine has been used as a sedative medication in doses of 5 to 6 mg/kg for children 1 to 6 years of age. Orally administered clonidine in a dose of 2 to 4 μg/kg has been demonstrated to cause sedation, decrease anesthetic requirements, and decrease the requirement for postoperative analgesics. Oral dexmedetomidine given at a dose of 2 μg/kg takes 60 to 90 minutes to affect sedation and anxiolysis; it produces bradycardia and sedation that persist beyond the duration of the anesthetic. Several regimens have been used for rectal induction, including methohexital 15 to 25 mg/kg. (See page 1239: Anxiolysis: Pharmacologic Sedation.)

27. C.   Mask induction of general anesthesia remains the most common induction technique for pediatric anesthesia in the United States. The incidence of bradycardia, hypotension, and cardiac arrest during mask induction is higher in infants younger than 1 year of age than in older children and adults. There is actually a small increase in MAC between birth and 6 months of age that represents the age of highest MAC. For sevoflurane, the change in MAC is marked, with a value of approximately 3.2% for young infants compared with 2.4% for young children. A right-to-left shunt slows the inhaled induction of anesthesia because the anesthetic concentration in the arterial blood increases more slowly. Desflurane has an unacceptable incidence of laryngospasm when used for inhalational induction. All inhalational anesthetics impair autoregulation, although sevoflurane does not significantly impair autoregulation in children ≤1.5 MAC. As in adults, hyperventilation restores autoregulation with isoflurane and sevoflurane. (See page 1220: Inhalational Anesthetics.)

28. E. The narrowest portion of the pediatric airway is at the level of the cricoid cartilage. Several formulas have been used for tube selection in children older than 1 year of age, the most common being (16 + age)/4. The size may also be estimated by comparing the size of the fifth digit or of a nostril. After the tube is in place, it should be checked to determine at what pressure air can escape around the tube. Air should leak out at no higher than 20 to 25 cm H_2O to minimize the risk of postextubation croup. Cuffed tubes may also be safely used in children by selecting a tube 0.5 mm smaller in internal diameter than the uncuffed choice. Care should be taken to check the pressure in the cuff to ensure that it does not exceed 20 cm H_2O. The length of a tube from the lips to mid-trachea in infants <1,000 g in weight is 6 cm; 1,000 to 3,000 g is 7 to 9 cm; in term neonates is 10 cm; and for infants and children, 10+ age (years) mm. (See page 1236: Induction of Anesthesia: Equipment.)

29. D. Spinal block is useful in preterm infants and neonates who require lower abdominal superficial surgery and wherein general anesthesia may worsen their underlying weaker respiratory status. When using bupivacaine for a caudal block, a 0.175% solution in a dose of 1 mL/kg is used, and if larger volumes are needed, 0.125% solution is recommended. When considering spinal anesthesia, it is important to note that the dural sac migrates cephalad during the first year of life, and in neonates, it is at S3; after age 1 year, it is at the S1 level. The sitting position may be especially helpful in neonates to maintain midline needle position and free flow of CSF. The catheter used for caudals is a #22 gauge for those ≤2 years or a #20 gauge for those >2 years. (See page 1247: Regional Anesthesia & Pain Management.)

CHAPTER 43

Anesthesia for Laparoscopic and Robotic Surgery

1. Robotic surgery improves upon conventional laparoscopy in all ways EXCEPT:

   A. Improved depth perception
   B. High-definition imaging
   C. Three-dimensional view
   D. Need for lower pneumoperitoneum pressures
   E. Intuitive instrument control

2. Robotic surgeries have disadvantages when compared to open procedures including:

   A. Use of the supine position
   B. Significantly prolonged operative time
   C. Longer hospital stays
   D. Higher rates of postoperative respiratory failure
   E. Limited application in most surgical subspecialties

3. Carbon dioxide is used to create a pneumoperitoneum rather than helium or nitrous oxide for all the following reasons EXCEPT:

   A. It is less soluble in blood.
   B. It is noncombustible.
   C. It has a larger margin of safety.
   D. It has decreased consequences if gas embolism occurs.
   E. It has a high capability for pulmonary excretion.

4. The standard of care for maximum intra-abdominal pressure to maintain during pneumoperitoneum is:

   A. 11 mm Hg
   B. 15 mm Hg
   C. 18 mm Hg
   D. 21 mm Hg
   E. 25 mm Hg

5. Which statement regarding the physiologic effects of laparoscopy is TRUE?

   A. They are well tolerated by all patients since the surgeries are noninvasive.
   B. The surgical procedure has little effect, because every procedure has the same level of pneumoperitoneum.
   C. It is simple to predict the effects.
   D. The anesthetic technique has the largest role in creating the physiologic effect.
   E. The physiologic effects depend on the interaction of many patient and surgical factors.

6. The cardiovascular changes of laparoscopy include:

   A. A decrease in systemic vascular resistance and a decrease in mean arterial pressure
   B. A decrease in systemic vascular resistance and an increase in mean arterial pressure
   C. No change in the systemic vascular resistance and an increase in mean arterial pressure
   D. An increase in systemic vascular resistance and no change in mean arterial pressure
   E. An increase in systemic vascular resistance and an increase in mean arterial pressure

7. Which of the following statements regarding the urinary system during laparoscopy is TRUE?

   A. Renal blood flow is increased.
   B. Urine output returns to normal around postoperative day number 2.
   C. The mechanical effect of the pneumoperitoneum is the only thing leading to the changes.
   D. The pneumoperitoneum causes neuroendocrine effects that help account for the changes.
   E. Urine output is usually maintained at normal rates.

8. Which of the following statements regarding the effect of laparoscopy on pulmonary function is FALSE?

   A. Total pulmonary compliance is unchanged.
   B. Higher peak airway pressures may be required.
   C. Functional residual capacity is reduced.
   D. The diaphragm is displaced.
   E. Patient positioning may lead to pulmonary changes.

9. How much does minute ventilation need to be increased to maintain normal $PaCO_2$s with carbon dioxide pneumoperitoneum?

   A. 20% to 30%
   B. 30% to 40%
   C. 40% to 50%
   D. 50% to 60%
   E. No change necessary

10. All of the following are reasons to minimize fluid in patients undergoing robotic prostatectomy EXCEPT:

    A. The head-down position can lead to facial edema.
    B. The long length of surgery increases laryngeal edema.
    C. Urine output is supranormal during this procedure.
    D. High urine outputs can interfere with the surgery.
    E. Traditional indicators of volume status are not reliable.

11. Which of the following statements regarding bradyarrhythmias during pneumoperitoneum is TRUE?

    A. Bradyarrhythmias rarely occur during laparoscopy.
    B. Bradyarrhythmias are caused by sympathetic output caused by peritoneal stretch.
    C. Bradyarrhythmias occurring during laparoscopy usually happen during deep anesthesia.
    D. Bradyarrhythmias during laparoscopy are benign and can be ignored.
    E. Bradyarrhythmias during laparoscopy are attributed to vagal tone following peritoneal stretch.

12. Treatment of hemodynamic dysfunction during laparoscopy includes all of the following EXCEPT:

    A. Release of the pneumoperitoneum
    B. Reducing the rate of fluid infusion
    C. Reducing the anesthetics
    D. Pharmacologic interventions aimed at correcting the problem
    E. Converting to an open procedure

13. Which of the following statements regarding subcutaneous emphysema is TRUE?

    A. Prolonged surgical time is not a risk factor for subcutaneous emphysema.
    B. The only way to diagnose subcutaneous emphysema is through rising ETCO$_2$.
    C. Immediate intervention is required once subcutaneous emphysema is diagnosed.
    D. Most subcutaneous emphysema resolves soon after the abdomen is deflated.
    E. All patients with the diagnosis of subcutaneous emphysema should have a chest x-ray postoperatively.

14. If a carbon dioxide embolism is suspected, in which position should the patient be placed?

    A. Left lateral decubitus with the head down
    B. Left lateral decubitus with the head up
    C. Right lateral decubitus with the head down
    D. Right lateral decubitus with the head up
    E. Trendelenburg

ANSWERS

1. D. Robotic surgery improves depth perception through high-definition, magnified, and three-dimensional view of the operative field, and provides intuitive instrument control that mimics natural hand and wrist movements, and eliminates surgeon tremor. The pneumoperitoneum necessary is the same for laparoscopic and robotic surgery. (See page 1258: Introduction.)

2. B. Robotic procedures can have significantly prolonged operative times and require patients be placed in extreme positions. Robotic surgery can be applied to virtually every surgical subspecialty (e.g., general, colorectal, head and neck, gynecologic, thoracic, and cardiac surgery). (See page 1258: Introduction.)

3. A. Laparoscopic procedures entail intraperitoneal insufflation of carbon dioxide (CO_2) to create a pneumoperitoneum that allows surgical exposure and manipulation. Carbon dioxide is used because it is noncombustible and more soluble in blood, which increases the safety margin, and decreases the consequences of gas embolism. Unlike nitrous oxide (N_2O), CO_2 does not support combustion and therefore, can be used safely with diathermy. Compared to helium, the high blood solubility of CO_2 and its capability for pulmonary excretion reduces the risk of adverse outcome in the event of gas embolism. (See page 1258: Surgical Techniques.)

4. B. It is standard of care to maintain the IAP below 15 mm Hg, because higher pressures can have significant physiologic consequences and can increase the incidence of intraoperative complications. (See page 1258: Surgical Techniques.)

5. E. The physiologic consequences of laparoscopy can be complex and depend on the interactions between the patient's pre-existing cardiopulmonary status and surgical factors such as the magnitude of IAP, degree of CO_2 absorption, alteration of patient position, and the type of surgical procedure. In addition, the anesthetic technique may influence the physiologic changes; however, these effects may be minimal with modern anesthetic technique. Of note, physiologic changes are well tolerated by most healthy patients; however, they could have adverse consequences in patients with limited cardiopulmonary reserve. (See page 1259: Physiologic Effects.)

6. E. The cardiovascular changes of laparoscopy include increases in systemic vascular resistance (SVR) and mean arterial pressure (MAP), which are caused by increased sympathetic output from CO_2 absorption and a neuroendocrine response to pneumoperitoneum. (See page 1259: Physiologic Effects, Cardiovascular Effects.)

7. D. The mechanical compressive and neuroendocrine effects of pneumoperitoneum may account for the reduc-

tion in renal blood flow, glomerular filtration, and urine output. However, the urine output generally normalizes following pneumoperitoneum deflation, with no consequent renal dysfunction. Nevertheless, there may be clinical implications in critically ill patients and those with renal dysfunction undergoing extensive laparoscopic procedures requiring prolonged pneumoperitoneum. (See page 1259: Physiologic Effects, Regional Perfusion.)

8. A. Changes in pulmonary function during laparoscopy include reduction in lung volumes and pulmonary compliance secondary to cephalad displacement of the diaphragm caused by increased IAP and patient positioning. Reduction in functional residual capacity (FRC) and total lung compliance results in basal atelectasis and increased airway pressures. In addition, the increase in minute ventilation required to avoid hypercarbia caused by systemic CO_2 absorption further increases peak airway pressures. (See page 1259: Physiologic Effects Respiratory and Gas Exchange Effects.)

9. A. The changes in pulmonary function (e.g., reduction in lung volumes, increase in peak inspiratory pressures, and decrease in pulmonary compliance) during laparoscopy may require intraoperative modification in mechanical ventilation. Typically, the minute ventilation needs to be increased by 20% to 30%, which could be achieved by increasing the respiratory rate while maintaining a constant tidal volume. (See page 1264: Anesthetic Management, Mechanical Ventilation.)

10. C. In patients undergoing robotic prostatectomy, fluid minimization is recommended, as steep head-down positioning for prolonged period may result in facial, pharyngeal, and laryngeal edema. Also, large fluid volumes can lead to high urine output and interfere with the surgical procedure. It is clear that traditional indicators used to guide fluid therapy (e.g., heart rate, arterial blood pressure, central venous pressures, and urine output) are not reliable. Urine output is reduced during laparoscopy, and its use to guide fluid therapy may lead to fluid overload. (See page 1264: Anesthetic Management, Fluid Management.)

11. E. Hemodynamic complications associated with laparoscopic procedures include dysrhythmias and alterations in arterial blood pressure (i.e., hypotension and hypertension). Bradyarrhythmias are attributed to increased vagal tone following peritoneal stretching, especially associated with "lighter" levels of anesthesia, while tachyarrhythmias may be due to hypercapnia as a result of intraperitoneal CO_2 insufflation. (See page 1266: Intraoperative Complications, Cardiopulmonary Complications.)

12. B. Treatment of hemodynamic dysfunction during laparoscopy should include confirmation that the IAP has not exceeded 15 mm Hg and that vascular injuries are ruled out, accompanied by supportive therapy including reduction in anesthetics, fluid administration, and pharmacologic interventions. In addition, hemodynamic instability in patients with a significant increase in SVR may require vasodilator therapy. After cardiopulmonary stabilization, cautious slow re-insufflation may be attempted using lower intra-abdominal pressures. However, with persistent signs of significant cardiopulmonary impairment, it may be necessary to convert to an open procedure. (See page 1266: Intraoperative Complications, Cardiopulmonary Complications.)

13. **D.**   Predictors of subcutaneous emphysema include operative time of greater than 200 minutes and use of 6 or more surgical ports. Subcutaneous emphysema is indicated by the development of crepitus. Increased CO_2 absorption may cause a sudden rise in $ETCO_2$. In most cases, no specific intervention is required and the subcutaneous emphysema resolves soon after the abdomen is deflated. However, if significant hypercarbia occurs despite aggressive hyperventilation, it may be necessary to temporarily deflate the abdomen to allow CO_2 elimination, followed by re-insufflation with lower IAP to prevent further extravasation of CO_2.

Development of late hypercarbia (i.e., in the recovery room) has been reported in patients with subcutaneous emphysema. Signs of hypercarbia in the postoperative period include somnolence, increased sympathetic output (i.e., increased heart rate and arterial blood pressure), and respiratory acidosis (and its consequences). If there is neck or face emphysema, a chest x-ray should be obtained in patients with cervical emphysema to "rule out" capnothorax or capnomediastinum. (See page 1266: Intraoperative Complications, Subcutaneous Emphysema.)

14. **A.**   If gas embolism is suspected, the abdomen should be deflated. Also, hyperventilation and rapid CO_2 washout should result in rapid absorption of the CO_2 embolus and facilitate reversal of hemodynamic impairment. In addition to aggressive cardiopulmonary resuscitation, the patient should be turned to the left lateral decubitus with a head-down position to allow the gas to rise into the apex of the right ventricle and prevent entry into the pulmonary artery. Hyperbaric oxygen and cardiopulmonary bypass have also been used to successfully treat symptomatic gas embolism. (See page 1266: Intraoperative Complications, Gas Embolism.)

Anesthesia and Obesity

1. Body mass index (BMI) is defined by which of the following?

A. Weight in pounds divided by height in inches
B. Weight in kilograms divided by height in square centimeters
C. Weight in pounds divided by height in square inches
D. Weight in kilograms divided by height in square meters
E. Weight in pounds divided by height in square centimeters

2. Which of the following statements regarding obesity is FALSE?

A. Visceral fat is particularly associated with cardiovascular disease and left ventricular dysfunction.
B. Morbid obesity is defined by a body mass index (BMI) above 40 kg/m^2.
C. Risks associated with obesity are related to the distribution of fat.
D. The effects of obesity are almost exclusively related to the cardiovascular system.
E. An android distribution is associated with increased oxygen consumption and increased incidence of cardiovascular disease.

3. Which of the following does not occur in obese patients?

A. Normal basal metabolic rate in relationship to body surface area
B. Decreased expiratory reserve volume and functional residual capacity (FRC) in the upright position
C. Normal closing capacity in the upright position, but abnormal in the supine position
D. Reduced chest wall and lung compliance
E. Normal lung compliance

4. Cardiovascular system changes that may occur with obesity include all of the following EXCEPT:

A. Mild-to-moderate hypertension
B. Accelerated increase in cardiac output in response to exercise or stress
C. Cardiomegaly with an elevated circulating blood volume
D. Impairment of diastolic function with elevated left ventricular end-diastolic pressure
E. Absence of accelerated atherosclerosis

5. Which of the following is FALSE?

A. Up to 50% of obese patients have clinically significant obstructive sleep apnea (OSA).
B. The apnea–hypopnea index qualifies the severity of OSA.
C. An apnea–hypopnea index of 10 signifies severe OSA.
D. Physiologic abnormalities from OSA include hypercapnia and pulmonary vasoconstriction.
E. Obesity hypoventilation (Pickwickian) syndrome occurs in up to 10% of morbidly obese patients.

6. Which of the following with respect to obesity and the gastrointestinal system and liver is FALSE?

A. There is delayed gastric emptying.
B. A positive correlation exists between obesity and esophageal erosions.
C. Weight loss does not significantly improve gastroesophageal reflux symptoms.
D. Fatty liver infiltrates of the liver are unlikely to result in significantly diminished capacity to metabolize drugs.
E. There is increased gastric acidity.

7. Which of the following statements regarding preoperative assessment of obese patients is TRUE?

A. Neck flexion may be compromised.
B. Serum evaluation of liver function studies for evidence of fatty liver infiltration is recommended.
C. Aspiration prophylaxis and antibiotic prophylaxis are not indicated.
D. Body mass index (BMI) correlates with the degree of difficulty of intubation.
E. Morbid obesity is not a risk factor for perioperative thromboembolic events.

8. Which of the following statements regarding anesthetic considerations for abdominal surgery in morbidly obese patients is FALSE?

   A. Invasive arterial pressure monitoring may be indicated for the super morbidly obese patient, even in the absence of cardiopulmonary disease.
   B. Supine positioning may cause ventilatory impairment and compression of the inferior vena cava and aorta.
   C. Prone positioning causes less respiratory compromise than the lateral decubitus position.
   D. Adequate preoxygenation is vital to preventing hypoxemia after loss of consciousness resulting from increased oxygen consumption.
   E. Positive end-expiratory pressure (PEEP) is the only ventilatory parameter that has consistently been shown to improve respiratory function in obese subjects.

9. Which of the following does not apply to the intraoperative anesthetic management of general anesthesia in obese patients?

   A. Consideration of an awake fiberoptic intubation should be given in all patients who meet the criteria for potential difficult intubation.
   B. Stacking is a useful positioning maneuver used to facilitate intubation.
   C. Myalgias are not frequently seen after administration of succinylcholine in morbidly obese patients.
   D. Smaller induction doses of medications are necessary in morbidly obese patients.
   F. Neck circumference is a good predictor of difficulty with intubation.

10. Which of the following statements regarding pharmacology in obese patients is TRUE?

   A. A drug that is mainly distributed to lean tissue should have the loading dose calculated on total body weight.
   B. Hyperlipidemia and an increase in concentration of α_1-acid glycoprotein may affect protein binding, leading to an increased free-drug concentration.
   C. Prolonged somnolence with thiopental is expected because of its highly lipophilic nature and large volume of distribution in obese patients.
   D. Prolonged somnolence with propofol is expected because of its highly lipophilic nature and large volume of distribution in obese patients.
   E. A normal prothrombin time with a prolonged partial thromboplastin time during orlistat treatment may reflect vitamin K deficiency.

11. Which of the following statements regarding the treatment of obesity is TRUE?

   A. The combination of phentermine and fenfluramine is a safe medical treatment for patients with a body mass index (BMI) above 30.
   B. Sibutramine inhibits the reuptake of norepinephrine to decrease appetite rather than increase satiety.
   C. Rhabdomyolysis occurs more commonly in morbidly obese patients undergoing open gastric bypass procedures compared with laparoscopic procedures.
   D. Bariatric surgery is considered the most effective treatment for morbid obesity.
   E. Lifestyle counseling is not an effective tool for long-term weight loss.

12. All of the following are true statements regarding intraoperative management of obese and morbidly obese patients EXCEPT:

   A. Operating room tables commonly have a maximum weight capacity of 200 kg.
   B. Obese patients are no more likely than nonobese patients to present with difficult mask ventilation and intubation.
   C. The head-up position provides the longest safe apnea period.
   D. Forearm measurements of blood pressure overestimate both systolic and diastolic blood pressure.
   E. Supine positioning causes ventilatory impairment and inferior vena cava and aortic compression.

ANSWERS

1. D. BMI is defined by weight in kilograms divided by height in square meters. (See page 1275: Definition and Epidemiology.)

2. D. Even modest obesity is associated with an increased risk of premature death or complications during the perioperative period. Visceral fat is particularly associated with cardiovascular disease and left ventricular dysfunction. Obesity and morbid obesity are associated with a BMI of 30 kg/m² or above and 40 kg/m² or above, respectively. Truncal distribution of fat, also called android distribution, is associated with increased oxygen consumption and an increased incidence of cardiovascular disease. Multiple physiologic systems are affected by obesity, such as the respiratory, cardiovascular, endocrine and metabolic, and gastrointestinal systems. (See pages 1275: Definition and Epidemiology, and 1276: Pathophysiology.)

3. C. In obesity, oxygen consumption and carbon dioxide production are increased, but the basal metabolic rate is normal because it is related to body surface area. A decreased expiratory reserve volume and a decrease in FRC occur in the upright position such that tidal volume may encroach upon the range of the closing capacity. This effect is exaggerated in the supine position. The results of this are ventilation–perfusion abnormalities, left-to-right shunting, and hypoxemia. Chest wall compliance is reduced in obesity, although lung compliance is unchanged. Respiratory functions, such as forced vital capacity, forced expiratory volume, and peak expiratory flows, are unchanged in obesity. As obesity increases, hypoventilation syndrome may occur. This is characterized by loss of hypercapnic drive, sleep apnea, hypersomnolence, and airway difficulties. This may progress to Pickwickian syndrome (hypercarbia, hypoxia, polycythemia, hypersomnolence, pulmonary hypertension, and biventricular failure). (See page 1276: Respiratory System.)

4. E. Arterial hypertension is associated with obesity. Mild-to-moderate hypertension with a 3- to 4-mm Hg increase in systolic and a 2-mm Hg increase in diastolic pressure occurs for every 10-kg weight gain. Cardiac output increases with exercise and stress. Cardiomegaly may occur, associated with an elevated circulating blood volume and cardiac output and hypertension. An accelerated increase in cardiac output occurs in response to exercise and stress in obese patients. Left ventricular wall stress leads to hypertrophy, reduced compliance, and impaired left ventricular filling (diastolic dysfunction) with elevated left ventricular end-diastolic pressure and pulmonary edema. Obesity accelerates atherosclerosis. (See page 1278: Cardiovascular and Hematologic Systems.)

5. C. Obese patients with upper airway obstructive syndrome can be classified into three categories: those with OSA, obstructive hypopnea syndrome, and upper airway resistance. Up to 50% of obese patients have significant OSA. OSA is defined as 10 seconds or more of total cessation of airflow five or more times per hour of sleep, despite continuous respiratory effort against a closed glottis in combination with a decrease in arterial oxygenation greater than 4%. The apnea–hypopnea index quantifies the severity of OSA. An index of above 30 signifies severe OSA, an index of 5 to 15 signifies mild OSA, and an index of 16 to 30 signifies moderate OSA. Physiologic abnormalities resulting from OSA include hypoxemia, hypercapnia, pulmonary and systemic vasoconstriction, and secondary polycythemia. These result in an increased risk of ischemic heart disease and cerebral vascular disease. Obesity hypoventilation (Pickwickian) syndrome results from long-term OSA and is seen in 5% to 10% of morbidly obese patients. It is a combination of obesity and chronic hypoventilation resulting in pulmonary hypertension and cor pulmonale. (See page 1276: Pathophysiology: Respiratory System.)

6. C. Gastric volume and acidity are increased, hepatic function is altered, and drug metabolism is adversely affected by obesity. Delayed gastric emptying occurs because of increased abdominal mass that causes antral distention, gastrin release, and a decrease in pH with parietal cell secretion. Weight loss significantly decreases gastroesophageal reflux symptoms. A positive correlation exists between obesity and frequent gastroesophageal reflux symptoms and erosions. Fatty infiltration of the liver reflects duration rather than the degree of obesity. Histologic and liver function abnormalities are seen in up to one-third of obese patients who have no evidence of concomitant liver disease, of which an increase in alanine aminotransferase is most frequently seen. No clear correlation exists between routine liver function tests and the capacity of the liver to metabolize drugs. (See page 1279: Gastrointestinal System.)

7. A. Evaluation of the airway is critical because of the numerous anatomic changes that could potentially result in difficulty intubating the obese patient. For example, flexion of the neck could result in difficulty because of excessive soft tissue. Submental fat may limit mouth opening. A large tongue, fleshy cheeks, redundant palate, and pharyngeal tissue may narrow the airway. However, BMI does not seem to have much influence on the difficulty of laryngoscopy. Neck circumference has been identified as the single best predictor of problematic intubation in morbidly obese patients. Liver function studies are not necessary, because they may not necessarily be indicative of fatty infiltration of the liver. Fatty infiltration of the liver reflects the duration rather than the degree of obesity. Despite histologic and enzymatic changes, no clear correlation exists between routine liver function tests and the capacity of the liver to metabolize drugs. All obese patients should receive aspiration prophylaxis and antibiotic prophylaxis. The incidence of wound infection is increased in obese patients. Morbid obesity is a known risk factor for perioperative thromboembolic events, including sudden death from acute pulmonary embolism. (See pages 1283: Preoperative Evaluation; 1279: Gastrointestinal System and 1283: Airway.)

8. **C.**   Invasive arterial pressure monitoring may be indicated for the super morbidly obese patient, not only for those patients with cardiopulmonary disease, but also for those patients in whom the noninvasive blood pressure cuff does not fit properly. Supine positioning causes ventilatory impairment and occlusion of the inferior vena cava and aorta. This may compromise venous return to the heart, with resultant hypotension. Prone positioning decreases functional residual capacity. In obese patients, care should be exercised to maintain freedom of abdominal movement and thus, prevent added detrimental effects on lung compliance, ventilation, and arterial oxygenation. Lateral decubitus positioning is favored over prone positioning whenever possible. Adequate preoxygenation is vital to prevent hypoxemia after loss of consciousness resulting from increased oxygen consumption. Positive end-expiratory pressure (PEEP), with or without recruitment maneuvers, is the only ventilatory parameter that has consistently been shown to improve respiratory function in obese subjects. (See pages 1285: Mechanical Ventilation and 1284: Intraoperative Considerations.)

9. **D.**   An awake fiberoptic intubation should be considered in all patients who are 75% over ideal body weight because of the greater incidence of difficulty with intubation. Neck circumference is the greatest predictor of problematic intubation. Myalgias are not frequently seen after succinylcholine administration in morbidly obese patients, so succinylcholine is acceptable to use for tracheal intubation. Stacking is a useful maneuver used to facilitate intubation so that the chin is at a higher level than the chest. The head-elevated laryngoscopy position (HELP) is a step beyond "stacking." The HELP position elevates the obese patient's head, upper body, and shoulders above the chest to the extent that an imaginary horizontal line connects the sternal notch to the external auditory meatus; this improves the laryngoscopy view. Larger induction doses may be required because obese patients have larger blood volumes, muscle mass, and cardiac output. Intra-arterial blood pressure monitoring may be necessary if proper fit of the blood pressure cuff is not possible. Profound muscle relaxation is important during laparoscopic bariatric procedures to facilitate ventilation and to maintain an adequate working space for visualization and safe manipulation of laparoscopic instruments. (See page 1284: Airway Management.)

10. **C.**   General pharmacokinetic principles dictate that drug dosing should take into account the volume of distribution for administration of the loading dose and the clearance of drug for the maintenance dose. A drug mainly distributed to lean tissues should have loading dose calculated on lean body weight. If a drug is equally distributed between adipose and lean tissue, dosing should be calculated based on total body weight. Hyperlipidemia and an increased concentration of α_1-acid glycoprotein may affect protein binding, leading to a decreased concentration of free drug. Prolonged somnolence may be expected with thiopental, because it is highly lipophilic and has a large volume of distribution in obese patients. Conversely, propofol is dosed as it is in nonobese patients; there is no difference in propofol's volume of distribution between obese and nonobese patients. Orlistat (OTC Alli, prescribed Xenical) or tetrahydrolipstatin, blocks the absorption of dietary fat by inhibiting lipases in the gastrointestinal tract. It leads to weight loss and improvement of blood pressure, fasting blood glucose levels, and lipid profile. A prolonged prothrombin time with a normal partial thromboplastin time during orlistat treatment may reflect vitamin K deficiency and this coagulopathy should be corrected 6 to 24 hours before elective surgery. (See page 1281: Pharmacology.)

11. **D.**   Medications used to treat obesity are formulated to decrease energy uptake, increase energy utilization, and decrease absorption of nutrients. The combination of phentermine and fenfluramine was popular until it became evident that it was associated with valvular heart disease and pulmonary hypertension. Sibutramine, a newer anti-obesity drug, inhibits reuptake of norepinephrine and increases satiety rather than decreasing appetite. It has no effect on release of serotonin, so it has not been associated with valvular heart disease. Bariatric surgery is the most effective treatment for morbid obesity. Procedures are classified as malabsorption, restrictive, or both. Malabsorption procedures (jejunoileal bypass and bilopancreatic diversion) are rarely used today. Restrictive procedures include vertical banded gastroplasty, adjustable gastric banding, and Roux-en-Y. Rhabdomyolysis is more common after laparoscopic procedures compared with open procedures. Long duration of surgery is a risk factor. Increased serum creatinine and creatinine phosphokinase or symptoms of buttocks, shoulder, or hip pain may be suggestive of rhabdomyolysis. (See page 1276: Management of Obesity: Medical Therapy.)

12. **B.**   Obesity may pose several challenges. Specially designed tables or two regular operating room tables may be required for the management of morbidly obese patients; regular operating room tables usually have a maximum weight limit of 200 kg. Obesity may cause a significant increase in oxygen consumption and cardiac output. The supine position causes ventilatory impairment and inferior vena cava and aortic compression in obese patients. Functional residual capacity (FRC) and oxygenation are further decreased with the supine position. Head-down positioning during laparoscopic procedures worsens FRC and should be avoided. The head-up position provides the longest safe apnea period during induction. Blood pressure measurements can be falsely elevated if the blood pressure cuff is too small. Cuffs with bladders, which encircle 75% of the entire upper arm, are preferable. Forearm measurements with a standard cuff overestimate both systolic and diastolic blood pressure. (See page 1284: Intraoperative Considerations Equipment and Monitoring.)

The Liver: Surgery and Anesthesia

1. All of the following statements regarding liver physiology are true EXCEPT:

   A. Hepatic blood flow equals approximately 100 mL/100 g/min.
   B. The hepatic artery supplies 25% of hepatic flow and nearly 50% of hepatic oxygen delivery.
   C. The liver generates approximately 25% of the body's lymph.
   D. The liver receives 25% of the cardiac output.
   E. The portal vein provides 75% of the total hepatic blood flow and 50% of its oxygen delivery.

2. All of the following are functions of the liver EXCEPT:

   A. Serving as a reservoir capable of accepting blood and then releasing it during periods of low blood volume
   B. Storing glucose as glycogen
   C. Synthesizing fats from proteins and carbohydrates
   D. 500 g/day of protein synthesis
   E. Toxic ammonia deamination

3. Which of the following blood clotting factors are not synthesized in the liver?

   A. II, III, and IV
   B. III, IV, and X
   C. III, IV, and V
   D. III, IV, and VIII
   E. I, II, and IV

4. Which of the following regarding bile is FALSE?

   A. Approximately 500 mL/day is produced by hepatocytes.
   B. The gallbladder holds 100 to 120 mL of bile in concentrated form.
   C. Cholestasis can result in steatorrhea and vitamin K deficiency.
   D. Cholecystokinin stimulates gallbladder contraction.
   E. Bile salts are needed for fat absorption.

5. Which of the following is true regarding laboratory evaluation of liver function?

   A. Aspartate aminotransferase (AST) is found in liver as well as nonhepatic tissues such as the heart, skeletal muscle, kidney, and brain.
   B. Fatty liver infiltration and chronic hepatic infections are associated with very high elevations in aspartate aminotransferase (AST) and alanine aminotransferase (ALT).
   C. The AST/ALT ratio is not helpful in differentiating alcoholic liver disease from viral liver disease.
   D. Serum alkaline phosphatase decreases with bile flow obstruction.
   E. Serum alkaline phosphatase is generated exclusively in the liver.

6. All of the following are true regarding hepatobiliary imaging EXCEPT:

   A. Plain radiography has a limited role in evaluation of hepatobiliary disease.
   B. Ultrasonography is the primary screening tool for hepatic disease, because it can penetrate air, allowing visualization of abdominal organs.
   C. Radioisotope scanning of the biliary tract remains an important tool in patients with suspected acute cholecystitis.
   D. Liver biopsy plays a key role in evaluation of otherwise unexplained abnormality of the liver enzymes in patients with or without hepatomegaly.
   E. Endoscopic retrograde cholangiopancreatography (ERCP) uses endoscopy to visualize the ampulla of Vater. It is the imaging technique of choice in patients with choledocholithiasis.

7. Features of acute liver failure include all of the following EXCEPT:

   A. It is defined as the appearance of encephalopathy with coagulopathy associated with liver dysfunction.
   B. Drug-related toxicity accounts for approximately 10% of acute liver failure.
   C. The illness has to be present for less than 26 weeks to be termed "acute."
   D. Acute liver illness may resolve spontaneously.
   E. Acetaminophen is the leading cause of drug-induced liver failure.

8. General measures to reduce cerebral edema include all of the following EXCEPT:

    A. Maintain the patient in 30-degree head-up position
    B. Maintain the head in neutral position
    C. Muscle relaxation for intubated patients
    D. Mannitol administration
    E. Impair venous return

9. Which of the following regarding acute hepatitis is FALSE?

    A. Diagnosis is made based on clinical signs and specific symptoms along with laboratory studies.
    B. Symptoms can include poor appetite and nausea.
    C. Signs can include a rash.
    D. The most common cause is one of the five identified viral hepatitides: A, B, C, D, and E.
    E. Hepatitis A is spread primarily through parenteral or mucosal exposure to infected blood or body fluids.

10. All of the following statements regarding massive hepatic necrosis after halothane exposure are true EXCEPT:

    A. The incidence of hepatic necrosis and death is 1 in 35,000 halothane anesthetics.
    B. Classic symptoms include fever, anorexia, malaise, rash, and subsequent jaundice.
    C. A proposed mechanism for halothane-associated hepatocellular injury is the combination of halothane degradation products and hypoxia.
    D. Prior exposure to halothane has no significance on the development of halothane hepatitis.
    E. Enflurane, isoflurane, and desflurane have been associated with inducing hepatic injury.

11. All of the following pregnancy-related conditions are common causes of liver disease in pregnancy EXCEPT:

    A. Hyperemesis gravidarum
    B. Intrahepatic cholestasis
    C. Preeclampsia
    D. Maternal–fetal blood Rh incompatibility
    E. Hemolysis, low platelet count, and elevated liver enzymes (HELLP syndrome)

12. The platelet range associated with mild HELLP syndrome (hemolysis low platelet count and elevated liver enzymes) is:

    A. 150,000 to 200,000/mm^3
    B. 100,000 to 150,000/mm^3
    C. 50,000 to 100,000/mm^3
    D. 25,000 to 50,000/mm^3
    E. <25,000/mm^3

13. Acute fatty liver of pregnancy is best managed by:

    A. Supportive measures
    B. Prompt delivery of the pregnancy
    C. Abdominal massage and manipulation
    D. Restriction of dietary fats
    E. Bed rest and intravenous hydration

14. What is the primary cause of thrombocytopenia associated with cirrhosis?

    A. Platelet consumption
    B. Reduction of thrombopoietin levels
    C. Bone marrow suppression
    D. Splenic sequestration
    E. Reduced levels of protein

15. Which of the following accurately describe the cardiovascular state of the cirrhotic patient?

    A. High cardiac output, high arterial blood pressure, and high systemic vascular resistance
    B. High cardiac output, low arterial blood pressure, and high systemic vascular resistance
    C. High cardiac output, low arterial blood pressure, and low systemic vascular resistance
    D. Low cardiac output, low arterial blood pressure, and high systemic vascular resistance
    E. Low cardiac output, low arterial blood pressure, and low systemic vascular resistance

16. Cirrhosis is characterized by:

    A. Normal platelet counts with impaired function
    B. Sodium wasting
    C. Autonomic dysfunction
    D. Preserved ability to increase cardiac output in response to exercise
    E. Normal procoagulant factors and impaired anticoagulant factors

17. With regard to hepatorenal syndrome, which has the longer untreated survival?

    A. Type 1
    B. Type 2
    C. Type 3
    D. Type 4
    D. Type 5

18. What is the accepted therapy for hepatorenal syndrome type I?

    A. Renal transplant
    B. Transjugular intrahepatic portal shunt
    C. Vasoconstrictors and intravascular volume expansion
    D. Lactulose
    E. Renal dialysis

19. What is the single best screening study for portopulmonary hypertension?

    A. CO diffusion imaging
    B. Pulmonary artery catheterization
    C. Epoprostenol trial
    D. Transthoracic echocardiography
    E. Chest CT Scan

20. Which of the following is NOT useful for reducing the production or increasing the excretion of ammonia?

    A. Neomycin
    B. Lactulose
    C. Metronidazole
    D. Rifaximin
    E. Protein restriction

21. In cirrhotic patients, albumin replacement therapy is generally recommended after how many liters of ascites drainage?

    A. 1 L
    B. 2 L
    C. 3 L
    D. 5 L
    E. 9 L

22. What is the normal range of the hepatic venous pressure gradient?

    A. 1 to 3 mm Hg
    B. 3 to 5 mm Hg
    C. 5 to 10 mm Hg
    D. 10 to 15 mm Hg
    E. 15 to 20 mm Hg

23. The acute management of acute variceal bleeding includes all of the following EXCEPT:

    A. Correction of coagulopathy
    B. Portal pressure reduction through pharmacology
    C. Endoscopic variceal ligation
    D. Volume resuscitation
    E. Maintaining hemoglobin above 12 mg/dL

24. Physical examination findings suggestive of active liver disease include all of the following EXCEPT:

    A. Spider angiomas
    B. Gynecomastia
    C. Ascites
    D. Testicular swelling
    E. Icterus

25. The medical optimization of cirrhotic patients undergoing surgery includes all of the following EXCEPT:

    A. Treatment of active infections
    B. Minimizations of vasoactive infusions
    C. Treating coagulopathy
    D. Allowing ascites to accumulate
    E. Optimizing central blood volume

26. What occurs to hepatic blood flow during neuraxial blocks above T5?

    A. It increases
    B. It decreases
    C. It remains unchanged

27. Which of the following volatile anesthetics is associated with the greatest decrease in hepatic blood flow at 1 MAC?

    A. Isoflurane
    B. Enflurane
    C. Sevoflurane
    D. Desflurane
    E. Isoflurane, enflurane, sevoflurane, and desflurane all equally affect hepatic blood flow at 1 MAC

28. How does one diagnose hepatic injury associated with volatile anesthesia?

    A. By identifying the rapid disappearance of bile ducts on fine-needle biopsies
    B. By trending serum alkaline phosphatase levels
    C. By correlating ultrasound to MRI imaging
    D. By exclusion of other causes
    E. By the appearance of microangiopathic hemolytic anemia

29. All of the following are factors of diminished clearance of pharmacologic agents by the failing liver EXCEPT:

    A. The increase in bile and bile salts
    B. Administration of drugs with extraction ratios greater than 0.7 during periods of low blood flow
    C. Administration of drugs with extraction ratios less than 0.3 during periods of low blood flow
    D. Administration of drugs with extraction ratios less than 0.3 during periods of low serum protein
    E. Administration of drugs intravenously in the setting of reduced plasma protein levels

30. Which of the following anesthetic induction agents have prolonged clearance times in cirrhotic patients compared to noncirrhotic patients?

    A. Ketamine
    B. Etomidate
    C. Diazepam
    D. Thiopental
    E. Propofol

31. In cirrhotic patients, what is the observed cardiovascular response to endogenous vasoconstrictors?

    A. It is exaggerated.
    B. It is diminished.
    C. It is unchanged.

32. All of the following are major indicators of intravascular albumin infusion in the treatment of cirrhotic patients EXCEPT:

    A. After paracentesis of more than 5 L
    B. Presence of spontaneous bacterial peritonitis
    C. Presence of hepatorenal syndrome type 1
    D. Presence of hepatorenal syndrome type 2
    E. With the goal prevention of renal impairment

33. All of the following can contribute to hepatic hypoxemia and postoperative jaundice EXCEPT:

    A. Pneumonia
    B. Polycythemia
    C. Hypoperfusion
    D. Fever
    E. Shock

ANSWERS

1. **C.**   Two large vessels, the hepatic artery, and the portal vein supply the liver. The liver receives approximately 25% of the cardiac output. Hepatic blood flow equals about 100 mL/100 g/min. The hepatic artery supplies 25% of the total hepatic blood flow but 50% of the oxygen supply. The portal vein supplies 50% of the oxygen supply and 75% of the total hepatic blood flow. The liver weighs approximately 1.4 to 1.8 kg, representing about 2% of the total body weight in adults. Since portal venous blood has already perfused the preportal organs, it is partially deoxygenated and is enriched with nutrients from the gastrointestinal tract. The liver generates approximately 50% of the body's lymph. (See page 1295: Hepatic Function in Health.)

2. **D.**   The liver has many physiologic functions, including regulation of blood coagulation, synthesis of hormones, erythrocyte breakdown, carbohydrate metabolism, lipid metabolism, amino acid metabolism, synthesis of proteins, and immunologic function. Due to the liver's ability to distend, it can accept or release blood, acting as a reservoir. The liver stores glucose as glycogen after hyperglycemia, after a carbohydrate meal. The liver synthesizes fats from protein and carbohydrates almost exclusively. The liver forms 15 to 50 g of protein per day and replaces the body's total protein content in several weeks. Ammonia is toxic and is deaminized in the liver. The liver inactivates corticosteroids, aldosterone, estrogen, androgens, insulin, and antidiuretic hormone. (See page 1295: Hepatic Function in Health.)

3. **D.**   All the blood clotting factors are synthesized in the liver with the exception of factor III (tissue thromboplastin), factor IV (calcium), and factor VIII (von Willebrand factor). (See page 1295: Hepatic Function in Health.)

4. **B.**   Approximately 500 mL of bile is produced per day and 35 to 50 mL of it is concentrated and stored in the gallbladder. When fat enters the duodenum, there is a release of the hormone cholecystokinin from the duodenal mucosa. Cholecystokinin causes the gallbladder to contract. Bile salts are needed for fat absorption and cholestasis can result in steatorrhea and vitamin K deficiency.

5. **A.**   Aspartate aminotransferase (AST) is found in liver as well as nonhepatic tissues such as the heart, skeletal muscle, kidney, and brain. Fatty liver infiltration and chronic hepatic infections are associated with mild (several fold) elevations in aspartate aminotransferase (AST) and alanine aminotransferase (ALT). The AST/ALT ratio is helpful in differentiating alcoholic liver disease in which the ratio is greater than 2, from viral liver disease in which the ratio is less than 1. Serum alkaline phosphatase increases with bile flow obstruction, and serum alkaline phosphatase may be generated from other tissues such as the placenta. (See page 1296: Assessment of Hepatic Function.)

6. **B.**   Plain radiography has a limited role in the evaluation of hepatobiliary disease. It is only useful for calcified or gas-containing lesions. Ultrasonography is the primary screening tool for hepatic disease, gallstones, and biliary tract disease. It is the best method for detecting gallstones and confirming extrahepatic obstruction. Its major limitations are its dependence on the operator's skill and its inability to penetrate bone and air, which may prevent complete examination of the abdominal organs. Radioisotope scanning of the biliary tract remains an important tool in patients with suspected acute cholecystitis. Radioisotopes that are cleared rapidly by hepatocytes and excreted into the bile permit rapid visualization of the biliary tract. This is helpful in diagnosing obstruction of the cystic duct. ERCP is the imaging choice in patients with choledocholithiasis. It uses endoscopy to visualize the ampulla of Vater and guide the insertion of a guidewire through the ampulla, permitting injection of contrast material into the pancreatic and common bile ducts. ERCP permits biopsy, brushing, balloon dilation, and stent insertion to relieve obstruction caused by tumors. Liver biopsy provides the only means of determining the precise nature of hepatic damage (necrosis, inflammation, steatosis, or fibrosis). It plays a key role in the evaluation of otherwise unexplained abnormalities of liver enzymes in patients with or without hepatomegaly. (See page 1297: Hepatobiliary Imaging and Liver Biopsy.)

7. **B.**   The most common causes for acute liver disease are drug toxicity and infection. Acute illnesses may resolve spontaneously, evolve into chronic disease, or result in acute liver failure. Acute liver failure is defined as appearance of encephalopathy together with coagulopathy in a patient without previous liver disease. Drug-related toxicity accounts for over half of the cases in the United States. Of these drug-related cases, over 80% are the result of acetaminophen ingestion. The illness has to have been less than 26 weeks in duration to satisfy the definition of acute liver failure. (See page 1297: Acute Liver Failure.)

8. **E.**   General measures to reduce cerebral edema include maintaining the patient in a 30-degree head-up position, and making sure the head is in neutral position so as not to impede venous return. Once a patient is intubated, muscle relaxants should be considered to minimize rises in intracranial pressure (ICP) from coughing, bucking, and shivering. Mannitol can be used to induce an osmotic diuresis, but may have limited utility in the patient with compromised renal function. (See page 1297: Acute Liver Failure.)

9. **E.**   The diagnosis of acute hepatitis is made on the basis of classic signs and symptoms, together with laboratory studies to assess liver damage and serologic assays. Symptoms can be nonspecific, such as fatigue, poor appetite, nausea, vomiting, and abdominal pain, and many infections are

subclinical. Signs may include jaundice, or a serum-sickness type presentation with fever, arthralgia or arthritis, and a rash that results from circulating hepatitis antigen–antibody complexes. Incubation periods can be several weeks to even months and patients may undergo surgery without awareness of illness. For this reason, viral hepatitis should be part of the differential diagnosis when there is any evidence of postoperative liver injury. The most common causes of acute viral hepatitis is, collectively, the five identified viral hepatitides: A (HAV), B (HBV), C (HCV), D (HDV or delta-virus), and E (HEV). HAV is spread primarily by the fecal–oral route or via contaminated food or water. (See page 1300: Acute Hepatitis.)

10. D. The incidence of fulminant hepatic necrosis and death associated with halothane is 1 in 35,000 anesthetics. The incidence of nonfatal hepatitis may be as high as 1 in 3,000 anesthetics. As a result of the National Halothane Study, the use of halothane dramatically decreased. Classic symptoms of volatile anesthetic-associated hepatitis include fever, anorexia, malaise, and rash. Jaundice appears 3 to 6 days later. The syndrome may occur after an uneventful anesthetic of short duration. Overt jaundice indicates severe disease and has a high mortality. The anesthetic agents enflurane, isoflurane, and desflurane have been associated with acute hepatic failure; however, the incidence of hepatitis attributed to them has been very small. (See page 1302: Drug Induced Liver Injury.)

11. D. Abnormalities in liver studies occur in 3% to 5% of pregnancies. Although many causes reflect underlying hepatic or biliary disease, the most common causes are one of five acute, pregnancy-related conditions: Hyperemesis gravidarum, intrahepatic cholestasis of pregnancy, preeclampsia, preeclampsia complicated by hemolysis, low platelet count and elevated liver enzymes (HELLP syndrome), and acute fatty liver of pregnancy. (See page 1303: Pregnancy-related Liver Diseases.)

12. B. Platelet count may be used to distinguish between mild, moderate, and severe HELLP(hemolysis, low platelet count, and elevated liver enzymes), with platelet counts of 100 to 150,000/mm³, 50 to 100,000/mm³, and <50,000/mm³, respectively. Severe HELLP syndrome is characterized by a platelet count of less than 50,000/mm³. Delivery of the pregnancy is the definitive therapy for HELLP syndrome. Up to 25% of patients may not present until the postpartum period. (See page 1303: Pregnancy-related Liver Diseases.)

13. B. Arrangements for rapid delivery should follow diagnosis of acute fatty liver of pregnancy, as recovery can only follow delivery. Recovery may be prolonged in patients who are severely ill upon presentation, and there is a role for transplantation in the patient who continues to deteriorate into acute liver failure after delivery. Acute fatty liver of pregnancy (AFLP) is the result of rapid microvesicular fatty infiltration of the liver, resulting in acute portal hypertension and encephalopathy. Although the exact mechanism of AFLP is unknown, there is an association

between it and abnormalities in the enzymes involved in β-oxidation of fatty acids. Symptoms of abdominal pain, nausea, headache, and vomiting, together with laboratory findings of elevated aminotransferases, bilirubin, and thrombocytopenia are similar to severe preeclampsia and HELLP syndrome. However, the AFLP patient additionally may have laboratory and clinical findings more unique to liver failure, such as hypoglycemia, elevated ammonia, asterixis, and encephalopathy. (See page 1303: Pregnancy-related Liver Diseases.)

14. D. Splenic sequestration is the primary cause of thrombocytopenia associated with cirrhosis. Thrombocytopenia is a well-known feature of cirrhosis. Estimates of incidence range from 30% to 64% of chronic cirrhosis patients, but platelet counts below 30,000/mm³ are rare. Since the liver is the primary site of thrombopoietin production, decreased levels of thrombopoietin contribute. Other factors include immunologic mechanisms, direct bone marrow suppression, and consumptive processes such as DIC. However, the primary cause is splenic sequestration in the setting of portal hypertension. Up to 90% of the platelet population may be sequestered in the spleen. Elevated levels of von Willebrand factor are felt to compensate for decreased platelet counts, augmenting the platelet–endothelial cell interaction on vessel walls. (See page 1304: Hemostasis.)

15. C. The cirrhotic patient typically has a hyperdynamic circulation, characterized by a high cardiac output, low arterial blood pressure, and low systemic vascular resistance. On examination, the patient is warm and appears well perfused despite systolic arterial pressures in the 80s and 90s. Although these patients have an elevated intravascular volume, this is not usually reflected in an elevated wedge pressure. This is due to sequestration of this volume into the massively dilated and collateralized splanchnic vascular bed, and the effective circulating volume is reduced. (See page 1305: Cardiac Manifestations.)

16. C. Autonomic dysfunction is a characteristic of the altered cirrhotic cardiovascular system. Chronotropic and hemodynamic incompetence in response to various challenges such as sustained handgrip, ice water hand submersion, Valsalva maneuver, and tilt table testing have demonstrated autonomic neuropathy in cirrhotic patients. In cirrhotic patients, platelet counts and function are diminished. Procoagulants and anticoagulants are synthesized in the liver and thus reduced in advanced liver disease. The hearts in cirrhotic patients have a diminished ability to increase cardiac output in response to exercise. The kidneys are characterized by sodium and free water retention in cirrhosis. (See page 1304: Cirrhosis and Portal Hypertension.)

17. B. There are two types of hepatorenal syndromes (HRS) described. Type 1 HRS is characterized by rapidly progressive renal failure with at least a doubling of serum creatinine over the course of 2 weeks in close proximity to a precipitating cause such as spontaneous bacterial peritonitis, sepsis, gastrointestinal bleeding, or surgical stress. Patients with type 1 HRS have a median survival of 2 to 4 weeks without therapy. Type 1 HRS is associated with failure of other organ systems and adrenal insufficiency. Type 2 HRS is more indolent. It may be a consequence of continuous and progressive activity of the circulatory homeostatic triad of the sympathetic, renin–angiotensin–aldosterone, and vasopressin systems, in an attempt to compensate for the progressive loss of effective circulating blood volume to the increasingly dilated splanchnic vasculature. Patients with type 2 HRS have a median survival of about 6 months. (See page 1306: Renal Dysfunction.)

18. C.   Vasoconstrictors and intravascular volume expansion are therapies for hepatorenal syndrome type I. Vasoconstrictors, such as arginine vasopressin (AVP) or its analogs, somatostatin or its analogs, and α-agonists such as norepinephrine and midodrine, combined with volume expansion have shown efficacy in reversing type 1 hepatorenal syndrome. Predictive factors of successful treatment include a starting creatinine <5 mg/dL, and a sustained rise in MAP from baseline throughout the 1- to 2-week course of treatment. More importantly, when therapy is withdrawn, recurrence is uncommon and occurs in <15% of patients. Liver transplantation is the definitive therapy for HRS. Placement of a transjugular intrahepatic portal shunt (TIPS) lowers portal pressures, and would be expected to decompress the splanchnic circulation, returning volume directly to the central circulation, but even when initially successful, there is a high rate of shunt stenosis and migration. (See page 1306: Renal Dysfunction.)

19. D.   Portopulmonary hypertension (PPHTN) is defined as pulmonary hypertension that exists in a patient who has portal hypertension with no other known cause. The single best screening study for PPHTN is the 2D transthoracic echocardiography (TTE). TTE allows estimation of RV systolic pressure (RVSP) by the velocity of the tricuspid regurgitant jet. Assuming no pulmonary arterial or valvular lesion, RSVP is a good estimate of pulmonary arterial systolic pressure. TTE also allows an estimation of CVP by caval changes with respiration, and evaluation of the RV for changes suggestive of elevated right-sided pressures such as RV dilation or hypokinesis, septal flattening, or moderate-to-severe tricuspid regurgitation. TTE screening has a sensitivity of 97% and a specificity of 77% in diagnosing moderate-to-severe PPHTN in patients undergoing pretransplantation workup. Right-sided cardiac catheterization is necessary, however, both to confirm elevated pressures and measure PVR. (See page 1308: Pulmonary Complications.)

20. E.   Hepatic encephalopathy (HE) is a serious reversible neuropsychiatric complication that is a feature of both chronic and acute liver disease. Its therapy is designed to either reduce the production of, or increase the excretion of ammonia. The nonabsorbable disaccharide lactulose has been the mainstay of therapy and remains the first-line drug for treating HE. Nonabsorbable antibiotics such as neomycin, metronidazole, and rifaximin are an alternative

to lactulose and work by inhibiting colonic growth of ammoniagenic bacteria. Although simple reduction in protein intake seems an intuitive solution, protein restriction may be harmful for cirrhotic patients who tend to have little nutritional reserve due to poor intake, and who have likely lost nutritional ground with every hospitalization. (See page 1309: Hepatic Encephalopathy.)

21. D.   Replacing albumin when ascitic fluid is drained is not well supported by randomized prospective trials. The reasons for using albumin replacement include preventing paracentesis-induced circulatory dysfunction, minimizing electrolyte disturbances, minimizing the nutritional impact of albumin loss, and preventing renal impairment. Current recommendations are that patients with drainage volumes <5 L do not need albumin replacement, and for larger volume paracentesis 6 to 8 g albumin/L may be considered. (See page 1311: Ascites.)

22. B.   A normal hepatic venous pressure gradient (HVPG) is 3 to 5 mm Hg. Patients with esophageal varices can be expected to have HVPGs of at least 10 to 12 mm Hg. Portal hypertension is diagnosed by measurement of the wedged hepatic venous pressure (WHVP). To correct for the contribution of increased intra-abdominal pressure from ascites, a free hepatic venous pressure or an inferior vena caval pressure should be subtracted from the measured WHVP to give the hepatic venous pressure gradient. (See page 1312: Varices.)

23. E.   Acute variceal bleed should be managed with a combination of volume resuscitation, correction of severe coagulopathy, pharmacologic manipulation of portal pressure, and endoscopic variceal ligation. Isolated volume replacement may lead to resistant or recurrent bleeding. The goal should be adequate resuscitation to maintain a hemoglobin level of 8 mg/dL and consideration of blood product transfusion to improve significant abnormalities in platelet count and INR. Elective intubation for airway protection is considered. Medications to reduce portal pressure include vasopressin and its analogs, and somatostatin and its analogs. Although β-blockers can reduce portal pressures, their effect on systemic pressures makes them undesirable in this setting. Early endoscopic variceal ligation in combination with pharmacotherapy is the preferred treatment for acute variceal bleed. (See page 1312: Varices.)

24. D.   Physical examination findings suggestive of active liver disease include icterus, palmar erythema, spider angiomas, gynecomastia, hepatosplenomegaly, ascites, testicular atrophy, petechiae, ecchymoses, and asterixis. (See page 1314: Hepatic Evaluation.)

25. D.   Medical management undertaken to optimize cirrhotic patients undergoing surgery should be directed toward treating active infection, minimizing vasoactive infusions, optimizing central blood volume and renal status while minimizing ascites, and improving encephalopathy and coagulopathy. However, there is little evidence to support specific goal-directed targets for preoperative care.

The perioperative risk depends more on the operative site and the degree of liver impairment than the anesthetic technique. (See page 1315: Perioperative Risk Associated with Liver Disease.)

26. B. Neuraxial blocks above T5 appear to reduce hepatic blood flow; this reduction in hepatic blood flow may not be reversed when block-related hypotension is corrected with catecholamines. (See page 1317: Selection of Anesthetic Technique.)

27. D. At anesthetic concentrations of 1 MAC, the listed volatile anesthetic agents produce very little reduction in hepatic blood flow except for desflurane, which appears to more substantially decrease hepatic blood flow at 1 MAC, causing a 30% reduction at this anesthetic depth. (See page 1317: Volatile Anesthetics.)

28. D. Since hepatic injury associated with volatile anesthesia does not have a pathognomic pathology, it is a diagnosis of exclusion. (See page 1317: Volatile Anesthetics.)

29. C. Bilirubin and bile acids can increase the unbound drug fraction by displacing drugs from protein binding sites. An increase in the free fraction of drug leads to enhanced effects and diminished hepatic clearance. The volume of distribution can increase with an increase in unbound drug. During periods of low hepatic blood flow, less amount of the circulating drug is remaining functional hepatocytes. The clearance of drugs with a low extraction ratio (less than 0.3) is influenced by hepatic enzyme induction, age, underlying type of hepatic pathology, and protein binding; however, it is not affected significantly by hepatic blood flow. Drugs with a high extraction ratio (greater than 0.7) have their clearance significantly affected by decreases in hepatic blood flow. (See page 1318: Pharmacokinetic and Pharmacodynamic Alterations.)

30. C. Benzodiazepines are an example of a drug with a low extraction ratio. As is commonly the case for drugs with low extraction ratios, the elimination half-life can be prolonged. As hepatic protein synthesis declines with advancing liver disease, the drug fraction bound to protein decreases. Since only the unbound drug is available for metabolism by hepatic enzymes, the elimination of benzodiazepines may be unaffected despite a reduction in intrinsic hepatic clearance. While ketamine, etomidate, propofol, and thiopental will have more pronounced pharmacodynamic effects, they are highly lipophilic and have high extraction ratios, and clearance is similar in cirrhotic to normal patients. (See page 1318: Pharmacokinetic and Pharmacodynamic Alterations.)

31. B. Patients with liver disease exhibit a reduced response to endogenous vasoconstrictors. This hyporesponsiveness to catecholamines may be modulated by the release of nitric oxide, prostacyclin, and other endothelial-derived factors in response to humoral and mechanical stimuli. (See page 1318: Vasopressors.)

32. D. In end-stage liver disease serum albumin function is quantitatively and qualitatively decreased. Albumin has three major indications in the treatment of cirrhotic patients: After large volume (5 L) paracentesis, the presence of spontaneous bacterial peritonitis to prevent renal impairment, and the presence of type 1 hepatorenal syndrome, where its use is beneficial in conjunction with splanchnic vasoconstrictors. (See page 1319: Volume Resuscitation.)

33. B. Hepatic hypoxemia can result from a number of causes including cardiopulmonary etiologies such as pneumonia, atelectasis, and heart failure. In addition, hypoperfusion (secondary to shock), anemia, or fever may provoke hepatic hypoxemia and postoperative jaundice. Surgery itself decreases hepatic blood flow. (See page 1320: Postoperative Liver Dysfunction.)

CHAPTER 46

Endocrine Function

1. Which of the following patients would not be hyperthyroid?

   A. A patient with elevated thyroxine (T_4) and elevated T_4-binding globulin levels
   B. A patient with elevated T_4 and elevated triiodothyronine (T_3)
   C. A patient with elevated T_4 and normal T_3
   D. A patient with elevated T_4 and low T_4-binding globulin
   E. A patient with normal T_4-binding globulin and elevated T_3

2. Which of the following statements regarding the uptake of radioactive iodine by the thyroid gland is FALSE?

   A. Radioactive iodine uptake (RAIU) is elevated in patients with hyperthyroidism.
   B. RAIU is decreased in cases of hyperthyroidism caused by thyroiditis.
   C. RAIU is increased by dietary deficiency of iodine.
   D. RAIU increases with corticosteroid use.
   E. No uptake of radioactive iodine may indicate thyroid malignancy.

3. Patients with mild to moderate hypothyroidism:

   A. Are at a significant risk of perioperative congestive heart failure
   B. Can be anesthetized safely without preoperative thyroid supplementation
   C. Should have urgent thyroid replacement before surgery if they have a history of coronary artery disease
   D. Are very sensitive to the effects of anesthetic drugs
   E. Are at a significant risk of postoperative ventilatory failure

4. Which of the following increases ionized serum calcium?

   A. Elevated serum albumin
   B. Alkalosis
   C. Acute hypomagnesemia
   D. Hypoparathyroidism
   E. Acute hyperphosphatemia

5. Regarding glucocorticoid physiology, which of the following statements is FALSE?

   A. Cortisol is the most potent endogenous glucocorticoid.
   B. Cortisol is the most potent regulator of adrenocorticotropic hormone (ACTH).
   C. The anti-inflammatory actions of cortisol relate to its effect in stabilizing lysosomes and promoting capillary integrity.
   D. Glucocorticoids facilitate free water clearance and stimulate hematopoiesis.
   E. Cortisol increases the killing potential of macrophages and monocytes.

6. Which statement about perioperative steroid replacement in patients who have received steroids is TRUE?

   A. Steroid replacement is not necessary with subarachnoid block or deep general anesthesia.
   B. Steroid replacement should always be given in supraphysiologic doses.
   C. Steroid replacement is not necessary if the patient is already steroid dependent.
   D. Steroid replacement in a low-dose regimen has been shown to be ineffective for most patients.
   E. There is no proven optimal regimen for steroid replacement in the perioperative period.

7. Which of the following statements regarding Conn's syndrome (primary hyperaldosteronism) is TRUE?

   A. It causes fatigue, hypertension, and hyperkalemia.
   B. Patients with Conn's syndrome have a high incidence of diastolic hypertension.
   C. Measuring plasma renin levels is not helpful in distinguishing primary from secondary hyperaldosteronism.
   D. Hyperaldosteronism is likely in edematous hypertensive patients with persistent hypokalemia.
   E. There is a decrease in renal sodium reabsorption.

8. Which of the following statements regarding pheochromocytoma is TRUE?

    A. Pheochromocytoma is a common adrenal cortical malignancy.
    B. Pheochromocytoma is a common cause of primary hypertension.
    C. Cardiovascular effects from pheochromocytoma are treated easily with deep anesthesia.
    D. Pheochromocytomas are not directly innervated, and catecholamine release is random.
    E. Pheochromocytoma is diagnosed easily and reliably by measurement of free catecholamines in the urine.

9. Which of the following statements regarding the perioperative anesthetic management of the patient with pheochromocytoma is TRUE?

    A. Patients who present with normotension do not require preoperative α-adrenergic blocking agents.
    B. Patients with pheochromocytoma who present with normotension typically need little medical management until the time of surgery.
    C. If α-adrenergic blocking agents have not been instituted before surgery, no special anesthetic induction technique is necessary.
    D. Although there is no clear advantage to one anesthetic technique over another, halothane should be avoided.
    E. Invasive monitoring is not required for patients whose blood pressures have been well controlled preoperatively.

10. Which of the following statements regarding type 1 diabetes mellitus is TRUE?

    A. Patients usually have normal insulin levels and significant insulin resistance in peripheral tissues.
    B. Patients are often treated with diet alone.
    C. Patients are frequently obese.
    D. Patients are prone to ketoacidosis.
    E. They may be effectively treated with oral hypoglycemic agents.

11. Which of the following statements regarding insulin is TRUE?

    A. The normal adult pancreas produces 200 to 300 U/day of insulin.
    B. The half-life of human insulin is 90 minutes.
    C. Hepatic dysfunction increases circulating insulin levels.
    D. Vagal stimulation decreases circulating insulin levels.
    E. α-adrenergic stimulation increases circulating insulin levels.

12. Regarding thyroid metabolism and function, which of the statements below is FALSE?

    A. Triiodothyronine (T_3) and thyroxine (T_4) are attached to the thyroglobulin protein and stored as colloid.
    B. Approximately 80% of T_3 is produced by the extrathyroidal deiodination of T_4.
    C. Most of the effects of thyroid hormones are mediated by the more potent and less protein-bound T_3.
    D. The half-life of T_3 is approximately 14 days.
    E. The degree to which T_3 and T_4 are protein bound in the circulation is the major factor influencing their activity and degradation.

13. Which of the following would be appropriate in the preoperative preparation of a patient with Graves' disease?

    A. Administration of potassium iodide for 7 to 14 days preoperatively
    B. A short-term course of thyroxine (T_4) supplementation
    C. Administration of propranolol for 1 month preoperatively
    D. Administration of propylthiouracil for 3 days preoperatively
    E. Radioactive iodine therapy is the recommended therapy for pregnant patients.

14. Which of the following statements regarding hyperparathyroidism is FALSE?

    A. Pregnant women with primary hyperparathyroidism should generally be treated with surgery.
    B. Treatment of hypercalcemia includes intravenous administration of normal saline and furosemide.
    C. Hypophosphatemia increases gastrointestinal absorption of Ca^{2+}, stimulates breakdown of bone, and impairs the uptake of Ca^{2+} by bone.
    D. The definitive diagnosis of primary hyperparathyroidism is made by RIA demonstration of an elevation in parathyroid hormone levels in the presence of hypercalcemia.
    E. Primary hyperparathyroidism is most commonly caused by a parathyroid carcinoma.

15. Which of the following statements regarding hypoparathyroidism is FALSE?

    A. The clinical features of hypoparathyroidism result from hypocalcemia.
    B. The cardiovascular manifestations are shortened QT interval and pericardial effusion.
    C. Neuronal irritability may cause seizures and muscle tetany.
    D. The Trousseau sign and the Chvostek sign are positive.
    E. Acute hypoparathyroidism may manifest as stridor or apnea.

16. Which of the following statements regarding mineralocorticoid physiology is TRUE?

    A. Angiotensin I is the most potent vasoconstrictor produced in the body.
    B. Angiotensin II directly stimulates the adrenal medulla to produce aldosterone.
    C. The renin–angiotensin system is the body's most important protector of volume status.
    D. Angiotensin I is altered enzymatically by converting enzyme primarily in the liver.
    E. Renin is the most potent mineralocorticoid produced by the adrenal gland.

17. Which of the following statements regarding Cushing's syndrome is FALSE?

    A. Most cases occur secondary to bilateral adrenal hyperplasia.
    B. Cushing's syndrome usually represents adrenal adenocarcinoma or a nonendocrine tumor when it occurs in older patients.
    C. Twenty-five percent of cases are caused by adrenal neoplasm.
    D. Cushing's syndrome may occur iatrogenically from steroid treatment of chronic illness.
    E. Most cases of Cushing's syndrome that occur spontaneously are associated with an anterior pituitary carcinoma.

18. Which of the following statements with respect to patients with Addison's disease is TRUE?

    A. The predominant cause of Addison's disease is autoimmune destruction of the adrenal gland.
    B. Patients with secondary forms of Addison's disease always have hyperpigmentation.
    C. Treatment includes replacement of mineralocorticoids and glucose.
    D. Diagnosis is confirmed by an increased adrenal response to adrenocorticotropic hormone (ACTH).
    E. Addison's disease results from an increased secretion of adrenal cortical hormones.

19. Which of the following statements regarding acute adrenal insufficiency is TRUE?

    A. It rarely, if ever, occurs in the perioperative period.
    B. Treatment consists primarily of fluid resuscitation.
    C. It usually requires continued steroid therapy for 4 to 6 weeks after the acute event.
    D. It may require the use of inotropes and invasive monitoring despite aggressive steroid treatment.
    E. It is rarely associated with physiologic stress.

20. Hypoaldosteronism:

    A. May be defined as failure to increase aldosterone production in response to adrenocorticotropic hormone (ACTH)
    B. Rarely occurs in patients with mild renal failure and long-standing diabetes mellitus
    C. Commonly presents with life-threatening hypokalemia and hypotension
    D. May be treated adequately with furosemide alone in patients with congestive heart failure
    E. Respiratory acidosis is frequently an early sign.

21. Which of the following statements regarding the preoperative preparation of a patient with pheochromocytoma is TRUE?

    A. Preoperative preparation is usually unnecessary if deep opioid anesthesia is planned.
    B. Phenoxybenzamine is a long-acting β-adrenergic blocker.
    C. Preoperative treatment usually is started with β-adrenergic blocking drugs to avoid reflex tachycardia when α-blocking drugs are added.
    D. Prazosin is a shorter-acting α-blocking agent that may be used in place of phenoxybenzamine.
    E. Prazosin is a noncompetitive presynaptic α_2- and postsynaptic α_1-blocker.

22. Which of the following statements regarding the pharmacologic therapy for pheochromocytoma is FALSE?

    A. Adrenergic blocking agents should not be given to pregnant patients.
    B. Acute hypertensive crises are best treated with short-acting drugs, such as sodium nitroprusside, esmolol, and phentolamine.
    C. Labetalol, a combination of α- and β-adrenergic antagonists, is an excellent second-line therapy.
    D. α-methyltyrosine is an agent used for reduction of catecholamine biosynthesis in situations in which surgery is contraindicated.
    E. The conversion of L-tyrosine to L-DOPA is the rate-limiting step in catecholamine biosynthesis.

23. All of the following are potential causes of diabetes mellitus EXCEPT:

    A. Cystic fibrosis
    B. Pancreatic surgery
    C. Pheochromocytoma
    D. Cushing's disease
    E. Addison's disease

24. Regarding treatment for diabetes, which statement is TRUE?

    A. Thiazolidinediones increase insulin secretion from the pancreas.
    B. Sulfonylureas inhibit β-cell insulin secretion.
    C. Amylin analogs suppress glucagon secretion and slow gastric emptying.
    D. Biguanides such as metformin decrease postprandial glucose absorption.
    E. Incretin mimetics increase insulin sensitivity.

25. All of the following options may be acceptable in the perioperative management of patients with diabetes mellitus EXCEPT:

    A. Maintain a continuous intravenous infusion of insulin.
    B. Give half the usual insulin dose preoperatively.
    C. Give insulin intraoperatively based on the level of measured glucose level.
    D. Do not give insulin.
    E. Routine administration of glucose containing intravenous fluids is recommended even if no insulin is administered.

26. Regarding anesthetic management of diabetes, which statement is FALSE?

    A. Sulfonylureas are known to have a cardioprotective effect.
    B. The "prayer sign" is associated with stiff joint syndrome and may predict difficult laryngoscopy.
    C. The standard glucose dosage for an adult patient is 5 to 10 g/hr (100–200 mL of 5% dextrose solution hourly).
    D. It is desirable to discontinue metformin preoperatively because it has been associated with severe lactic acidosis.
    E. Peripheral nerves are more vulnerable to pressure or stretch injuries.

27. Which of the following statements regarding nonketotic hyperosmolar coma is TRUE?

    A. Patients often present with extremely high blood sugar concentrations and volume overload.
    B. It usually occurs in "brittle" diabetics.
    C. Cerebral edema may result in delayed recovery of mental status.
    D. The mainstay of treatment is high-dose intravenous insulin by continuous infusion.
    E. Decreased plasma viscosity leads to increased surgical bleeding.

28. Which of the following statements regarding patients with diabetic ketoacidosis is TRUE?

    A. The serum potassium level will always be low.
    B. The total body potassium level will always be high.
    C. With appropriate treatment, the serum potassium level will tend to increase toward the normal range.
    D. All patients with ketoacidosis, except those with acute renal failure, should be given intravenous potassium supplementation.
    E. Acidosis causes a shift of potassium ions into the cells.

29. Concerning the anterior pituitary, which of the following is FALSE?

    A. About 20% to 30% of acromegalic patients are difficult to intubate.
    B. An unusually small epiglottis in a patient with acromegaly makes them more prone to aspiration.
    C. Impotence in men and secondary amenorrhea in women are early manifestations of panhypopituitarism.
    D. Sheehan's syndrome occurs after postpartum hemorrhagic shock.
    E. Vasopressin is secreted by the posterior pituitary.

30. Hypoglycemia in patients undergoing general anesthesia:

    A. Is diagnosed easily by recognition of the usual signs and symptoms
    B. Causes effects that may be misinterpreted as light anesthesia
    C. Rarely occurs in diabetic patients who receive insulin perioperatively
    D. Is rare in diabetic patients with renal insufficiency
    E. Is defined as a serum glucose level below 90 mg/dL

31. Which of the following statements regarding the posterior pituitary is FALSE?

    A. It is composed of terminal nerve endings that extend from the ventral hypothalamus.
    B. It secretes vasopressin.
    C. It secretes antidiuretic hormone (ADH).
    D. It secretes oxytocin.
    E. It secretes growth hormone.

32. Which of the following statements regarding vasopressin is TRUE?

    A. It promotes the reabsorption of sodium from the thick ascending limb of the loop of Henle.
    B. Serum levels decrease with increasing osmolality.
    C. It functions to relax vascular smooth muscle.
    D. It may increase circulating von Willebrand factor.
    E. It is released by the anterior pituitary.

33. Which of the following statements regarding diabetes insipidus is TRUE?

    A. It may occur after intracranial trauma.
    B. Urine output is highly concentrated.
    C. Symptoms include hyponatremia.
    D. There is an excessive secretion of antidiuretic hormone (ADH).
    E. It can be caused by elevated levels of vasopressin.

ANSWERS

1. A. Elevations in T_4-binding globulin concentration are the most common cause of hyperthyroxinemia in euthyroid patients. Elevations of T_4, T_3, or both in the presence of an elevated thyroid hormone–binding rate, all indicate hyperthyroidism. (See page 1328: Tests of Thyroid Function.)

2. D. Radioactive iodine is generally taken up by normally functioning thyroid tissue. Uptake is under the control of thyroid-stimulating hormone (TSH), and factors that decrease TSH, such as corticosteroid use, decrease RAIU. Hyperfunctioning thyroid tissue increases RAIU activity, but malignant or nonfunctioning tissue decreases RAIU. (See page 1328: Radioactive Iodine Uptake.)

3. B. Several studies have shown that patients with mild-to-moderate hypothyroidism may be anesthetized safely without preoperative supplementation and are not at an increased risk for perioperative complications. Patients with a history of coronary artery disease or unstable angina may have symptoms precipitated by supplementation with thyroxine, and replacement therapy should be delayed until the postoperative period. (See page 1331: Treatment and Anesthetic Considerations.)

4. C. Acute hypomagnesemia causes increases in parathyroid hormone release and serum ionized calcium. An increase in serum albumin levels increases the total serum calcium, as well as calcium binding, and subsequently results in a lowered free or ionized calcium level. Acute hyperphosphatemia and alkalosis lower ionized calcium. (See page 1331: Calcium Physiology.)

5. E. Actually, cortisol antagonizes leukocyte migration inhibition factor, thus reducing white cell adherence to vascular endothelium and diminishing leukocyte response to local inflammation. Phagocytic activity does not decrease, but the killing potential of macrophages and monocytes is diminished. Other diverse actions include the facilitation of free water clearance, maintenance of blood pressure, a weak mineralocorticoid effect, promotion of appetite, stimulation of hematopoiesis, and induction of liver enzymes. The anti-inflammatory actions of cortisol relate to its effect in stabilizing lysosomes and promoting capillary integrity. (See page 1334: Glucocorticoid Physiology.)

6. E. Since acute adrenal crisis is life threatening and there is relatively little risk in providing steroid coverage for isolated periods of stress, most clinicians empirically administer supplemental steroids to all patients who have received steroid replacement for 1 to 2 weeks during the previous 6 to 12 months. However, they may not be necessary in all cases. There is no proven optimal regimen for perioperative steroid replacement. A low-dose regimen (125 mg of hydrocortisone in 24 hours) has been shown to be equally effective compared with the more traditional use of supra-physiologic doses. (See page 1337: Steroid Replacement during the Perioperative Period.)

7. B. Possibly as many as 1% of unselected hypertensive patients have primary hyperaldosteronism (Conn's syndrome). The increase in renal sodium reabsorption and extracellular volume expansion is partly responsible for the high incidence of diastolic hypertension in these patients. Hypersecretion of the major adrenal mineralocorticoid aldosterone increases the renal tubular exchange of sodium for potassium and hydrogen ions. This leads to hypertension, hypokalemic alkalosis, skeletal muscle weakness, and fatigue. The diagnosis of primary or secondary hyperaldosteronism should be entertained in nonedematous hypertensive patients with persistent hypokalemia who are not receiving potassium-wasting diuretics. There is an increase in renal sodium reabsorption in these patients. The measurement of plasma renin levels is useful in distinguishing primary from secondary hyperaldosteronism. (See page 1336: Mineralocorticoid Excess.)

8. D. Pheochromocytoma is the only important disease process associated with the adrenal medulla. These tumors, which are not innervated directly, produce, store, and secrete catecholamines. Although pheochromocytomas occur in fewer than 1% of hypertensive patients, it is important to aggressively evaluate patients with clinically suspected symptoms, because surgical excision is curative in more than 90% of patients. Most deaths in patients with pheochromocytoma are from cardiovascular causes. Malignant spread occurs in approximately 10% of cases. The most common screening tests are measurements of catecholamine metabolites, vanillylmandelic acid, and unconjugated norepinephrine in the urine. However, urinary levels are not always elevated to a significant degree. (See page 1339: Pheochromocytoma.)

9. D. Occasionally, a patient with pheochromocytoma may present without hypertension. These patients are noted to be difficult to manage on an outpatient basis because of the fear of clinically significant orthostatic hypotension with α-blockade therapy. Because of the unpredictable and potentially lethal nature of the patient's response to the stress of anesthesia and surgery, all patients presenting for pheochromocytoma surgery should receive preoperative α-blocking therapy. When this is not possible, sodium nitroprusside infusions are often initiated in anticipation of the marked blood pressure elevations that may occur with laryngoscopy and surgical stimulation. Although there is no clear advantage of any one anesthetic technique, drugs that are known to liberate histamine should be avoided. Halothane should also be avoided because it sensitizes the myocardium to catecholamines and predisposes to ventricular irritability. Invasive monitors are used in most adult patients. (See page 1341: Perioperative Anesthetic Management.)

10. D. Diabetes is often divided into two broad types: Type 1, or insulin-dependent diabetes mellitus, and type 2, or non–insulin-dependent diabetes mellitus. Patients with type 1 diabetes typically experience the onset of disease in early life. Consequently, this form is also referred to as juvenile-onset diabetes. Generally, patients with type 1 diabetes are not obese, have an abrupt onset of the disease, and have very low levels of circulating insulin. Treatment of these patients requires insulin. Patients with type 1 diabetes are prone to becoming ketotic and are likely to develop end-organ complications of diabetes. (See page 1342: Diabetes Mellitus.)

11. C. Insulin is metabolized in the liver and kidneys. In patients with hepatic dysfunction, the loss of gluconeogenesis and the prolongation of insulin effect increase the risk of hypoglycemia. Normal production of insulin in adults is equivalent to 40 to 50 U/day. The half-life of insulin in the circulation is only a few minutes. Insulin release is related to a number of events. First, and most important, is the direct effect of glucose to stimulate insulin release. The mechanism involves interaction with hormones from the gastrointestinal tract released during enteral feeding. An increase in insulin release results from vagal stimulation. Insulin release is also caused by β-adrenergic stimulation as well as α-adrenergic blockade. (See page 1343: Physiology.)

12. D. The half-life of T_3 is 24 to 30 hours. The half-life of T_4 in the circulation is 6 to 7 days. After organification, monoiodotyrosine or diiodotyrosine is coupled enzymatically by thyroid peroxidase to form either T_3 or T_4. These hormones are attached to the thyroglobulin protein and stored as colloid in the gland. The release of T_3 and T_4 from the gland is accomplished through proteolysis from the thyroglobulin and diffusion into the circulation. Approximately 80% of T_3 is produced by the extrathyroidal deiodination of T_4, and 20% is produced by direct thyroid secretion. Most of the effects of thyroid hormones are mediated by the more potent and less protein-bound T_3. The degree to which these hormones are protein bound in the circulation is the major factor influencing their activity and degradation. (See page 1327: Thyroid Metabolism and Function.)

13. A. The combination of propranolol and potassium iodide every 8 hours for 7 to 14 days may be used to ameliorate cardiovascular symptoms and to reduce the circulating concentration of T_4 and triiodothyronine (T_3). Although propylthiouracil is also an effective treatment, it would require 6 to 8 weeks to render the patient euthyroid. Patients with Graves' disease already have elevated levels of T_4 and should not be given T_4 supplements. Radioactive iodine therapy is an effective treatment for some patients with thyrotoxicosis. However, it should not be administered to patients who are pregnant because it crosses the placenta and may destroy the fetal thyroid. (See page 1331: Treatment and Anesthetic Considerations.)

14. E. Primary hyperparathyroidism is most commonly caused by a benign parathyroid adenoma (90% of cases) or hyperplasia (9%) and very rarely by a parathyroid carcinoma. Primary hyperparathyroidism may also exist as part of a multiple endocrine neoplastic (MEN) syndrome. Hyperplasia usually involves all four glands. Although most patients with primary hyperparathyroidism have hypercalcemia, most are asymptomatic at the time of diagnosis. When symptoms occur, they usually result from the hypercalcemia that accompanies the disease. Primary hyperparathyroidism occurring during pregnancy is associated with a high maternal and fetal morbidity rate (50%). The placenta allows the fetus to concentrate calcium, promoting fetal hypercalcemia and leading to hypoparathyroidism in the newborn. Pregnant women with primary hyperparathyroidism should generally be treated with surgery. Emergency treatment of hypercalcemia is undertaken before surgery when the serum Ca^{2+} concentration exceeds 15 mg/dL (7.5 mEq/L). Lowering the serum Ca^{2+} concentration is initially accomplished by expanding the intravascular volume and establishing a sodium diuresis. This is achieved with the intravenous administration of normal saline and furosemide. (See page 1332: Hyperparathyroidism.)

15. B. The clinical features of hypoparathyroidism result from hypocalcemia. Neuronal irritability and skeletal muscle spasms, tetany, or seizures reflect a reduced threshold of excitation. The Chvostek sign is a contracture of the facial muscles produced by tapping the facial nerve. The Trousseau sign is contraction of the fingers and wrist after application of a blood pressure cuff inflated above the systolic pressure for approximately 3 minutes. Both the Chvostek sign and the Trousseau sign indicate hypocalcemia. The acute onset of hypocalcemia after thyroid or parathyroid surgery may manifest itself as stridor and apnea. (See page 1334: Clinical Features and Treatment.)

16. C. Angiotensin II, not angiotensin I, is the most potent vasopressor produced in the body. It directly stimulates the adrenal cortex to produce aldosterone. The renin–angiotensin system is the body's most important protector of volume status. The major regulators of aldosterone release are the renin–angiotensin system and serum potassium. The juxtaglomerular apparatus that surrounds the renal afferent arterioles produces renin in response to decreased perfusion pressures and sympathetic stimulation. Renin splits the hepatic precursor angiotensinogen to form the decapeptide angiotensin I, which is then altered enzymatically by converting enzyme (primarily in the lung, not the liver) to form the octapeptide angiotensin II. Aldosterone is the most potent mineralocorticoid produced by the adrenal gland. Aldosterone binds to receptors in the sweat glands, the alimentary tract, and the distal convoluted tubule of the kidney. (See page 1335: Mineralocorticoid Physiology.)

17. E. Cushing's syndrome may be caused either by overproduction of cortisol by the adrenal cortex or by exogenous glucocorticoid therapy. Most cases of Cushing's syndrome that occur spontaneously result from bilateral adrenal hyperplasia secondary to adrenocorticotropic hormone (ACTH) production by an anterior pituitary microadenoma. The primary overproduction of cortisol is caused by an adrenal neoplasm in 20% to 25% of patients. When

Cushing's syndrome occurs in patients older than 60 years, the most likely causes are adrenal adenocarcinoma or ectopic ACTH produced from a nonendocrine tumor. An increasingly common cause of Cushing's syndrome is the prolonged administration of exogenous glucocorticoids used to treat various illnesses. (See page 1335: Glucocorticoid Excess [Cushing Syndrome].)

18. **A.** Addison's disease results from a lowered secretion of adrenal cortical hormones. At present, the most frequent cause of Addison's disease is autoimmune destruction of the adrenal gland. Primary Addison's disease causes hyperpigmentation as ACTH levels increase in response to low cortisol levels. Secondary forms of the disease result from low levels of ACTH, and these patients never have hyperpigmentation. The diagnosis of primary adrenal insufficiency is unequivocally confirmed by the failure of the adrenal gland to respond to exogenously administered ACTH. Treatment of the disease involves glucocorticoid (e.g., prednisone or hydrocortisone) and mineralocorticoid (e.g., fludrocortisone) replacement. (See page 1336: Adrenal Insufficiency.)

19. **D.** Acute adrenal insufficiency is usually precipitated by sepsis, trauma, or surgical stress. Immediate therapy is mandatory regardless of the cause and consists of fluid and electrolyte resuscitation, and steroid replacement. Steroid replacement is continued during the first 24 hours, and if the patient is stable, the steroid dose reduction begins on the second day. If the patient continues to be hemodynamically unstable after adequate fluid resuscitation, inotropic support and invasive monitoring may be necessary. (See page 1331: Treatment and Anesthetic Considerations.)

20. **D.** Mineralocorticoid insufficiency may occur for various reasons and is commonly seen in patients with mild renal failure and long-standing diabetes. It results from a failure to increase aldosterone production in response to salt restriction or volume contraction. Most patients present with hypotension, hyperkalemia that may be life threatening, and metabolic acidosis (as a result of impaired sodium and potassium exchange). Patients may be treated with mineralocorticoid replacement. An alternative approach in patients with pre-existing hypertension or congestive heart failure involves administering furosemide alone or in combination with mineralocorticoid. (See page 1338: Mineralocorticoid Insufficiency.)

21. **D.** A dramatic reduction in perioperative mortality in patients undergoing surgery for pheochromocytoma has been achieved with the introduction of α-antagonists preoperatively. β-adrenergic blockade is often added after α-blockade has been established. β-blockers should not be given until adequate α-blockade is achieved to avoid the possibility of unopposed α-mediated vasoconstriction. Phenoxybenzamine is a long-acting, noncompetitive, presynaptic α_2- and postsynaptic α_1-blocker. Prazosin is a postsynaptic α_1-blocking agent with a shorter half-life than phenoxybenzamine. Both drugs have been used successfully in the preoperative preparation of patients

with pheochromocytoma. (See page 1336: Anesthetic Considerations.)

22. **A.** Acute hypertensive crises are best treated with intravenous infusions of short-acting drugs. These include phentolamine, nitroprusside, and esmolol. Labetalol is a β-antagonist with α-blocking activity that is an effective second-line medication. α-Methyltyrosine inhibits the enzyme tyrosine hydroxylase, which is the rate-limiting step in catecholamine biosynthesis. This medication is currently reserved for patients with metastatic disease and those in whom surgery is contraindicated. Unrecognized pheochromocytoma during pregnancy may be life threatening to the mother and the fetus. Although the safety of adrenergic blocking agents during pregnancy has not been established, these agents probably improve fetal survival. (See page 1336: Anesthetic Considerations.)

23. **E.** Diabetes can be a secondary result of a disease that damages the pancreas. Examples include pancreatic surgery, chronic pancreatitis, cystic fibrosis, and hemochromatosis. Diabetes may also result from one of the endocrine diseases that produce a hormone that opposes the action of insulin. Examples include glucagonoma, pheochromocytoma, and acromegaly. An increased effect of glucocorticoids from Cushing's disease or from steroid therapy may also oppose the effect of insulin and may thereby elicit clinical diabetes. (See page 1343: Classification.)

24. **D.** Whereas amylin analogs (pramlintide [Symlin]) suppress glucagon secretion and slow gastric emptying, incretin mimetics (exenatide [Byetta]), as the name implies, emulate natural incretin hormones (glucagon-like peptide 1, glucose-dependent insulinotropic polypeptide), increase insulin production, inhibit glucagon secretion, and decrease glucose absorption. Rosiglitazone (Avandia) and pioglitazone (Actos) are thiazolidinediones that increase insulin sensitivity. α-Glucosidase inhibitors (acarbose, miglitol) decrease postprandial glucose absorption. Metformin is a biguanide that decreases hepatic glucose output and enhances the sensitivity of both hepatic and peripheral tissues to insulin. Sulfonylureas (glyburide, glipizide, glimepiride) and glinides (repaglinide, nateglinide) enhance β-cell insulin secretion. (See page 1331: Treatment and Anesthetic Considerations.)

25. **E.** There is no consensus about the optimal way to manage perioperative metabolic changes in diabetic patients. For some diabetic patients, the best method of management is to not give insulin. For short procedures in nonstressed patients, particularly if they are not receiving insulin on a long-term basis, they may have enough endogenous insulin production to maintain a reasonable glucose balance in the unfed state. (See page 1347: Perioperative Glycemic Control.)

26. **A.** Laryngoscopy may be difficult in up to 40% of juvenile patients with diabetes mellitus presenting for renal transplantation. This may be because of diabetic stiff joint syndrome, a frequent complication of type 1 diabetes, leading

to decreased mobility of the atlanto-occipital joint. The "prayer sign," which is an inability to approximate the palmar surfaces of the interphalangeal joints, is associated with stiff joint syndrome and may predict difficult laryngoscopy. The standard glucose dosage for an adult patient is 5 to 10 g/hr (100–200 mL of 5% dextrose solution hourly). Fasting patients will not have postprandial hyperglycemia. Sulfonylureas should be held while the patient is NPO (nothing per mouth) to decrease the risk of hypoglycemia and because they interfere with the cardioprotective effect of ischemic preconditioning. Metformin should probably also be held, especially if there is a risk of decreased renal function because of a risk of lactic acidosis. Another area of patient monitoring that is extremely important in diabetic patients is positioning on the operating table. Injuries to the limbs or nerves are more likely in patients who arrive in the operating room already compromised by diabetic peripheral vascular disease or neuropathy. The peripheral nerves may already be partially ischemic and therefore more vulnerable to pressure or stretch injuries. (See page 1335: Anesthetic Management.)

27. **C.** An occasional elderly patient with minimal or mild diabetes may present with remarkably high blood glucose levels and profound dehydration. Such patients usually have enough endogenous insulin activity to prevent ketosis. Marked hyperosmolarity may lead to coma and seizures with increased plasma viscosity, producing a tendency to intravascular thrombosis. It is characteristic of this syndrome that the metabolic disturbance responds quickly to rehydration and small doses of insulin. With rapid correction of hyperosmolarity, cerebral edema is a risk, and recovery of mental acuity may be delayed after the blood glucose level and circulating volume have been normalized. (See page 1350: Hyperosmolar Nonketotic Coma.)

28. **D.** Potassium replacement is a key concern in patients with diabetic ketoacidosis. Because of the hyperglycemia-induced osmotic diuresis, the total body's potassium stores are reduced. However, acidosis by itself causes a shift of potassium ions out of the cell. Thus, the serum potassium concentration may be normal or even slightly elevated while the patient remains acidotic. As soon as the metabolic acidosis is corrected, the potassium ions shift back into cells. Consequently, the serum potassium concentration may decline acutely. Therefore, early and vigorous potassium replacement is required in these patients. (Patients with renal failure are an exception.) (See page 1350: Diabetic Ketoacidosis.)

29. **B.** Acromegaly in adult patients may pose several problems for anesthesiologists. Hypertrophy occurs in skeletal, connective, and soft tissues. The tongue and epiglottis are enlarged, making the patient susceptible to upper airway obstruction. The incidence of difficult intubation is 20% to 30%, and it may be clinically unpredictable. Impotence in men and secondary amenorrhea in women are early manifestations of panhypopituitarism. Panhypopituitarism after postpartum hemorrhagic shock (Sheehan's syndrome) is caused by necrosis of the anterior pituitary gland. Vasopressin (antidiuretic hormone) and oxytocin are the two principal hormones secreted by the posterior pituitary. (See page 1351: Anterior Pituitary.)

30. **B.** Hypoglycemia is the most feared clinical occurrence when dealing with diabetic patients and is almost impossible to diagnose in unconscious patients. With hypoglycemia, a reflex catecholamine release produces overt sympathetic hyperactivity, causing tachycardia, diaphoresis, and hypertension. In anesthetized patients, the signs of sympathetic hyperactivity can be misinterpreted as inadequate or light anesthesia. Hypoglycemia is more likely to occur in diabetic surgical patients with renal insufficiency in whom the action of insulin and oral hypoglycemic agents may be prolonged. An avoidable cause of inadvertent hypoglycemia is the administration of insulin to a patient who is not receiving sufficient caloric input. Clinically significant hypoglycemia is defined by Whipple's triad: (1) Symptoms of neuroglycopenia, (2) simultaneous blood glucose concentration <40 mg/dL, and (3) relief of symptoms with glucose administration. (See page 1351: Hypoglycemia.)

31. **E.** The posterior pituitary, or neurohypophysis, is composed of terminal nerve endings that extend from the ventral hypothalamus. The two hormones it secretes are vasopressin (also called ADH) and oxytocin. (See page 1352: Posterior Pituitary.)

32. **D.** Antidiuretic hormone (ADH, also called vasopressin because it constricts vascular smooth muscle) promotes reabsorption of free water by increasing the cell membrane's permeability to water. The target sites for ADH are the collecting tubules of the kidneys. The primary stimulus for ADH release is an increase in serum osmolality. ADH may also promote hemostasis through an increase in the level of circulating von Willebrand factor. (See page 1352: Vasopressin.)

33. **A.** Diabetes insipidus results from inadequate secretion of ADH. Failure to secrete an adequate amount of ADH results in polydipsia, hypernatremia, and a high output of poorly concentrated urine. This disorder usually occurs after destruction of the pituitary gland by intracranial trauma, infiltrating lesions, or surgery. (See page 1352: Diabetes Insipidus.)

CHAPTER 47

Anesthesia for Otolaryngologic Surgery

1. The most serious complication of tonsillectomy is postoperative hemorrhage. Approximately 75% of postoperative tonsillar hemorrhages occur within how many hours of surgery?

   A. 1
   B. 6
   C. 12
   D. 24
   E. 48

2. All of the following statements regarding emesis after tonsillectomy are true EXCEPT:

   A. It occurs in about 30% to 65% of patients.
   B. It may result from central stimulation of the chemoreceptor trigger zone.
   C. It is sometimes responsive to meperidine.
   D. It may be avoided by decompressing the stomach before extubation.
   E. It may be treated with 0.10 to 0.15 mg/kg of intravenous ondansetron.

3. All of the following statements regarding negative pressure pulmonary edema are true EXCEPT:

   A. It is associated with a decrease in pulmonary hydrostatic pressure.
   B. It is caused by the sudden relief of a previously obstructed airway.
   C. Intrapleural pressure in an obstructed airway may reach −30 cm H_2O.
   D. It may be prevented by the application of continuous positive airway pressure.
   E. It is associated with diffuse bilateral infiltrates on chest radiographs.

4. The most common cause of stridor in infants is:

   A. Peritonsillar abscess
   B. Foreign body obstruction
   C. Laryngomalacia
   D. Croup
   E. Epiglottitis

5. Regarding the pain associated with tonsillectomy, which of the following statements is TRUE?

   A. It is usually less severe when intraoperative hemostasis is achieved with laser and electrocautery rather than with sharp surgical dissection and ligation of blood vessels.
   B. It is usually less severe than after adenoidectomy.
   C. Its severity is often reduced when the peritonsillar space is infiltrated with local anesthetic.
   D. Its occurrence may be reduced with the intraoperative use of corticosteroids.
   E. It is usually related to underlying infection.

6. A Le Fort III fracture:

   A. Passes above the floor of the nose but involves the lower third of the nasal septum
   B. Crosses the medial wall of the orbit, including the lacrimal bone
   C. Passes through the base of the nose and the orbital plates
   D. Is a horizontal fracture of the maxilla
   E. Always involves a fracture of the cribriform plate of the ethmoid bone

7. A rigid bronchoscope with an internal diameter of 3 mm would have an external diameter of approximately:

   A. 3.5 mm
   B. 4 mm
   C. 5 mm
   D. 6 mm
   E. 7 mm

8. All are true for anesthesia for nasal surgeries EXCEPT:

   A. Detailed cardiovascular history during preoperative evaluation is imperative.
   B. Relative hypotension is desirable.
   C. Patient should be positioned in the reverse Trendelenburg position.
   D. Inhalation anesthesia clearly is preferable for maintenance of anesthesia.

9. All are true regarding anesthesia for ear tube insertions EXCEPT:

    A. It is commonly performed for chronic serous otitis in toddlers.
    B. It requires the creation of an opening in the tympanic membrane.
    C. Premedication with a short-acting benzodiazepine may prove useful.
    D. Cases are often performed in children despite concomitant symptoms of URI.

10. Which of the following regarding bronchoscopy is FALSE?

    A. Premedication with glycopyrrolate may be useful.
    B. The size of the bronchoscope selected is based on the external diameter of the tracheal tube.
    C. High fresh gas flow rates and a large tidal volume are typically used for ventilation.
    D. Typically the expiratory time is set higher than usual.

11. Which of the following regarding peritonsillar abscesses is FALSE?

    A. They are most commonly located below the laryngeal inlet.
    B. They usually do not interfere with ventilation by mask.
    C. They usually do not impair vocal cord visualization.
    D. They often require surgical intervention.

12. According to most guidelines, all of these patients undergoing adenotonsillectomy should be admitted for inpatient management EXCEPT:

    A. A 10-year-old child with Down syndrome
    B. A healthy 1-year-old child
    C. A 7-year-old child with a peritonsillar abscess
    D. A 15-year-old patient with a mild upper respiratory infection

13. Which of the following statements about middle ear surgery is FALSE?

    A. Patient positioning carries the risk of C1–C2 subluxation in the pediatric population as a result of laxity of the cervical spine ligaments.
    B. Maintenance of relative hypotension may be requested to reduce intraoperative bleeding.
    C. Nitrous oxide should be avoided during procedures involving tympanic grafts.
    D. Dissection during surgery carries the potential for injury to the third cranial nerve.

14. All are true about epiglottitis EXCEPT:

    A. It is caused by *Haemophilus influenzae* type B.
    B. Symptoms include sudden onset of fever, dysphagia, and a muffled voice.
    C. It is associated with a characteristic "steeple sign" appearance on radiologic examination.
    D. Treatment usually involves establishing a definitive airway.

15. All are true regarding laryngotracheobronchitis, EXCEPT:

    A. Symptoms usually include low-grade fever, inspiratory stridor, and a barking cough.
    B. It is associated with a characteristic "steeple sign" appearance on radiologic examination.
    C. It is caused by *Haemophilus influenzae* type B.
    D. Severe cases often respond to nebulized racemic epinephrine.

16. All are true regarding the use of laser for airway surgery, EXCEPT:

    A. The energy emitted by the CO_2 laser is absorbed by water in the tissues and blood.
    B. The CO_2 laser may cause retinal injury.
    C. The neodymium:yttrium-aluminum-garnet (Nd:YAG) laser has more limited penetrance than the CO_2 laser.
    D. Standard polyvinyl chloride (PVC) endotracheal tubes are flammable.

17. Findings in a patient with foreign body aspiration do not include which of the following?

    A. Refractory wheezing
    B. Stridor
    C. Tachypnea
    D. Fever
    E. Erythema

18. All are true regarding obstructive sleep apnea (OSA) syndrome in children EXCEPT:

    A. The STOP questionnaire can be used to screen patients.
    B. High BMI is a risk factor for developing OSAS.
    C. It may be associated with cardiovascular and hemodynamic comorbidities.
    D. It is a risk factor for metabolic syndrome.

19. Which of the following is true regarding jet ventilation?

    A. A continuous flow of oxygen is maintained under constant pressure.
    B. Oxygen–air mix is used as the carrier gas to drive gas flow.
    C. Inhalational anesthesia is used to maintain intraoperative anesthesia.
    D. Pneumomediastinum is a potential complication.

20. Which of the following is true regarding maxillofacial trauma?

    A. Anatomically, the angle of the mandible is least likely to fracture.
    B. Le fort 1 fracture is a pyramidal fracture crossing the medial wall of the orbit.
    C. It is associated with cervical spine injury, more common at C6–C7.
    D. Almost all high-impact injuries are associated with major additional injuries.

ANSWERS

1. B. Approximately 75% of postoperative tonsillar hemorrhages occur within 6 hours of surgery. Most of the remaining 25% occur within the first 24 hours of surgery, although bleeding may not be noted until the sixth postoperative day. About two-thirds of postoperative bleeding originates from the tonsillar fossa, 27% occurs in the nasopharynx, and 7% involves both regions. (See page 1357: Tonsillectomy and Adenoidectomy > Complications.)

2. C. The incidence of postoperative emesis after tonsillectomy is approximately 30% to 65%. The exact cause is unclear but is probably multifactorial. Potential causative factors include irritant blood in the stomach, impaired gag reflex resulting from inflammation and edema, and central nervous stimulation of the chemoreceptor trigger zone as a result of gastric distention. Management of postoperative nausea and vomiting commonly includes administration of ondansetron, dexamethasone, or both. The use of meperidine for postoperative pain control has been shown to exacerbate symptoms, especially in children. (See page 1357: Tonsillectomy and Adenoidectomy > Complications.)

3. A. Negative pressure pulmonary edema is a rare but serious condition caused by the sudden relief of a previously obstructed airway. Under normal circumstances, intrapleural pressures range from −2.5 to −10 cm H_2O during inspiration. In the presence of airway obstruction, the intrapleural pressure may reach −30 cm H_2O. Rapid relief of airway obstruction results in a decrease in airway pressure, an increase in venous return, and an increase in pulmonary hydrostatic pressure. The net result is the development of pulmonary edema. Mild cases may be asymptomatic. However, in serious cases, the condition is marked by the appearance of frothy pink fluid in the endotracheal tube, decreased O_2 saturation, wheezing, dyspnea, and tachypnea. A chest radiograph illustrating diffuse, usually bilateral, interstitial pulmonary infiltrates, combined with an appropriate clinical history, supports the diagnosis. (See page 1357: Tonsillectomy and Adenoidectomy > Complications.)

4. C. Laryngomalacia is the most common cause of stridor in infants. Laryngomalacia is most often secondary to a long epiglottis that prolapses posteriorly as well as prominent arytenoid cartilages with redundant aryepiglottic folds that obstruct the glottic opening during inspiration. Symptoms usually present shortly after birth. Peritonsillar abscess, foreign body obstruction, croup, and epiglottitis are also potential but less common causes of stridor in this age group. (See page 1363: Stridor, Table 47-2: Causes of Stridor, Table 47-3: Clinical component of the evaluation of patients with stridor.)

5. D. Pain after tonsillectomy is often severe in contrast to the minimal discomfort usually associated with adenoidectomy. An increase in pain medication requirements has been noted in patients in whom intraoperative hemostasis

is achieved using laser or electrocautery as opposed to sharp surgical dissection and ligation of blood vessels. Intraoperative administration of corticosteroids appears to be somewhat effective at reducing postoperative pain by decreasing edema formation. In contrast, injection of local anesthetic into the peritonsillar space has not been associated with a decrease in postoperative pain. (See Page 1357: Tonsillectomy and Adenoidectomy > Complications.)

6. C. The Le Fort III fracture parallels the base of the skull, passing through the base of the nose and ethmoid as well as the orbital plates. The Le Fort III fracture may, but does not always, involve fracture of the cribriform plate. In the course of his studies, Le Fort determined the common lines of fracture of the midface. The Le Fort I fracture is a horizontal fracture of the maxilla, passing above the floor of the nose but involving the lower third of the septum and mobilizing the palate, maxillary alveolar process, lower third of the pterygoid plates, and parts of the palatine bones. The Le Fort II fracture crosses the medial wall of the orbit, involving the lacrimal bone, passes beneath the zygomaticomaxillary suture, crosses the lateral wall of the antrum, and passes through the pterygoid plates. (See page 1369: Maxillofacial Trauma.)

7. C. Bronchoscopes are sized based on their internal diameter. Their external diameters are significantly greater than those of endotracheal tubes of similar size. Whereas the external diameter of a rigid bronchoscope with an internal diameter of 3 mm is 5 mm, the external diameter of a comparably sized endotracheal tube is 4.3 mm. (See page 1363: Bronchoscopy and Table 47-4: Comparison of external diameter of standard endotracheal tubes versus rigid bronchoscopy.)

8. D. Since current practice involves the instillation of vasoconstrictors that can be systemically absorbed, it is important to take a detailed preoperative cardiovascular history of coronary artery disease and arrhythmias. Systemic absorption of topical vasoconstrictors may exacerbate arrhythmias and cause hypertension. To achieve optimal visualization, bleeding is kept to a minimum by the use of vasoconstrictors and by maintaining relative hypotension. For the same reasons, the head is elevated at least 15 degrees during positioning to facilitate venous drainage. Many providers now prefer the use of TIVA since it has been shown to reduce blood loss and improve visualization better than inhalation anesthesia. (See page 1367: Nasal Surgery.)

9. C. Children with chronic and repeated attacks of serous otitis media may benefit from plastic tube placement in the middle ear to drain the accumulated serous fluid. This usually requires creation of a small opening in the tympanic membrane (myringotomy). This is a relatively short procedure and therefore premedication is not usually recommended because even short-acting sedatives can outlast the duration of surgical procedure. Most children with middle ear infection have concomitant upper respiratory infection (URI) and most of the times the eradication of middle ear fluid can resolve the URI. Based on clinical experience and current evidence, most practitioners do not recommend cancelling patients with concomitant URI, provided endotracheal anesthesia is not warranted. (See page 1361: Ear surgery > Myringotomy and Tube Insertion.)

10. **B.** An intravenously administered antisialagogue like glycopyrrolate as a premedication may be particularly useful to decrease secretions prior to bronchoscopy. This ensures that secretions in the airway do not compromise the view through the bronchoscope. While selecting a bronchoscope, it is the internal diameter which matters, and not the external diameter, because the external diameter may be significantly greater than an endotracheal tube of the same size. Typically, the ventilation of the patient through a bronchoscope requires high fresh gas flows and large tidal volumes along with high inspired concentrations of the inhalation agent to compensate for leaks around the bronchoscope. When using manual ventilation, it is imperative to ensure that the exhalation time is prolonged and adequate to allow enough time for the lungs to passively recoil fully and prevent air trapping. (See page 1363: Bronchoscopy.)

11. **A.** Peritonsillar abscess, previously known as quinsy tonsil, is a serious consequence of tonsillar infection and is usually located in the lateral pharynx above the glottis and laryngeal inlet. It does not typically interfere with mask ventilation or vocal cord visualization, and frequently requires surgical drainage. (See page 1357: Tonsillectomy and Adenoidectomy > Complications.)

12. **D.** According to most guidelines, patients who should be admitted to the hospital after adenotonsillectomy include children aged 3 years and younger, and patients with anatomic and medical conditions that may lead to increased risk of bleeding (e.g., abnormal coagulation profile, bleeding diathesis) or airway obstruction (e.g., craniofacial abnormality, achondroplasia, or Treacher Collins, Crouzon, Goldenhar, or Down syndrome). A patient for whom surgery is being performed because of the presence of an acute peritonsillar abscess, would also warrant postoperative inpatient monitoring. However, an otherwise healthy child older than 3 years of age with a mild upper respiratory infection need not routinely be admitted unless the patient did not meet discharge criteria in the recovery room. (See pages 1357: Tonsillectomy and Adenoidectomy > Complications and 1362: Table 47-1, Tonsillectomy and Adenoidectomy Inpatient guidelines.)

13. **D.** For middle ear surgeries, in order to gain access to the surgical site, the head is positioned on a rest which may be lower than the operative table. Further, extreme degrees of lateral rotation may be requested to facilitate surgical exposure which may produce tension on the heads of the sternocleidomastoid muscles. The laxity of the ligaments of the cervical spine, as well as immaturity of the odontoid process in children, make them especially prone to C1–C2

subluxation during these extremes of positioning. Bleeding must be kept to a minimum during surgery of the small structures of the middle ear, and maintenance of relative hypotension is often effective at minimizing bleeding. In addition, injection of concentrated epinephrine solution in the area of the tympanic vessels helps minimize bleeding by causing vasoconstriction. The middle ear and sinuses are air-filled, nondistensible cavities. An increase in the volume of gas contained within these structures results in an increase in pressure. Nitrous oxide diffuses along a concentration gradient into the air-filled middle ear spaces more rapidly than nitrogen moves out. During procedures in which the eardrum is replaced or a perforation is patched, nitrous oxide should be discontinued before the application of the tympanic membrane graft to avoid pressure-related displacement. Ear surgery often involves surgical dissection near the facial nerve (cranial nerve VII), thus placing it at risk of being injured if not properly identified and protected. Cranial nerve III, the oculomotor nerve, innervates the extrinsic muscles of the eye and is not encountered during typical dissections for middle ear surgery. (See page 1362: Middle Ear and Mastoid.)

14. **C.** Acute epiglottitis is most commonly caused by *H. influenza* Type B infection. Characteristic signs and symptoms of acute epiglottitis include sudden onset of fever, dysphagia, drooling, a thick muffled voice, and preference for the sitting position with the head extended and leaning forward. Retractions, labored breathing, and cyanosis may be observed when obstruction is present. If the clinical situation allows, oxygen should be administered by mask, and lateral radiographs of the soft tissues in the neck may be obtained. Thickening of the aryepiglottic folds as well as swelling of the epiglottis may be noted, producing a classic "thumb sign." In contrast, narrowing of the airway column producing the "steeple sign" on radiographic examination is seen in patients with laryngotracheobronchitis (croup). Management of epiglottitis involves establishing a definitive airway as soon as feasible, and the endotracheal tube chosen should be at least 1 size (0.5 mm) smaller than would normally be chosen. (See page 1364: Pediatric Airway Emergencies > Epiglottitis.)

15. **C.** Laryngotracheobronchitis, or croup, occurs in children 6 months to 6 years of age, where the child presents with low-grade fever, inspiratory stridor, and a "barking" cough. The onset is more insidious than that of epiglottitis. Radiologic examination confirms the diagnosis: A subglottic narrowing of the airway column secondary to circumferential soft tissue edema that produces a characteristic "steeple sign." It is usually viral in origin. Management includes cool, humidified mist and oxygen therapy usually administered in a tent for mild to moderate cases. More severe cases are accompanied by tachypnea, tachycardia, and cyanosis that may respond to racemic epinephrine administered by a nebulizer. (See page 1364: Pediatric Airway Emergencies > Laryngotracheobronchitis.)

16. **C.** CO_2 laser, the most widely used in medical practice, particularly in airway surgeries, emits energy which is absorbed by water contained in the blood and tissues.

Since human tissue is approximately 80% water, laser energy absorbed rapidly increases the temperature, thus denaturing protein and causing vaporization of the target tissue. Because of this absorption, the CO_2 laser does not penetrate deeply (0.01 mm) and may thus cause injury to the cornea, sparing the retina. The Nd:YAG laser, on the other hand, has a deeper penetration than the CO_2 laser and therefore caries the risk of retinal injury and scarring if misdirected. All standard PVC endotracheal tubes are flammable and may ignite and vaporize when in contact with the laser beam because of which specifically designed laser tubes are used to secure the airway. (See page 1366: Laser Surgery of the Airway.)

17. **E.**   Patients with foreign body aspiration may have coughing, choking, refractory wheezing, stridor, tachypnea, and fever. (See page 1364: Pediatric Airway Emergencies > Foreign Body Aspiration.)

18. **A.**   Adults with obstructive sleep apnea syndrome (OSAS) are usually screened prior to surgery by the STOP questionnaire to prevent airway obstruction during sleep. In children, the results of this questionnaire are not reliable and screening is more complicated. Increased Body Mass Index (BMI) is a predisposing physical characteristic that increases the risk of OSAS. Children with OSAS have cardiovascular and hemodynamic comorbidities that usually include an altered regulation of blood pressure and sympathetic activity. Pulmonary hypertension is also a well-described comorbidity. Obese children are more prone to develop a metabolic syndrome characterized by insulin resistance, dyslipidemia, and hypertension. (See page 1358: Sleep Disordered Breathing and Obstructive Sleep Apnea.)

19. **D.**   Jet ventilation involves intermittent bursts of oxygen delivered under pressure via a bronchoscope. Continuous flow of oxygen is not achieved during jet ventilation. Oxygen rather than oxygen–air mix should be used as the carrier gas to compensate for intermittent and suboptimal ventilation during jet ventilation. Inhalational anesthesia is best avoided because the delivery of the agent may be interrupted leading to varying anesthetic depths. Intermittent bursts of oxygen under high pressure coupled with inadequate exhalation may lead to rupture of alveolar blebs or bronchi causing pneumothorax or pneumomediastinum. (See Page 1363: Bronchoscopy.)

20. **C.**   The angle of mandible, ramus, and condyles are most susceptible to fractures as the cortex of the mandible is thinner on the posterior margin. The body of the mandible at the level of first molar is also a common site of fracture. Le fort I fracture is not a pyramidal fracture involving the orbit, rather a horizontal fracture of the maxilla passing above the floor of the nose. Current literature reports a 5.5% incidence of associated cervical spine injury, with the C6–C7 level being most commonly affected (50%), followed by C2 (31%). Current evidence suggests that high velocity, high-impact injuries are frequently associated with concomitant major and minor additional injuries other than maxillofacial trauma; however, the reported incidence is about 31% to 32% of each major and minor injury. (See page 1369: Maxillofacial Trauma.)

CHAPTER 48

Anesthesia for Ophthalmologic Surgery

1. When considering the anatomy of the eye, all of the following statements are correct, EXCEPT:

    A. The sphenoid and zygomatic bones are integral parts of the orbit.
    B. Blood supply to the eye is achieved by means of both internal and external carotid arteries.
    C. The iris dilator is sympathetically innervated while the iris sphincter is parasympathetically innervated.
    D. The trochlear nerve supplies the lateral rectus muscle.
    E. The motor innervation of the eye and its adnexa are supplied by the oculomotor, trochlear, abducens, and facial nerves.

2. Which of the following statements about aqueous humor is TRUE?

    A. It is entirely formed in the posterior chamber.
    B. The formation process entails active transport of sodium.
    C. Aqueous humor is iso-osmolar to plasma.
    D. Carbonic anhydrase is solely responsible for active secretion in the posterior chamber.
    E. Obstruction of venous return to the right side of the heart does not affect intraocular pressure (IOP).

3. Which of the following statements with respect to intraocular pressure (IOP) is FALSE?

    A. Once the globe is open to atmospheric pressure, increases in IOP are insignificant.
    B. Changes in venous pressure contribute more significantly to IOP than changes in arterial pressure.
    C. External pressure on the eye or extraocular muscle contraction, scleral rigidity, and changes in intraocular contents are important regulators of IOP.
    D. Balance between aqueous humor production and outflow is the most important determinant in maintaining IOP.
    E. Intravenous mannitol can be used to lower intraocular pressure.

4. Which statement regarding the relationship between intraocular pressure (IOP) and glaucoma is FALSE?

    A. IOP above 22 mm Hg is considered abnormal.
    B. Vomiting may increase the IOP by as much as 40 mm Hg.
    C. Open-angle glaucoma results from sclerosis in the trabecular system and responds to epinephrine and selective β-blockers.
    D. Closed-angle glaucoma is an acute process that responds well to atropine.
    E. Laryngoscopy and tracheal intubation may elevate IOP.

5. Which of the following statements regarding neuromuscular blocking drugs is FALSE?

    A. In contrast to depolarizing drugs, nondepolarizing neuromuscular blocking drugs lower intraocular pressure (IOP).
    B. Succinylcholine (Sch) causes an average increase in IOP of approximately 8 mm Hg.
    C. No technique consistently and completely blocks the ocular hypertensive response to Sch administration.
    D. Sch should be used only with extreme reluctance in any ocular surgery because of the high probability of causing eye injury.
    E. Sch causes an increase in IOP that dissipates within minutes.

6. Decreased intraocular pressure (IOP) is associated with all of the following EXCEPT:

    A. Sevoflurane
    B. Elevated body temperature
    C. Trimethaphan
    D. Sorbitol
    E. Glycerin

7. Which of the following statements regarding the oculocardiac reflex is FALSE?

    A. It may be triggered by pressure on the globe or a retrobulbar block.
    B. If the oculocardiac reflex occurs, the procedure may continue without pausing if the patient has been premedicated with an anticholinergic agent.
    C. The efferent limb is the vagus.
    D. Atropine premedication may have an abortive action on this effect.
    E. The oculocardiac reflex dissipates within seconds after cessation of eye manipulation.

8. Which of the following statements is TRUE?

   A. Treatment of patients with glaucoma with echothiophate poses minimal implications for general endotracheal anesthesia.
   B. Intraocular phenylephrine should be used with caution in patients with coronary artery disease.
   C. Cocaine used as a topical anesthetic in ocular surgery can lead to hypertension that is best treated by β-blockade.
   D. Cyclopentolate administration is associated with miosis.
   E. Intraocular sulfur hexafluoride administration requires minimal changes in the general anesthetic technique.

9. Concerns regarding sympathomimetics, anticholinergics and β-blockers used for intraocular surgery include all of the following EXCEPT:

   A. Adrenergic agents are associated with mydriasis.
   B. In patients with glaucoma, scopolamine should generally be used in lieu of atropine.
   C. Small amounts of intraocular phenylephrine may have deleterious systemic effects.
   D. Timolol may cause bronchospasm.
   E. Topical β-blockers should be used with caution in patients with congestive heart failure.

10. Regarding retrobulbar and peribulbar blocks, which of the following is TRUE?

    A. The oculocardiac reflex occurs solely with peribulbar block.
    B. It is not possible to anticipate the risk of global interruption during retrobulbar block.
    C. The onset of action for peribulbar block is quicker.
    D. There have been no reported cases of brainstem anesthesia with peribulbar block.
    E. When performing needle orbital blocks, the patient should be instructed to gaze in the opposite direction.

11. Which of the following techniques with regard to anesthetic considerations in ophthalmologic surgery is FALSE?

    A. MAC is a common technique and can be used in all adult eye surgeries.
    B. LMA is an acceptable method of airway management in patients without significant aspiration risk.
    C. Although a low risk procedure, standard ASA monitoring guidelines should be applied to the patient undergoing cataract surgery.
    D. Patients in which cough during extubation could be disastrous may benefit from intravenous lidocaine administration.
    E. Multimodal administration of antiemetics is often indicated in eye surgeries.

12. Which of the following statements regarding ocular injury is TRUE?

    A. Corneal abrasions are the most common cause of anesthesia-related ocular injury.
    B. Protective goggles need not be worn once the patient is anesthetized for laser surgery.
    C. Orange tinted protective goggles can be used with most laser devices.
    D. All antiseptics may be used to clean the periorbital area.
    E. Corneal abrasions are associated only with visual blurring.

13. Which of the following statements regarding postoperative blindness is FALSE?

    A. Retinal ischemia can be induced by an ill-fitting mask.
    B. Prolonged cases in the prone position have an associated risk of postoperative blindness as high as 1%.
    C. There is a strong male predominance associated with anterior and posterior ischemic optic neuropathy .
    D. All forms of postoperative blindness are irreversible.
    E. Risk factors for postoperative blindness may include type and duration of surgery, positioning, and fluid administration.

14. A 27-year-old man is brought to the emergency room after sustaining a motor vehicle accident. Massive bleeding and visible damage to the right orbit are noticed during assessment. Surgical intervention is mandatory. Which of the following statements is INCORRECT?

    A. Succinylcholine (Sch) may be safely used to secure the airway.
    B. Awake intubation is an acceptable alternative for securing the airway.
    C. Additional injuries (e.g., cranial fractures, airway injury) must be included in the anesthesia assessment.
    D. Retrobulbar block offers the advantage of local anesthesia without the need of airway manipulation, which could trigger increases in the intraocular pressure (IOP).
    E. Administration of intravenous lidocaine, 1.5 to 2 mg/kg before tracheal extubation may be helpful in attenuating coughing.

15. A 4-month-old boy is scheduled for elective strabismus corrective surgery. Which of the following statements regarding strabismus surgery in INCORRECT?

    A. Strabismus may be acquired secondary to cataracts.
    B. Succinylcholine may interfere with strabismus surgery.
    C. Patients with strabismus may have an increased risk of malignant hyperthermia.
    D. Nonsteroidal anti-inflammatory agents are reasonable to use in patients having strabismus surgery.
    E. If the oculocardiac reflex occurs during strabismus surgery it should be immediately treated with atropine.

ANSWERS

1. D. The walls of the orbit are composed of the frontal, zygomatic, greater wing of the sphenoid, maxilla, palatine, lacrimal, and ethmoid bones. Blood supply to the eye and orbit is by means of branches of both the internal and external carotid arteries. Venous drainage of the orbit is accomplished through the multiple anastomoses of the superior and inferior ophthalmic veins. Venous drainage of the eye is achieved mainly through the central retinal vein. All of these veins empty directly into the cavernous sinus. The covering of the eye is composed of three layers: The sclera, uveal tract, and retina. The sensory and motor innervations of the eye and its adnexa are as follows: A branch of the oculomotor nerve supplies a motor root to the ciliary ganglion, which in turn supplies the sphincter of the pupil and the ciliary muscle; the trochlear nerve supplies the superior oblique muscle; the abducens nerve supplies the lateral rectus muscle; the facial nerve supplies the frontalis and the upper eyelid orbicularis; and the lower branch supplies the orbicularis of the lower eyelid. (See page 1374: Ocular Anatomy.)

2. B. Two-thirds of the aqueous humor is formed in the posterior chamber by the ciliary body in an active secretory process involving both the carbonic anhydrase and the cytochrome oxidase systems. The remaining third is formed by passive filtration of aqueous humor from the vessels on the anterior surface of the iris. At the ciliary epithelium, sodium is actively transported into the aqueous humor in the posterior chamber. Bicarbonate and chloride ions passively follow the sodium ions. This active mechanism causes the osmotic pressure of the aqueous to be many times greater than that of plasma. Aqueous humor flows from the posterior chamber through the pupillary aperture into the anterior chamber, and then the aqueous flows into the peripheral segment of the anterior chamber and exits the eye through the trabecular network, the Schlemm canal, and the episcleral venous system. A network of connecting venous channels eventually leads to the superior vena cava and right atrium. Thus, obstruction of venous return at any point from the eye to the right side of the heart impedes aqueous drainage, elevating IOP accordingly. (See page 1375: Ocular Physiology.)

3. A. Increase in IOP pressure with an open globe can lead to prolapse of the iris and lens, and loss of vitreous. With chronic hypertension, adaptive compression of vasculature by the choroid as a result of increased IOP will reduce the afferent flow and serves as a feedback mechanism of establishing intraocular euvolemia. Scleral rigidity leads to decreased globe compliance and increased IOP. Likewise, hardening or enlargement of the lens can result in anterior displacement and narrowing of the trabecular meshwork, decreasing aqueous humor drainage. Anterior displacement is usually gradual although sudden displacement can lead to acute-angle closure glaucoma. Balance between production and outflow of aqueous humor is the most important determinant of IOP by the formula IOP = K $[(O_{Paq} - O_{Ppl}) + CP]$, where K is the coefficient of outflow, O_{Paq} is the osmotic pressure of aqueous humor, O_{Ppl} is the osmotic pressure of plasma, and CP is the capillary pressure. Mannitol augments the intravascular oncotic pressure and decreases aqueous humor production and thus the IOP. Dehydration can be adventitious as it increases plasma oncotic pressure and decreases intravascular volume, both of which reduce IOP. Similarly, mydriasis is generally avoided as it affects aqueous humor outflow. (See page 1376: Maintenance of Intraocular Pressure and Figure 51-1.)

4. D. IOP normally varies between 10 and 22 mm Hg. IOP exceeds not only tissue pressure by 2 to 3 mm Hg but also intracranial pressure by as much as 7 to 8 mm Hg. Straining, vomiting, or coughing may increase IOP by as much as 40 mm Hg. Three main factors influence IOP: External pressure on the eye by the contraction of the orbicularis oculi muscle and the tone of the extraocular muscles, venous congestion of orbital veins (as may occur with vomiting and coughing), and changes in intraocular contents (lens, vitreous, intraocular tumor, blood, or aqueous humor). Laryngoscopy and tracheal intubation may also elevate IOP, even without any visible reaction to intubation, although the effect is exaggerated when the patient coughs. Topical anesthetization of the larynx may attenuate the hypertensive response to laryngoscopy, but it does not reliably prevent associated increases in IOP. With open-angle glaucoma, the elevated IOP exists with an anatomically open anterior chamber angle; it is thought that sclerosis of trabecular tissue results in impaired aqueous filtration and drainage. Treatment consists of medication to produce miosis and trabecular stretching. Closed-angle glaucoma is characterized by movement of the peripheral iris into direct contact with the posterior corneal surface, mechanically obstructing aqueous outflow. Atropine premedication in the dose range used clinically has no effect on IOP in either open- or closed-angle glaucoma. (See page 1376: Maintenance of Intraocular Pressure.)

5. D. Neuromuscular blocking drugs have both direct and indirect actions on IOP. If paralysis of the respiratory muscles is accompanied by alveolar hypoventilation, the latter secondary effect may supervene to increase IOP. In contrast to nondepolarizing drugs, the depolarizing drug Sch elevates IOP by an average of 8 mm Hg. Changes in extraocular muscle tone do not contribute significantly to the increase in IOP observed after Sch administration. Various methods have been advocated to prevent Sch-induced elevations in IOP. Although some attenuation of the increase results, no technique consistently and completely blocks the ocular hypertensive response. The efficacy of pretreatment with nondepolarizing drugs is controversial. Sch, if unaccompanied by pretreatment with a nondepolarizing neuromuscular blocking drug, is relatively contraindicated in patients with penetrating ocular wounds and should not be given for the first time after the eye has been opened. Nonetheless, it no longer is valid to recommend that Sch be used only with extreme reluctance in ocular surgery. Clearly, any Sch-induced increment in IOP is usually dissipated before surgery is started. (See page 1378: Neuromuscular Blocking Drugs.)

6. **B.**   Hypoventilation, as well as administration of carbon dioxide, elevates IOP. Virtually all central nervous system depressants, including neuroleptics, opioids, and induction agents (e.g., barbiturates, etomidate, and propofol) lower IOP. Inhalation anesthetics reportedly cause dose-related decreases in IOP. Hypothermia lowers IOP. On initial consideration, hypothermia may be expected to increase IOP because of the associated increase in viscosity of aqueous humor. However, hypothermia is linked with decreased formation of aqueous humor and with vasoconstriction; the net result is a reduction in IOP. Ganglionic blockers such as trimethaphan significantly lower IOP in normal subjects despite mydriasis. Intravenous administration of hypertonic solutions such as dextran, urea, mannitol, and sorbitol elevate plasma osmotic pressure, decreasing aqueous humor formation and reducing IOP. Glycerin decreases IOP, although it is less predictable than mannitol. (See page 1377: Effects of Anesthesia and Adjuvant Drugs on Intraocular Pressure.)

7. **B.**   The oculocardiac reflex is triggered by pressure on the globe and traction on the extraocular muscles, the conjunctiva, or the orbital structures. The reflex may also be elicited by performance of a retrobulbar block. Although the most common manifestation of the oculocardiac reflex is sinus bradycardia, a wide spectrum of cardiac dysrhythmias may occur, including junctional rhythm, ectopic atrial rhythm, atrioventricular blockade, ventricular bigeminy, multifocal premature ventricular contractions, wandering pacemaker, idioventricular rhythm, asystole, and ventricular tachycardia. Hypercarbia and hypoxemia are thought to augment the incidence and the severity of the oculocardiac reflex. The most common manifestation of this reflex is bradycardia. The afferent limb is trigeminal, and the efferent limb is the vagus. This reflex has a higher incidence in children. Various maneuvers to abolish or obtund the oculocardiac reflex have been promulgated. None of these have been consistently effective, safe, and reliable. Complete vagolytic blockade in adults mandates 2 to 3 mg (0.03–0.05 mg/kg) of atropine. In pediatric patients, preanesthetic administration of 0.02 mg/kg of atropine or 0.01 mg/kg of glycopyrrolate may be considered due to increase in vagal tone. Since the peak effect of intramuscular atropine occurs approximately 30 minutes after administration, it is not surprising that studies with the usual routine dose have shown inconsistent protection against the oculocardiac reflex. If a cardiac dysrhythmia appears, the surgeon should be asked to cease operative manipulation. Next, the patient's anesthetic depth and ventilatory status should be evaluated. Commonly, the heart rate and rhythm return to baseline within 20 seconds after institution of these measures. (See page 1379: Oculocardiac Reflex.)

8. **B.**   Drugs absorbed from the conjunctiva enter the systemic venous circulation, and drugs passing through the nasolacrimal duct may be absorbed via the nasal mucosa. Phenylephrine eye drops produce pupillary dilation and capillary decongestion. Side effects, although rare, have been reported, including hypertension, headache, tachycardia, and tremulousness. In patients with coronary artery disease, severe myocardial ischemia, cardiac dysrhythmias, and even myocardial infarction have been reported following administration of 10% phenylephrine drops. Similarly, patients with cerebral aneurysms may have an increased risk of cerebral hemorrhage following administration of phenylephrine at this concentration. Echothiophate is a long-acting anticholinesterase miotic that lowers IOP and may prolong the action of succinylcholine. In addition, a delay in metabolism of ester local anesthetics should be expected. Cocaine is occasionally used in ophthalmologic surgery for its powerful vasoconstrictive effects, and should be avoided in patients with significant hypertension and those taking tricyclic antidepressants or monoamine oxidase inhibitors. In patients receiving significant amounts of cocaine, sympathomimetics, phenylephrine, and epinephrine should be avoided as well as β_2 specific blockers; labetalol should be used because of its α- and β-blockade and prolonged duration of action. Cocaine-induced chest pain/myocardial ischemia should be treated with nitroglycerin. Cyclopentolate is a mydriatic with side effects that include central nervous system toxicity that is manifested by dysarthria, disorientation, and frank psychotic reactions. Intraocular sulfur hexafluoride has been used for retinal detachment surgery to facilitate reattachment mechanically. Nitrous oxide should be terminated 15 minutes before gas injection to prevent expansion of intravitreous gas bubble. If the patient requires general anesthesia after this procedure, nitrous oxide should be avoided for 10 days. (See page 1380: Anesthetic Ramifications of Ophthalmic Drugs.)

9. **B.**   Atropine doses of 0.4 mg given parenterally have exquisitely minimal intraocular absorption while scopolamine has a greater mydriatic effect and should generally be avoided in patients at risk for closed-angle glaucoma. Intraocular phenylephrine relieves capillary congestion and causes papillary dilation but can lead to significant hypertension and produce myocardial ischemia or rupture of cerebral aneurysms leading to hemorrhage. Timolol, a nonselective β-blocker can be absorbed in significant quality and should be avoided in patients with obstructive airway disease, congestive heart failure, and heart blocks other than first degree. Life-threatening asthmatic crises have been reported after the administration of timolol drops to some patients with chronic, stable asthma. Betaxolol is β_1-specific and oculoselective, and has minimal pulmonary effects, but should be used with caution in patients with heart block greater than first degree, sinus bradycardia, cardiogenic shock, or myocardial failure. (See page 1380: Anesthetic Ramifications of Ophthalmic Drugs.)

10. **D.**   Since the late 1980s, peribulbar block has become increasingly popular. The advantages of this technique include its safety and the fact that an eyelid block is usually superfluous because the relatively large volume of injected

local anesthetic usually diffuses into the eyelids. Two injections are required, one placed inferotemporally and one between the supraorbital notch and trochlea. The onset is usually slower than with retrobulbar blockade and may be delayed for as long as 15 to 20 minutes, and requires a larger volume of anesthetic. Another disadvantage of peribulbar blockade is that pressure on the globe is required to distribute the local anesthetic. However, no cases of either retrobulbar hemorrhage or brainstem anesthesia have been documented associated with peribulbar block. Both retrobulbar and peribulbar blocks are associated with the oculocardiac reflex. The patient should be instructed to maintain gaze in the neutral position as a supranasal gaze was found to stretch the optic nerve in the path of the needle, increasing the risk of needle-associated nerve trauma during retrobulbar injection. A recessed globe, history of scleral buckling and myopia, which relates to an increase in the anterior–posterior dimension of the eye, provides an increased risk of globe interruption during a needle block. Patients for cataract surgery will generally undergo preoperative ultrasound for the determination of appropriate replacement lens size. An axial length of >26 mm that can be identified by ultrasound confers a greater risk. (See pages 1381: Preoperative Evaluation and 1383: Retrobulbar and Peribulbar Blocks.)

11. A. MAC, with or without drug administration, can be used in many eye surgeries, but is generally avoided in the pediatric population and in open eye surgeries where movement can be catastrophic. LMA is safe to use during ocular surgeries and provides a unique advantage of less increase in IOP associated with laryngoscopy and tracheal intubation, with the benefit of less bucking and coughing during emergence. Although low risk, the use of standard monitoring including electrocardiogram and oxygen saturation are necessary to identify oculocardiac reflex and possible brainstem anesthesia resulting from orbital blocks. In patients where extubation-associated coughing and postoperative vomiting can lead to major IOP increases, pre-extubation intravenous lidocaine, 1.5 to 2 mg/kg, can be given. Opioids associated with postoperative vomiting should be avoided and prophylactic administration of multimodal antiemetics, possibly in conjunction with a propofol total intravenous anesthesia technique, should be considered. (See page 1388: Sections, General Principles of Monitored Anesthesia Care and Anesthetic Management in Specific Situations.)

12. A. Corneal abrasions are the most common ocular complication of general anesthesia. Patients report foreign body sensation, pain, tearing, and photophobia; the pain is generally associated with eye blinking. Eyes should be taped shut immediately following induction and prior to mask ventilation and laryngoscopy. Spills into the eye are a source of chemical injury. The FDA has reported serious damage resulting from Hibiclens, a 4% chlorhexidine gluconate solution. Goggles must be worn at all times when a laser is in use in the operating room. The goggles must have the appropriate tint corresponding to the wavelength they intend to block. CO_2 lasers, argon, Nd:YAG, and Nd:YAG-KTP require the use of clear,

orange, green, and orange-red tinted goggles, respectively. (See pages 1393: Sections, Postoperative Ocular Complications and Principles of Laser Therapy.)

13. D. Retinal ischemia can be associated with ill-fitting anesthesia masks, hypotension, large volumes of sulfur hexafluoride in the presence of nitrous oxide, impaired intraocular venous drainage, or elevated IOP. Patients in prone position are at an increased risk for pressure on the globes, especially if large volumes of crystalloids are administered. Prone positioning may be associated with a risk of postoperative visual loss as high as 1%. Anterior ischemic optic neuropathy (AION) can result from hypo or lack of perfusion to the anterior portion of the optic nerve resulting in painless visual loss that may not be immediately apparent. Posterior ischemic optic neuropathy (PION) is caused by reduced oxygen delivery to the retrolaminar portion of the optic nerve. Symptoms may be delayed for several days and are often bilateral, suggesting involvement of the optic chiasm; they may result in permanent impairment. Risk factors for AION and PION include: Surgery exceeding 6 hours, blood loss exceeding 1 L, lower percent colloid administration, obesity, and the use of a Wilson frame. A strong male predominance has been observed in both AION and PION. Cortical blindness occurs following injury rostral to the optic chiasm. Risk factors include systemic disease, CABG, and profound hypotension. Recovery, although prolonged, may be considerable. (See page 1393: Section Postoperative Ocular Complications.)

14. D. The anesthesiologist involved in caring for a patient with a penetrating eye injury and a full stomach confronts special challenges. The anesthesiologist must weigh the risk of aspiration against the risk of blindness in the injured eye that could result from elevated IOP and extrusion of ocular contents. As in all cases of trauma, attention should be given to the exclusion of other injuries, such as skull and orbital fractures, intracranial trauma associated with subdural hematoma formation, and the possibility of thoracic or abdominal bleeding. Although regional anesthesia is often a valuable alternative for the management of trauma patients who have recently eaten, such an option is not available for patients with penetrating eye injuries. Retrobulbar blockade is ill advised because extrusion of intraocular contents may ensue via pressure generated by local anesthetic infiltration. Even though it is conceivable that a well-conducted, extremely smooth awake intubation after topical anesthesia may not increase IOP, it seems much more probable that the coughing and straining that will occur will result in increased IOP. Sch offers the distinct advantages of swift onset, superb intubating conditions, and a brief duration of action. If administered after careful pretreatment with a nondepolarizing drug and an induction agent, Sch typically produces only a modest increase in IOP. Intravenous lidocaine, 1.5 to 2 mg/kg, may be given just prior to tracheal extubation and is helpful in attenuating coughing. (See page 1388: Anesthetic Management of Specific Situations: Open-Eye, Full Stomach.)

15. E. Infantile strabismus occurs within the first 6 months of life and is often observed in the neonatal period.

Although most patients with strabismus are healthy, the incidence of strabismus is increased in those with central nervous system dysfunction. Strabismus may be acquired secondary to oculomotor nerve trauma or to sensory abnormalities such as cataracts or refractive aberrations. Patients with strabismus or ptosis may have an increased incidence of malignant hyperthermia. This observation is due to the fact that people susceptible to malignant hyperthermia often have areas of skeletal muscle weakness or other musculoskeletal abnormalities. Succinylcholine can be used but must be given more than 20 minutes before forced ductal testing, a technique to evaluate for mechanical restriction of the extraocular muscles. The use of atropine affords some protection against elicitation of the oculocardiac reflex; however, administration during active oculocardiac reflex can trigger dangerous cardiac dysrhythmias. For this reason, many anesthesiologists routinely premedicate children scheduled for strabismus surgery with intravenous atropine. Strabismus surgery is associated with significant pain that can be treated with nonsteroidal anti-inflammatory drugs. One study recommends ketorolac in doses of 0.75 mg/kg as an alternative to morphine, noting a much lower incidence of nausea and vomiting. (See page 1390: Strabismus Surgery.)

CHAPTER 49

The Renal System and Anesthesia for Urologic Surgery

1. Which of the following statements is TRUE regarding the renal system?

   A. Renal pain sensation is conveyed to the spinal cord via the T6 to T9 nerve roots.
   B. Bladder stretch sensation is transmitted by sympathetic fibers from the T11 to L2 nerve roots.
   C. The kidneys receive about 25% of the total cardiac output.
   D. Increasing the chloride delivery to the juxtaglomerular apparatus induces the release of renin.
   E. Prostaglandins cause constriction of renal arterioles reducing renal blood flow during times of stress.

2. Which of the following measures is NOT an effective strategy in preventing radiocontrast-induced acute kidney injury?

   A. Prophylactic administration of N-acetylcysteine
   B. Avoidance of concurrent NSAID administration
   C. Appropriate prehydration before the administration of radiocontrast
   D. Delaying elective surgery until the effects of radiocontrast media have resolved
   E. Utilizing smaller total radiocontrast doses

3. Which of the following is believed responsible for blindness after transurethral resection of the prostate (TURP)?

   A. Sorbitol
   B. Glycine
   C. Mannitol
   D. Urea
   E. Glycogen

4. Which of the following blood tests best predicts the development of acute renal failure (ARF) in critically ill patients?

   A. Creatinine clearance (CrCl)
   B. Urine sodium concentration (U_{Na})
   C. Serum creatinine (Cr)
   D. Fractional excretion of sodium (FE_{Na})
   E. Oliguria

5. Which of the following anesthetic agents does NOT have altered pharmacodynamics significant enough to warrant alterations in dosing in patients with end-stage renal disease (ESRD)?

   A. Thiopental
   B. Dexmedetomidine
   C. Midazolam
   D. Isoflurane
   E. Meperidine

6. Causes for increased release of antidiuretic hormone (ADH) include which of the following?

   A. Decreased extracellular sodium
   B. Decreased extracellular osmolality
   C. Increased atrial filling pressures
   D. Arterial baroreceptor stimulation by hypotension
   E. Increased intravascular volume

7. Which of the following statements regarding anesthesia and renal function is FALSE?

   A. Methoxyflurane and possibly enflurane are consistently the only agents that produce clinically relevant renal damage.
   B. Spinal anesthesia is the safest anesthetic for the kidney.
   C. Most renal injuries during anesthesia are caused by physiologic perturbations.
   D. Anesthesia does not directly affect renal hormonal control.
   E. In general, most anesthetics do not directly harm the kidney.

8. Alterations in drug administration in patients with chronic renal failure is NOT required for which of the following alterations in homeostasis?

   A. Alteration in the increase of F_A/F_I for inhaled agents
   B. Alterations in protein binding
   C. Alterations in elimination half-life for various compounds
   D. Alterations in volume of distribution
   E. Alterations in renal drug excretion

9. Electrocardiographic (ECG) changes are NOT associated with which of the following?

   A. Hypocalcemia
   B. Hypercalcemia
   C. Hypernatremia
   D. Hypermagnesemia
   E. Hypokalemia

10. What is the single most reliable predictor of postoperative renal dysfunction?

    A. Pre-existing renal disease
    B. Preoperative hypovolemia
    C. Congestive heart failure
    D. Cirrhosis
    E. Advanced age

11. During cardiac surgery, proven techniques to prevent renal injury include which of the following?

    A. Dopamine
    B. Mannitol
    C. Furosemide
    D. Fenoldopam
    E. Avoidance of hypovolemia and hypotension

12. Qualities of the ideal irrigation solution for transurethral resection of the prostate (TURP) do NOT include which of the following?

    A. Isotonic
    B. Electrically conductive
    C. Nonhemolytic
    D. Osmotically active
    E. Transparent

13. Which of the following statements regarding regional anesthesia and transurethral resection of the prostate (TURP) is TRUE?

    A. A T12 sensory level is required to prevent sensation of an overly distended bladder.
    B. Epidural anesthesia is the regional technique of choice for TURP.
    C. Regional anesthesia may improve detection of TURP syndrome symptoms.
    D. Regional anesthetics have been shown to reduce mortality compared with general anesthesia.
    E. Regional anesthesia is associated with a decrease in the amount of irrigating solution absorbed.

14. Which of the following statements regarding shock-wave lithotripsy is FALSE?

    A. Minimal immersion techniques are devoid of cardiovascular and pulmonary derangements.
    B. Pregnancy is a contraindication.
    C. Patients are at risk of contusion from the shock wave.
    D. Pacemakers are an absolute contraindication to lithotripsy.
    E. The risk of kidney injury increases with increased sound pulse counts.

15. Which of the following is FALSE regarding patients with renal cell carcinoma?

    A. Surgery is the treatment of choice.
    B. Postoperative pain is significant after open radical nephrectomy, often requiring multimodal therapy.
    C. There is an increased incidence of deep venous thrombosis (DVT).
    D. Patients undergoing open radical nephrectomy are prone to hemodynamic instability.
    E. Less than 1% of these patients have tumor extension into the renal vein.

16. Endovascular repair of an abdominal aortic aneurysm is gaining in popularity compared with the open approach. Which of the following statements regarding the endovascular approach is FALSE?

    A. Typically, hemodynamic alterations are reduced.
    B. Long-term incidences of renal failure or insufficiency are lower than with an open approach.
    C. The risk of atheroembolism is unchanged.
    D. Patients typically experience less postoperative pain.
    E. Patients may be exposed to substantial amounts of radiocontrast dye.

ANSWERS

1. C. The kidneys receive about 25% of the total cardiac output despite making up only about 0.4% of the total body weight. Pain originating from the kidneys is transmitted to the spinal cord via the T10 and T11 nerve roots. Bladder stretch sensation is transmitted through the parasympathetic system originating from the S2 to S4 segments. A decrease in renal blood flow decreases the GFR, which decreases chloride delivery to the juxtaglomerular apparatus. This decrease in chloride delivery triggers the release of renin. Prostaglandins cause renal arteriole dilation that maintains renal blood flow during times of stress. (See page 1401: Renal Anatomy and Physiology.)

2. A. The concept that prophylactic administration of N-acetylcysteine can prevent radiocontrast-induced nephropathy has largely been abandoned. Measures that can prevent or reduce renal injury associated with radiocontrast media include prehydration, the use of smaller doses of radiocontrast, and the withholding of other nephrotoxic agents including NSAIDs. Radiocontrast-induced renal injury starts within 24 to 48 hours of administration and peaks within 3 to 5 days. Elective surgery should be postponed after the administration of radiocontrast agents until the renal insult has resolved. (See page 1409: Nephrotoxins and Perioperative Acute Kidney Injury).

3. B. All of these substances (except for glycogen) are used as osmotic agents in TURP procedures. Glycine is the only agent that directly produces transient blindness. It is believed that blindness is a result of glycine action as an inhibitory neurotransmitter. (See page 1428: Irrigating Solutions and Transurethral Resection Syndrome.)

4. C. Serum creatinine is the most effective blood test for reflecting change in renal filtration and predicting renal outcome, even during the perioperative period. Although poor urine output (<400 mL urine/24 hrs) may reflect hypovolemia or impending "prerenal" failure, the majority of perioperative renal failure episodes develop in the absence of oliguria. CrCl is a predictor of imminent renal failure but requires a multi-hour urine sample. Estimates of glomerular filtration rate can be made by determining CrCl from urine and blood creatinine tests. U_{Na}^+ reflects resuscitative fluids being used. Fractional excretion of sodium (FE_{Na}) does not serve as an early indicator of ARF. It can differentiate prerenal from renal causes of ARF after the condition is established. (See page 1404: Clinical Assessment of the Kidney.)

5. D. Thiopental, midazolam, and dexmedetomidine all undergo significant protein binding. This binding is reduced in ESRD, resulting in a larger free fraction of the drug. This requires an altered dosing scheme for these medications. Isoflurane pharmacodynamics are not affected by renal failure. Meperidine is not recommended for use in patients with poor renal function, partly because of its neurotoxic, renally excreted metabolite, normeperidine. (See page 1411: Induction Agents and Sedatives.)

6. D. ADH is released by the posterior pituitary gland in response to increased extracellular sodium or increased osmolality. It is also released during times of hypotension through receptors in the atria and the arterial tree. ADH release results in increased free water absorption at the distal and the collecting tubules. By increasing the quantity of free water absorbed, the elevated sodium and osmolality levels are diluted, and hypovolemia is abated. ADH release can also be released in response to reductions in intravascular volume. (See page 1403: Tubular Reabsorption of Sodium and Water.)

7. B. In general, an anesthetic is not injurious to the renal system; an exception is methoxyflurane. During the metabolism of this drug, free fluoride is released, which can cause renal injury. Enflurane and sevoflurane also generate free fluoride; however, the quantity released is substantially less than with methoxyflurane, and enflurane and sevoflurane have not consistently caused clinically relevant renal injury. No comparative studies have demonstrated superior renal protection or improved renal outcome with general versus regional anesthesia. Most renal injuries occur secondary to physiologic perturbations as a result of surgery, as well as complications such as hypoxia, hypovolemia, and hypotension. Anesthetics do not directly alter renal hormonal regulation. (See page 1411: Anesthetic Agents in Renal Failure.)

8. A. The pharmacokinetics of most enteral and parenteral medications is altered in patients with chronic renal failure (with the exclusion of alveolar uptake of inhaled anesthetic agents). There is an increase in the volume of distribution for water-soluble drugs, resulting in lower concentration of a drug given as a single bolus. Reduced excretion of the parent drug and any of its active metabolites results in prolonged duration of action for a number of agents. Protein binding is typically reduced in chronic renal failure, resulting in a larger free fraction (which produces the effects). There is no alteration in alveolar uptake in patients with chronic renal failure (as long as they are not in congestive heart failure). (See page 1411: Drug Prescribing in Renal Failure.)

9. C. Hyponatremia is the most commonly occurring electrolyte disorder. Symptoms rarely occur unless sodium values are <125 mmol/L, and these include a spectrum ranging from anorexia, nausea, and lethargy to convulsions, dysrhythmias, coma, and even death due to osmotic brain swelling. There are no specific EKG changes noted with hypernatremia. Clinical manifestations of hypokalemia include ECG changes (flattened T waves, U waves, prodysrhythmic state) and skeletal muscle weakness. QT interval shortening and dysrhythmias are associated with both hypercalcemia and hypocalcemia. In more extreme cases of hypermagnesemia, flaccid skeletal muscle paralysis, hyporeflexia, bradydysrhythmias, and cardiac arrest may occur. (See page 1406: Electrolyte Disorders.)

10. A. The single most reliable predictor of postoperative renal dysfunction is preoperative renal dysfunction. Other risk factors include cardiac dysfunction, sepsis, volume depletion, and hepatic failure. By itself, advanced age is not predictive of postoperative renal dysfunction. (See pages 1408: Prerenal Azotemia and 1408: Acute Kidney Injury.)

11. E. Numerous agents (including ANP, dopamine, fenoldopam, insulin-like growth factor 1, mannitol, or furosemide) have been used intraoperatively without success in attempts to protect the kidney during cardiac surgery. In general, maintenance of adequate intravascular volume and blood pressure are the only proven preventive measures that can be taken to preserve renal function. (See page 1415: High-risk Surgical Procedures.)

12. B. TURP involves the use of a fiber-optic scope and an electrocautery loop to resect the prostate from inside the lumen of the urethra. To clear the resected material and blood, an irrigating solution is infused. This irrigating solution must be optically clear and nonconductive toward electricity (because the cautery unit will be in direct contact with fluid). During resection, the fluid used during irrigation is absorbed by the open veins within the prostate, so the fluid must be isotonic and nonhemolytic. Unipolar cautery requires osmotically active fluid and each of these solutes is associated with its own side effect profile. Newer technologies for TURP such as laser and bipolar cautery do not require these osmotically active solutes. (See page 1428: Irrigating Solutions and Transurethral Resection Syndrome.)

13. C. Regional anesthesia is used extensively for TURP procedures. There is no difference in mortality between patients receiving general anesthesia and those receiving regional anesthetics. Spinal anesthesia is the technique of choice if a regional technique is selected because spinal anesthesia provides a more reliable block than epidural anesthesia. If a patient selects a regional block for TURP, the anesthesiologist must anesthetize to the T10 level to block sensation from an over distended bladder. Since patients are awake during regional anesthesia, there is an increased likelihood that the TURP syndrome symptoms will be detected earlier. Regional anesthesia's decrease in venous pressure may increase the amount of irrigating solution absorbed during the procedure. (See page 1426: Transurethral Resection and Surveillance Procedures.)

14. D. Lithotripsy involves crushing renal calculi with an externally generated shock wave. Early lithotripsy machines transferred the shock wave to the patient by immersing the patient in a water bath. The water transferred the shock wave effectively because tissue and water have similar acoustic properties. Immersion in the water bath may lead to significant physiologic changes, including increased central venous pressure, vasodilation, decreased vital capacity, and decreased functional residual capacity. The new minimal immersion techniques are devoid of physiologic derangements. Small patients are at risk of pulmonary contusions because their lungs lie within the path of the shock wave. Pacemakers were once believed to be a contraindication for lithotripsy, but a review of shock-wave lithotripsy treatments in pacemaker-dependent patients found a low (<1%) incidence of major pacemaker complications. Pregnancy is a contraindication to lithotripsy. The risk of kidney injury and subcapsular hematoma increases with increased pulse counts. (See page 1432: Shock Wave Lithotripsy.)

15. E. Renal cell carcinoma is the most common malignancy of the kidney. Surgical excision is the mainstay of treatment because renal cancer is refractory to nonsurgical therapies (chemotherapy and radiation). Patients undergoing open radical nephrectomy are prone to hemodynamic instability, not only from blood loss but also because of compression of the inferior vena cava secondary to positioning or surgical compression. Patients having open resections often experience significant postoperative pain, and the use of multimodal therapies, including epidural analgesia, may be helpful. Renal tumors may also be associated with a hypercoagulable state. Sudden intraoperative clot formation has been reported. Tumor thrombus extension into the renal vein or more proximal vasculature can occur in 4% to 10% of patients. (See page 1417: Radical Nephrectomy.)

16. B. Endovascular procedures to repair abdominal aortic aneurysms typically produce fewer hemodynamic alterations and because of the smaller incisions, produce less postoperative pain. The incidence of renal complications is similar to open approaches. Endovascular procedures do not have a lower incidence of long-term renal insufficiency/failure. This is probably because of the similar risk of atheroembolism and because of the significant quantity of radiographic contrast dye used during the procedure. (See page 1415: High-risk Surgical Procedures.)

50

Anesthesia for Orthopedic Surgery

1. Which of the following statements regarding peripheral nerve block for the foot is TRUE?

   A. The saphenous, sural, and peroneal nerves are branches of the femoral nerve, which may be blocked at the knee level.
   B. If anesthesia is provided by an ankle block, surgery using a midleg or thigh tourniquet must be limited to 90 minutes.
   C. Induction or "setup" time is consistently reduced compared with an intrathecal injection.
   D. Clonidine may be used to prolong surgical anesthesia.
   E. Prolonged block delays postanesthesia care unit and hospital discharge times.

2. All of the following apply to microvascular surgery EXCEPT:

   A. To avoid compromising blood flow to a replanted limb, phenylephrine should not be used to maintain systemic blood pressure.
   B. Maintenance of blood flow through anastomoses may be achieved with vasodilators and an increase in the perfusion pressure.
   C. Dextran and papaverine may be used to preserve blood flow.
   D. An epidural catheter placement may improve the perfusion.
   E. Hypothermia may have a deleterious effect.

3. Which of the following statements regarding patients with scoliosis is TRUE?

   A. Scoliosis that requires surgery is usually the result of a neuromuscular disorder.
   B. Resting hypercapnia is the best indicator of the need for postoperative ventilatory support.
   C. They may have associated cyanotic heart disease.
   D. They should be managed with hemodilution or controlled hypotension but never both.
   E. Moderate, controlled hypotension is complicated by thrombosis and therefore is not usually beneficial.

4. Which of the following statements regarding neurophysiologic monitoring is TRUE?

   A. Motor-evoked potentials (MEPs) are commonly monitored during spine surgery.
   B. The anesthetic technique of choice when MEPs are being monitored is a nitrous–narcotic–relaxant technique.
   C. Somatosensory-evoked potentials (SSEPs) monitor motor function only in areas of the spinal cord supplied by the anterior spinal artery.
   D. SSEP waveforms may be altered by acute nerve injury, hypercarbia, hypoxia, or hypotension.
   E. Volatile anesthetics commonly produce a dose-related increase in SSEP amplitude.

5. Risk factors for fat embolism syndrome include all of the following EXCEPT:

   A. Generally 20 to 40 years of age
   B. Male gender
   C. Disorders of lipid metabolism
   D. Rheumatoid arthritis
   E. Intramedullary instrumentation

6. In conducting an anesthetic technique for orthopedic hip surgery, the following should be taken into consideration:

   A. The fracture table offers the advantages of easy maintenance of traction and radiographic images.
   B. An isobaric intrathecal technique cannot be used.
   C. Using a regional technique often worsens the blood loss during surgery.
   D. Calcium channel blockers are contraindicated for deliberate hypotension.

7. Which of the following statements regarding procedures for the upper extremity is TRUE?

   A. Regional anesthesia may increase blood loss as well as lower the incidence of thromboembolism.
   B. Prolonged regional block often delays hospital discharge.
   C. Venous air embolism is uncommon.
   D. Neuropraxia is rare and occurs most commonly at the level of an axillary block.

8. Which of the following statements regarding infraclavicular block for surgery at the elbow is TRUE?

    A. It is not preferred in outpatients because of the risk of pneumothorax.
    B. Patients must have postoperative chest radiography to identify pneumothorax.
    C. It is most reliable for surgery above the proximal humerus.
    D. A pneumothorax of 10% should be treated with a chest tube.

9. Which of the following statements regarding continuous brachial plexus anesthesia is FALSE?

    A. It may reduce postoperative vasospasm after limb replantation.
    B. A continuous indwelling catheter may be inserted using interscalene, infraclavicular, or axillary techniques.
    C. Infusion via a continuous indwelling catheter can produce profound analgesia in the major nerve distributions.
    D. There are several long-term benefits with a single injection regional anesthetic technique compared with a general anesthetic.

10. Knee surgery in which a tourniquet will be used requires anesthesia of all of the following EXCEPT:

    A. Femoral nerve
    B. Lateral femoral cutaneous nerve
    C. Sciatic nerve
    D. Iliohypogastric nerve

11. Which of the following statements regarding the use of regional anesthesia for orthopedic surgery in children is FALSE?

    A. It carries the same advantages for adults, including decreased nausea and vomiting, and decreased time to discharge.
    B. Regional techniques are often technically difficult to perform in the pediatric population.
    C. Brachial plexus block may be facilitated with a nerve stimulator.
    D. Regional techniques are readily adaptable and often underused.

12. Which of the following statements regarding patients with spinal shock is TRUE?

    A. They should never receive succinylcholine because of the potential for hyperkalemia.
    B. Hyperventilation and resultant hypocarbia can improve blood flow and "protect" an ischemic spinal cord tissue.
    C. Spinal shock is short lived and usually improves within 24 to 48 hours.
    D. Spinal shock may mask ongoing hypovolemic shock.

13. Which of the following statements regarding a "wake-up test" is TRUE?

    A. Up to 60% of patients will have a recall of the test.
    B. It can be safely and easily performed.
    C. It is an accurate test with very few false-negative results.
    D. Patients who do experience recall frequently describe it as intensely painful.

14. Which of the following statements regarding the use of limb tourniquets is TRUE?

    A. The tourniquet overlap should always be placed directly over the neurovascular bundle to reduce the likelihood of nerve injury.
    B. When selecting a tourniquet, the width of an inflated cuff should be greater than 50% of the limb diameter.
    C. Cuff pressure must be maintained at no less than 200 mm Hg more than the patient's systolic blood pressure.
    D. The duration of a safe tourniquet time is generally considered to be 180 to 200 minutes.

15. Which of the following statements is TRUE?

    A. The optimal treatment of a patient with suspected fat embolism syndrome includes stabilization of long bone fractures.
    B. Autonomic hyperreflexia occurs in approximately 20% of patients after recovery from spinal shock as a consequence of a high spinal cord injury.
    C. Nitrous oxide should be increased to at least 66% before the use of methyl methacrylate.
    D. Reduction of intraoperative blood pressure during total hip arthroplasty resulting from central neuraxial blockade probably does not reduce blood loss during total hip arthroplasty.

16. Which of the following statements regarding spinal cord injury is FALSE?

    A. A high thoracic lesion (T1–T3) results in respiratory failure unless artificial pulmonary ventilation is used.
    B. A T4 lesion will cause loss of abdominal and intercostal support, leading to long-term difficulties in respiration.
    C. A lesion at C7 can lead to a vital capacity reduction of up to 60%.
    D. There is a higher rate of infection in patients with a spinal cord lesion.

17. Which of the following is TRUE regarding spinal shock?

    A. The root cause of spinal shock is grossly exaggerated sympathetic vascular tone below the site of the lesion.
    B. Bradycardia is seen in spinal shock from a T2 lesion.
    C. Tachycardia is seen in spinal shock from a C5 lesion.
    D. Autonomic instability should be managed with stabilizing fluid boluses.
    E. Monitoring of CVP should be performed for fluid management in a patient with a T6 lesion.

18. Which of the following is TRUE regarding autonomic hyperreflexia?

    A. The syndrome is characterized by severe paroxysmal hypertension with tachycardia (baroreceptor reflex), dysrhythmias, and cutaneous vasoconstriction.
    B. Thirty-five percent of patients exhibit autonomic hyperreflexia when there has been complete cord transection above T5.
    C. The exaggerated supraspinal inhibition allows the sympathetic outflow below the lesion to react to the stimulus unopposed.
    D. Many patients with spinal injuries and autonomic hyperreflexia will report characteristic headaches with bladder distention.
    E. If autonomic hyperreflexia occurs, it should be treated by removal of the stimulus, deepening anesthesia, and administration of direct-acting vasoconstrictors.

19. The following statement regarding upper extremity surgery is FALSE:

    A. Radial nerve palsy is identified in over 15% of patients with humeral shaft fractures.
    B. The most common level of nerve injury is at the level of the brachial plexus trunks, which is the level at which an interscalene block is performed.
    C. Less than 5% of patients undergoing total shoulder arthroplasty have a documented postoperative neurologic deficit.
    D. Up to 10% of patients present with a nerve injury to the brachial plexus which resolves in 3 to 4 months.

20. Which of the following statements concerning elbow surgery is FALSE?

    A. Infraclavicular and supraclavicular approaches to the brachial plexus are most reliable.
    B. Supraclavicular and infraclavicular blocks have a higher risk of pneumothorax than other brachial plexus blocks.
    C. Postblock pneumothorax may not become evident until it occurs 6 to 12 hours after hospital discharge.
    D. Chest tube placement is advised for a pneumothorax involving >8% of lung volume.

21. Which of the following statements concerning surgery to the ankle and foot is TRUE?

    A. Innervation of the foot is provided by the femoral nerve (via the sural nerve) and by the sciatic nerve (via the posterior tibial, and deep and superficial peroneal nerves).
    B. Inflation of a thigh tourniquet for longer than 15 to 20 minutes necessitates a general or neuraxial anesthetic, regardless of surgical site.
    C. Placement of an indwelling catheter is the standard for most minor foot and ankle surgeries.
    D. Prolonged peripheral or plexus blockade provides excellent pain relief, and reduces the risk of accidental nerve trauma outside the hospital environment.

22. The following is FALSE regarding venous thromboembolism:

    A. Without prophylaxis, venous thrombosis develops in 10% to 20% of orthopedic patients, and 1% to 10% show clinical or laboratory evidence of pulmonary embolism.
    B. The incidence of fatal pulmonary embolism is highest in patients who have undergone surgery for hip fracture.
    C. Most orthopedic cases other than acute spinal cord injury and major joint replacement do not warrant anticoagulation prophylaxis.
    D. Venous thromboembolism is a major cause of death after surgery or trauma to the lower extremities.

23. Which of the following is TRUE regarding pediatric orthopedic surgery?

    A. Regional anesthesia is not recommended for use in the pediatric population.
    B. Intravenous regional (Bier) block is contraindicated in the pediatric population due to local anesthetic toxicity.
    C. Coexisting neuromuscular conditions may predispose pediatric orthopedic patients to latex allergies or malignant hyperthermia.
    D. Regional anesthetic procedures are technically challenging to be performed on children because the anatomy is inconsistent as compared to adults.

24. Which of the following is FALSE regarding microvascular surgery?

    A. Hypothermia is utilized in microvascular surgical patients in order to better preserve the tissue.
    B. Volatile anesthetics are potent vasodilators and can increase tissue blood flow 200% to 300%, even at typical expired anesthetic concentrations.
    C. Direct-acting vasodilating agents produce vasodilation but do not prevent vasospasm because of direct surgical stimulation.
    D. Nitroprusside has been shown to reduce perfusion in a microvascular free flap.
    E. Regional anesthetic techniques have no effect on vasospasm in the replanted (denervated) tissue.

25. Which of the following is FALSE regarding surgery of the shoulder?

    A. In the beach chair position, venous air embolism occurs at a rate of 10% to 15%, due to the fact that the operative site is higher than the heart.
    B. The Bezold–Jarisch reflex has been described in awake, sitting patients undergoing shoulder surgery under an interscalene block.
    C. The interscalene block can result in a 25% loss of pulmonary function.
    D. Interscalene or supraclavicular blockade alone can provide appropriate surgical anesthesia for shoulder surgeries.

ANSWERS

1. D. Innervation of the foot is provided by the femoral nerve (via the saphenous nerve) and by the sciatic nerve (via the posterior tibial, sural, deep peroneal, and superficial peroneal nerves). Central neuraxial blockade and peripheral nerve blocks at the upper leg, knee, or ankle are appropriate regional anesthetic techniques for foot surgery. Selection of the regional technique is based on the surgical site, the use of a calf or thigh tourniquet, the degree of weight bearing or ambulation, and the need for postoperative analgesia. For example, inflation of a thigh tourniquet for more than 15 to 20 minutes typically necessitates a general or neuraxial anesthetic; otherwise, "solid" block of the femoral, sciatic, obturator, and lateral femoral cutaneous nerves is required. Often patients undergoing lower extremity peripheral techniques may be discharged directly from the operating room to the outpatient nursing station, reducing recovery time and charges. The use of long-acting local anesthetics and the addition of epinephrine or clonidine allow prolongation of postoperative analgesia. However, additional onset time is required with bupivacaine and ropivacaine; this may translate into a longer "induction time." (See page 1451: Surgery to the Ankle and Foot.)

2. A. Microvascular surgery includes both replantation, the reattachment of a completely severed body part, and revascularization, the re-establishment of blood flow through a severed body part. Most replantation surgeries involve the upper extremity. Blood flow may be improved by increasing the perfusion pressure, preventing hypothermia, and using vasodilators and sympathetic blockade. Microvascular perfusion pressure depends on both adequate intravascular volume and oncotic pressure. It has not been established that the use of phenylephrine to support blood pressure jeopardizes blood flow to the tissue being replanted. Body temperature is also a determinant of blood flow. Hypothermia not only results in peripheral vasoconstriction but also causes sympathetic activation, shivering, increased oxygen demand, a leftward shift of the oxygen–hemoglobin dissociation curve, and altered coagulation. Therefore, hypothermia must be prevented in patients undergoing microvascular surgery. Regional anesthetic techniques provide sympathectomy and vasodilation to the proximal (innervated) segment of an extremity but have no effect on vasospasm in the replanted (denervated) tissue. Antithrombotics (heparin), fibrinolytics (streptokinase, urokinase, low–molecular-weight dextran), and smooth muscle relaxants (papaverine, local anesthetics) are also used to preserve blood flow in microvascular anastomoses. A combination of general and continuous regional anesthesia allows prolonged intraoperative anesthesia and postoperative analgesia, reduces the amount of inhalational agent, and increases the patient's acceptance of lengthy surgical procedures. However, regardless of the anesthetic technique, conditions that stimulate vasospasm or vasoconstriction, such as pain, hypotension, and hypovolemia, should be avoided. (See page 1452: Microvascular Surgery.)

3. C. Idiopathic scoliosis represents 75% to 90% of scoliosis cases. The remaining 10% to 25% of cases are associated with neuromuscular diseases and congenital abnormalities, including congenital heart disease, trauma, and mesenchymal disorders. Vital capacity appears to be a reliable prognostic indicator of perioperative respiratory reserve. Postoperative ventilation is most likely required for patients with a vital capacity of less than 40% of predicted vital capacity. Scoliosis is also associated with congenital heart conditions, including mitral valve prolapse, coarctation, and cyanotic heart disease, suggesting a common embryonic insult or collagen defect. Normovolemic hemodilution combined with induced hypotension and autotransfusion may decrease or eliminate the need for homologous transfusion. Moderate induced hypotension (reduction of systolic pressure 20 mm Hg from baseline or lowering mean arterial pressure to 65 mm Hg in normotensive patients) has been shown to decrease blood loss, reduce transfusion requirements by 50%, and shorten operating times. (See page 1442: Scoliosis.)

4. D. Although the use of MEPs remains limited, SSEP monitoring is widely accepted. However, somatosensory stimulation follows the dorsal column pathways of proprioception and vibration, pathways supplied by the posterior spinal artery. Conversely, MEPs monitor motor pathways that are supplied by the anterior spinal artery. MEPs are not routinely monitored because they are technically more difficult to use. Muscle relaxants cannot be used in patients undergoing MEP monitoring. It is critical to note that postoperative paraplegia has occurred in at least one patient with preserved SSEP monitoring intraoperatively. Numerous variables are known to alter SSEP waveforms. In addition to neural injury, SSEPs are altered by hypercarbia, hypoxia, hypotension, and hypothermia. All of the volatile anesthetics produce a dose-related decrease in the amplitude and an increase in the latency of SSEPs. (See page 1445: Spinal Cord Monitoring.)

5. C. Fat embolism syndrome is associated with multiple traumatic injuries and surgery involving long bone fractures. Risk factors include all genders between 20 and 30 years of age, hypovolemic shock, intramedullary instrumentation, rheumatoid arthritis, cemented total hip arthroplasty, and bilateral total knee surgery. The incidence of fat embolism syndrome in isolated long bone fractures is 3% to 4%, and mortality associated with this condition is significant (10%–20%). (See page 1454: Fat Embolus Syndrome.)

6. A. Whereas the lateral decubitus position is frequently used to facilitate surgical exposure for total hip replacement, a fracture table is often used for repair of femur fractures. In transferring the patient from the supine to lateral decubitus position, care must be taken to maintain the patient's head and shoulders in a neutral position. The fracture table affords two advantages: Maintenance of traction on the fractured extremity, allowing manipulation for closed reduction and fixation, and access to the fracture site for radiography in several planes. The patient must be carefully monitored for hemodynamic changes during positioning, whether he or she is under regional or general anesthesia. Regional anesthetic techniques are well suited to procedures involving the hip. Central neuraxial blockade is commonly used. Both hypobaric and isobaric spinal anesthetic solutions are effective. Epidural blockade also provides excellent surgical anesthesia, allowing for prolonged anesthesia as well as postoperative analgesia. Regional anesthetic techniques reduce blood loss in patients undergoing hip surgery. Deliberate hypotension may also be used with general anesthesia as a means of reducing surgical blood loss. Diltiazem, nitroprusside with and without captopril, β-blockers, and nitroglycerin have also been used to induce hypotension. (See page 1449: Surgery to the Hip.)

7. **C.** Regional anesthetics offer several advantages over general anesthetics in patients undergoing orthopedic procedures, including improved postoperative analgesia, decreased incidence of nausea and vomiting, less respiratory and cardiac depression, improved perfusion via sympathetic block, reduced blood loss, and decreased risk of thromboembolism. Although prolonged blockade of the lower extremities interferes with ambulation and therefore may delay outpatient discharge, persistent upper extremity block is not a contraindication to hospital discharge. Theoretically, venous air embolism may occur during surgical procedures to the shoulder because the operative site is higher than the heart; however, this complication has not been reported in the literature. Four percent of patients undergoing total shoulder arthroplasty have a documented postoperative neurologic deficit, including 3% of patients with injury to the brachial plexus. The level of injury is at the level of the nerve trunks, which is the level at which an interscalene block is performed, making it impossible to determine the origin of the nerve injury (surgical vs. anesthetic). Most of these nerve injuries represent a neuropraxia; 90% of them resolve in 3 to 4 months. (See page 1449: Surgery to the Upper Extremities.)

8. **A.** Surgical procedures to the distal humerus, elbow, and forearm are commonly performed using regional anesthetic techniques. Infraclavicular and supraclavicular approaches to the brachial plexus are the most reliable and provide consistent anesthesia to the four major nerves of the brachial plexus: Median, ulnar, radial, and musculocutaneous. It does not include the intercostobrachial nerve, which needs to be blocked for procedures at or above the elbow. However, the small but definite risk of pneumothorax associated with supraclavicular and infraclavicular blocks makes these approaches less suitable for outpatient procedures. Typically, the pneumothorax becomes evident 6 to 12 hours after hospital discharge. Therefore, postoperative chest radiography is not always helpful. Although chest tube placement is advised for pneumothorax greater than 20% of lung volume, the lung may also be reexpanded with a small Teflon catheter under fluoroscopic guidance, eliminating the need for hospital admission. The axillary approach to the brachial plexus eliminates the risk of pneumothorax and reliably provides adequate anesthesia for surgery near the elbow. (See page 1448: Surgery to the Elbow.)

9. **D.** Continuous infusion of local anesthetic solution, such as bupivacaine 0.125%, prevents vasospasm and increases circulation after limb replantation or vascular repair. More concentrated solutions of bupivacaine result in complete sensory block and allow early joint mobilization after painful surgical procedures to the elbow. Brachial plexus catheters may be inserted using interscalene, infraclavicular, and axillary approaches. However, the axillary approach is the most common. Overall, there are early but no long-term benefits with the use of a single injection regional anesthetic technique compared with a general anesthetic. However, placement of an indwelling perineural catheter results in more substantial and lasting benefits, including avoidance of hospital admission and readmission, decreased opioid-related side effects, decreased sleep disturbance, and improved rehabilitation. (See page 1448: Continuous Brachial Plexus Anesthesia.)

10. **D.** Surgical anesthesia for operative procedures on the knee, in which a tourniquet will be used, requires blockade of the femoral, lateral femoral cutaneous, obturator, and sciatic nerves that innervate the leg. The iliohypogastric nerve innervates above both the surgical and tourniquet sites. (See page 1450: Total Knee Arthroplasty.)

11. **B.** Pediatric patients present with a variety of orthopedic conditions, including congenital deformities, traumatic injuries, infections, and malignancies. Anesthetic management of pediatric orthopedic patients involves not only the usual pediatric patient considerations, such as airway management, fluid replacement, and maintenance of body temperature, but also the unique concerns associated with orthopedic surgery. Often regional anesthetic procedures are technically easier to perform on children because their relative lack of subcutaneous tissue facilitates both identification of bony and vascular landmarks and spread of local anesthetic. The advantages of regional anesthesia in children are similar to those in adults and include earlier ambulation and hospital discharge, decreased incidence of nausea and vomiting, and prolonged postoperative analgesia. However, pediatric patients are often not considered candidates for regional techniques. Neural blockade may be initiated after induction of general anesthesia and before surgical incision, to provide possible preemptive analgesia, or on completion of the surgical procedure, to extend the duration of postoperative analgesia. Blockade of the brachial plexus is usually accomplished with perivascular, sheath, or nerve stimulator techniques in children younger than 7 years of age because elicitation of paresthesias is regarded as uncomfortable (and therefore unacceptable) by younger pediatric patients. (See page 1453: Pediatric Orthopedic Surgery.)

12. **D.** In spinal shock, hyperventilation should be avoided because hypocarbia decreases spinal cord blood flow. Spinal shock may persist from a few days to 3 months. It is

usually safe to administer succinylcholine for the first 48 hours. Spinal shock may mask underlying hypovolemic shock. (See page 1441: Surgery to the Spine.)

13. C.   If there is satisfactory movement of the hands, but not the feet, during a wake-up test, the distraction on the rod is released one notch, and the test is repeated. Increasing the blood pressure and blood volume may be attempted to increase spinal cord perfusion. Recall of the event occurs in up to 20% of patients and is rarely viewed as unpleasant. It is important to describe what will transpire to the patient before surgery, so anxiety will be minimized if the patient is fully awake. The "wake-up test" is associated with few false-negative results, that is, it is extremely rare for a patient who was neurologically intact when awakened intraoperatively to have a neurologic deficit upon completion of the procedure. However, certain hazards of the "wake-up test" do exist and include recall, pain, air embolism, dislocation of spinal instrumentation, and accidental tracheal extubation or removal of intravenous and arterial lines. Since the "wake-up test" requires patient cooperation, it may be difficult to perform on young children and mentally challenged patients. (See page 1445: Spinal Cord Monitoring.)

14. B.   The cuff should be large enough to circle the limb comfortably to ensure uniform pressure. The point of overlap should be placed 180 degrees from the neurovascular bundle because there is some area of decreased compression at the overlap point. The width of the inflated cuff should be greater than 50% of the limb diameter. Pressure is usually maintained by compressed gas (air or oxygen) and must be monitored continually while the tourniquet is in use. Before tourniquet inflation, the limb should be elevated for about 1 minute and tightly wrapped with an elastic bandage distally to proximally to ensure exsanguination. Limb tourniquets are relatively contraindicated when infection or a tumor is present. Opinions differ as to the pressure required in tourniquets to prevent bleeding. Leg tourniquets are often pressurized more than arm tourniquets on the theory that larger limbs require more pressure than smaller limbs. In general, a cuff pressure of 100 mm Hg above a patient's measured systolic pressure is adequate for the thigh, and 50 mm Hg above systolic pressure is adequate for the arm, with the understanding that if hypertensive episodes occur, the cuff pressure should be increased. The duration of safe tourniquet inflation is generally considered to be 2 hours. (See page 1453: Tourniquets.)

15. A.   Appropriate intervention for fat embolism entails early surgical stabilization of fracture sites, aggressive respiratory support, and reversal of possible aggravating factors (e.g., hypovolemia). After recovery from spinal shock, 85% of patients exhibit autonomic hyperreflexia when there has been complete cord transection above T5. The syndrome is characterized by severe paroxysmal hypertension with bradycardia, arrhythmias, and cutaneous vasoconstriction below and vasodilation above the level of the injury. Methyl methacrylate is often injected under pressure, and it is theorized that air embolism may be one of the causes of hypotension that may accompany injection of cement; thus, nitrous oxide should be discontinued several minutes before this point. Multiple studies have demonstrated reduced intraoperative blood loss during total hip arthroplasty completed under central neuraxial blockade compared with general anesthesia. (See pages 1449: Surgery to the Lower Extremities; 1442: Autonomic Hyperreflexia; 1454: Fat Embolus Syndrome; and 1454: Methyl Methacrylate.)

16. A.   Ventilatory impairment increases with higher levels of spinal injury. A high cervical lesion that includes the diaphragmatic segments (C4–C5) results in respiratory failure, and death occurs unless artificial pulmonary ventilation is used. Lesions between C5 and T7 cause significant alterations in respiratory function, owing to the loss of abdominal and intercostal support. The indrawing of flaccid thoracic muscles during inspiration produces paradoxical respirations, resulting in a vital capacity reduction of 60%. Inability to cough and effectively clear secretions results in atelectasis and infection. (See page 1441: Spinal Cord Injuries.)

17. B.   During spinal shock, there is loss of sympathetic vascular tone below the injury. If the cardioaccelerator fibers (T1 through T4) are damaged, bradycardia results. Therefore, hemorrhagic shock may not produce a compensatory tachycardia in these patients; the rate may remain at 40 to 60 beats per minute. Monitoring of central venous or pulmonary artery pressures may be necessary for fluid management in a patient with a high cervical lesion. Autonomic instability should be treated with vasoconstrictors, vasodilators, and positive chronotropic drugs as needed. (See page 1441: Spinal Cord Injuries.)

18. D.   After recovery from spinal shock, 85% of patients exhibit autonomic hyperreflexia when there has been complete cord transection above T5. The syndrome, which can also occur with injuries at lower levels, is characterized by severe paroxysmal hypertension with bradycardia (baroreceptor reflex), dysrhythmias, cutaneous vasoconstriction below, and vasodilation above, the level of the injury. The episode is typically precipitated by distention of the bladder or rectum, but can be induced by any noxious stimulus. Many patients with spinal injuries and autonomic hyperreflexia will report characteristic headaches with bladder distention. The lack of supraspinal inhibition allows the sympathetic outflow below the lesion to react unopposed to the stimulus. If autonomic hyperreflexia occurs, it should be treated by removal of the stimulus, deepening anesthesia, and administration of direct-acting vasodilators. (See page 1441: Spinal Cord Injuries.)

19. D.   Four percent of patients undergoing total shoulder arthroplasty have a documented postoperative neurologic deficit, including 3% of patients with injury to the brachial plexus. The level of injury is at the level of the nerve trunks, which is the level at which an interscalene block is performed, making it impossible to determine the etiology of the nerve injury (surgical vs. anesthetic). Radial nerve palsy is identified in up to 18% of patients with humeral shaft fractures. (See page 1447: Surgery to the Shoulder and Upper Arm.)

20. D. Infraclavicular and supraclavicular approaches to the brachial plexus are the most reliable and provide consistent anesthesia to the four major nerves of the brachial plexus: Median, ulnar, radial, and musculocutaneous. However, the small but definite risk of pneumothorax associated with supraclavicular and infraclavicular blocks usually makes this approach unsuitable for outpatient procedures. Typically, the pneumothorax occurs 6 to 12 hours after hospital discharge; therefore, a postoperative chest radiograph is not helpful. Chest tube placement is advised for pneumothorax >20% of lung volume, the lung may also be re-expanded with a small Teflon catheter under fluoroscopic guidance, eliminating the need for hospital admission. (See page 1448: Surgery to the Elbow.)

21. B. Innervation of the foot is provided by the femoral nerve (via the saphenous nerve) and by the sciatic nerve (via the posterior tibial, sural, and deep and superficial peroneal nerves). Inflation of a thigh tourniquet for longer than 15 to 20 minutes necessitates a general or neuraxial anesthetic, regardless of surgical site; otherwise, "solid" block of the femoral, sciatic, obturator, and lateral femoral cutaneous nerves is required. Placement of an indwelling catheter is indicated for major foot and ankle surgery, and allows for superior and prolonged analgesia with minimal opioid-related side effects.

Prolonged peripheral or plexus blockade provides excellent pain relief; however, the risk of accidental nerve trauma in an anesthetized extremity is theoretically higher outside the hospital environment. (See page 1451: Surgery of the Ankle and Foot).

22. A. Venous thromboembolism is a major cause of death after surgery or trauma to the lower extremities. Without prophylaxis, venous thrombosis develops in 40% to 80% of orthopedic patients, and 1% to 28% show clinical or laboratory evidence of pulmonary embolism. The incidence of fatal pulmonary embolism is highest in patients who have undergone surgery for hip fracture. For patients undergoing major joint replacement, administration of low—molecular-weight heparin (LMWH), warfarin, fondaparinux, or rivaroxaban is recommended. Similar recommendations are made for patients with acute spinal cord injury. Conversely, other orthopedic patients are considered low risk, and no pharmacologic prophylaxis is warranted. (See page 1454: Venous Thromboembolism).

23. C. Coexisting neural and muscular conditions may predispose pediatric orthopedic patients to latex allergy (e.g., myelomeningocele) and malignant hyperthermia. Children older than 7 years of age may tolerate a primary regional anesthetic technique, whereas younger children may benefit from a general or combination of regional/ general anesthesia. Often, regional anesthetic procedures are technically easier to perform on children because the relative lack of subcutaneous tissue facilitates identification of bony and vascular landmarks as well as spread of local anesthetic solutions. Intravenous regional (Bier) block is particularly useful in the pediatric population for limited procedures such as closed reduction of forearm fractures. (See page 1453: Pediatric Orthopedic Surgery.)

24. A. Hypothermia must be prevented in microvascular surgical patients. All the volatile anesthetics are potent vasodilators and can increase tissue blood flow 200% to 300%, even at typical expired anesthetic concentrations. Direct-acting vasodilating agents, such as sodium nitroprusside, trimethaphan, and hydralazine, produce vasodilation but do not prevent vasospasm because of direct surgical stimulation. Nitroprusside has been shown to reduce perfusion in a microvascular free flap. Regional anesthetic techniques provide sympathectomy and vasodilation to the proximal (innervated) segment of an extremity, but have no effect on vasospasm in the replanted (denervated) tissue. (See page 1452: Microvascular Surgery.)

25. A. With careful positioning and appropriate sedation, interscalene or supraclavicular blockade alone can provide excellent surgical anesthesia. Severe hypotension and bradycardia (e.g., Bezold–Jarisch reflex) have been reported in awake, sitting patients undergoing shoulder surgery under an interscalene block. In theory, VAE may occur during surgical procedures to the shoulder because the operative site is higher than the heart, but the incidence is low. Due to the potential for ipsilateral diaphragmatic paresis and 25% loss of pulmonary function, interscalene block is contraindicated in patients with severe pulmonary disease. (See page 1447: Surgery of the Shoulder and Upper Arm.)

Transplant Anesthesia

1. Which of the following statements concerning transplant immunology is FALSE?

   A. Transplant recipients who are not seropositive for cytomegalovirus (CMV) should receive CMV-negative blood.
   B. Interleukin-2 (IL-2) is involved in T-cell activation.
   C. Calcineurin enhances transcription of IL-2.
   D. The major blood group antigens are not potent transplant antigens.
   E. T lymphocytes play a major role in the immune response to a transplanted organ.

2. Which of the following statements concerning renal transplantation is FALSE?

   A. Cadaveric grafts can be safely transplanted after 24 hours of cold ischemia time.
   B. Intraoperative administration of insulin likely is effective in diabetic patients with elevated glucose concentrations during transplantation.
   C. Regional anesthesia for kidney transplantation is often contraindicated.
   D. Inhaled anesthetic techniques are better at preserving (graft) renal flow than intravenous techniques.
   E. Patients undergoing cadaveric transplants are more prone to pulmonary edema.

3. Which of the following is not a major anesthetic consideration during liver transplantation?

   A. Hypothermia
   B. Hypovolemia
   C. Hypocalcemia
   D. Metabolic alkalosis
   E. Reperfusion syndrome

4. Which of the following statements concerning organ transplantation in children is FALSE?

   A. Biliary atresia is the most common indication for pediatric liver transplantation.
   B. Children have a lower rate of successful renal transplantation than adults.
   C. Small children receiving large grafts may have respiratory compromise with abdominal closure.
   D. Hyperacute rejection does not occur because of the immaturity of the immune system and the absence of antibodies to various antigens.
   E. ABO-incompatible transplantation is contraindicated in the pediatric population.

5. The maximum tolerable cold ischemia time for a kidney that is being transported for transplantation is ___ hour(s).

   A. 1
   B. 3
   C. 12
   D. 36
   E. 60

6. Which of the following statements pertaining to brain-dead patients is FALSE?

   A. Flat electroencephalogram is consistent with brain death.
   B. There is absence of spinal reflexes in all brain-dead patients.
   C. Adrenergic surges just after brain death can cause ischemia and ischemia–reperfusion injuries.
   D. Brain death is associated with hemodynamic instability, which can negatively impact donor organ function.
   E. Transcranial Doppler as well as traditional or isotope angiography are used to confirm the clinical examination and lack of circulation to the brain.

7. Which of the following statements concerning lung transplantation is TRUE?

   A. Diabetes and hypertension are contraindications to lung transplantation.
   B. The age limit for single-lung transplantation is 55 years.
   C. Left-sided endobronchial double-lumen tubes are typically preferred for right as well as left transplants.
   D. Patients are not screened for malignancy.
   E. Hepatitis B and hepatitis C are not contraindications to lung transplantation.

8. Which of the following statements concerning glucocorticoids is FALSE?

   A. They produce glucose intolerance.
   B. They may cause hypertension.
   C. They may cause weight gain.
   D. They facilitate cytotoxic T-cell expression.
   E. They may cause gastrointestinal ulceration.

9. Which of the following statements concerning azathioprine is FALSE?

   A. Cardiac arrest and upper airway edema have been reported complications.
   B. Pancytopenia is a side effect.
   C. The S phase of the cell cycle is affected.
   D. The M phase of the cell cycle is affected.
   E. The intravenous dose is about half the oral dose.

10. Which of the following statements concerning cyclosporine is FALSE?

    A. It may exacerbate risk factors for coronary artery disease.
    B. It is nephrotoxic.
    C. It may cause hypertension.
    D. It may induce ischemic vascular disease.
    E. It does not interfere with the duration of nondepolarizing muscle relaxants.

11. Which of the following statements concerning monoclonal and polyclonal antibodies is TRUE?

    A. OKT3 antibody does not affect T cells.
    B. OKT3 may cause generalized weakness, fever, chills, and hypotension.
    C. Antilymphocyte globulin administration is not specific for lymphocytes.
    D. They do not contain human constant regions in the immunoglobulin.
    E. They should be avoided in patients with acute transplant rejection.

12. Which of the following statements concerning the recipient during renal transplantation is FALSE?

    A. After the first anastomosis is started, diuresis is initiated with mannitol and furosemide.
    B. Nonsteroidal anti-inflammatory drugs (NSAIDs) should be avoided in renal transplant recipients.
    C. The donor should be kept relatively volume depleted to minimize the kidney's work of filtration.
    D. Recipient iliac artery and vein are usually used for graft vascularization.
    E. Tight blood glucose control (80–110 mg/dL) is a reasonable anesthetic management goal during renal transplantation.

13. Which of the following statements pertaining to the anhepatic stage of orthotopic liver transplantation is FALSE?

    A. This phase begins when the liver is functionally excluded from the circulation.
    B. Arm lymphedema, but not air embolism, may be associated with venovenous bypass.
    C. Most patients can be managed without venovenous bypass.
    D. Venovenous bypass improves venous return.
    E. Venous return decreases by 50% to 60% with complete caval clamping.

14. Which of the following is the least likely to occur upon unclamping the new liver after vascular anastomosis?

    A. Hypertension
    B. Hypotension
    C. Bradycardia
    D. T-wave elevation
    E. Ventricular arrhythmias

15. Which of the following may be effective therapy for a patient with severe, irreversible pulmonary hypertension?

    A. Heterotopic heart transplant
    B. Orthotopic heart transplant
    C. Heart–lung transplant
    D. Left ventricular assist device (LVAD)
    E. None of the above

16. Which of the following statements concerning heart transplantation is TRUE?

    A. The pulmonary artery catheter is withdrawn from the surgical field after caval cannulation.
    B. Residual native atrial tissue may continue to have electrical activity, which would be seen as three P waves on the EKG.
    C. Isoproterenol is frequently used to decrease graft heart rate.
    D. Although the donor heart is denervated, normal physiologic feedback loops controlling inotropy and chronotropy are not lost.
    E. Ischemic time for the donor heart starts with aortic cross-clamp during the harvest and ends with removal of the cross-clamp from the recipient aorta.

17. In regards to attempts to induce hemodynamic changes, the transplanted heart responds poorly to all of the following medications/maneuvers EXCEPT:

    A. Ephedrine
    B. Carotid massage
    C. Isoproterenol
    D. Laryngoscopy
    E. Valsalva maneuver

18. Which of the following statements pertaining to pancreas–kidney transplantation is FALSE?

    A. Patients with type I diabetes who have frequent metabolic complications but preserved renal function should still undergo simultaneous pancreas–kidney grafts.
    B. Proper donor selection and targeted antibiotic coverage leads to better graft survival after isolated pancreas transplant.
    C. Close intraoperative blood glucose monitoring and control is important.
    D. These transplant recipient patients should undergo preoperative cardiac evaluation.
    E. End-organ complications of type 1 diabetes are the focus of the preoperative assessment of pancreas transplant recipients.

19. In regards to corneal transplantation, which of the following is FALSE?

    A. Corneas are the most common organs transplanted in the United States.
    B. This surgery must be performed under general anesthesia.
    C. Diuretics and fluid restriction may be necessary to prevent edema.
    D. Maintaining low intraocular pressure is a major intraoperative anesthetic goal.
    E. The most common cause of graft loss in the first year after corneal transplantation is rejection of corneal allografts.

ANSWERS

1. **D.** The antigens on the tissue's cell surface induce an immunologic reaction. T lymphocytes play a primary role in the immune response and allograft destruction. The major blood group antigens (ABO) are particularly potent transplant antigens. Calcineurin enhances transcription of T-cell IL-2. "Humanized" antibodies are directed against a portion of the IL-2 receptor and work by blocking IL-2–mediated T-cell activation. Since recipients are immunosuppressed, a diagnosis of occult infection (e.g., tuberculosis) should be excluded. For the same reason, it is standard to order CMV-negative blood for transfusion for seronegative recipients. (See pages 1464: Immunosuppressive Agents and 1466: Renal Transplantation.)

2. **D.** Cadaveric grafts can be safely transplanted after 24 hours of cold ischemia time and up to 36 hours, allowing scheduling of preoperative dialysis. In general, concerns over uremic platelet dysfunction and residual heparin from preoperative dialysis have limited the use of regional anesthesia for kidney transplantation. The major anesthetic consideration is maintenance of renal blood flow. No data are available to determine whether inhaled or intravenous techniques are better at preserving (graft) renal flow. For patients with diabetes, intraoperative administration of insulin to normalize blood glucose has not been formally studied for improving outcome. However, recent studies in patients in intensive care units suggest that outcome is significantly improved when glucose is tightly controlled. Therefore, optimal management of glucose (80–110 mg/dL) seems a reasonable anesthetic goal during renal transplantation. (See page 1466: Renal Transplantation.)

3. **D.** Loss of ascitic fluid and persistent bleeding may lead to hypovolemia and associated oliguria during liver transplantation. Metabolic acidosis may result from poor perfusion; it tends to persist in the absence of hepatic metabolic function. Rapid blood replacement may cause citrate-induced hypocalcemia. Preparation of fluid-warming units, gas circuit humidifiers, warming blankets, and non-conductive wraps for the head and extremities is essential for optimal preservation of normothermia. Sodium bicarbonate and calcium are given just before unclamping to counteract the effects of potassium on the heart. The original descriptions of reperfusion syndrome emphasized (often severe) hypotension and bradycardia with portal reperfusion. (See pages 1472: Pediatric Liver Transplantation and 1484: Pediatric Heart Transplantation.)

4. **E.** Although ABO-incompatible transplantation is contraindicated in the adult population, it is more successful in pediatric recipients. Hyperacute rejection does not occur because of the immaturity of the immune system and the absence of antibodies to various antigens, including blood group antigens. Pediatric renal transplantation is associated with somewhat lower rates of success than adult transplantation, with vascular thromboses of the grafts more common in young children. Small children receiving large grafts may have respiratory compromise with abdominal closure. Biliary atresia is the most common indication (43%) for pediatric liver transplantation. (See page 1466: Renal Transplantation.)

5. **D.** A cadaver allograft may be transplanted semi-electively because the tolerable ischemic time for kidneys is up to 36 hours. (See page 1466: Renal Transplantation: Preoperative Considerations.)

6. **B.** The legal and medical brain death criteria differ from state to state, but all states require cessation of both cerebral and brainstem functions. Brain-dead patients may have intact spinal reflexes, and therefore, they may require neuromuscular blockade during organ procurement. A flat electroencephalogram is consistent with brain death. Transcranial Doppler as well as traditional or isotope angiography are used to confirm the clinical examination and lack of circulation to the brain. Brain death is associated with hemodynamic instability as well as wide swings in hormone levels, systemic inflammation, and oxidant stress, all of which negatively impact donor organ function. Furthermore, adrenergic surges just after brain death can cause ischemia and ischemia–reperfusion injuries. (See page 1460: Anesthetic Management of Organ Donors—Brain-dead Donors.)

7. **C.** Since the right upper lobe bronchial orifice is relatively close to the origin of the main bronchus, left-sided endobronchial double-lumen tubes have been recommended for both right and left single-lung transplants as well as for bilateral-lung transplants. As for other transplants, patients are screened for malignancy (e.g., mammography, Pap test, and colonoscopy). Systemic disease processes such as diabetes and hypertension are not considered contraindications as long as they are clinically stable and medically optimized; however, chronic viral diseases are contraindications to transplantation. In the past, specific age limits were recommended for lung transplantation recipients, but current guidelines list age >65 years as a relative contraindication to transplantation. (See page 1473: Lung Transplantation.)

8. **D.** Corticosteroids disrupt the expression of many cytokines in T cells, antigen-presenting cells, and macrophages. Well-known side effects are hypertension, diabetes, hyperlipidemia, weight gain (including Cushingoid features), and gastrointestinal ulceration. (See page 1465: Corticosteroids.)

9. **D.** Azathioprine is hydrolyzed in blood to 6-mercaptopurine, a purine analog and metabolite with the ability to incorporate into DNA during the S phase of the cell cycle. Since DNA synthesis is a necessary prerequisite to mitosis, azathioprine exerts an antiproliferative effect. Azathioprine's major side effect is repression of bone marrow cell cycling,

which may cause pancytopenia. Cardiac arrest and severe upper airway edema are rare complications. The intravenous dose is about half the oral dose. (See page 1466: Other Immunosuppressive Drugs.)

10. E. Although rare, cyclosporine may prolong the action of pancuronium. Complications of cyclosporine use include hypertension (often requiring therapy), hyperlipidemia, ischemic vascular disease (including in heart recipients), diabetes, and nephrotoxicity. Ischemic cardiac disease is the leading cause of death in kidney transplant recipients, partly because of the underlying disease that preceded transplantation, but the use of calcineurin inhibitors may exacerbate risk factors for coronary artery disease. (See page 1465: Calcineurin Inhibitors.)

11. B. Antilymphocyte globulin is a polyclonal antibody that seems to diminish the availability of activated T lymphocytes and T-cell proliferation. They have a long history of use in treating acute transplant rejection and for the induction of immunosuppression. OKT3 antibody is directed against a component of the T-cell receptor complex and affects immunosuppression by blocking T-cell function. Acute administration of OKT3 in awake patients (especially in the first administration) may result in generalized weakness, fever, chills, and some hypotension. More severe hypotension, bronchospasm, and pulmonary edema have also been reported. (See page 1466: Polyclonal and Monoclonal Antibodies Immunosuppressive Drugs.)

12. C. The major anesthetic consideration is maintenance of renal blood flow. No data are available to determine whether inhaled or intravenous techniques are better at preserving (graft) renal flow. Therefore, typical hemodynamic goals during transplantation are systolic pressure above 90 mm Hg, mean systemic pressure above 60 mm Hg, and central venous pressure above 10 mm Hg. These goals are usually achieved without use of vasopressors by using isotonic fluids and adjusting anesthetic doses. The donor volume should be maintained. The recipient iliac artery and vein are used for renal graft vascularization. After the first anastomosis is started, a diuresis is initiated (mannitol and furosemide are often both given). It is recommended that NSAIDs be avoided in renal transplant recipients. Since tight glucose control after kidney transplant is associated with less rejection and diabetics with poorly controlled glucose levels after transplantation have increased mortality, tight blood glucose control (80–110 mg/dL) is thought to be a reasonable anesthetic management goal during renal transplantation. (See page 1466: Renal Transplantation-intraoperative Protocols.)

13. B. During the anhepatic stage, which begins when the liver is functionally excluded from the circulation, many centers use venovenous bypass. This helps to avoid drastic decreases in venous return and relieves venous congestion in the lower body, bowel, and kidneys. With complete vena cava cross-clamp, venous return decreases by 50% to 60%, often resulting in hypotension. Venovenous bypass does have the potential for complications including arm lymphedema and air embolism as well as vascular injury.

Most patients can be managed without venovenous bypass by using some volume loading. (See page 1468: Liver Transplantation--Coagulation Management.)

14. A. The original descriptions of reperfusion syndrome emphasized (often severe) hypotension (not hypertension) and bradycardia with portal reperfusion. Now with flushing techniques that precede reperfusion and changes in preservation solution, bradycardia is uncommon. Typically, reperfusion is associated with hypotension (a further decrease of already low systemic vascular resistance and increase in cardiac output), which may or may not require treatment. Portal unclamping may result in an increase in serum potassium. T waves may become elevated after unclamping. Ventricular arrhythmias, bradyarrhythmias, and severe hypotension may also occur. (See page 1468: Liver Transplantation—Coagulation Management.)

15. D. Pulmonary hypertension is associated with increased perioperative mortality. Although reversible pulmonary hypertension may be an indication for transplantation, severe, irreversible pulmonary hypertension is a contraindication to transplantation. Patients with irreversible pulmonary hypertension may be candidates for LVAD insertion as definitive therapy or as a bridge to transplantation. Totally implantable artificial hearts are not currently used because of technical issues. Heterotopic heart transplantation has been virtually abandoned. Bilateral sequential lung transplant has largely replaced heart–lung transplantation combined with advances in the pharmacologic management of pulmonary hypertension and right ventricular failure. (See pages 1477: Heart Transplantation and 1477: Heart–Lung Transplant [Adult and Pediatric].)

16. E. Ischemic time for the donor heart starts with aortic cross-clamp during the harvest and ends with removal of the cross-clamp from the recipient aorta. During heart transplantation, a long, sterile sheath should cover the pulmonary artery catheter so it may be pulled back before (not after) caval cannulation, and the catheter can be readvanced after removal of the superior caval cannula. Residual native atrial tissue may continue to have electrical activity, which would be seen as two (not three) P waves on the EKG. Isoproterenol is used frequently to increase (not decrease) heart rate because of its direct effects on cardiac β-receptors. Use of temporary epicardial pacing is sometimes needed until isoproterenol has had adequate time to reach maximal effect. Since the donor heart is denervated, normal physiologic feedback loops controlling inotropy and chronotropy are lost. (See page 1477: Heart Transplantation.)

17. C. The transplanted heart cannot respond to indirect-acting agents, such as ephedrine, or the autonomic effects of carotid massage, the Valsalva maneuver, or laryngoscopy. β effects (not α effects) of epinephrine and norepinephrine are exaggerated in heart transplant recipients. Isoproterenol is the mainstay of chronotropic therapy in these patients. The denervated heart does not compensate in reflex fashion for hemodynamic changes induced by regional anesthetics. (See page 1484: Management of Transplant Patients for Nontransplant Surgery.)

18. A.   The majority of pancreas transplants (about 75%) are done as simultaneous pancreas/kidney transplants from a single deceased donor; however, patients with type I diabetes who have preserved renal function usually undergo independent pancreas grafts. Proper donor selection and targeted antibiotic coverage leads to better graft survival after isolated pancreas transplant. The preoperative assessment of pancreas transplant recipients focuses on the end-organ complications of type 1 diabetes, and these patients also undergo a cardiac assessment. Intraoperatively, close attention to the control of blood glucose is indicated to protect newly transplanted β cells from hyperglycemic damage. (See page 1473: Pancreas and Islet Transplantation.)

19. B.   Corneas are the most common organs transplanted in the United States. Corneal transplants can be performed under local anesthesia and intravenous sedation; general anesthesia usually is not required. Intraoperatively, maintaining low intraocular pressure is a major anesthetic goal, and occasionally, diuretics and intravenous fluid restriction may be needed to prevent edema. The most common cause of graft loss in the first year after transplantation is rejection of corneal allografts. (See page 1466: Corneal Transplantation.)

Trauma and Burns

1. Which of the following statements regarding airway management in trauma patients is FALSE?

   A. Blind passage of a nasopharyngeal airway should be avoided if a basilar skull fracture is suspected.
   B. A cuffed supraglottic airway provides protection against pulmonary aspiration of gastric contents.
   C. Cricothyrotomy is contraindicated in patients younger than 12 years of age and in patients suspected of having laryngeal trauma.
   D. The esophageal–tracheal combitube has been associated with esophageal lacerations.

2. For trauma patients with head or neck injuries, which of the following statements is FALSE?

   A. Insertion of supraglottic airways will result in no cervical spine movement.
   B. Two percent to four percent of blunt trauma patients have cervical spine injuries.
   C. Head injury patients with low GCS scores are more likely to have neck injuries.
   D. Serious airway compromise may develop within a few hours in up to 50% of patients with major penetrating facial injuries.
   E. The presence of cartilaginous fractures or mucosal abnormalities of the airway necessitates performing an awake intubation.

3. Considerations in the management of patients with tension pneumothorax or flail chest injury should include all of the following EXCEPT:

   A. Immediate treatment for tension pneumothorax should be done with the insertion of a 14G angiocatheter via the second intercostal space on the midclavicular line.
   B. A flail chest injury results in impaired respiratory mechanics, so intubation and mechanical ventilation are the primary treatments of choice.
   C. Classic symptoms of tension pneumothorax include cyanosis, tachypnea, hypotension, and neck vein distention.
   D. Contusion of the underlying lung with increased elastic recoil and work of breathing is the main cause of respiratory insufficiency in flail chest.
   E. Effective pain relief, by itself, can improve respiratory function.

4. Which of the following statements regarding manual in-line immobilization (MILI) of the cervical spine is FALSE?

   A. Two operators in addition to the laryngoscopist are needed.
   B. Cephalad traction should be used because it aligns the head in a neutral position.
   C. MILI produces a higher incidence of inadequate visualization during direct laryngoscopy.
   D. Part of the cervical hard collar may be removed after MILI.
   E. Both shoulders should be stabilized by holding them against the table or stretcher.

5. Which of the following statements regarding resuscitation in trauma is TRUE?

   A. Tamponade is the most common cause of shock in patients with chest trauma.
   B. Resuscitation with 2,000 mL of isotonic fluids over 15 minutes will not permit estimation of the severity of hemorrhage.
   C. The base deficit, blood lactate level, and probably sublingual PCO_2 ($SLPCO_2$) are the most useful and practical markers of organ perfusion that can be used to set the goals of resuscitation in trauma patients.
   D. Intraosseous cannulation has many severe side effects.
   E. Intraosseous cannulation should not be used in children younger than 5 years old.

6. Which one of the following statements regarding the management of patients with head injuries is FALSE?

   A. After the initial traumatic event, a leading cause of morbidity is the progression of secondary injury resulting from tissue hypoxia.
   B. A maximally dilated and unresponsive pupil suggests uncal herniation under the falx cerebri.
   C. The most important therapeutic maneuvers are aimed at maintaining cerebral perfusion pressure and O_2 delivery.
   D. A reduction in intracranial pressure with pentobarbital is an effective means of cerebral protection and should be instituted in all instances of head injury.
   E. The Glasgow Coma Scale (GCS) is a valuable tool in the evaluation of head-injured patients.

7. Which of the following statements regarding abdominal injuries is FALSE?

   A. Traumatic herniation after diaphragmatic injury is more common on the left side than on the right side.
   B. A focused assessment with sonography for trauma (FAST) scan requires one-third of the time the conventional approach requires.
   C. Laparoscopy is an excellent screening tool in patients with abdominal trauma.
   D. Significant intra-abdominal bleeding is typically accompanied by considerable changes in abdominal girth.
   E. Diagnosis with FAST requires the presence of intra-peritoneal fluid.

8. Of the following methods of intraoperative monitoring for trauma patients, which single monitor is the most necessary before surgery?

   A. Right radial intra-arterial catheter (A-line)
   B. Urine output
   C. Central venous pressure (CVP) monitoring
   D. Transesophageal echocardiography (TEE)
   E. Esophageal temperature monitoring

9. Which statement regarding resuscitation during trauma is FALSE?

   A. Patients with burns of greater than 30% of the total body surface area develop resistance to most nondepolarizing muscle relaxants.
   B. The current recommendation for administration of hydroxyethyl starch ("hespan") should not exceed 20 mL/kg over 24 hours.
   C. Patients with hemorrhagic shock often exhibit bradycardia and respond readily to catecholamine infusions.
   D. Hypothermia leads to impaired O_2 release from red blood cells because of a leftward shift of the O_2 dissociation curve.
   E. Hypothermia and acidosis increase likelihood of a coagulopathy.

10. The Brain Trauma Foundation and the American Association of Neurological Surgeons recommend the maintenance of all of the following therapeutic interventions EXCEPT:

   A. PaO_2 greater than 95 mm Hg
   B. Mean arterial pressure (MAP) greater than 80 mm Hg
   C. Cerebral perfusion pressure (CPP) between 50 and 70 mm Hg
   D. Head-of-bed elevation greater than 30 degrees
   E. Initiating maintenance of $PaCO_2$ between 25 and 30 mm Hg within the first 24 hours

11. Which statement regarding neck and chest injuries is FALSE?

   A. Signs of airway injury include respiratory distress, subcutaneous crepitus, and laryngeal tenderness.
   B. First rib fractures are an indication of severe underlying trauma.
   C. The most definitive test for pneumothorax in supine patients is computed tomography (CT).
   D. After placement of a thoracostomy tube, drainage of 200 mL of blood and collection of more than 50 mL/hr are indications for thoracotomy.
   E. Sternal fractures usually are not associated with serious trauma to the thoracic or abdominal viscera.

12. Which of the following statements regarding pelvic and extremity injuries is FALSE?

   A. After pelvic fracture, retroperitoneal hematomas may lead to respiratory difficulty because of pressure on the diaphragm.
   B. Angiographic embolization is indicated to treat arterial bleeding after pelvic fracture.
   C. Open fractures of the extremities should be repaired within 6 hours to reduce the likelihood of sepsis.
   D. Immediate surgery is indicated for suspected extremity compartment syndrome when intracompartmental pressure exceeds 15 cm H_2O.
   E. Compartment syndrome is frequently characterized by severe pain in the affected extremity.

13. All of the following statements regarding burns are true EXCEPT:

   A. Fourth-degree burns involve muscle, fascia, and bone, and thus necessitate complete excision, leaving the patient with limited function.
   B. Full-thickness burns involving more than 10% of the total body surface area are considered major burns.
   C. Sources of airway compromise after burns include upper airway edema from fluid resuscitation and copious, thick secretions.
   D. Since swelling of the airway after thermal injury is only minimal in children, intubation is often not necessary in pediatric patients.
   E. In burn patients, fluid resuscitation may aggravate respiratory obstruction.

14. Which statement regarding carbon monoxide and cyanide poisoning is TRUE?

   A. Methylene blue is the main treatment for cyanide toxicity.
   B. The classic cherry red color of the blood commonly occurs at carboxyhemoglobin (HbCO) concentrations ≥10%.
   C. Patients with an HbCO level of ≥30% at admission are recommended for hyperbaric O_2 therapy.
   D. In burn victims, CO inhalation is always associated with smoke.
   E. Carbon monoxide causes right-shifting of the hemoglobin dissociation curve.

15. Which statement regarding the management of burn injuries is FALSE?

    A. Fluid flux in burn patients is enhanced by increased intravascular hydrostatic and interstitial osmotic pressures and decreased interstitial hydrostatic pressure.
    B. The hematocrit in burn patients should be kept above 30%.
    C. Fluid resuscitation is essential in the early care of burn patients with injuries of more than 15% of the total body surface area.
    D. Smaller burns can be managed with replacement at 150% of the calculated maintenance rate.
    E. Crystalloid solutions are preferred for resuscitation during the first day after a burn injury.

16. What serum creatinine kinase level (U/L) is most associated with renal failure in a patient with crush injury?

    A. 5,000
    B. 500
    C. 4,000
    D. 3,000
    E. 900

17. Which of the following accurately describes signs and symptoms of abdominal compartment syndrome?

    A. Decreased peak airway pressures
    B. Polyuria
    C. A tense, severely distended abdomen
    D. Intravesical pressure <20 mm Hg
    E. Low CO_2 levels

18. Prothrombin Complex Concentrate contains the following factors EXCEPT:

    A. XII
    B. VII
    C. X
    D. IX
    E. II

19. In patients with pulmonary contusions, which of the following statements is FALSE?

    A. Low tidal volumes, positive end-expiratory pressure (PEEP), and low plateau pressures decrease the likelihood of acute respiratory distress syndrome (ARDS)-related lung injury.
    B. Airway pressure release ventilation (APRV) may provide improved V/Q matching.
    C. Double-lumen tubes may be used to provide differential lung ventilation.
    D. High-frequency jet ventilation (HFJV) may enhance oxygenation in life-threatening hypoxemia.
    E. Neck vein distention is almost always present, and tracheal deviation is almost always appreciated, in a patient with tension pneumothorax.

20. Secondary brain injury (after initial traumatic brain injury) may occur as a result of all of the following EXCEPT:

    A. Hypotension
    B. Hypoxemia
    C. Anemia
    D. Hyperglycemia
    E. Hypertension

ANSWERS

1. B. The cuffed oropharyngeal airways and laryngeal mask airway provide for an adequate airway but do not necessarily protect against gastric aspiration in trauma patients. Blind passage of a nasopharyngeal airway in a patient with a basilar skull fracture may result in entry into the anterior cranial fossa and is therefore contraindicated with this injury. Cricothyrotomy is contraindicated in patients younger than 12 years old and in patients suspected of having laryngeal trauma. Permanent laryngeal damage may occur in young patients, and uncorrectable airway obstruction may occur in patients with laryngeal trauma. The esophageal–tracheal combitube is an acceptable airway alternative. It is not, however, without complications, such as esophageal laceration and its sequelae, including pneumothorax, pneumomediastinum, and subcutaneous emphysema. (See page 1491: Airway Evaluation and Intervention.)

2. A. Supraglottic intubating airways with or without the aid of FOB can be used, but neck movement with these devices appears to be comparable to that produced by conventional laryngoscopes. Overall, 2% to 4% of blunt trauma patients have cervical spine (C-spine) injuries, of which 7% to 15% are unstable. The most common causes include high-speed motor vehicle accidents, falls, diving accidents, and gunshot wounds. Head injuries, especially those with low Glasgow Coma Scores (GCS) and focal neurologic deficits, are likely to be associated with C-spine injuries. Serious airway compromise may develop within a few hours in up to 50% of patients with major penetrating facial injuries or multiple trauma as a result of progressive inflammation or edema resulting from liberal administration of fluids. The presence of cartilaginous fractures or mucosal abnormalities necessitates awake intubation with a fiber optic bronchoscope or awake tracheostomy. (See pages 1493: Cervical Spine Injury; 1496: Cervical Airway Injuries; 1491: Airway Evaluation and Intervention; and 1495: Direct Airway Injuries.)

3. B. Evidence suggests that liberal use of mechanical ventilation in the presence of a flail chest or pulmonary contusion increases the rate of pulmonary complications and mortality and prolongs the hospital stay. A flail chest results from comminuted fractures of at least three adjacent ribs or rib fractures with associated costochondral separation or sternal fracture. Without significant gas exchange abnormalities, chest wall instability alone is not an indication for ventilatory support. Effective pain relief by itself can improve respiratory function and often avoids the need for mechanical ventilation. Tension pneumothorax can be manifested by cyanosis, tachypnea, hypoxia, and neck vein distention. The definitive treatment is chest tube placement with suction (tube thoracostomy). The emergency treatment of tension pneumothorax, however, may require insertion of a 14G angiocatheter (needle thoracostomy) via the second intercostal space at the midclavicular line on the affected side. (See pages 1497: Management of

Breathing Abnormalities and 1497: Thoracic Airway Injuries.)

4. B. Stabilization of the head, neck, and torso in the neutral position for airway management in patients whose cervical spines are yet to be cleared is best accomplished by manual in-line immobilization (MILI). This is best accomplished by having two operators in addition to the physician who is managing the airway. The first operator stabilizes and aligns the head in the neutral position without applying cephalad traction, and the second operator stabilizes both shoulders by holding them against the table or stretcher. The anterior portion of the hard collar, which limits mouth opening, may be removed after immobilization. In-line stabilization, however, decreases the visibility of the larynx in a significant proportion of patients. Almost all airway maneuvers, including jaw thrust, chin lift, head tilt, and oral airway placement, result in some degree of cervical spine movement. (See page 1506: Initial Evaluation: Airway Management.)

5. C. Hemorrhage is the most common cause of traumatic hypotension and shock. Other sources include abnormal pump function, pericardial tamponade, pre-existing cardiac disease, pneumothorax or hemothorax, and spinal cord injury. Response to fluids aids in the assessment of hypovolemia. Administration of 2 L of lactated Ringer's solution over 15 minutes in adults should normalize the vital signs if hemorrhage is mild (10%–20% blood volume), transiently improve moderate hemorrhage (20%–40% blood volume), and have no response in patients with severe hemorrhage (>40% blood volume). Some of the proven markers of organ perfusion can be used during early management to set the goals of resuscitation. Of these, the base deficit, blood lactate level, and probably sublingual PCO_2 ($SLPCO_2$) are the most useful and practical tools during all phases of shock. Intraosseous cannulation is an acceptable form of vascular access in children younger than 5 years and has a low incidence of complications. (See page 1498: Management of Shock.)

6. D. Of all the possible secondary insults to the injured brain, decreased oxygen delivery as a result of hypotension and hypoxia has the greatest detrimental impact. Therefore, rapid diagnosis and treatment of head injury are paramount. Every effort should be made to support the blood pressure with fluids and vasopressors (preferably phenylephrine, which does not constrict the cerebral vessels) and ensure adequate oxygenation before the unconscious patient is evaluated. The GCS is a valuable tool in the evaluation of head-injured patients and provides a standard means of evaluating the patient's neurologic status. Physical signs of brain injury include motor dysfunction, which, in turn, includes ocular motor abnormalities such as unresponsive pupils. Management of head-injured patients should be aimed at maintaining cerebral perfusion and O_2 delivery. Decreasing intracranial pressure is a major step in this process. High-dose barbiturates (e.g., pentobarbital), however, are of no routine value and are used only for refractory intracranial pressure elevation. A maximally dilated and unresponsive pupil suggests uncal herniation under the falx cerebri and compression of the oculomotor nerve by the medial portion of the temporal lobe. (See page 1502: Early Management of Specific Injuries: Head Injury.)

7. D. Laparoscopy is an excellent screening tool in abdominal trauma patients. An analysis showed that it avoided laparotomy in 63% of patients and missed only 1% of injuries. It is also possible to repair diaphragmatic, bladder, and solid organ injuries with this technique. FAST requires one-third of the time as the conventional approach. FAST is operator dependent, has good specificity but moderate sensitivity, can diagnose injuries associated with intraperitoneal fluid but not those without it, and cannot determine the severity of organ injury. The liver protects the right side of the diaphragm, so traumatic herniation is more common on the left side. Absence of abdominal distention does not rule out intra-abdominal bleeding; at least 1 L of blood can accumulate before the smallest change in girth is apparent, and the diaphragm can also move cephalad, allowing further significant blood loss without any change in abdominal circumference. (See page 1512: Diaphragmatic Injury and Abdominal and Pelvic Injuries.)

8. A. Intra-arterial blood pressure monitoring allows beat-to-beat data acquisition and sampling for blood gases. A relatively stable patient may rapidly decompensate when the abdomen or chest is open. Thus, arterial blood pressure monitoring is valuable for therapeutic decisions. The radial artery is the vessel of choice in abdominal and chest trauma in which the aorta may be cross-clamped, making a femoral or dorsalis pedis cannula nonfunctional. The right radial artery is preferred in cases of chest trauma in which cross-clamping of the descending aorta may result in occlusion of the left subclavian artery. CVP monitoring is often unnecessary in young, healthy patients, but this approach can guide fluid replacement in elderly patients and when myocardial damage is likely. Delaying emergent surgery to place a central venous line is rarely indicated unless a large-bore catheter is needed for volume resuscitation. CVP measurements are subject to error in the presence of decreased ventricular compliance or pulmonary contusion, and systolic pressure variation and stroke volume estimates based on the arterial pressure tracing appear to correlate best with intravascular volume status. Urine output is routinely monitored as an indicator of organ perfusion, hemolysis, skeletal muscle destruction, and urinary tract integrity after trauma. Its reliability for monitoring perfusion is decreased by prolonged shock prior to surgery and osmotic diuresis caused by administration of mannitol or radiopaque dye. TEE provides valuable diagnostic information, including right and left ventricular volumes, ejection fraction, and the presence of tamponade and wall motion abnormalities. Visualization of fat and air entry into the right side of the heart and monitoring ventricular volume are added benefits. Despite this, TEE probe

insertion before surgery is typically not critical. (See page 1518: Monitoring.)

9. C. Confusion may arise concerning whether a patient is experiencing hemorrhagic shock or neurogenic shock. Indeed, a trauma patient may experience both types of shock simultaneously. However, the hallmark of neurogenic shock is that patients exhibit bradycardia and readily respond to fluids and catecholamine infusions. Flaccid areflexia, loss of rectal sphincter tone, paradoxical respiration, and bradycardia in a hypovolemic patient suggest the diagnosis. Hemorrhagic shock usually manifests with tachycardia and hypotension. Burns of greater than 30% of the total body surface area lead to resistance to all nondepolarizing muscle relaxants, with the possible exception of mivacurium, beginning at approximately 1 week and peaking around 5 to 6 weeks after injury. Current dosing recommendations for hydroxyethyl starch are to give no more than 20 mL/kg over 24 hours. This is because of potential coagulation abnormalities resulting from reduced platelet function, reduced fibrinogen levels, reduced factor VIII, and reduced von Willebrand factor. Patients with hypothermia have a left shift of the O_2 dissociation curve, which impairs tissue oxygenation. One of the principal goals during early management of hemorrhaging trauma victims is to avoid the development of acidosis, hypothermia, and coagulopathy. Both acidosis and hypothermia are major factors in the induction of coagulopathy. (See pages 1520: Anesthetic and Adjunct Drugs; 1523: Burns; and 1523: Intraoperative Management: Management of Intraoperative Complications: Persistent Hypotension, Hypothermia, and Coagulation Abnormalities.)

10. E. The Brain Trauma Foundation and the American Association of Neurological Surgeons have published evidence-based guidelines for the treatment of head-injured patients. The most important therapeutic maneuvers in these patients are aimed at normalizing intracranial pressure (ICP), CPP, and oxygen delivery. Primary therapy includes normalization of the systemic blood pressure (mean blood pressure > 80 mm Hg) and maintaining the PaO_2 above 95, the ICP below 20 to 25 mm Hg, and the CPP at 50 to 70 mm Hg. Maintaining the CPP above 70 mm Hg (the former standard) is no longer advised because it may be associated with an increased incidence of adult respiratory distress syndrome. The patient is kept at 30 degrees of head elevation, sedation and paralysis are given as necessary, and cerebrospinal fluid is drained through a ventriculostomy catheter, if available. Until about 1995, hyperventilation to a $PaCO_2$ of 25 to 30 mm Hg was a mainstay of therapy of patients with head injury. However, brain ischemia, which is probably the most threatening consequence of head injury, is likely to occur during the first 6 hours after trauma even when the CPP is maintained above the generally recommended 50 to 70 mm Hg. This hypoperfusion seems to be caused largely by increased cerebral vascular resistance, which may be enhanced by hyperventilation. However, some degree of hyperventilation may be necessary for short periods in patients who have severe injuries and elevated ICP that does not respond to normal ventilation and diuretics, although this should not be used during the first 24 hours after injury. (See page 1502: Head Injury.)

11. **D.** Respiratory distress, cyanosis, and stridor are obvious signs of airway injury. Other signs that strongly suggest airway injury are dysphonia, hoarseness, cough, hemoptysis, air bubbling from the wound, subcutaneous crepitus, laryngeal tenderness, pneumothorax, and hemothorax. First rib fractures, because of the high amount of injury required for fracture, indicate severe underlying trauma, particularly to the aorta, subclavian vessels, heart, brain, or spinal cord. Likewise, scapula fractures suggest severe thoracic injury, particularly cardiac and lung injuries. Paradoxically, sternal fractures are usually not associated with serious trauma to the thoracic or abdominal viscera. Upright plain radiographs provide the best opportunity for detection of pleural air. This position, however, may be impossible or contraindicated in some trauma patients. Although chest radiography and an ultrasonography may complement each other, CT is the most definitive radiologic test for detecting pneumothorax. Initial drainage of 1,000 mL of blood or collection of above 200 mL/hr for several hours after thoracostomy, is an indication for thoracotomy. Additional indications are a "white lung" appearance on the anteroposterior chest radiograph, a continuous major air leak from the chest tube, and evidence of pericardial tamponade. (See page 1508: Neck Injury, Chest Wall Injury, and Pleural Injury.)

12. **D.** Pelvic fractures may often result in significant bleeding, but the bleeding tends to be venous in nature and often tamponades itself. Arterial bleeding, in turn, may lead to large retroperitoneal hematomas and thus respiratory difficulty. Thus, angiography and embolization are indicated for treatment of arterial bleeding. Delayed fracture repair is associated with an increased risk of sepsis, pneumonia, deep venous thrombosis, and cerebral complications of fat embolism. Therefore, fixation should occur as soon as possible. In particular, open fractures should be repaired within 6 hours to reduce the risk of sepsis. Compartment syndrome, which is characterized by severe pain in the affected extremity, should be recognized early, so emergency fasciotomy can be effective in preventing irreversible muscle and nerve damage. The definitive diagnosis is made by measuring compartment pressures. Pressures exceeding 40 cm H_2O are an indication for immediate surgery. (See page 1513: Fractures of the Pelvis and Extremity Injuries.)

13. **D.** The pediatric airway can be greatly compromised by even minimal amounts of swelling because of its small diameter. Prophylactic intubation may often be required in children who are suspected of having an inhalational injury even though they are not yet in respiratory distress. Burns are classified as first, second, third, and fourth degree. First- and second-degree burns are partial thickness, and third- and fourth-degree burns are full thickness. Fourth-degree burns are the most severe and leave the patient with the highest likelihood of decreased function. Major burns include the following: (1) Full-thickness burns of more than 10% of the total body surface area; (2)

partial-thickness burns of more than 25% of the total body surface area in adults and more than 20% of the total body surface area at extremes of age; (3) burns involving the face, hands, feet, or perineum; (4) inhalational, chemical, or electrical burns; and (5) burns in patients with severe pre-existing medical conditions. In the upper airway, glottic and periglottic edema as well as copious, thick secretions may produce respiratory obstruction; this may be aggravated by fluid resuscitation even in the absence of significant inhalation injury. (See page 1514: Burns and Airway Complications.)

14. **C.** Carbon monoxide interferes with mitochondrial function and produces tissue hypoxia by shifting the hemoglobin dissociation curve to the left. The ultimate effect is impaired release of O_2 to tissues. This effect can be offset by high concentrations of inspired O_2. The classic cherry red color of blood occurs at an HbCO concentration of above 40%, but this may be obscured by coexistent hypoxia and cyanosis. Therefore, HbCO concentration by co-oximetry is the most sensitive indicator of carbon monoxide toxicity. The most effective treatment to date for carbon monoxide toxicity is hyperbaric O_2 therapy. An HbCO level of 30% or more is an indication for this therapy. Cyanide toxicity may also accompany smoke inhalation in victims of fires within a closed space. Specific treatments for cyanide toxicity include amyl nitrate, sodium nitrite, and thiosulfate. The half-life of cyanide, however, is short (~1 hour), so removal from the toxic environment and treatment with O_2 are often all that are necessary to reduce cyanide levels. (See page 1515: Carbon Monoxide Toxicity and Cyanide Toxicity.)

15. **B.** Fluid flux in burn patients is enhanced by increased intravascular hydrostatic and interstitial osmotic pressures and decreased interstitial hydrostatic pressure. Intravascular volume may be restored with either crystalloid or colloid solutions. Crystalloid solutions are preferred for resuscitation during the first day after a burn injury; leakage of colloids during this phase may increase edema. Fluid resuscitation is essential in the early care of burn patients with injuries of more than 15% of the total body surface area; smaller burns can be managed with replacement at 150% of the calculated maintenance rate and careful monitoring of fluid status. Patients often tolerate a decreased hematocrit after a burn injury. Transfusion is usually not initiated until the hematocrit is below 15% to 20% in healthy patients, approximately 25% in healthy patients who need extensive procedures, and 30% or more in patients with a history of pre-existing cardiac disease. (See page 1516: Fluid Replacement.)

16. **A.** The cause of renal failure in crush syndrome is probably rhabdomyolysis-induced myoglobin release into the circulation. Serum creatinine kinase (CK) levels increase in these patients; levels above 5,000 U/L are associated with renal failure. The differentiation of myoglobinuria from hemoglobinuria may be determined by examination of spun urine; a clear supernatant suggests myoglobin, whereas a rose color indicates hemoglobin. The traditional prophylaxis for renal failure after rhabdomyolysis includes

fluids, mannitol, and bicarbonate. However, more recent data suggest that bicarbonate and mannitol are ineffective. (See page 1528: Acute Renal Failure.)

17. **C.** Clinically, a tense, severely distended abdomen, raised peak airway pressure, CO_2 retention, and oliguria should direct the clinician to measure the intravesical pressure via a Foley catheter, which reflects the intra-abdominal pressure. Values >20 to 25 mm Hg may indicate inadequate organ perfusion and necessitate abdominal decompression, which, if delayed, may result in progression to multi-organ failure and death. (See page 1528: Abdominal Compartment Syndrome.)

18. **A.** Prothrombin Complex Concentrate (PCC, Factor IX complex) contains factors II, VII, IX, and X. In the trauma setting, it is used for rapid reversal of vitamin K antagonist oral anticoagulants (warfarin), especially in patients with intracranial bleeding. A similar effect can be obtained by administering FFP, but at a much slower rate and a larger infused volume; however, there is a smaller risk of viral transmission.

19. **E.** Indications for tracheal intubation and mechanical ventilation in patients with pulmonary contusion include respiratory insufficiency or failure despite adequate analgesia, clinical evidence of severe shock, associated severe head injury or injury requiring surgery, airway obstruction, and significant pre-existing chronic pulmonary disease. PEEP with low tidal volumes (6–8 mL/kg) and low inspiratory alveolar or plateau pressures should be used to decrease the likelihood of ARDS if ventilation is controlled. In intubated, spontaneously breathing patients, airway pressure releases ventilation, in which spontaneous breathing is superimposed on mechanical ventilation by intermittent sudden, brief decrease of continuous positive airway pressure, provides improved V/Q matching and systemic blood pressure, lower sedation requirements, greater O_2 delivery, and shorter periods of intubation. Patients with severe, unilateral pulmonary contusion unresponsive to these measures may be treated by differential lung ventilation via a double-lumen endobronchial tube. In bilateral severe contusions with life-threatening hypoxemia, HFJV may enhance oxygenation and cardiac function, which may be compromised by concomitant myocardial contusion or ischemia. Although cyanosis, tachypnea, hypotension, neck vein distention, tracheal deviation, and diminished breath sounds on the affected side are the classic signs of tension pneumothorax, neck vein distention may be absent in hypovolemic patients and tracheal deviation may be difficult to appreciate. (See page 1497: Thoracic Airway Injuries: Management of Breathing Abnormalities.)

20. **E.** Approximately 40% of deaths from trauma are caused by head injury, and even a moderate brain injury may increase the mortality rate of patients with other injuries. In nonsurvivors, progression of the damaged area beyond the directly injured region (i.e., secondary brain injury) can be demonstrated at autopsy. The primary objective of the early management of patients with brain trauma is to prevent or alleviate the secondary injury process that may follow any complication that decreases the oxygen supply to the brain, including systemic hypotension, hypoxemia, anemia, increased intracranial pressure, acidosis, and possibly hyperglycemia (serum glucose > 200 mg dL^{-1}). (See page 1493: Head, Open Eye, and Contained Major Vessel Injuries.)

Emergency Preparedness for and Disaster Management of Casualties from Natural Disasters and Chemical, Biologic, Radiologic, Nuclear, and High-Yield Explosive (CBRNE) Events

1. Which of the following facts about smallpox is FALSE?

   A. Infection is spread mainly via aerosolized droplets.
   B. Requires only 10 to 100 organisms to cause infection.
   C. Mortality after infection is as high as 50%.
   D. A rash develops as one of the first signs of infection.
   E. There is a predilection for the pox lesions to occur on the distal extremities and face.

2. The following facts about *Bacillus anthracis* (anthrax) are true EXCEPT:

   A. *Bacillus anthracis* must be finely ground so that spores may deposit themselves in the terminal bronchioles and alveoli.
   B. The lethal dose in 50% of humans (LD50) for anthrax is 1,000 spores.
   C. Anthrax may be aerosolized or sprayed as a means for terrorists to spread infection.
   D. Inhalation type anthrax is the most common form.
   E. An influenza-like prodrome occurs followed by dyspnea, cyanosis, hemoptysis, stridor, and chest pain.

3. The following facts about *Yersinia pestis* (plague) are true EXCEPT:

   A. The organism is viable for only 60 minutes after being dispersed.
   B. Rodents and fleas are the natural hosts for *Y. pestis*.
   C. There are two types of plague: Bubonic and pneumonic.
   D. The bubonic plague is also known as the "Black Death."
   E. Avoidance of illness may be accomplished by early vaccination.

4. The following facts about *Francisella tularensis* (Tularemia) are true EXCEPT:

   A. Humans acquire tularemia after being bitten by an infected deerfly or tick bite.
   B. Mortality of tularemia is in excess of 50%.
   C. As few as 10 to 50 organisms can invade the body.
   D. A vaccination of attenuated whole organism was available in the past.
   E. Cutaneous ulceration develops at the site of infection entry.

5. The following facts about *Clostridium botulinum* (botulism) are true EXCEPT:

   A. Death develops after a spastic paralysis occurs leading to respiratory failure.
   B. Botulinum is the most potent toxin known to humans.
   C. Treatment includes the use of antitoxin.
   D. Mortality rate is approximately 5% to 10%.
   E. Acetylcholine is involved in botulism's mechanism of action.

6. With regard to hemorrhagic fevers, which of the following is INCORRECT?

   A. They are transferred via rodent/insect reservoirs.
   B. They are RNA-based viruses.
   C. Ribavirin is a treatment for these viruses.
   D. This group comprises at least 18 viruses.
   E. Vaccinations are available for most of these viruses.

7. Terrorist groups have considered viral hemorrhagic fevers as potential weapons. This family of viruses includes all of the following EXCEPT:

   A. Marburg virus
   B. Dengue virus
   C. Arenaviruses
   D. Filoviruses
   E. Picornaviruses

8. Which of the following characteristics are not shared by hemorrhagic fevers?

   A. They cause DIC.
   B. Incubation periods are measured in days.
   C. Mortality rate can be 60%.
   D. There are vaccines available for yellow fever, hantavirus, and dengue fever.
   E. The hemorrhagic fevers are single-stranded RNA viruses.

9. Nuclear radiation presents an obvious health and safety concern. Which of the following is TRUE regarding presentation of a patient following exposure of high-dose ionizing radiation?

   A. Epithelial tissue will become saturated with bilious pigment.
   B. Radioactive iodine can accumulate in the thyroid.
   C. The bone marrow begins to overproduce plasma cells.
   D. Radiation accumulating in the blood–brain barrier will cause hallucinations.
   E. Cesium-137 will replace iron in hemoglobin, causing anemia.

10. Which of the following statements regarding ionizing radiation is TRUE?

    A. Chest radiographs lead to 50 to 100 mrem of exposure annually.
    B. CT scans can give 10 to 20x the amount of radiation as a chest film.
    C. Potassium iodide can attenuate most of the radiation-induced thyroid effects if given within 72 hours of exposure.
    D. Treatment is largely supportive, as these patients will develop acute radiation syndrome manifested by bleeding and sepsis.
    E. The use of macrophage-stimulating factor is essential for treating radiation sickness in the first 24 hours after exposure.

11. Which of the following is FALSE regarding radiation damage to humans?

    A. Patients who present with nausea, vomiting, diarrhea, and fever are likely to have severe acute radiation syndrome.
    B. With 0.75 to 1 Gy of exposure, hypotension, erythema, and CNS dysfunction can manifest weeks after the exposure.
    C. Hematopoietic syndrome (severe lymphoid and bone marrow suppression) results from exposure to 1 to 2 Gy.

    D. Hematopoietic syndrome may lead to death within weeks of the exposure event.
    E. Long-term effects include thyroid cancer and psychological injury.

12. With regard to disaster management in a nuclear crisis, the following statement is FALSE:

    A. As part of the containment process, to the extent possible patients should be decontaminated at the site.
    B. Removal of clothing is critically important, as material-emitting radiation can remain on a person's clothing.
    C. Chelation therapy that has been recommended includes calcium diethylenetriamine pentaacetic acid (DTPA).
    D. For individuals with a contaminated GI tract, selective decontamination has not been proven useful.
    E. "Dirty wounds" should be closed, cleaned, debrided, excised, and observed.

13. With regard to radiation exposure, the following is FALSE:

    A. 1 Bq = 1 disintegration per second.
    B. The Curie (Ci) is the SI measure of human exposure to radiation.
    C. The rad is the energy deposited by any type of radiation to any type of tissue or material. 1 rad = 0.01 Gy.
    D. The Gray is the SI unit for the energy deposited by any type of radiation, in joules per kilogram. 1 Gy = 100 rad.
    E. 100 rem = 1 sievert (Sv).

14. Which of the following biologic agents are listed as human warfare category C?

    A. Q-fever
    B. Equine encephalitic virus
    C. Cholera
    D. Rhinovirus
    E. Variola

15. Which of the following biologic agents are listed as category A?

    A. Anthrax
    B. Cholera
    C. Encephalitis
    D. Shigella
    E. Burkholderia mallei

16. Choose the correct answer with respect to the management of disasters associated with large casualties.

    A. Most residency program directors feel that anesthesiologists are well prepared to manage the large number of patients from a mass casualty event.
    B. Each type of disaster is unique and lacks common related principles.
    C. Anesthesiologists should not be expected to provide assistance during such emergencies.
    D. Nongovernmental organizations (NGOs) list anesthesia providers as tertiary healthcare workers needed to manage mass casualty events.
    E. Anesthesiologists possess the skills to manage a variety of scenarios, which accompany natural or man-made disasters.

17. All the following statements regarding terrorist use of weapons of mass destruction are true EXCEPT:

    A. Sarin is the most commonly used nerve agent.
    B. In dealing with acts of terrorism, geography is helpful in anticipating what type of event might occur.
    C. Anthrax and small pox are the most commonly used biologic agents.
    D. The most dangerous biologic agents have high lethality and infectivity.
    E. "Dirty" bombs are the most likely source of radiation used by terrorists.

18. A mass casualty incident:

    A. Would be a nuclear explosion in a populated area
    B. Results in a number of patients that the community healthcare system has the resources to treat
    C. Usually overwhelms a community's hospital emergency rooms
    D. Is always handled in an organized fashion without confusion
    E. Is worse than an event

19. The department of Health and Human Services (DHHS):

    A. Is maintained on a local state level
    B. Funds and equips several medical surgical teams (MSuRT) for disaster
    C. Created and maintains a National Disaster Medical System (NDMS)
    D. Was established as a response to the earthquake in Haiti in 2010
    E. Maintains over 300 MSuRTs

20. Which of the following regarding Disaster Medical Assistance Teams (DMAT) is FALSE?

    A. It is maintained by the DHHS.
    B. It sets up teams that are self-sustaining for at least 72 hours.
    C. A DMAT is supposed to train one weekend a month.
    D. It has the ability to mobilize rapidly.
    E. A DMAT has the capacity to perform surgical procedures.

21. The Joint Commission:

    A. Does not recognize the fact that hospitals have limited resources to respond to catastrophic events
    B. Published the "White Pater" in 2003 to help communities develop strategies for managing casualties
    C. Published mandatory guidelines for emergency community preparedness
    D. Requires hospitals to have monthly drills of their emergency preparedness
    E. Does not monitor hospitals' emergency preparedness procedures

22. Anesthesia providers can best utilize their skills in the management of healthcare delivery during a disaster in all the following EXCEPT:

    A. Assist in triage outside the hospital
    B. To assist in decontamination
    C. Performing surgical procedures
    D. To assist in ventilator management
    E. To assist with vascular access

23. Which of the following statements regarding triage classification is TRUE?

    A. As time passes, triage officers become more conservative and try to save as many victims as possible even if it means devoting major resources to a given patient.
    B. Delayed care patients are usually transported to an area separate from the ED where they can be provided comfort care.
    C. Immediate care victims must be treated within an 8-hour window.
    D. The expectant care triage group is not expected to survive.
    E. Triage patients are classified into six groups overall.

24. Therapy is not typically required if these symptoms accompany the agent responsible for the casualty:

    A. Explosive agent: Normal SpO_2 and intact tympanic membranes
    B. Radiation agent: Nausea within 6 hours of exposure
    C. Radiation agent: Abnormal leukocyte counts 48 hours after exposure
    D. Biologic agents: Fever, rash or dyspnea
    E. Chemical (nerve) agents: Bronchospasm or arrhythmia

25. The toxicity of the nerve agents depends on all of the following EXCEPT:

    A. The compound delivered
    B. The dose delivered
    C. The time of exposure
    D. Whether they are G series nerve agents since these are more toxic than V series agents

26. Signs of excessive acetylcholine include all of the following EXCEPT:

    A. Copious secretions
    B. Mydriasis
    C. Arrhythmias
    D. Bronchospasm
    E. Death

27. Nerve agents are similar to which of the following compounds?

    A. Antihistamines
    B. Organophosphate insecticides
    C. Antipsychotics
    D. Steroids
    E. Anticholinergics

28. Treatment for victims exposed to hydrogen cyanide includes:

    A. Vasodilators
    B. Sodium nitroprusside
    C. Sodium thiosulfate
    D. Steroids

29. Treatment for nerve agent poisoning includes all of the following EXCEPT:

    A. Atropine
    B. 2-PAM Chloride
    C. Benzodiazepines
    D. Glycopyrrolate

ANSWERS

1. D. Small pox is a highly contagious and potentially deadly weapon as an increasing number of people no longer carry immunity and in general, most civilians are no longer vaccinated. Forty percent to eighty percent of persons exposed to smallpox will develop disease. Smallpox is highly infective requiring only 10 to 100 organisms to infect an individual. After infection occurs, a prodrome develops which consists of malaise, headache, backache, and an onset of fever up to 40°C. The fever decreases over 3 to 4 days and a rash then develops. This is in contrast to chickenpox, where the rash develops at the same time as the fever. Unlike chickenpox, smallpox has a predilection for the distal extremities and face although no region is spared. Smallpox is spread mostly by aerosolization of droplets, which are inhaled; however, linens that come into contact with pustules can carry disease. (See page 1542: Biologic: Smallpox.)

2. D. *Bacillus anthracis* is a gram-positive, spore-forming bacillus, transmitted to humans following contact with contaminated animals. Anthrax must be ground finely to allow for passage into the terminal bronchioles and alveoli. The lethal dose in 50% of humans (LD50) for anthrax is 1,000 spores. Three types of primary anthrax exist: Cutaneous, inhalation, and gastrointestinal, with 95% being the cutaneous form. Anthrax may be aerosolized or sprayed as a means for terrorists to spread infection. Initially a flu-like prodrome occurs with fever, myalgia, malaise, and a nonproductive cough with or without chest pain. The patient appears to improve for a few days, and then dyspnea, cyanosis, hemoptysis, stridor, and chest pain ensue. Dyspnea is an ominous sign, and usually followed by death in 1 to 2 days. (See page 1542: Biological: Plague.)

3. E. *Yersinia pestis* is a nonmotile, gram-positive bacillus. Rodents and fleas are the natural hosts; however, soil can become contaminated, serving as a source of infection. The organism is viable for only 60 minutes after being dispersed. With bubonic plague, there is a 2- to 6-day incubation period, then a sudden onset of fever, chills, weakness, and headache. Painful swelling, or buboes, occurs in the lymph nodes in the groin, neck, or axilla. Twenty-five percent of patients have pustules, papules, or skin lesions near the buboes. Without treatment, patients become septic, develop cyanosis and peripheral tissue gangrene, leading to the term "Black Death." Patients infected with bubonic plague may seed their lungs leading to a highly contagious aerosolization of *Y. pestis* known as pneumonic plague. Mortality of plagues is over 50%. Treatment with antibiotics is available although no vaccination is currently available. (See page 1542: Biological: Plague.)

4. B. *Francisella tularensis* is a gram-negative pleomorphic rod. Infection is acquired after a bite from an infected animal, deerfly, or tick. Infection can also be brought about by ingestion of infected food or via aerosolization. Cutaneous ulcers develop at the site of entry. As few as 10 to 50 organisms can invade the body via hair follicles or mini-abrasions. Incubation is 2 to 6 days, at which time skin swelling and ulceration occur, eventually leading to a black scar. Inhalation tularemia is a possible threat. Following an incubation period of 3 to 5 days, fever, pharyngitis, bronchitis, pneumonia, pleuritis, and hilar lymphadenopathy ensue. Mortality rate of pneumonic tularemia is approximately 5% to 15%. An attenuated whole organism vaccination was formerly available. Treatment for tularemia is antibiotics. (See page 1542: Biological: Tularemia.)

5. A. *Clostridium botulinum's* threat as a biologic weapon is due to its ability to cause neuroparalysis. The live organism is not infectious; however, the gram-positive anaerobic spores, found in soil and agricultural products, may be deadly. Ingested toxins are distributed from the gastrointestinal tract or lungs into the blood. The toxins migrate to cholinergic nerve endings and block release of acetylcholine. This leads to a progressively worsening weakness and flaccid paralysis, starting at the extremities and progressing to respiratory muscle failure. Botulism is the most deadly toxin known to humans with an LD100 of only 1 pg. After ingestion, an incubation period of between 2 hours and 8 days occurs. Patients then become progressively weaker and complain of diplopia, dysarthria, dysphagia, and dyspnea leading to paralysis. There is also a muscarinic blockade resulting in decreased salivation, ileus, and urinary retention. Toxins can be removed by gastric lavage, cathartic, and with enemas. Antitoxin can be used and speeds recovery. Mortality is approximately 5% to 10%. (See page 1542: Biological: Botulism.)

6. E. Numerous viral hemorrhagic fevers exist, most notably: Hantavirus, ebola virus, and dengue and yellow fever. This group, comprised of at least 18 viruses, is made up of RNA-based viruses. This group causes a typical viral prodrome after inoculation through the dermis or following inhalation of viral particles. They are transferred via rodent/insect reservoirs. The virus replicates in lymphoid cells and has an incubation period that ranges from 2 to 18 days. This can lead to sepsis, septic shock, capillary leak resulting in pulmonary edema, thrombocytopenia, and disseminated intravascular coagulation (DIC). Fatality rate ranges from 2% to 60%. A specific antiviral therapy has not been established; however, treatment with ribavirin, interferon alpha, and hyperimmune globulin are often administered. A live, attenuated vaccine is available for yellow fever; however, a vaccine is not available for the other causes of hemorrhagic fever. (See page 1542: Biological: Hemorrhagic Fevers.)

7. E. There are a number of viral hemorrhagic fevers that are listed as category A agents, including the arenaviruses (lassa fever and others), bunyaviruses (hanta), flaviviruses (dengue), and filoviruses (ebola and marburg). Picornaviruses are not hemorrhagic in nature (however, they can cause flu-like symptoms and even poliomyelitis-like symptoms similar to the poliovirus). (See page 1545: Hemorrhagic Fevers.)

8. D. The viruses are single-stranded, ribonucleic acid (RNA) viruses which have a rodent or insect reservoir. The incubation period is within several days of contact or inhalation of the agent, at which time patients present with fever, myalgia, and evidence of a capillary leak (systemic leak or pulmonary edema), thrombocytopenia, and disseminated intravascular coagulation (DIC). The fatality rate, depending on the specific virus used is anywhere from 2% to 60%. There are no specific antiviral therapies for this class of viruses. There is a live attenuated virus vaccine for yellow fever, but there are none for any of the other agents. (See page 1545: Hemorrhagic Fevers.)

9. B. Potassium iodide is indicated to protect the thyroid gland from taking up iodine-131. Other expected injuries include radiation burns, bone marrow suppression, destruction of the lining of the gastrointestinal (GI) tract, GI bleeding with translocation of bacteria, infection, sepsis, septic shock, and death. Radiation does not accumulate in the "blood–brain barrier." Cesium-137 is a component of nuclear fallout, but does not replace iron in red blood cells. Ionizing radiation primarily functions by creation of free-radical molecules, which can then cause cross-linking of other molecules. (See page 1545: Radiation—Nuclear.)

10. D. Potassium iodide can attenuate most of the radiation-induced thyroid effects, but must be given as quickly as possible because after 24 hours, there is little protective effect. Treatment is largely supportive, as these patients will develop acute radiation syndrome manifested by bleeding and sepsis. Granulocyte–macrophage colony-stimulating factor and thrombopoietin or interleukin 11, though postulated, have not been proven to be of benefit. A chest radiograph leads to 5 to 10 mrem of exposure, whereas a CT scan can give up to 5,000 mrem—significantly more than 20x that of a chest film! (See page 1545: Radiation—Nuclear.)

11. C. Patients who present with nausea, vomiting, diarrhea, and fever are likely to have severe acute radiation syndrome. Hypotension, erythemia, and CNS dysfunction will manifest later. "Short-term" effects such as these, however, may not appear until days to weeks after the exposure, depending on the amount of exposure (as little as 0.75–1 Gy), whereas hematopoietic syndrome (severe lymphoid and bone marrow suppression) results from exposure to 3 to 6 Gy. Long-term effects include thyroid cancer and psychological injury. (See page 1545: Radiation—Nuclear.)

12. E. Dirty wounds should not be closed. As part of the containment process, to the extent possible, patients should be decontaminated at the site. Removal of clothing is critically important. Beta and gamma rays and neutrons will be gone unless there is still material emitting this radiation on a person's clothing. Chelation therapy has been recommended, including calcium diethylenetriamine pentaacetic acid (DTPA) as an initial dose and then zinc DTPA. For individuals with a contaminated GI tract, selective decontamination may be helpful, though again this has not been documented to be of benefit in this situation. (See page 1545: Radiation—Nuclear.)

13. B. The Curie is the traditional measure of radioactivity, as measured by radioactive decay. 1 Ci = 2.7×10^{10} disintegrations per second. The Sievert is the SI unit for measurement of human exposure to radiation, in joules per kilogram. 1 Sv = 100 rem. 1 Bq = 1 disintegration per second. The rad is the energy deposited by any type of radiation to any type of tissue or material. 1 rad = 0.01 Gy. The Gray is the SI unit for the energy deposited by any type of radiation, in joules per kilogram. 1 Gy = 100 rad. (See page 1547: Table 4.)

14. B. Equine encephalitic viruses are amongst the only category C agents listed. Category C agents are emerging pathogens that might be engineered for biologic warfare. (See page 1543: Table 3.)

15. A. Anthrax is the only category A agent listed. The others are category B agents. Category A agents are those weapons that are highly contagious and fit all the characteristics of a relatively ideal biologic agent. These include hemorrhagic fever viruses. Category B agents are relatively easy to disseminate but have low mortality rates. (See page 1543: Table 3.)

16. E. Most residency program directors would agree that anesthesiologists are well prepared to manage individual patients but are lacking when it comes to education in managing the numbers of patients that might arise from a mass casualty event. There are certain principles that are common to all such events. Independent of their etiology, and as a group, anesthesiologists are as well prepared if not better prepared, to assist their communities in planning for and in caring for patients from a disaster. Nongovernmental organizations (NGOs) place anesthesia providers at the top of the list of healthcare workers who are needed to manage the sequelae of natural disaster and mass casualty events. (See page 1536: Introduction.)

17. B. In dealing with acts of terrorism, geography is not helpful in anticipating what might occur, but that is not to say that one cannot anticipate what to expect. One can learn from experience: Terrorists have been successful in their minds' eyes with improvised explosive devices (IEDs), and even in those situations in which IEDs were not used, terrorists have chosen to use certain weapons of mass destruction (WMDs) more often than others. For example, if they were to choose a chemical agent, a nerve agent is most likely, and amongst those sarin has been the agent of choice. Similarly, amongst biologic agents, anthrax, which was used in 2001, or smallpox, would be the most likely choice because of the high lethality and infectivity associated with those two agents. Twice in the past 20 years, "dirty" bombs have either been planned or planted (and fortunately not used), so such a device would be the most likely source of radiation used by terrorists. (See page 1536: Introduction.)

18. **B.** A mass casualty incident is one that results in a number of patients that the community healthcare system has the resources to treat, despite turmoil and confusion. A mass casualty event is one that overwhelms the hospital or the community's healthcare system. (See page 1536: Introduction.)

19. **C.** In September 2011, the United States Department of Homeland Security published its first edition of a 111-page document: National Preparedness Goal. Of note, is that within the "Response" section, medical response is one of eleven for which the government has planned a response which is under the auspices of the Department of Health and Human Services (DHHS). The DHHS created and maintains a National Disaster Medical System (NDMS). Unfortunately, the system has not been adequately established and maintained. As highlighted by the US response to the earthquake in Haiti in 2010, the DHHS maintains only three International Medical Surgical Teams (IMSuRT). (See page 1537: Government Plan.)

20. **E.** Another team that the Department of Health and Human Services (DHHS) maintains in its National Disaster Medical System (NDMS) in addition to the IMSuRT is the DMAT (Disaster Medical Assistance Team)—a team that can rapidly mobilize and whose goal is to set up and be staffed with physicians, nurses and other support personnel, emergency facilities, and pharmaceutical dispensaries geographically as close as possible to a disaster. The teams are supposed to be self-sustaining for at least 72 hours before they require outside logistics. Just as the reserve military forces do, the DMAT is supposed to train one weekend a month. Not many surgeons or anesthesiologists have joined the DMAT, as the team does not have the capacity to perform surgical procedures. (See page 1537: Government Plan.)

21. **B.** In 2003, the Joint Commission published its "Health Care at the Crossroads: Strategies for Creating and Maintaining Community-wide Emergency Preparedness Systems." The white paper has not been updated but emergency preparedness is one of the "standards" the Joint Commission uses to certify hospitals. The Joint Commission recognizes that there has been a change in healthcare delivery in the United States over the last several years and decades, reflective of similar problems faced worldwide, that has left the healthcare system underfunded with limited resources and ever-increasing demand. Despite the best effort of law enforcement, fire and rescue teams, and emergency medical agencies, hospitals will continue to play a vital role in helping communities respond to catastrophic events. The Joint Commission was proactive in recognizing that, "It is no longer sufficient to develop disaster plans and dust them off if a threat appears imminent. Rather a system of preparedness across communities must be in place everyday." (See page 1538: NGOs' Plan.)

22. **C.** Some areas that anesthesia providers can assist in management of healthcare delivery during a disaster include: (1) Assisting in triage outside the hospital, (2) assisting in decontamination, (3) assisting with vascular access or airway management, and (4) assisting in ventilator management in the ICU or in overflow areas of the hospital. (See page 1538: NGOs' Plans.)

23. **D.** If assigned to triage patients, the anesthesiologist will be expected to classify patients into four groups—those requiring immediate care, delayed care, first aid, and expectant care. The latter group includes those expected to survive, or, because of the number of patients arriving, those for whom there are not adequate personnel or resources to adequately resuscitate without jeopardizing the lives of many more patients who would not receive the care they require and for whom the prognosis is more favorable. Experience has taught that initially triage officers are "conservative": They try to save as many as possible, but over days, if not hours, they gain experience and become better at identifying patients for whom resources exist to improve outcome. (See page 1539: Triage.)

24. **A.** Depending on which agent is involved in a mass casualty, the following lists symptoms which require medical intervention or therapy:
    a. Chemical (nerve) agents: If only headache, miosis, rhinorrhea, and lacrimation after exposure then a patient can be decontaminated and dismissed. Patients with dyspnea, bronchospasm, or arrhythmias will require treatment with atropine.
    b. Biologic agents: Fever, rash, dyspnea, and cough.
    c. Radiation/nuclear: Nausea within 6 hours of exposure: Because of the prevalence for those with this symptom, check leukocyte count, dismiss, and have the patient return in 48 hours for a repeat check—if no change in count, no therapy indicated.
    d. Explosive: If tympanic membranes intact and SpO_2 within normal limits, then other injuries are unlikely. (See page 1539: Role of Anesthesiologist in Mass Casualties.)

25. **D.** The toxicity of the nerve agents depends on the compound delivered, the dose that is delivered (LC), and the time (t) that an individual is exposed to that dose. G series agents are known as nonpersistent, whereas the V agents are persistent (in the environment) and are 10 times more toxic than the G agents. VX is the only agent ever fielded by the United States. (See page 1540: Chemical; Nerve Agents; Treatment.)

26. **B.** Similar to organophosphate insecticides and to the anticholinesterase drugs anesthesiologists use daily, nerve agents inhibit acetylcholinesterase. This inhibition results in excessive amounts of acetylcholine (the reason an anticholinergic agent such as atropine or glycopyrrolate is administered any time we inject an anticholinesterase such as neostigmine) at preganglionic muscarinic and postganglionic muscarinic and nicotinic receptors, leading to copious secretions, miosis, arrhythmias, bronchospasm, tonic muscle contractions, respiratory paralysis, seizures, and death. Similar to managing the side effects of neostigmine, a cholinergic agent and competitive muscarinic blockers (i.e., atropine or glycopyrrolate) are administered to

attenuate and block the muscarinic side effects of the agents. (See page 1540: Chemical, Nerve Agents.)

27. B.   Nerve agents inhibit acetylcholinesterase, similar to organophosphate insecticides and to the anticholinesterase drugs anesthesiologists use daily. Similar to managing the side effects of neostigmine, a cholinergic agent and competitive muscarinic blockers (i.e., atropine or glycopyrrolate) are administered to attenuate and block the muscarinic side effects of the agents.

28. C.   The third and final class of chemical toxins is considered the blood agents—hydrogen cyanide and cyanogen chloride. Because of the instability of the latter, hydrogen cyanide is more likely to be used by terrorists in a closed environment as an aerosol. Again, anesthesiologists are familiar with this class of substances because of the clinical use of sodium nitroprusside as an intravascular vasodilator, which results in cyanide as a metabolite. Cyanide inhibits cellular respiration by interrupting the oxidative electron transfer process in mitochondria. The treatment for cyanide toxicity is similar to what we anesthesiologists would do for someone who had an accidental overdose of sodium nitroprusside: Intravenous thiosulfate and supportive care including tracheal intubation, ventilation with 100% oxygen, and inotropes and vasopressors to stabilize the cardiovascular system.

29. D.   Depending on the extent of exposure, treatment is different. For minimal exposure, often seen with brief exposure to nerve agent vapor, patients may complain of headache and tightness in the chest and manifest miosis, rhinorrhea, and salivation. Individuals must be removed from further exposure, clothing removed, topical atropine applied to the eye if pain is significant, and wet decontamination if there was any liquid exposure. With moderate exposure, the same signs are present, but now the patient demonstrates more severe rhinorrhea, complains of dyspnea, and on examination, there is evidence of bronchospasm and muscle fasciculation. Patients with moderate (and severe) poisoning require treatment with atropine and 2-PAM chloride intramuscularly. Casualties again must have their clothing removed and if they were exposed to liquid nerve agent, they need to go through a wet decontamination process. With severe exposure, the same symptoms as mentioned above are present, but now the patient manifests severe respiratory compromise, flaccid paralysis, incontinence, arrhythmias, and convulsions. After decontamination the patient will require repetitive doses of intravenous atropine, along with intramuscular 2-PAM chloride, benzodiazepines to treat the seizures (caused by the muscarinic effects of the nerve agents within the CNS), and intubation and mechanical ventilation depending on the degree of respiratory compromise. (See page 1540: Chemical, Nerve, Treatment.)

CHAPTER

54

Postanesthesia Recovery

1. The greatest postanesthesia care unit (PACU) cost is for:
   A. Disposable items
   B. Antiemetics
   C. Routine diagnostic testing
   D. Staffing
   E. Respiratory therapy

2. Postoperative patient triage decisions should be based on:
   A. Ambulatory versus inpatient status
   B. Potential for postoperative complications
   C. Age
   D. American Society of Anesthesiologists (ASA) classification
   E. Insurance coverage

3. Disadvantages of intramuscular opioid administration (compared with intravenous administration) include all of the following EXCEPT:
   A. Unpredictable uptake
   B. Larger dose requirements
   C. Shortened onset
   D. Pain on administration
   E. Risk of hematoma formation

4. Which of the following statements regarding epidural opioid analgesia is FALSE?
   A. Serotonin antagonists may be used to treat side effects.
   B. It improves outcomes after urologic procedures.
   C. The addition of clonidine enhances analgesia.
   D. It is a useful technique for controlling pain after gastroplasty surgery.
   E. Immediate and delayed respiratory depression results from vascular uptake and cephalad spread in CSF.

5. Which statement regarding hypoxemia in the postanesthesia care unit (PACU) is TRUE?
   A. Hypoxemia rarely occurs after regional anesthesia.
   B. Children with adenotonsillar hypotrophy are at increased risk for hypoxemia.
   C. The incidence of hypoxemia in postoperative patients breathing room air in the PACU is low.
   D. The cost of providing supplemental oxygen is prohibitive.
   E. The use of oxygen prevents hypoxemia.

6. Which of the following is not a cause of hyponatremia?
   A. Intravenous administration of excess free water
   B. Use of sodium-free irrigating solutions
   C. Excess use of salt-wasting diuretics such as furosemide
   D. Syndrome of inappropriate antidiuretic hormone secretion
   E. Prolonged attempts of induction of labor with oxytocin

7. Which statement regarding adjuncts used for postoperative analgesia is TRUE?
   A. Rofecoxib administration provides a secondary cardioprotective benefit.
   B. Ketorolac administration may decrease cardiac ischemic events.
   C. Ibuprofen and acetaminophen are ineffective when they are administered orally before surgery.
   D. Agonist–antagonist analgesics are the best adjuncts to supplement analgesia.
   E. The use of clonidine is limited by bradycardia.

8. Which of the following statements regarding postoperative pain control in the postanesthesia care unit (PACU) is TRUE?

    A. Intravenous opioid loading is unnecessary before starting intravenous patient-controlled analgesia (PCA).
    B. Addition of clonidine to epidural infusions reduces the side effects of epidural opioids.
    C. Epidural analgesia always improves surgical outcomes.
    D. The use of intrawound continuous-flow catheters increases the length of hospital stay.
    E. Alternative modalities such as hypnosis or transcutaneous nerve stimulation are very effective in controlling surgical pain.

9. The most common sign of myocardial ischemia in the postanesthesia care unit (PACU) is:

    A. ST-T wave changes on the electrocardiogram (ECG) or monitor
    B. Diaphoresis
    C. Angina
    D. Dyspnea
    E. Tachycardia

10. Patients with obstructive sleep apnea (OSA) should be monitored with pulse oximetry until the oxygen saturation remains above ____ on room air while sleeping.

    A. 85%
    B. 90%
    C. 92%
    D. 95%
    E. 99%

11. According to the American Society of Anesthesiologists (ASA) and the Cardiac Anesthesia/Surgery Societies, patients who are not bleeding, are stable, and are euvolemic can tolerate a hemoglobin as low as:

    A. 6 g/dL
    B. 7 g/dL
    C. 8 g/dL
    D. 9 g/dL
    E. 10 g/dL

12. Which of the following is not a risk factor for postoperative apnea in preterm infants?

    A. Preoperative hematocrit
    B. Type of anesthetic
    C. Postconceptual age
    D. Weight
    E. Active/recent URI

13. Laryngospasm that occurs during emergence can be overcome by:

    A. Applying positive pressure by mask and deepening sedation with propofol but should usually avoid succinylcholine
    B. Only applying positive pressure by mask
    C. Applying positive pressure by mask, deepening sedation with ketamine and, if obstruction persists giving an intubating dose of succinylcholine
    D. Avoidance of positive pressure by mask, and a small dose of propofol
    E. Applying positive pressure by mask, deepening sedation with propofol and, if obstruction persists, giving a small dose of intravenous succinylcholine

14. The level of postoperative care a patient requires is determined by all of the following EXCEPT:

    A. Underlying illness
    B. Duration and complexity of anesthesia and surgery
    C. Risk of postoperative complications
    D. The inhalation anesthetic used
    E. Comorbidities

15. Upon arrival in the postanesthesia care unit (PACU), each patient assessment should include all of the following EXCEPT:

    A. Heart rhythm
    B. Temperature
    C. Ventilatory rate
    D. Capnography
    E. Blood pressure

16. Which of the following statements concerning postoperative pain management is FALSE?

    A. Appropriate postoperative pain management helps control hypertension and tachycardia.
    B. A tachycardic patient with low blood pressure should be treated aggressively with opioids.
    C. Sufficient analgesia is the desired endpoint, even if large doses of opioids are necessary.
    D. Short-acting opioids are useful to expedite discharge and minimize nausea in ambulatory settings, although duration of analgesia can be a problem.
    E. Disadvantages of intramuscular administration include larger dose requirements, delayed onset, and unpredictable uptake in hypothermic patients.

17. Discharge criteria for the postanesthesia care unit (PACU) include:

    A. Observation for at least 60 minutes after the last intravenous opioid is administered
    B. Achieving of normal body temperature
    C. Monitoring of oxygen saturation for 45 minutes after discontinuation of supplemental oxygen
    D. The presence of airway reflexes to prevent aspiration
    E. The patient must be able to void independently

18. Which of the following statements concerning upper airway edema is TRUE?

    A. It often leads to complete obstruction of the airway.
    B. Endotracheal intubation should be avoided.
    C. It is unrelated to C1 esterase inhibitor deficiency.
    D. It should be treated with emergency jet ventilation as soon as possible.
    E. It may be exacerbated by laryngoscopy.

19. Which of the following should not be used to acutely treat postoperative wheezing?

    A. IV steroids
    B. Aerosolized epinephrine
    C. Intramuscular terbutaline
    D. Ipratropium bromide
    E. Intravenous epinephrine infusion

20. All of the following medications are known to potentiate neuromuscular relaxation EXCEPT:

    A. Propanolol
    B. Intravenous phenytoin (Dilantin)
    C. Digoxin
    D. Furosemide
    E. Antibiotics

21. Which of the following tests reliably predicts recovery of airway protective reflexes?

    A. A negative inspiratory pressure of 25 cm H_2O or less
    B. Sustained head lift for 10 seconds
    C. Return of train-of-four (TOF) response to preoperative levels
    D. A forced vital capacity of 10 to 12 mL/kg
    E. None of the above

22. Pulmonary dead space increases with all of the following EXCEPT:

    A. Pulmonary embolism
    B. Endotracheal intubation
    C. Pulmonary hypotension
    D. Decreased cardiac output
    E. TRALI

23. Increased CO_2 production in the postanesthesia care unit (PACU) may be caused by all of the following EXCEPT:

    A. Shivering
    B. Infection
    C. Parasympathetic nervous system activity
    D. Hyperalimentation
    E. Malignant hyperthermia

24. Which of the following is not a proven effective treatment for postoperative hypoxemia?

    A. Incentive spirometry
    B. Semi-sitting position
    C. Continuous positive airway pressure (CPAP) by mask
    D. Endotracheal intubation without CPAP
    E. Reverse Trendelenburg position

25. Which of the following is not known to worsen ventilation–perfusion matching?

    A. An increase in pulmonary artery pressure
    B. A decrease in pulmonary artery pressure
    C. Impaired hypoxic pulmonary vasoconstrictive reflex
    D. An increase in the percentage of inspired oxygen
    E. Vasoconstrictors

26. All of the following regarding aspiration of gastric contents is true EXCEPT:

    A. It typically results in bacterial tracheal bronchitis.
    B. It may rapidly progress to acute respiratory distress syndrome (ARDS) and pulmonary edema.
    C. It can cause transient laryngospasm.
    D. It often causes an increase in pulmonary dead space.
    E. It can cause pulmonary edema.

27. All of the following should be done for patients who aspirate a large amount of gastric contents EXCEPT:

    A. Should be intubated and undergo suctioning before the administration of positive-pressure ventilation
    B. Should have tracheal pH ascertained and bicarbonate solutions instilled to increase the pH in the trachea to above 7.4
    C. Should be observed for 24 to 48 hours with serial temperature, white blood cell count, chest radiography, and arterial blood gas (ABG) measurements
    D. Should receive frequent pulse oximetry monitoring
    E. Should undergo immediate lateral head positioning and suction of airway

28. Treatment of patients with significant aspiration and resultant hypoxemia includes:

    A. Administration of furosemide
    B. Administration of high-dose steroids
    C. Aggressive fluid restriction
    D. Positive end-expiratory pressure (PEEP) mechanical ventilation
    E. Prophylactic antibiotics

29. Risk factors for corneal abrasion include all of the following EXCEPT:

    A. Prone positioning
    B. Head or neck surgery
    C. Lateral positioning
    D. Wearing mascara
    E. Short intraoperative period

30. The following statements concerning hypothermia and shivering in the postanesthesia care unit (PACU) are true EXCEPT:

    A. Severe shivering may increase CO_2 production by more than 100%.
    B. Myocardial ischemia and ventilatory failure may occur secondary to severe shivering.
    C. Intensity of shivering may be accentuated by inhalation anesthetic-related tremor.
    D. Meperidine is an effective treatment for postoperative shivering.
    E. Nonshivering thermogenesis is effective in adults.

31. Potential causes for prolonged unresponsiveness after anesthesia include all of the following EXCEPT:

    A. Pseudocholinesterase deficiency
    B. Hypoglycemia
    C. Hyperthermia
    D. Residual inhalation anesthetic
    E. Hypothermia

32. All of the following regarding hearing impairment after anesthesia and surgery are true EXCEPT:

    A. It usually requires intervention before its resolution.
    B. It occurs in 8% to 16% of patients after dural puncture for spinal anesthesia.
    C. It can be caused by eustachian tube inflammation and otitis secondary to endotracheal intubation.
    D. It is often related to disruption of the round window or tympanic membrane rupture.
    E. It is relatively common.

ANSWERS

1. D. The greatest PACU cost is for staffing. The mix of nursing staff (e.g., amount of training, experience, salaries, and benefit levels), the number of patients per caregiver, and the duration of PACU stay all determine an overall personnel cost per admission. Routine postoperative diagnostic testing increases costs for securing and processing tests, as well as for professional interpretation. Use of routine therapies such as oxygen, antiemetic therapy, and respiratory therapy increases the expenditure per patient for drugs and disposable items and may add to the staffing resources required per patient. (See page 1556: Value and Economics of the Postanesthesia Care Unit.)

2. B. Patients must be carefully evaluated to determine which level of postoperative care is most appropriate. Triage should be based on clinical condition and the potential for complications that require intervention. Alternatives to postanesthesia care unit (PACU) care must be used in a nondiscriminatory fashion. Triage should not be based on age, ASA classification, ambulatory versus inpatient status, or type of insurance. A wide margin of safety and applicable PACU standards should be preserved when appropriate. (See page 1557: Postanesthestic Triage.)

3. C. Disadvantages of the intramuscular route include larger dose requirements, delayed onset, and unpredictable uptake in hypothermic patients. The risk of hematoma formation is another consideration in anticoagulated patients. (See page 1558: Postoperative Pain Management.)

4. B. Epidural opioid analgesia is effective after thoracic and abdominal procedures because it helps to wean patients with obesity or chronic obstructive pulmonary disease from mechanical ventilation. Immediate and delayed ventilatory depression may occur related to vascular uptake and cephalad spread in cerebrospinal fluid, respectively. Nausea and pruritus are troubling side effects. Whereas nausea resolves with antiemetics, pruritus often responds to naloxone infusion. Addition of local anesthetic or clonidine enhances analgesia and decreases the risk of side effects from epidural opioids. Whether epidural analgesia improves surgical outcomes remains debatable. (See page 1558: Postoperative Pain Management.)

5. B. The incidence of hypoxemia in postoperative patients is high. In one study of PACU patients placed on room air, 30% of patients younger than 1 year old, 20% of those 1 to 3 years old, 14% of those 3 to 14 years old, and 7.8% of adults had their hemoglobin saturations decrease to below 90%. Perioperative hypoxemia occurs more frequently in children with respiratory infections or chronic adenotonsillar hypertrophy. Hypoxemia occurs frequently after regional anesthesia. Use of oxygen neither consistently prevents hypoxemia nor addresses underlying causes. The cost of supplemental oxygen is minimal, the inconvenience to patients is minor, and the overall risk is small. (See page 1568: Supplemental Oxygen.)

6. C. Postoperative hyponatremia occurs when excess free water is infused during surgery or sodium-free irrigating solution is absorbed by prostatic sinuses during transurethral prostate resection. Free-water retention may also be caused by inappropriate antidiuretic hormone secretion or prolonged induction of labor with oxytocin. Therapy for hyponatremia includes administration of normal saline and intravenous furosemide to promote renal wasting of free water in excess of sodium. (See page 1572: Hyponatremia.)

7. B. Perioperative oral or intravenous administration of cyclooxygenase-2 (COX-2) inhibitors offers promising adjuvant therapy to augment postoperative analgesia. Unfortunately, recent concerns about negative cardiac side effects of these agents led to the withdrawal of rofecoxib and clouded the overall appropriateness of this approach. Ibuprofen and acetaminophen are effective when administered orally before surgery. The antiplatelet properties of ketorolac may decrease cardiac ischemic events in patients with coronary artery disease. Agonist–antagonist analgesics offer little advantage. The use of clonidine to supplement analgesia is effective but may be limited by hypotension. (See page 1558: Postoperative Pain Management.)

8. B. Intravenous opioid loading in the PACU is important for a smooth transition to intravenous PCA. Addition of local anesthetic or clonidine enhances analgesia and decreases the risk of side effects from epidural opioids, although local anesthetics add risk of hypotension or motor block. Whether epidural analgesia improves surgical outcomes is debatable. Continuous-flow catheters with pressure delivery systems of local anesthetics have been used intrawound to reduce pain and opioid requirements, increase patient satisfaction, and reduce the length of hospital stay. Modalities such as guided imagery, hypnosis, transcutaneous nerve stimulation, music, massage, and acupuncture have limited utility for controlling surgical pain. (See page 1558: Postoperative Pain Management.)

9. E. In the PACU, it is a rare event for a patient to complain de novo of chest pain. The most common sign of myocardial ischemia is tachycardia. Tachycardia is often a reaction to, not necessarily the cause of, myocardial ischemia. The ECG may show classic ST-T wave elevation or depression depending on lead placement and the area of ischemia. But the lack of ST-T wave elevation does not rule out coronary artery disease. (See page 1562: Cardiovascular Complications.)

10. B. In May 2003, the American Society of Anesthesiologists (ASA) Task Force on Perioperative Management of Patients with Obstructive Sleep Apnea issued guidelines based on the ASA scoring system for OSA and classifying patients as having mild, moderate, or severe OSA based on the apnea–hypopnea index. Patients who use continuous positive airway pressure or noninvasive positive-pressure ventilation should continue to use these therapies. Regarding monitoring, there is agreement among the task force consultants that pulse oximetry should be used until the patient's oxygen saturation remains above 90% on room air while sleeping. The use of telemetry for monitoring pulse oximetry, electrocardiography, or ventilation may be beneficial in reducing adverse postoperative events and should be used on a patient need basis. (See page 1567: Obstructive Sleep Apnea.)

11. A. Recent works from the ASA and the cardiac anesthesia and surgery societies (Society of Thoracic Surgeons and Society of Cardiovascular Anesthesiologists) have published guidelines for transfusion and blood management. It is now well accepted that patients who are stable, not bleeding, and euvolemic can tolerate a hemoglobin of 6 g/dL. (See page 1567: Anemia.)

12. D. The risk for apnea after anesthesia in preterm infants depends on the type of anesthetic, postconceptual age, and preoperative hematocrit. Children with active or recent upper respiratory infection are more prone to breath-holding, severe cough, and arterial desaturations below 90% during recovery, especially if they have a history of reactive airway disease or secondhand smoke exposure or have undergone intubation and/or airway surgery. (See page 1563: Inadequate Respiratory Drive.)

13. E. During emergence, stimulation of the pharynx or vocal cords by secretions, blood, foreign matter, or extubation may precipitate laryngospasm. The laryngeal constrictor muscles occlude the tracheal inlet and reduce gas flow. Patients are at higher risk if they smoke, are chronically exposed to smoke, have irritable airway conditions, have copious secretions, or have undergone upper airway surgery. Laryngospasm can usually be overcome by providing gentle positive pressure (10–20 mm Hg) in the oropharynx with 100% oxygen. Prolonged laryngospasm is relieved with a small dose of succinylcholine (e.g., 0.1 mg/kg) or deepening sedation with propofol. An intubating dosage of succinylcholine should not be used to break postoperative laryngospasm, especially if the alveolar partial pressure of oxygen (PaO_2) is decreased by hypoventilation. As little as 5 to 10 mg of succinylcholine can break the laryngospasm. (See page 1563: Increased Airway Resistance.)

14. D. For both ambulatory and inpatient surgery, the level of postoperative care a patient requires is determined by the comorbidities present, the degree of the underlying illness, the duration and complexity of the anesthesia and surgery (but not specifically the inhalational agent used), and the risk of postoperative complications. Using a less intensive postanesthesia setting for selected patients may reduce the cost of the surgical procedure and may allow the facility to divert scarce postanesthesia care unit resources to patients with greater needs. (See page 1557: Levels of Postanesthetic Care.)

15. D. Every patient admitted to a PACU should have heart rate and rhythm, systemic blood pressure, and ventilatory rate recorded. Capnography is necessary only for patients receiving mechanical ventilation or those at risk for compromised ventilatory function. Assessment every 5 minutes for the first 15 minutes and every 15 thereafter is a prudent minimum. Temperature should be documented at least on admission and discharge, along with the level of consciousness, airway patency, and skin color. (See page 1558: Admission to the Postanesthesia Care Unit.)

16. B. Relief of surgical pain with minimal side effects is a primary goal of PACU care. Improving patient comfort and relief of pain reduces sympathetic nervous system response, helping to control postoperative hypertension and tachycardia. Analgesics may precipitate hypotension in hypovolemic patients who rely on sympathetic activity for cardiovascular homeostasis such as tachycardic patients with normal or low blood pressure. Sufficient analgesia is the desired clinical endpoint for all patients, even if large doses of opioids are necessary. Short-acting opioids are useful to expedite discharge and minimize nausea in ambulatory settings, although duration of analgesia can be a problem. Disadvantages of intramuscular administration include larger dose requirements, delayed onset, and unpredictable uptake in hypothermic patients. (See page 1558: Postoperative Pain Management.)

17. D. Before discharge from the PACU, each patient should be sufficiently oriented to assess his or her physical condition and to summon assistance upon discharge. Airway reflexes and motor function must be adequate to prevent aspiration. Blood pressure, heart rate, and indices of peripheral perfusion should be relatively constant for at least 15 minutes. Achieving normal body temperature and voiding are not absolute requirements. Patients should be observed for at least 15 minutes after the last intravenous opioid or sedative is administered. Oxygen saturation should be monitored for 15 minutes after discontinuation of supplemental oxygen to detect hypoxemia. (See page 1560: Discharge Criteria.)

18. E. Acute extrinsic upper airway compression must be relieved if possible. If the obstruction is fixed, emergency tracheal intubation may become necessary. However, airway manipulation is fraught with danger. Even minor trauma from intubation attempts may convert a partially obstructed airway into a totally obstructed airway. Complete obstruction from airway edema is rare. Edema is often resolved by nebulized racemic epinephrine. Small doses of corticosteroid have also been effective. An acute airway emergency may be precipitated if tracheal intubation or face mask ventilation cannot be accomplished. In these cases, cricothyroidotomy and emergency jet ventilation are the treatments of choice. However, these should be attempted after endotracheal intubation has failed. Patients with C1 esterase inhibitor deficiency can develop severe angioneurotic edema after even slight trauma to the airway. (See page 1563: Increased Airway Resistance.)

19. A. The treatment of small airway resistance is directed at the underlying cause. Patients often respond well to their existing regimens of albuterol or other inhalers. Intramuscular or sublingual terbutaline may be added. If ventilation is still compromised or is unduly labored, an aminophylline loading dose and maintenance infusion may be administered.

Bronchospasm resistant to β-sympathomimetic medication may improve with an anticholinergic medication such as atropine or ipratropium. If bronchospasm is life threatening, an intravenous epinephrine infusion usually yields profound bronchodilation. Administration of steroid therapy offers little acute improvement, but may prevent later recurrence. (See page 1563: Increased Airway Resistance.)

20. **C.** Medications that potentiate neuromuscular relaxation include some antibiotics, furosemide, propranolol, and acutely administered (intravenous) phenytoin. Conversely, long-term phenytoin use increases the dose requirements for nondepolarizing neuromuscular blocking agents. (See page 1564: Neuromuscular and Skeletal Problems.)

21. **E.** A forced vital capacity of 10 to 12 mL/kg and an inspiratory pressure of 25 cm H_2O or less imply that the strength of ventilatory muscles is adequate to sustain ventilation. The ability to sustain head elevation in a supine position is a rough index of muscular recovery. Tactile TOF assessment accurately assesses the patient's ability to ventilate. However, none of these clinical endpoints reliably predicts recovery of the airway protective reflexes. (See page 1564: Neuromuscular and Skeletal Problems.)

22. **B.** Any decrease in pulmonary blood flow, as would be caused by pulmonary embolism pulmonary hypotension, decreased cardiac output, or TRALI causes an increase in physiologic dead space. Upper airway dead space (anatomic dead space) has been shown to be reduced by approximately 75% after endotracheal intubation and almost eliminated by tracheostomy. (See page 1565: Increased Dead Space).

23. **C.** In the PACU, metabolic rate and CO_2 production may increase by as much as 40%. Shivering, high work of breathing, infection, sympathetic nervous system activity, and rapid carbohydrate metabolism during intravenous hyperalimentation also accelerate CO_2 production. Malignant hyperthermia generates CO_2 production many times greater than normal. (See page 1565: Increased Carbon Dioxide Production.)

24. **D.** In the PACU, conservative measures to improve lung volume such as assuming a semi-sitting or reverse Trendelenburg position often produce lasting improvements in oxygenation. Incentive spirometry and mask CPAP both increase functional residual capacity and improve ventilation–perfusion matching, resulting in improved oxygenation. Intermittent positive-pressure breathing techniques are probably not effective. Endotracheal intubation without CPAP results in a progressive reduction of functional residual capacity and ventilation–perfusion mismatching that may actually worsen arterial hypoxemia. (See page 1566: Distribution of Ventilation.)

25. **E.** Increased pulmonary artery pressure may interfere with ventilation–perfusion matching by increasing blood flow to less dependent (and less ventilated) portions of the lung as well as by increasing flow through the bronchial circulation and pulmonary arterial venous anastomoses. Reduction in pulmonary artery pressures may also change ventilation–perfusion matching by compromising perfusion to the nondependent lung. Inhalation anesthetics, nitroprusside, vasodilators, and other medications impair hypoxic pulmonary vasoconstriction; this partially explains the increase in the alveolar–arterial oxygen gradient associated with general anesthetics. The effects of anesthetics on hypoxic pulmonary vasoconstriction persist into the recovery period. An increased inspired O_2 fraction may interfere with ventilation–perfusion matching in patients with acute lung disease, perhaps resulting from interference with hypoxic pulmonary vasoconstriction or promotion of reabsorption atelectasis. (See page 1566: Distribution of Perfusion.)

26. **A.** Cough, mild tracheal irritation, or transient laryngospasm are immediate sequelae after aspiration of gastric contents during vomiting or regurgitation. Large-volume aspiration can predispose to infection, small airway obstruction, or pulmonary edema. Aspiration of gastric contents during vomiting or regurgitation causes chemical pneumonitis that is characterized initially by diffuse bronchospasm, hypoxemia, and atelectasis. This may rapidly progress to ARDS and pulmonary edema. Occlusion or destruction of the pulmonary microvasculature is often evident, resulting in increased pulmonary vascular resistance and increased dead space. Bacterial infection rarely results. Advancing age, in the absence of coexisting disease, is not a risk factor for aspiration. (See page 1568: Perioperative Aspiration.)

27. **B.** Patients who aspirate a large amount of gastric contents should be observed for 24 to 48 hours for the development of aspiration pneumonitis. Observation includes serial temperature checks, white blood cell counts with differential, chest radiography, and ABG determinations. Fluffy infiltrates may appear on the chest radiograph within 24 hours of the event. If a large aspiration has occurred, the patient should first undergo immediate lateral head positioning and suction of airway, then the trachea should be intubated, and suctioning should be performed before institution of positive-pressure ventilation (to avoid widely disseminating any aspirated material into the distal airways). Instillation of saline or alkalotic solutions is not recommended. Bacterial infection does not necessarily occur after aspiration, and prophylactic antibiotics are thus not recommended. In fact, they may promote colonization by resistant organisms. (See page 1568: Perioperative Aspiration.)

28. **D.** If significant aspiration causes hypoxemia, increased airway resistance, consolidation, or pulmonary edema, then institution of supplemental oxygen, continuous positive airway pressure, or mechanical ventilation with PEEP may be necessary. Pulmonary edema is usually secondary to increased capillary permeability and should not be treated with diuretics. Hypovolemia from fluid losses into the lung may necessitate aggressive fluid infusion. High-dose steroids yield little improvement of long-term outcome after aspiration. (See page 1568: Perioperative Aspiration.)

29. E.   Corneal abrasions occur more frequently in elderly patients, after long procedures, with lateral or prone positioning, and after head or neck surgery. Corneal injury can occur during emergence in the PACU from patients rubbing their eyes, if a rigid oxygen face mask rides up on the eye, or if the eye is rubbed with a pulse oximeter probe and from eye make-up (particularly mascara) being rubbed in the eyes. (See page 1572: Ocular Injuries and Visual Changes.)

30. E.   Nonshivering thermogenesis is ineffective in adults. Postoperative shivering is uncomfortable and increases the risk of accidental trauma. Moreover, severe shivering may increase oxygen consumption and CO_2 production by 200%. This increases cardiac output and minute ventilation; myocardial ischemia or ventilatory failure may result. The intensity of postoperative shivering is sometimes accentuated by inhalation anesthetic-related tremors. Meperidine is a particularly effective treatment for postoperative shivering. (See page 1574: Hypothermia and Shivering.)

31. C.   Residual sedation from inhalation anesthetics is a frequent cause of prolonged unconsciousness, particularly after long procedures, in obese patients, and when high inspired concentrations are continued through the end of surgery. Profound residual neuromuscular paralysis may mimic unconsciousness by precluding any motor response to stimuli. This may occur after gross overdose, if reversal agents are omitted, in patients with unrecognized neuromuscular disease, and in patients with phase II blockade (caused by either excessive succinylcholine administration or pseudocholinesterase deficiency). Hypothermia (<33°C) impairs consciousness and increases the depressant effect of medications. A serum glucose level should be evaluated to rule out hypoglycemia. (See page 1574: Persistent Sedation.)

32. A.   Hearing impairment after anesthesia and surgery is relatively common. Although impairment is often subclinical, patients sometimes experience decreased auditory acuity, tinnitus, or roaring. The incidence of detectable hearing impairment is particularly high after dural puncture for spinal anesthesia (8%–16%), and it varies with the needle size, needle type, and patient age. Impairment can be unilateral or bilateral and usually resolves spontaneously. Hearing loss is often related to disruption of the round window or rupture of the tympanic membrane. (See page 1573: Hearing Impairment.)

Critical Care Medicine

1. Which of the following is not used in the management of severe sepsis and septic shock?

   A. Empiric broad-spectrum antibiotics within 1 hour of diagnosis and reassessment of appropriate therapy upon availability of microbiology results
   B. Vasopressin as an adjunct vasopressor for a target mean blood pressure of 65 mm Hg
   C. Pulmonary artery catheterization in patients with acute lung injury
   D. Fluid challenges to achieve adequate filling pressures, and a reduction of rate of fluids with rising filling pressures and no improvement in tissue perfusion

2. Decreased brain tissue oxygen pressure ($PbrO_2$) measurements may occur as a result of all of the following EXCEPT:

   A. Increase in intracranial pressure (ICP)
   B. Arterial oxygen desaturation
   C. Barbiturate coma
   D. Hyperventilation

3. All of the following statements regarding therapies that lower intracranial pressure (ICP) are accurate EXCEPT:

   A. Propofol causes systemic hypotension and decreases cerebral metabolism, resulting in a coupled decline in cerebral blood flow (CBF) with a consequent decrease in ICP.
   B. Although barbiturates are effective at reducing ICP, their routine use in patients with traumatic brain injury (TBI) does not appear beneficial and may actually result in excess mortality in patients with diffuse brain injury.
   C. Although neuromuscular blockade may result in a lowering of ICP, the routine prolonged intensive care unit (ICU) use of neuromuscular blockade is discouraged.
   D. Hyperventilation effectively reduces ICP by reducing CBF, and prophylactic hyperventilation has proven to be beneficial in TBI.

4. Which of the following statements regarding the management of cerebral vasospasm after subarachnoid hemorrhage (SAH) is TRUE?

   A. There is a good correlation between the transcranial Doppler (TCD) velocities and angiographic findings, especially for the posterior circulation.
   B. The calcium channel blocker nimodipine is effective primarily because it reduces the frequency of angiographic vasospasm compared with a placebo-treated group.
   C. Prophylactic "triple-H" therapy is one of the proven mainstays of management for cerebral ischemia associated with SAH-induced vasospasm.
   D. Patients treated within 6 to 12 hours after the development of ischemic symptoms with the use of balloon angioplasty have better results than those receiving delayed intervention.

5. Ventilator-induced lung injury (VILI) or ventilator-associated lung injury (VALI) is associated with the following features EXCEPT:

   A. Histologically, the features seen are diffuse alveolar damage and increased microvascular permeability.
   B. VILI is associated with the systemic release of inflammatory mediators.
   C. Tidal volume selection based on actual body weight improves mortality.
   D. Tidal volumes as low as 4 cc/kg may be appropriate to avoid VILI.

6. All of the following statements regarding acute respiratory distress syndrome (ARDS) are true EXCEPT:

   A. Pulmonary injury is not the only trigger for the syndrome.
   B. The mortality rate is approximately 30% to 40%.
   C. Positive end-expiratory pressure (PEEP) is a useful adjunct in maintaining oxygenation.
   D. Late in the syndrome, increasing inspired O_2 resolves the hypoxia more effectively than does PEEP.

7. Which of the following statements is TRUE regarding tissue plasminogen activator (TPA) administration in patients with an acute ischemic stroke?

   A. Treatment is uniformly effective when administered any time within 3 hours of the onset of symptoms.
   B. It reduces mortality.
   C. Direct intra-arterial administration is more effective than systemic administration.
   D. Patients should not be treated with any other anticoagulants within 24 hours after receiving TPA.

8. Strategies that help(s) prevent the development of auto-PEEP in patients with chronic obstructive pulmonary disease (COPD) include all of the following EXCEPT:

   A. Reducing tidal volumes to 6 to 8 mL/kg
   B. Permissive hypercapnia and resultant respiratory acidosis
   C. Prolonged expiratory phase of ventilation
   D. Limiting inspired O_2 concentration

9. Regarding glucose management in critically ill patients, all of the following are true EXCEPT:

   A. Hyperglycemia is associated with increased risk of postoperative infection.
   B. The blood glucose level is a risk factor for mortality in diabetic patients admitted with acute myocardial infarction.
   C. Patients in the intensive care unit (ICU) may have elevated blood glucose levels because of total parenteral nutrition (TPN) or steroid administration.
   D. Elevated blood glucose levels in patients with traumatic brain injury (TBI) are expected and do not require intervention.

10. All of the following statements regarding sedation with propofol for patients with traumatic brain injury (TBI) are true EXCEPT:

    A. Propofol improves mortality resulting from improved intracranial pressure (ICP) regulation.
    B. Prolonged administration of high-dose propofol may produce lactic acidosis and death.
    C. Propofol may decrease cerebral perfusion pressure (CPP) because of hemodynamic instability.
    D. Propofol improves cerebral metabolic O_2 balance better than benzodiazepines.

11. Septic shock is associated with all of the following EXCEPT:

    A. Vulnerable intestinal villi, because of their counter-current circulation
    B. Insufficient splanchnic circulation resulting in thrombocytopenia
    C. Reduction in splanchnic intramucosal pH
    D. Metabolic acidosis even with sufficient levels of O_2 delivery

12. All of the following statements are true regarding the use of norepinephrine in shock EXCEPT:

    A. Its effects are mediated through α- and β-adrenoreceptors.
    B. In volume-resuscitated individuals, norepinephrine improves renal perfusion.
    C. Norepinephrine should be administered at the first sign of sepsis because early intervention may prevent progression to profound septic shock.
    D. Norepinephrine may produce a reduction in lactate levels by improving perfusion.

13. Vasopressin used for the management of septic shock is associated with all the following EXCEPT:

    A. Significant increase in the systemic vascular resistance (SVR)
    B. Significant increase in the heart rate
    C. In patients with hepatorenal syndromes, improved urinary output
    D. Generally unaffected pulmonary vascular resistance (PVR)

14. Ventilator-associated pneumonia (VAP) is associated with all of the following features EXCEPT:

    A. Reduced incidence with gastric acid suppression therapy
    B. Reduced incidence with strict hand washing, oral care, and the head-up position
    C. Higher mortality risk with late-onset VAP than early-onset VAP
    D. Early-onset VAP is generally caused by different organisms than late-onset VAP

15. Which of the following statements about dexmedetomidine is FALSE?

    A. It is an α_2-adrenergic receptor agonist.
    B. It has some analgesic effects.
    C. It produces sedation without inducing unresponsiveness.
    D. It is approved by the Food and Drug Administration (FDA) for prolonged sedation.

16. Nutritional supplementation in the intensive care unit (ICU):

    A. Should be started 36 to 48 hours after ICU admission
    B. Is facilitated by raising the head of the bed to 30 to 40 degrees
    C. Is equally effective via enteral and parenteral routes
    D. Requires postpyloric positioning of feeding tubes

17. Advantages of the Glasgow Coma Scale (GCS) in patients with traumatic brain injury (TBI) include all EXCEPT:

    A. It provides an objective method of measuring the level of consciousness.
    B. It has high intra- and inter-rater reliability across observers with a wide variety of experience.
    C. It is accurate even when only the partial score is used, such as in patients with endotracheal intubation whose verbal responses cannot be assessed.
    D. It is a powerful predictor of poor outcome from TBI.

18. The pulmonary artery catheter (PAC):

   A. Improves mortality in elderly, high-risk surgical patients

   B. Needs further research to establish utility in critically ill patients

   C. Can guide supraphysiologic resuscitation to improve outcomes

   D. Improves survival in acute respiratory distress syndrome (ARDS)

19. Catheter-related bloodstream infections (CRBSI) may be reduced by:

   A. Skin cleansing with chlorhexidine

   B. Using catheters coated with antibiotics

   C. Using the jugular vein preferentially

   D. Routine catheter replacement at 3 or 7 days

20. Interventions in the processes of critical care that have been shown to improve outcomes as adopted by the Leapfrog Initiative include all of the following EXCEPT:

   A. Management or co-management by intensivists who are present at all times

   B. Intensivists that can—at least 95% of the time—return ICU pages within 5 minutes

   C. Management or co-management by intensivists who provide clinical care exclusively in the ICU

   D. Utilization of procedural checklists

ANSWERS

1. C. The initiation of empiric broad-spectrum antibiotics within 1 hour of diagnosis and reassessment of appropriate therapy upon availability of microbiology results is part of the 6-hour sepsis management bundle promoted by the Surviving Sepsis Campaign. Norepinephrine and dopamine are first-line vasopressors, with vasopressin serving as an adjunct vasopressor for a target mean blood pressure of 65 mm Hg. Fluid challenges are indicated to achieve adequate filling pressures, and a reduction of rate of fluids is recommended with rising filling pressures and no improvement in tissue perfusion. Pulmonary artery catheterization has not been shown to improve fluid management in patients with acute lung injury. (See page 1591: Section: Table on Management of Severe Sepsis and Septic Shock.)

2. C. $PbrO_2$ measurements are performed by introducing a small, oxygen-sensitive catheter into the brain tissue. The device monitors a very local area of the brain tissue, and this technique is increasingly used for evaluation of cerebral oxygenation (normal $PbrO_2$ values: 25–30 mm Hg). Monitoring may be performed in relatively undamaged parts of the brain or, preferably, in the penumbra region of an intracerebral lesion. Various studies have shown that an increase in ICP, a decrease in CPP or arterial oxygenation, and hyperventilation may result in decreased $PbrO_2$. Studies have demonstrated improvement in $PbrO_2$ after red blood cell transfusion, during barbiturate coma, and after decompressive hemicraniectomy. (See page 1583: Section: Brain Tissue Oxygenation.)

3. D. Hyperventilation effectively reduces ICP by reducing CBF. However, the role that hyperventilation should play in routine management of patients with TBI is not clear. Primarily, this is related to concerns that hyperventilation may lead to critically low CBF, resulting in worsening cerebral ischemia. In small, randomized trials, prophylactic hyperventilation has not proven to be beneficial in TBI. In contrast, it has been proposed that "optimized hyperventilation" in the presence of "luxury perfusion" (excess CBF) may increase global cerebral oxygen metabolism and help normalize global cerebral glucose extraction. Based on the available evidence, prolonged or prophylactic hyperventilation should be avoided after severe TBI, especially in the first 24 hours after the injury. Propofol rapidly penetrates the central nervous system and has rapid elimination kinetics. Propofol causes systemic hypotension and decreases cerebral metabolism, resulting in a coupled decline in CBF, with consequent decrease in ICP. The use of high-dose propofol to control refractory intracranial hypertension is not recommended, and barbiturates should be considered if ICP is not controlled by moderate doses of propofol. The mechanisms by which barbiturates exert their cerebroprotective effect appear to be mediated by a reduction in ICP via alteration in vascular tone, reduction of cerebral metabolic rate, and inhibition of free radical peroxidation. Although barbiturates are effective at reducing ICP, their routine use in patients with TBI does not appear beneficial and may actually result in excess mortality in patients with diffuse brain injury. This effect may in part relate to the profound cardiovascular depressant effects of barbiturates. Although neuromuscular blockade may result in a decrease in ICP, the routine use of neuromuscular blockade is discouraged because its use has been associated with a longer ICU course, a higher incidence of pneumonia, and a trend toward more frequent sepsis without any improvement in outcome. (See page 1583: Section: Traumatic Brain Injury.)

4. D. Interventional neuroradiology with the use of balloon angioplasty may reverse or improve vasospasm-induced neurologic deficits. Patients treated within 6 to 12 hours after the development of ischemic symptoms have better results than those receiving delayed intervention. The risks of angioplasty include intimal dissection, vessel rupture, ischemia, and infarction. Hypervolemic, hypertensive, and hemodilution ("triple-H") therapy is one of the mainstays of treatment for cerebral ischemia associated with SAH-induced vasospasm despite the lack of evidence for its effectiveness, especially for its prophylactic use. There is no consensus with regard to the goals of therapy, and it is unclear which component of this therapy is necessary or sufficient to treat vasospasm. The calcium channel blocker nimodipine (60 mg orally q4h for 21 days) is recognized as effective prophylaxis for cerebral vasospasm and improvement in neurologic outcome (reduction of cerebral infarction and poor outcome) and mortality from cerebral vasospasm in patients with SAH (level I evidence). Although angiographic studies do not demonstrate a difference in the frequency of vasospasm compared with a placebo-treated group, the benefits of nimodipine have been attributed to a cytoprotective effect related to the reduced availability of intracellular calcium and improved microvascular collateral flow. Transcranial Doppler has been used to identify and quantify cerebral vasospasm on the basis that velocity profiles increase as the diameter of the vessel decreases. There is a poor correlation between the TCD velocities and angiographic findings, especially for the posterior circulation. (See page 1585: Section: Subarachnoid Hemorrhage.)

5. C. VILI or VALI refers to microscopic injury to the lung caused by overdistention ("volutrauma") and cyclic reopening of alveoli ("atelectrauma"). VALI has been well demonstrated in numerous experimental models and is histologically similar to the features seen in acute lung injury (ALI) of other causes, with diffuse alveolar damage and increased microvascular permeability. In addition, VALI is associated with the systemic release of inflammatory mediators that may contribute to multiple organ failure. Clinically, patients believed to be at risk for VALI are those with abnormally low recruitable lung volumes, particularly those with ALI and acute respiratory distress syndrome (ARDS). Thus, a "lung-protective" ventilatory strategy using low tidal volume ventilation has been proven to save lives when applied to patients with ALI and ARDS. In summary, although tidal volumes of 10 to 12 mL/kg (predicted body weight) may still be indicated for some patients, in most cases, an initial tidal volume of 8 mL/kg is probably appropriate, and volumes as low as 4 mL/kg may be appropriate in some cases. In addition, because lung volumes correlate with height rather than weight, tidal volume selection should be based on predicted or ideal body weight rather than actual weight to avoid lung overdistention. (See page 1593: Section: Acute Respiratory Failure.)

6. D.   ARDS arises from various underlying pathophysiologic perturbations, such as sepsis, trauma, hypotension, pneumonia, aspiration, and amniotic fluid embolism. The syndrome arises from a loss in alveolar capillary integrity, which results in the leakage of plasma and red blood corpuscles into the alveoli. Leukoaggregation on the endothelial surface and proliferation of type II pneumocytes also occur. Clinically, ARDS and acute lung injury (ALI) are characterized by reduced static thoracic (lung and chest wall) compliance and severe impairment of gas exchange, including high intrapulmonary shunt and dead space fraction. There is a large increase in the arterial–alveolar (A–a) gradient for O_2, and the patient complains of dyspnea and is tachypneic with increased work of breathing. Initially, increased inspired O_2 improves oxygenation, but as the shunt fraction increases and the work of breathing overwhelms the patient, positive-pressure ventilation will have to be instituted. PEEP is the mainstay of treatment to improve oxygenation. Since the disease process is one of shunt, PEEP helps recruit nonventilated alveoli and thereby reduces the A–a gradient. PEEP also reduces pulmonary water and decreases the work of breathing. The treatment of ALI and ARDS is largely supportive and includes aggressive treatment of inciting events, avoidance of complications, and mechanical ventilation. Mortality associated with ARDS has decreased substantially over the past 20 years and is currently in the 30% to 40% range overall. (See page 1593: Section: Acute Respiratory Failure and Clinical Manifestations.)

7. D.   TPA must be administered within 3 hours of the onset of symptoms of cerebral occlusion to be effective. Even within the 3-hour window, the benefits of TPA appear to be greater the sooner the treatment is started. Administration does not reduce mortality, but it does improve neurologic outcome. Regional or local intra-arterial administration of a thrombolytic agent within 6 hours of symptom onset demonstrates a high recanalization rate, but a potential limitation to the use of intra-arterial treatment is the time required to mobilize a team to perform angiography (level II evidence). However, direct arterial injection has yet to be proven more effective than peripheral systemic administration. After TPA has been administered, no other anticoagulants or antiplatelet agents can be administered within 24 hours of treatment because doing so would increase the risk of bleeding and increase mortality. (See page 1586: Section: Acute Ischemic Stroke.)

8. D.   In patients with obstructive lung disease (asthma and COPD), limitation of expiratory flow leads to air trapping

and the development of intrinsic PEEP or auto-PEEP. To reduce the occurrence of auto-PEEP, tidal volume should be limited to 6 to 8 mL/kg. The expiratory phase of ventilation should be made as long as possible to facilitate alveolar emptying. Both of the foregoing strategies may result in insufficient ventilation, and respiratory acidosis may occur. This produces minimal physiologic effects and should be tolerated. O_2 concentration in the inspired mixture does not affect auto-PEEP. (See page 1593: Section: Principles of Mechanical Ventilation.)

9. D.   Increased blood glucose levels in critically ill patients result from diabetes, TPN, and steroid administration as well as from stroke or trauma to the central nervous system. Hyperglycemia results from increased glucose production and insulin resistance caused by inflammatory and hormonal mediators that are released in response to injury. Hyperglycemia is associated with increased risk of postoperative infection (wound and otherwise) and poor outcome in patients with stroke or TBI. In addition, the blood glucose level is a risk factor for mortality in diabetic patients admitted with acute myocardial infarction. An elevated glucose level in patients with brain trauma is a harbinger of poor outcome and should be treated to reduce mortality and morbidity. (See page 1597: Section: Glucose Management in Critical Illness.)

10. A.   Sedation of neurologically impaired patients should typically be achieved with short-acting sedatives to allow for frequent assessment of neurologic status. Although no studies have investigated the effect of sedation on outcome, a common practice is to provide sedation with propofol or benzodiazepines in patients after TBI. Both agents have favorable effects on cerebral oxygen balance, although propofol is more potent in this regard. Propofol produces rapidly reversible sedation that reduces cerebral metabolic demand and coupled blood flow. This, in turn, results in a reduction of ICP, which improves CPP. In inadequately resuscitated individuals, propofol may produce hypotension, which would result in a worsening of CPP. Prolonged high-dose administration of propofol (>80 μg/kg/min and >24 hours) may produce lactic acidosis and death (propofol infusion syndrome). Sedation-mediated alterations in CPP and reduced cerebral O_2 requirements have not produced a reduction in mortality. (See page 1583: Section: Traumatic Brain Injury.)

11. B.   Septic shock is a form of distributive shock associated with activation of the systemic inflammatory response. The hemodynamic profile of septic shock is influenced by several sepsis-induced physiologic changes, including hypovolemia and vasodilation, in addition to cardiac depression. Microcirculation is altered, and metabolic needs are increased. The ability of tissues to extract and use oxygen may be impaired. Thus, metabolic acidosis may be present despite normal levels of oxygen transport. Intestinal villi have a countercurrent flow that makes them susceptible to low flow states. These alterations result in insufficient blood flow to the intestinal mucosa, which produces localized acidosis. This flow can be indirectly measured (intramucosal pH and PCO_2), and hemodynamic therapy may be altered to improve splanchnic oxygenation. Decreased splanchnic circulation does not cause thrombocytopenia. (See page 1589: Section: Septic Shock.)

12. C. Norepinephrine's effects are mediated through α- and β-adrenoreceptors. Norepinephrine produces an increase in systolic blood pressure with variable effects on cardiac output and heart rate. In septic individuals, intravascular volume expansion is the first line of therapy. If patients remain persistently hypotensive despite volume expansion and markers of adequate preload, the use of vasopressors is indicated. Norepinephrine increases systemic vascular resistance, which improves splanchnic blood flow and decreases lactate levels. In patients who are septic and euvolemic, norepinephrine increases renal blood flow. In all cases, norepinephrine should not be administered to improve hemodynamics before fluid administration has been attempted. (See page 1591: Section: Management of Shock with Vasopressors or Inotropes.)

13. B. Vasopressin is a potent vasoconstrictor when administered in low doses to patients in shock, particularly those with distributive shock caused by sepsis or hepatic failure and those with circulatory failure after cardiopulmonary bypass. Vasopressin administration results in significant increase in systemic blood pressure with little or no effect on cardiac output, heart rate, or pulmonary vascular resistance. At low doses, it does not affect renal blood flow, and in the hepatorenal syndrome, it increases urinary output. (See page 1591: Section: Management of Shock with Vasopressors or Inotropes.)

14. A. VAP occurs typically in two forms: Early, which is a low-mortality form, and late, a high-mortality form. The early form of VAP is caused by *H. influenzae, S. pneumoniae,* and methicillin-sensitive *S. aureus.* Late-onset VAP is associated with virulent organisms such as methicillin-resistant *S. aureus, Pseudomonas aeruginosa,* and *Acinetobacter* spp. Whereas late-onset VAP has a high mortality rate, early-onset VAP has almost no mortality rate. Precautions, including thorough hand washing, oral care, and a head-up position, may reduce its incidence. Acid suppression therapy increases the risk of VAP because of gastric bacterial overgrowth. (See page 1601: Section: Ventilator-associated Pneumonia.)

15. D. Dexmedetomidine is an α_2-adrenergic receptor agonist like clonidine, which produces sedation and mild analgesia. It does not produce respiratory depression. The sedation it creates allows the patient to be responsive when stimulated. The drug is expensive and is currently approved only for 24 hours of use. (See page 1599: Section: Sedation of Critically Ill Patients.)

16. B. Enteral nutrition should be started as early as possible after admission to the ICU. Early feeding (within 4 hours) resulted in less organ dysfunction than delayed (36 hours) initiation. Parenteral nutrition is inferior to enteral nutrition. Patients who receive enteral nutrition have a lower infection risk and reduced translocation and nitrogen imbalance compared with patients receiving parenteral nutrition. The location of the feeding tube does not affect mortality, ICU length of stay, or development of pneumonia. Elevating the head of the bed may reduce aspiration. (See page 1599: Section: Nutrition in Critically Ill Patients.)

17. C. The GCS is the most widely used clinical measure of injury severity in patients with TBI. The advantages of this scale are that it provides an objective method of measuring consciousness, it has high intra- and inter-rater reliability across observers with a wide variety of experience, and it has an excellent correlation with outcome. However, the GCS score is unmeasurable in up to 25% to 45% of patients at admission and is inaccurate when only the partial score is used, such as in patients with endotracheal intubation whose verbal responses cannot be assessed. TBI qualifies as severe when the GCS score is 8 or less after cardiopulmonary resuscitation. The predictive value of the GCS score at admission is about 69% for good neurologic outcome and 76% for unfavorable outcome. After 7 days, these figures approximate 80% for both favorable and unfavorable outcome. (See page 1583: Section: Diagnosis and Management of the Most Common Types of Neurologic Failure: Traumatic Brain Injury.)

18. B. Despite the theoretical benefits of the PAC, few data support a positive effect on mortality or other substantive outcome variables. There was no benefit to therapy directed by PAC over standard therapy in elderly, high-risk surgical patients requiring intensive care. More recently, the FACTT (Fluid and Catheter Treatment Trial) conducted in a large cohort of approximately 1,000 ARDS patients assigned to receive PAC- or central venous catheter-guided therapy did not find any survival or organ function differences between the two groups but did find twice as many catheter-related complications (mostly dysrhythmias) in PAC-monitored patients. A large, randomized, prospective study of the therapeutic strategy known as supraphysiologic resuscitation to defined endpoints (cardiac index > 4.5 L/min, DO_2 > 600 mL/m^2/min, and VO_2 > 170 mL/m^2/min) in patients with septic and surgical- or trauma-related shock found that this approach was associated with increased mortality in patients with septic shock. (See page 1587: Section: Functional Hemodynamic Monitoring.)

19. A. CRBSI is more likely when placement occurs under emergency conditions and is reduced by the use of strict aseptic technique with full barrier precautions. This includes preinsertion hand washing, the use of a full gown and gloves, and the use of a large barrier drape. In addition, skin cleansing with chlorhexidine is more effective than cleansing with other agents. These simple interventions should be considered as standards of care and are recommended by the Centers for Disease Control and Prevention. Catheter-related infection is insertion site dependent, increasing in frequency from subclavian to internal jugular to femoral vein sites, respectively. Catheter-related infection and bacteremia increase with the duration of catheterization, particularly for durations of longer than 2 days. However, routine catheter replacement at 3 or 7 days does not reduce the incidence of infection and results in increased mechanical complications. Thus, routine guidewire exchange of catheters is not recommended. Catheters coated with either antiseptics (chlorhexidine and silver sulfadiazine) or antibiotics (rifampin and minocycline) reduce bacterial colonization of catheters but have not been consistently shown to reduce bacteremia or other morbidities. (See page 1600: Section: Complications in the Intensive Care Unit: Detection, Prevention, and Therapy.)

20. **A.** The Leapfrog Group is a coalition of over 150 purchasers and providers of healthcare benefits, including large companies such as General Motors, Motorola, and Merck, and insurers such as Aetna. The stated goal of the Leapfrog Group is to improve healthcare, in particular by reducing deaths due to medical error. To accomplish this mission, the group formulated the Leapfrog Initiative, which includes a series of "safety standards" that healthcare providers (largely hospitals) should strive for if they are to provide care for Leapfrog Group employees. Prompted by the data associating intensivists with improved outcomes, the Leapfrog Initiative included an ICU Physician Staffing (IPS) standard that promotes the continuous involvement of intensivists in the care of critically ill patients. This includes management or co-management by intensivists during daytime hours, ready availability via paging (within 5 minutes), ready availability (within 5 minutes) of Fundamentals of Critical Care Support (FCCS)-trained effectors at the bedside, and efforts to reduce errors of omission by utilizing checklists during procedures and patient rounds. (See page 1582: Section: Processes of Care in the Intensive Care Unit.)

Acute Pain Management

1. Which of the following is not a characteristic of epidurally administered lipophilic opioids?

   A. Primarily supraspinal mechanism of action
   B. Quick onset
   C. Short duration
   D. Slow systemic uptake

2. End results of the surgical stress response include all of the following EXCEPT:

   A. Hyperglycemia
   B. Poor wound healing
   C. Positive nitrogen balance
   D. Impaired immunocompetence

3. The safety of epidural administration of which of the following adjuvant medications has not yet been determined and is therefore not recommended for use?

   A. Clonidine
   B. Ketamine
   C. Alfentanil
   D. Hydromorphone

4. The circulating levels of which of the following hormones is not increased postoperatively?

   A. Insulin
   B. Glucagon
   C. Antidiuretic hormone
   D. Growth hormone
   E. Cortisol

5. Which of the following statements concerning the analgesia provided by intrathecal clonidine is FALSE?

   A. A commonly utilized epidural solution is in a concentration of 2 μg/mL.
   B. It may cause hypotension and bradycardia.
   C. It interacts synergistically with opioids and local anesthetics.
   D. It has been proven efficacious for orthopedic surgeries.
   E. It produces respiratory depression comparable to that produced by morphine.

6. Which of the following statements concerning nonopioid analgesics is FALSE?

   A. Intravenous acetaminophen has been introduced in the United States.
   B. Acetaminophen is associated with impaired platelet function and gastrointestinal (GI) ulceration.

   C. Dexmedetomidine is a highly selective α_2-agonist that does not depress respiration.
   D. Gabapentin is effective for neuropathic pain syndrome and postoperative pain.

7. Which of the following statements is not associated with increased risk of nephrotoxicity in the perioperative period?

   A. Hypovolemia
   B. Congestive heart failure
   C. Concomitant morphine use
   D. Chronic renal insufficiency

8. All of the following have opioid-sparing properties and may be used in the perioperative period to attenuate excessive sedation induced by opioids, EXCEPT:

   A. Acetaminophen
   B. Nonsteroidal anti-inflammatory drugs (NSAIDs)
   C. N-methyl-D-aspartate (NMDA) receptor antagonists
   D. Gabapentin
   E. Capsaicin

9. All of the following practices maximize the success of preemptive analgesia EXCEPT:

   A. The chosen technique should include the entire surgical field.
   B. The anesthetic depth should block all nociceptive input during surgery.
   C. Analgesia should include the surgical and postsurgical time periods.
   D. Patients with chronic pain should be selected preferentially.
   E. It involves NMDA receptor blockade.

10. Which of the following statements regarding strategies for acute pain management is FALSE?

   A. The majority of postoperative pain is nociceptive in nature.
   B. Neuropathic pain may be a result of accidental nerve injury secondary to cutting, entrapment, or compression.
   C. Neuropathic pain only follows a dermatomal distribution in the postoperative period.
   D. Nociceptive pain typically responds best to N-methyl-D-aspartate (NMDA) agonists.
   E. Opioids and nonsteroidals are the mainstay of treatment in the postoperative period.

11. Which of the following statements regarding nonsteroidal analgesics is FALSE?

    A. Their effects are mediated via prostaglandin inhibition.
    B. They have an opioid-sparing effect.
    C. There is potential for less nausea and vomiting.
    D. It provides more effective analgesia than intravenous opioids.
    E. Ketorolac can be administered in doses of 15 to 30 mg.

12. The benefits of continuous peripheral nerve block (CPNB) include all of the following, EXCEPT:

    A. Prolonged postoperative analgesia
    B. Facilitated discharge from the hospital
    C. Fewer opioid-related side effects
    D. Greater patient satisfaction
    E. Absence of neurologic complications

13. Cyclooxygenase (COX) exists as two separate isomers, COX-1 and COX-2. Which of the following statements regarding these isomers is TRUE?

    A. COX-2 is the constitutive form.
    B. COX-1 is the inducible enzyme form.
    C. COX-1 does not mediate hemostasis.
    D. COX-2 mediates pain and fever.
    E. COX-2 can be safely administered to patients undergoing orthopedic procedures.

14. All of the following statements regarding the administration of opioid analgesics are true, EXCEPT:

    A. Opioid-induced hyperalgesia (OIH) is a rare phenomenon.
    B. Patients with OIH become suddenly more sensitive to pain despite continued treatment with opioids.
    C. Tolerance rarely develops to the constipating effects of opioids.
    D. N-methyl-D-aspartate (NMDA) receptor antagonists may abolish OIH.
    E. All opioids equally produce OIH.

15. Which of the following statements regarding methadone is TRUE?

    A. It is poorly absorbed from the gastrointestinal (GI) tract.
    B. Its use is not cost effective for long-term analgesia.
    C. It inhibits serotonin reuptake.
    D. Its elimination is primarily through liver.
    E. It produces NMDA receptor antagonism.

16. Which of the following statements regarding the performance of ultrasound-guided nerve blocks is FALSE?

    A. Continuous peripheral nerve blocks (CPNB) have been shown to provide pain control that is superior to pain control supplied by opioids.
    B. Hemorrhagic complications (as opposed to neurologic deficits) appear to be the predominant risk associated with the performance of peripheral nerve blockade in anticoagulated patients.
    C. With ultrasound guidance, the endpoint for injection has become real-time observation of hydrodissection.
    D. Even with ultrasound, motor stimulation is required for successful interscalene block.
    E. Factors such as type of anesthetic, surgery, and individual patient risk factors contribute to morbidity from CPNB.

17. Chronic pain is characterized by all of the following, EXCEPT:

    A. It is defined as pain without apparent biologic value that has persisted beyond the normal tissue healing time.
    B. It is often associated with depression and anxiety.
    C. Antiarrhythmics and anticonvulsants may be used for treatment.
    D. Associated psychiatric diagnoses may include hypochondriasis.
    E. Chronic pain patients usually continue their opioids throughout their lives.

18. Which of the following statements concerning epidural anesthesia with opioids is TRUE?

    A. Compared with fentanyl, morphine produces a more segmental block.
    B. Hydrophilic opioids have a slower onset and longer duration.
    C. Fentanyl may provide adequate analgesia after thoracotomy if it is infused at the L3–L4 level.
    D. Hydromorphone has a reduced incidence of pruritus compared with morphine.
    E. Fentanyl produces analgesia in the epidural space only via spinal mechanisms.

19. All of the following are accepted techniques to reduce anxiety in children, EXCEPT:

    A. Parental counseling
    B. Distraction techniques
    C. Game playing
    D. Book reading
    E. Pharmacologic premedication

20. Which of the following statements regarding pediatric acute pain management is TRUE?

    A. Evaluation of pain intensity is easier than in the adult population.
    B. Parental behavior and attitudes do not impact a child's behavior during anesthetic induction.
    C. Patient-controlled analgesia (PCA) by proxy poses no risk to infants provided it is parent controlled.
    D. There is risk associated with epidural analgesia related to systemic toxicity.
    E. Peripheral nerve blockade is usually done with the patient fully awake to avoid neuronal injury.

ANSWERS

1. D. In general, the epidural administration of hydrophilic opioids tends to have a slow onset, a long duration, and a mechanism of action that is primarily spinal in nature. The epidural administration of lipophilic opioids, on the other hand, has a quick onset, a short duration, and a mechanism of action that is primarily supraspinal, secondary to rapid systemic uptake. (See page 1626: Methods of Analgesia: Neuraxial Analgesia.)

2. C. Surgical stress causes release of cytokines and precipitates adverse neuroendocrine and sympathoadrenal responses, resulting in detrimental physiologic responses, particularly in high-risk patients. The increased secretion of the catabolic hormones cortisol, glucagon, growth hormone, and catecholamines, and the decreased secretion of the anabolic hormones insulin and testosterone characterize the neuroendocrine response. The end result of this is hyperglycemia and a negative nitrogen balance; the consequences include poor wound healing, muscle wasting, fatigue, and impaired immunocompetence. (See page 1617: The Surgical Stress Response.)

3. B. The safety of epidurally administered ketamine has not been determined, so routine use cannot be recommended at this time. (See page 1626: Methods of Analgesia: Neuraxial Analgesia.)

4. A. The surgical stress response to pain includes an increase in the level of circulating catecholamines, cortisol, angiotensin II, glucagon, growth hormone, and antidiuretic hormone, as well as a decrease in the levels of anabolic hormones (testosterone and insulin). The overall metabolic effects are gluconeogenesis, hyperglycemia, a negative nitrogen balance, and sodium and water retention. The magnitude of the neuroendocrine and cytokine response to surgery correlates with the degree of tissue injury and with overall outcome. (See page 1617: The Surgical Stress response.)

5. E. Clonidine (2 μg/mL) can be combined with an opioid and a local anesthetic and is usually infused at a rate of 5 to 20 μg/hr. Side effects that limit its clinical usefulness include hypotension, bradycardia, and sedation (not respiratory depression). An epidural infusion consisting of ropivacaine 0.2%, fentanyl 5 μg/mL, and clonidine 2 μg/mL infused at a rate of 3 to 7 mL/hr following a total knee arthroplasty has been reported to cause no significant sedation in this dose range. Clonidine is synergistic with local anesthetics and opioids. (See page 1626: Methods of Analgesia: Neuraxial Analgesia.)

6. B. Acetaminophen is not associated with the impaired platelet function and GI ulceration that are seen with many nonsteroidal anti-inflammatory drugs. Intravenous acetaminophen (Ofirmev) was released in the United States in November of 2010. The drug is available as a 1 g (1,000 mg/100 mL) infusion that does not require reconstitution, and can be infused through a peripheral IV over 15 minutes. Dexmedetomidine is a highly selective α_2-agonist that does not depress respiration. Gabapentin is effective for neuropathic pain syndrome and postoperative pain. (See page 1623: Non-opioid Analgesic Adjuncts.)

7. C. The risk of nephrotoxicity is increased in patients with hypovolemia, congestive heart failure, and chronic renal insufficiency. Morphine does not cause nephrotoxicity and it does not increase the risk of nonsteroidal anti-inflammatory drug (NSAID)-induced nephrotoxicity. NSAIDs have been proven effective in the treatment of postoperative pain when used with opioids, but may cause renal injury. (See page 1623: Non-opioid Analgesic Adjuncts.)

8. E. Excessive sedation may respond to a change in the opioid. Use of a multimodal analgesic technique, which incorporates the use of a regional anesthetic (e.g., epidural or peripheral nerve blockade), an NSAID, acetaminophen or other nonopioid analgesics such as an NMDA receptor antagonist, or an α_2-δ subunit calcium channel ligand will have an opioid-sparing effect, which should attenuate opioid-induced sedation. NSAIDs are opioid sparing and may significantly decrease the incidence of opioid-related side effects such as postoperative nausea and vomiting and sedation. Gabapentin and pregabalin are α_2-δ subunit calcium channel ligands. Although capsaicin has substance P inhibition properties there are no studies showing its usefulness in the perioperative period. (See page 1626: Patient-controlled Analgesia.)

9. D. Although the use of preemptive analgesia is certainly enticing, its clinical benefit in humans has received mixed reviews. For preemptive analgesia to be successful, three critical principles must be adhered to: The depth of analgesia must be adequate enough to block all nociceptive input during surgery, the analgesic technique must be extensive enough to include the entire surgical field, and the duration of analgesia must include both the surgical and postsurgical time periods. Patients with pre-existing chronic pain tend to respond poorly to preemptive techniques because of pre-existing sensitization of the nervous system. Theoretically, preemptive analgesia is achieved by preventing NMDA receptor activation in the dorsal horn that is associated with wind-up, facilitation, central sensitization expansion of receptive fields, and long-term potentiation, all of which can lead to a chronic pain state. (See page 1617: Preventive Analgesia.)

10. C. Although the majority of postoperative pain is nociceptive in character, a small percentage of patients may experience neuropathic pain postoperatively. It is critical to recognize this fact because patients with neuropathic pain are at increased risk of progressing to a chronic pain state. Neuropathic pain may be the result of accidental nerve injury secondary to cutting, traction compression, or entrapment. There may be a delay in the onset of the pain, and it may follow a nondermatomal distribution. Nociceptive pain responds best to opioids, nonsteroidal anti-inflammatory drugs, para-aminophenols, and regional anesthesia techniques. Patients with neuropathic pain, on the other hand, may benefit from the addition of nonopioid analgesic adjuvants such as the NMDA receptor antagonists, α_2-agonists, and the α_2-δ subunit calcium channel ligands. (See page 1617: Acute Pain Management.)

11. **D.** NSAIDs have proven effective in the treatment of postoperative pain. In addition, they are opioid sparing and can significantly decrease the incidence of opioid-related side effects such as postoperative nausea and vomiting and sedation. Unlike the opioids, NSAIDs exhibit a "ceiling effect" with respect to maximum analgesic effects. Parenteral NSAIDs such as ketorolac are commonly employed as part of a multimodal approach for acute perioperative pain management. The optimal dose of ketorolac for postoperative pain control is 15 to 30 mg intravenously every 6 to 8 hours, not to exceed 5 days. The dose should be decreased in patients with renal failure. (See page 1623: Nonopioid analgesic adjuncts.)

12. **E.** Single-injection techniques are limited in duration but continuous peripheral nerve block (CPNB) techniques can extend the benefits of peripheral nerve blockade well into the postoperative period. CPNB has proven to be an effective technique for postoperative pain management; it is superior to opioid analgesia with fewer opioid-related side effects and rare neurologic and infectious complications. The benefits of CPNB in the ambulatory setting include prolonged postoperative analgesia, facilitated discharge from the hospital, fewer opioid-related side effects, and greater patient satisfaction. (See page 1629: Peripheral Nerve Blockade.)

13. **D.** The therapeutic benefit of nonsteroidal anti-inflammatory drugs is believed to be mediated through the inhibition of COX enzymes, types I and II, which convert arachidonic acid to prostaglandins. COX-1 is the constitutive enzyme that produces prostaglandins, which are important for general "housekeeping" functions such as gastric protection and hemostasis. COX-2, on the other hand, is the inducible form of the enzyme that produces prostaglandins that mediate pain, inflammation, fever, and carcinogenesis. The effect of COX-2 inhibitors on bone fusion following orthopedic procedures continues to be controversial, and no recommendations can be made at this time. (See page 1623: Non-opioid Analgesic Adjuncts.)

14. **E.** Opioid-induced hyperalgesia (OIH) is a relatively rare phenomenon whereby patients who are receiving opioids suddenly and paradoxically become more sensitive to pain despite continued treatment with opioids. Evidence suggests that OIH is more likely to develop after administration of high doses of phenanthrene opioids such as morphine. Changing the opioid to a phenyl piperidine derivative such as fentanyl may thwart OIH. Evidence also suggests that coadministration of an NMDA receptor antagonist may abolish opioid-induced tolerance (OIT)

and OIH. OIT rarely develops to the constipating effects of opioids. A peripherally acting μ-receptor antagonist that has negligible systemic absorption, alvimopan, attenuates opioid-induced constipation and shortens postoperative ileus and length of hospital stay. (See page 1619: Opioid Analgesics.)

15. **E.** Methadone is a relatively inexpensive synthetic opioid considered to be a "broad-spectrum" opioid because it is a μ-receptor agonist, an N-methyl-D-aspartate antagonist, and an inhibitor of monoamine transmitter reuptake, making it potentially useful for treatment of neuropathic pain. The drug is well absorbed from the GI tract, with a reported bioavailability of approximately 80%. The drug is extensively metabolized in the liver by the cytochrome P450 (CYP450) system to inactive metabolites, which are cleared in the bile and urine, and unlike with morphine, it is generally not necessary to adjust the dosage of methadone in patients with renal insufficiency. (See page 1619: Opioid Analgesics.)

16. **D.** Single-injection peripheral nerve blockade has been shown to provide pain control that is superior to that of opioids with fewer side effects. Single-injection techniques are limited in duration, but CPNB techniques may extend the benefits of peripheral nerve blockade well into the postoperative period. CPNB has proven to be an effective technique for postoperative pain management, which is superior to opioid analgesia with fewer opioid-related side effects and rare neurologic and infectious complications. Although bleeding complications may be associated with the placement of CPNB catheters, the actual risks related to this technique are not well defined. Hemorrhagic complications, rather than neurologic deficits, appear to be the predominant risk associated with the performance of peripheral nerve blockade in anticoagulated patients. If a perioperative nerve injury occurs, it is incumbent upon the physician to determine which combination of anesthetic, surgical, and patient risk factors are involved in any nerve injury and not assume a priori that the regional anesthetic is the culprit. A recent study of interscalene block has confirmed that regardless of motor response, as long as the needle tip is positioned between the two most lateral nerve structures, a successful blockade of the plexus will be achieved. The endpoint for injection of local anesthetic has now become real-time observation of hydrodissection rather than motor stimulation. (See page 1629: Peripheral Nerve Blockade.)

17. **E.** Chronic pain is defined as "pain without apparent biologic value that has persisted beyond the normal tissue healing time usually taken to be 3 months" (International Association for the Study of Pain) and "pain of a duration or intensity that adversely affects the function or well-being of the patient" (American Society of Anesthesiologists). Chronic pain is often associated with anxiety and depression, which may require treatment with various anxiolytics, antidepressants, anticonvulsants, and antiarrhythmic and skeletal muscle relaxants in addition to opioids. Symptoms unique to chronic pain include tight musculature, limited range of motion, lack of energy, sleep

disturbance, irritability, and social withdrawal. Associated psychiatric diagnoses include hypochondriasis and psychosis. Although the goal of opioid therapy for chronic pain is improvement of pain, function, and quality of life, unacceptable opioid side effects and concerns about adverse hormonal effects and immune modulation from long-term exposure can cause patients to abandon therapy. (See page 1638: Perioperative Pain Management of the Opioid-dependent Patient.)

18. **D.**   Various opioids, including agonist–antagonist agents, may be used via the epidural route. Lipophilic agents, such as fentanyl, tend to provide a greater segmental analgesic effect; therefore, the epidural catheter should be sited in a position to cover the dermatomes included in the surgical field. Morphine is more hydrophilic and thus can be infused at a lower lumbar level and still provide analgesia for upper abdominal and thoracic procedures. Hydrophilic opioids have a slower onset and longer duration of action. Hydromorphone is associated with less incidence of pruritus and nausea than morphine. Epidurally administered opioids have the distinct advantage of producing analgesia without causing significant sympatholytic effect or motor blockade. Analgesia occurs by way of a spinal mechanism and through a supraspinal mechanism following systemic adsorption. (See page 1627: Neuraxial Analgesia.)

19. **D.**   Good evidence suggests that the level of preoperative anxiety and stress adversely impacts postoperative pain and recovery from surgery. A number of methods can be used to reduce preoperative anxiety in children. They include preoperative parental education and counseling about the operative experience; distraction techniques, including videos and music; handheld video games; game playing with the support of the family or child life specialists; and parental presence coupled with oral midazolam administration to ease the anxiety associated with the transition to the induction of anesthesia. As parental behavior and attitudes can be major determinants of a child's behavior during the inhalational induction of anesthesia, the anesthesiologist is obliged to counsel and inform parents as to the importance of modulating their fear and anxiety should they want to be present during anesthetic induction. (See page 1641: Special Considerations in the Perioperative Pain Management of Children.)

20. **D.**   Acute pain management in children undergoing surgery or invasive procedures offers several specific and unique challenges for anesthesiologists. Assessment of the degree of pain is often more difficult in children because of their poor communication ability and their emotional responses. Parental behavior and attitudes may be major determinants of a child's behavior during the inhalational induction of anesthesia and the perioperative period. Despite a parent's potential ability to help with assessment of pain, PCA by proxy is a safety risk because there is no complete assurance that parents will be competent in assessing the intensity of their children's pain or be able to regulate the bolus dosages to avoid opioid overdosage. Regarding epidural anesthesia, serious risk is associated with epidural analgesia in children related to the systemic toxicity of the local anesthetic and the need to place the epidural under general anesthesia. The use of stimulating needles permits the anesthesiologist to place the injection after the child is anesthetized. As the child is unresponsive, it is important that the initial injection meets no resistance in order to avoid intraneural injection. (See page 1641: Special Considerations in the Perioperative Pain Management of Children.)

Chronic Pain Management

1. Which nerve fibers mediate the "second," or protopathic, pain response?

    A. Aα
    B. Aβ
    C. Aδ
    D. C
    E. None of the above

2. The "wind-up" phenomenon involves which of the following nerve fibers?

    A. Aβ
    B. B
    C. Aδ
    D. C
    E. Aγ

3. Which of the following statements regarding the spinothalamic tract (STT) is FALSE?

    A. STT neurons relay nociceptive input from the spinal cord.
    B. Axons of the STT ascend primarily in the contralateral and anterolateral tracts of the spinal cord.
    C. Axons of the STT terminate in the posterior complex of the thalamus.
    D. STT neurons are primarily located in lamina VIII.
    E. STT neurons relay nociceptive input to supraspinal levels.

4. Which of the following chemical mediators is not typically released after injury?

    A. Substance P
    B. Serotonin
    C. Bradykinin
    D. Histamine
    E. Insulin

5. Which of the following is considered an excitatory amino acid?

    A. Arginine
    B. Valine
    C. Glutamate
    D. Bradykinin
    E. Histamine

6. Which of the following statements regarding chronic regional pain syndrome (CRPS) is FALSE?

    A. CRPS type I and type II exhibit the same symptoms except there is a preceding nerve injury in CRPS II.
    B. Risk factors for the development of CRPS include prior trauma, prior surgery, and work-related injuries.
    C. There typically is a close relationship between the severity of the symptoms and the severity of the inciting injury.
    D. Signs and symptoms include spontaneous pain, hyperalgesia, and allodynia as well as trophic, sudomotor, and vasomotor abnormalities.
    E. It is more common in females.

7. Which of the following statements regarding diabetic painful neuropathy (DPN) is FALSE?

    A. Symptoms include burning pain; deep, aching pain; electrical or stabbing sensations; paresthesias; and hyperesthesia.
    B. It often is helped by anticonvulsants and tricyclics.
    C. The incidence of diabetic neuropathy increases with the duration of diabetes, age, and the degree of hyperglycemia.
    D. Peripheral neuropathy is seen in <20% of patients with insulin-dependent diabetes.
    E. The incidence increases with increased hyperglycemia.

8. Which of the following statements regarding herpes zoster is FALSE?

    A. After resolution of an acute episode of herpes zoster, some patients develop a persistent pain known as postherpetic neuralgia (PHN).
    B. Neuraxial local anesthetics and methylprednisolone, given during the acute stage of herpes zoster, may prevent the development of postherpetic neuralgia.
    C. Antiviral agents such as acyclovir, famciclovir, and valacyclovir may hasten the healing of the rash and reduce the duration of viral shedding.
    D. It commonly affects thoracic dermatomes.
    E. The mainstay of treatment for PHN is serial neuraxial injection.

9. Which of the following statements regarding tricyclic anti-depressants (TCAs) is FALSE?

   A. Side effects include sedation and dry mouth.
   B. Urinary retention is attributable to activation of muscarinic receptors.
   C. Sleep pattern improvement is usually prompt after initiation of these drugs.
   D. Nortriptyline is equally effective as amitriptyline but has a better side effect profile.
   E. They reduce the reuptake of norepinephrine and serotonin.

10. Which of the following statements regarding cancer pain is FALSE?

   A. Up to 25% of patients with cancer who are in active treatment and up to 90% of patients with advanced cancer experience significant pain.
   B. Opioids are the mainstay of treatment.
   C. Neurolytic blocks should be considered when oral pharmacologic agents fail to effectively control pain.
   D. Intrathecal opioids should be considered when oral pharmacologic agents fail to effectively control pain.
   E. Behavioral and psychological management are not meaningful components of cancer pain control.

11. Which of the following is FALSE about spinal cord stimulation (SCS)?

   A. It is based on the gate control theory, wherein the SCS opens the gate to inhibitory C fiber pathways at the dorsal horn.
   B. Analgesia may be brought about by alteration of the sympathetic tone.
   C. A trial period is often indicated before a permanent stimulator is placed.
   D. Complications include nerve and spinal cord injury, infection, hematoma, and lead breakage or migration.
   E. SCS impacts pain transmission via the substantia gelatinosa.

12. Which of the following statements concerning celiac plexus block is FALSE?

   A. Needles are placed just anterior to the body of L1.
   B. Injections are performed with 5 mL of 50% alcohol.
   C. Orthostatic hypotension is a potential side effect.
   D. More than 75% of patients with upper abdominal cancer experience good to excellent pain relief.
   E. Patients may develop paraplegia.

13. Which of the following statements regarding intrathecal drug delivery systems (IDDS) is FALSE?

   A. IDDS allows direct administration of drugs near the spinal cord receptors, bypassing the blood–brain barrier.
   B. High testosterone levels are seen with IDDS usage.
   C. Complications include infection, bleeding, respiratory depression, pump malfunction, catheter failure, and peripheral edema.
   D. It may cause formation of an inflammatory mass.
   E. A trial injection is often advisable.

14. Which of the following statements regarding interventional pain therapies is FALSE?

   A. Discography is to evaluate the symptoms of discogenic pain, which includes radicular back pain that is worse in the standing or sitting position.
   B. Kyphoplasty is associated with a lower rate of cement extravasation than vertebroplasty.
   C. Minimally invasive lumbar decompression (MILD) involves thinning of the posterior longitudinal ligament.
   D. MILD is indicated for neurogenic claudication.
   E. In intradiscal electrothermal therapy (IDET), the electrode is gradually heated to 90°C for 4 minutes.

ANSWERS

1. **D.** Aδ and C fibers are nociceptors that both respond to painful stimuli but mediate different aspects of pain sensation. Aδ fibers are fast-conducting fibers involved in the "first," or epicritic, pain response, which is localized and characterized as sharp or pricking. C fibers are slow-conducting fibers that are involved in the "second," or protopathic, pain response, which is poorly localized and characterized as burning or dull. (See page 1646: Anatomy, Physiology, and Neurochemistry of Somatosensory Pain Processing: Primary Afferents and Peripheral Stimulation.)

2. **D.** The "wind-up" phenomenon involves C fibers. (See page 1646: Anatomy, Physiology, and Neurochemistry of Somatosensory Pain Processing: Transition from Acute to Persistent Nociception.)

3. **D.** STT cells are the primary relay cells that provide nociceptive information from the spinal cord to the supraspinal levels. The axons of the STT transcend up the spinal cord primarily in the contralateral and anterolateral tracts, where they terminate in the posterior complex of the thalamus, including the ventral posterior lateral and ventral posterior medial nuclei. STT cells that receive input are located in various laminae (I, IV, V, VII, and X). (See page 1646: Anatomy, Physiology, and Neurochemistry of Somatosensory Pain Processing: Neurobiology of Ascending Pathways.)

4. **E.** Numerous chemical mediators are released after injury. These substances include bradykinin, serotonin, prostaglandins, leukotrienes, histamine, and substance P. Bradykinin, which is released locally after tissue injury, is capable of evoking pain on intradermal injection. (See page 1646: Anatomy, Physiology, and Neurochemistry of Somatosensory Pain Processing: Primary Afferents and Peripheral Stimulation.)

5. **C.** Considerable evidence suggests that excitatory amino acids such as glutamate and aspartate are the principal neurotransmitters responsible for activation of dorsal horn neurons after noxious stimulation. (See page 1646: Anatomy, Physiology, and Neurochemistry of Somatosensory Pain Processing: Neurochemistry of Peripheral Nerve and the Dorsal Root Ganglion.)

6. **C.** Previous trauma, nerve injury, surgery, work-related injuries, and female sex are known risk factors for the development of CRPS, a syndrome of spontaneous pain, hyperalgesia, allodynia, autonomic dysfunction, and dystrophy. The severity of the symptoms may not correlate with the intensity of the inciting injury. The International Association for the Study of Pain has further differentiated CRPS into two types: CRPS I and CRPS II ("causalgia"). The clinical features of CRPS type II are the same as in CRPS type I except there is a preceding nerve injury in CRPS II. (See page 1657: Neuropathic Pain Syndromes: Complex Regional Pain Syndrome.)

7. **D.** Diabetic peripheral neuropathy is present in up to 65% of patients with insulin-dependent diabetes. The incidence increases with the duration of diabetes, age, and the degree of hyperglycemia. Symptoms include burning pain; deep, aching pain; electrical or stabbing sensations; paresthesias; and hyperesthesia. Management includes both tight glucose control and pharmacologic agents such as anticonvulsants (gabapentin, pregabalin), tricyclic antidepressants (amitriptyline, nortriptyline), serotonin norepinephrine reuptake inhibitors (duloxetine, milnacipran), opioids, and tramadol. (See page 1657: Neuropathic Pain Syndromes: Diabetic Painful Neuropathy.)

8. **E.** Herpes zoster most commonly involves the thoracic and the trigeminal dermatomes, with the ophthalmic division of the trigeminal nerve being the second most common. Persistent pain lasting more than 3 months after the resolution of the rash is known as PHN. Antiviral agents have been advocated for management of acute stage of the disease and have been shown to hasten the healing of the rash, reduce the duration of viral shedding, and may also decrease the incidence and duration of PHN. Injection of neuraxial local anesthetics and methylprednisolone, when performed 3 to 4 times during the acute stage of herpes zoster, may prevent the development of postherpetic neuralgia. However, the mainstay of treatment for PHN is pharmacologic management which includes anticonvulsants, opioids, and antidepressants. (See page 1657: Neuropathic Pain Syndromes: Herpes Zoster and Postherpetic Neuralgia.)

9. **B.** The most popular explanation for the analgesic property of TCAs is reuptake inhibition of serotonin and norepinephrine, which increases the level of these neurotransmitters in the brainstem and spinal cord. Nortriptyline is equally effective as amitriptyline but has a better side effect profile. Although the antidepressant and pain-relieving effects are often delayed in onset, the improvement in sleep patterns provided by these drugs usually occurs promptly, often with the initial dose. TCA inhibition at histaminic, muscarinic, and nicotinic receptors results in the common occurrence of side effects of sedation, dry mouth, and urinary retention. (See page 1659: Pharmacologic Management: Antidepressants.)

10. **E.** Up to 25% of patients with cancer who are in active treatment and up to 90% of patients with advanced cancer experience significant pain. The management of cancer pain should be multifaceted, including antineoplastic treatment, pharmacologic management, interventional management, behavioral and psychological management, and ultimately, hospice care. The mainstay of treatment is opioids, with up to 70% to 95% of patients experiencing relief when appropriate guidelines are followed. When failure of pharmacologic agents occurs, neurolytic blocks and intrathecal opioids may be used. (See page 1658: Cancer Pain.)

11. A. The effects of SCS are based on the gate control theory, in which increasing the input of large nerve fibers would close the "gate" at the substantia gelatinosa of the dorsal horn of the spinal horn from transmitting information of painful stimuli to the brain. In ischemic pain, the analgesia may be secondary to alteration of the sympathetic tone which improves the oxygen supply-and-demand balance. Placement of a permanent stimulator is preceded by a trial period to confirm its efficacy. Complications of SCS include nerve and spinal cord injury, infection, hematoma, and lead breakage or migration. (See page 1663: Interventional Techniques: Spinal Cord Stimulation.)

12. B. In a meta-analysis of 21 retrospective studies, it has been reported that 89% of 1,145 patients who underwent celiac plexus block for pain of upper abdominal cancer had good to excellent pain relief in the first 2 weeks after the block; partial to complete pain relief continued in 90% of the patients as of the 3-month interval. Complications from a celiac plexus block include orthostatic hypotension, interscapular back pain, retroperitoneal hematoma, reactive pleurisy, hiccups, hematuria, transient diarrhea, abdominal aortic dissection, transient motor paralysis, and paraplegia. The retrocrural technique for percutaneous injection of the celiac plexus involves bilateral placement of the block needle just anterior to the body of L1 and posterior to the aorta and diaphragmatic crura. Thirty to forty milliliters of the neurolytic agents (50% alcohol or 6%–10% phenol) are used for the retrocrural approach and anterocrural approach. (See page 1658: Cancer Pain: Neurolytic Blocks for Visceral Pain from Cancer.)

13. B. Intradermal drug delivery systems (IDDS) may be used in situations in which oral or transdermal opioids are ineffective at reasonable doses or when they cause unacceptable side effects. IDDS allows direct infusion of drugs near the spinal cord receptors, thus bypassing the blood–brain barrier and allowing a decreased equianalgesic dose to be given with a decrease in side effects and adverse events. A trial period is recommended before an intrathecal pump is permanently placed. The trial can be performed through the intrathecal or epidural space via single-shot, intermittent bolus or continuous infusion, either on an outpatient or inpatient basis. Complications of IDDS may include infection, bleeding, respiratory depression, pump malfunction, catheter failure, hormonal dysfunction, peripheral edema, and the formation of an inflammatory mass. IDDS is associated with decreased testosterone levels and small gonads, which may be treated with hormonal replacement therapy. (See page 1663: Interventional Techniques: Intrathecal Pumps.)

14. C. Discography is a technique to evaluate back pain of discogenic origin. The symptoms of discogenic pain are nonspecific and include nonradicular back pain that is worse in the standing or sitting position. The neurologic examination is usually normal including the straight-leg raise. Compared to vertebroplasty, kyphoplasty is associated with a lower rate of cement extravasation because of the higher viscosity of the PMMA that is used, the lower injection pressure employed, and the inflatable bone trap that seals pathways for cement leakage. Minimally invasive lumbar decompression (MILD) involves limited percutaneous laminotomy and thinning of the ligamentum flavum to increase the critical diameter of the stenosed spinal canal, thus alleviating pain due to neurogenic claudication. Intradiscal electrothermal therapy (IDET) is a procedure in which a thermal resistance catheter is placed in the disc and heated to 90°C for 4 minutes. Heat causes the collagen of the annulus fibrosis to contract. (See page 1663: Interventional Techniques: Discography, IDET, MILD, Vertebroplasty and Kyphoplasty.)

Cardiopulmonary Resuscitation

1. Which of the following statements is FALSE?

   A. During single rescuer CPR, the 2010 AHA guidelines recommend that chest compressions be initiated before ventilation attempts.
   B. The most common electrocardiogram patterns found in witnessed, adult, sudden cardiac arrest are pulseless electrical activity and asystole.
   C. Within the hospital, the operating room is the site where CPR is most successful.
   D. Interrupting chest compressions to perform intubations or defibrillations has been shown to reduce survival rates.
   E. Optimum outcome from ventricular fibrillation is more likely to be obtained if defibrillation is applied within 8 minutes of arrest.

2. All of the following statements are correct EXCEPT:

   A. Current evidence suggests that using atropine does not improve outcome in bradysystolic or asystolic arrest.
   B. The half-life of epinephrine during CPR is longer than the half-life of vasopressin.
   C. Amiodarone has β-adrenergic, α-adrenergic, calcium, potassium, and sodium blocking properties.
   D. If administration of calcium is indicated, calcium chloride is preferable to calcium gluconate.
   E. Current recommendations for use of sodium bicarbonate include arrests associated with severe preexisting metabolic acidosis, hyperkalemia, tricyclic antidepressants overdose, and phenobarbital overdose.

3. Considering foreign body obstruction, all the following statements are true EXCEPT:

   A. Blind finger sweeps in the mouth of the patient has a high failure rate.
   B. Total airway obstruction by a foreign body is characterized by rasping or wheezing respirations, and the inability to cough.
   C. Abdominal thrusts should be performed in the supine position only if the patient is unconscious.
   D. Sternal thrusts are an alternative to abdominal thrusts in a pregnant or massively obese patient.
   E. Placing the patient in a head-down position (such as leaning over the chair) may be effective in relieving obstruction.

4. Which of the following doses is not correct for adult use in cardiac arrest?

   A. Sodium bicarbonate: 1 mEq/kg
   B. Epinephrine: 1 mg repeated every 3 to 5 minutes
   C. Amiodarone: Single 150 mg IV bolus over 10 minutes
   D. 10% calcium chloride: 2 to 4 mg/kg
   E. Vasopressin: 40 units

5. All of the following statements regarding patient ventilation during cardiac arrest are true EXCEPT:

   A. Mouth-to-mouth or mouth-to-nose ventilation provides a CO_2 concentration of 4% and an oxygen concentration of 17%.
   B. Partial airway obstruction by the tongue and pharyngeal tissue is a major etiology of high airway pressures and gastric insufflation.
   C. Esophageal opening pressures during cardiac arrest are likely similar to those of an anesthetized patient—approximately 20 cm H_2O.
   D. During CPR in adults and one-rescuer CPR in children, current recommendations are two breaths after every 30 compressions.
   E. Tidal volumes with a self-inflating resuscitation bag and mask are often greater than with mouth-to-mouth or mouth-to-mask ventilation.

6. All the following statements regarding the adequacy of circulation are correct EXCEPT:

   A. The critical coronary perfusion pressure is associated with a diastolic pressure of 40 mm Hg or above.
   B. Administration of sodium bicarbonate will elevate end-tidal CO_2 levels, making it inaccurate for assessing adequacy of CPR.
   C. Unlike the native beating heart, coronary perfusion during CPR occurs during both systole and diastole.
   D. CO_2 excretion during CPR even with an endotracheal tube in place is flow dependent, not ventilator dependent.
   E. End-tidal CO_2 levels will return to baseline within 3 to 5 minutes after administering sodium bicarbonate.

7. Which of the following statements is FALSE?

   A. Vasopressin can be administered through an endotracheal tube.

   B. Resuscitation medications given through an endotracheal tube should be diluted in doses 2.5 times higher than what is given intravenously.

   C. The efficacy of epinephrine use for cardiac arrest results from its strong β-adrenergic stimulus.

   D. Current evidence suggests that epinephrine is similarly efficacious as vasopressin during CPR.

   E. Medications delivered through an antecubital peripheral intravenous line may reach their sites of action more reliably than medications delivered through a femoral venous line.

8. All of the following statements are true EXCEPT:

   A. Blood gases during CPR would show arterial respiratory acidosis and venous respiratory alkalosis with a markedly elevated arteriovenous CO_2 difference.

   B. Mixed alveolar CO_2 (end-tidal CO_2) during CPR shows a poor correlation with arterial CO_2 due to decreased pulmonary blood flow, but does correlate well with cardiac output.

   C. During CPR the victim's head should be level with the heart for adequate brain perfusion.

   D. Adult chest compressions should depress the sternum by at least 2 in., 100 times per minute, allowing for complete chest recoil during relaxation phases.

   E. There are no antiarrhythmic drugs that have been shown to be superior to electrical defibrillation.

9. All of the following statements regarding the mechanism and physiology of cardiopulmonary resuscitation (CPR) are true EXCEPT:

   A. The cardiac pump mechanism assumes that sternal compression increases intraventricular pressures.

   B. The thoracic pump mechanism assumes that sternal compression increases pressures in all intrathoracic structures equally.

   C. When properly performed, CPR distributes approximately 60% of blood flow to organs above the diaphragm, and 40% to organs below the diaphragm.

   D. During experimental closed-chest massage, cardiac output is reduced to 10% to 33% of normal.

   E. During CPR, cerebral perfusion is 50% to 90% of normal, while myocardial perfusion is 20% to 50% of normal.

10. Each of the following statements concerning defibrillation are true EXCEPT:

   A. If fibrillation is not seen on the ECG, take time to check the trace from the second lead or from a different position of paddle electrodes before deciding against defibrillation.

   B. Some shortcomings of current AEDs include: Requiring up to 90 seconds to analyze rhythm, not recognizing low-amplitude VF, and misinterpreting pacemaker spikes for QRS complexes.

   C. Low-amplitude and high-frequency fibrillatory waveforms are less likely to be associated with successful resuscitation, and more likely to convert to asystole following defibrillation.

   D. Paddles should be applied with a pressure of 11 kg.

   E. Joules = watts × seconds.

11. All of the following statements are true EXCEPT:

   A. Higher-energy shocks are associated with increased incidence of atrioventricular blocks.

   B. The recommended initial defibrillation dose for children is 2 J/kg.

   C. Current evidence suggests that using an initial dose of ≤200 J with biphasic waveform defibrillators is comparable to using 300 J.

   D. With biphasic defibrillators, adults with a higher body mass index should receive defibrillation at the higher end of the 2 to 4 J/kg range.

   E. When using a monophasic waveform defibrillator, a single shock of 360 J should be used.

12. Which of the following statements is FALSE?

   A. Chest compressions should be immediately performed after defibrillation without pausing to check a pulse or analyze ECG rhythm.

   B. Positive pressure ventilation during CPR can adversely affect survival.

   C. Mean arterial pressure after resuscitation should be kept between 90 and 110 mm Hg because of severely attenuated cerebral autoregulation.

   D. Pediatric arrests commonly present as asystole and PEA, and are usually caused by progressive problems with airway and ventilation.

   E. When untreated VF has been occurring for over 4 minutes, there will be improved outcomes if defibrillation is initiated before chest compressions.

13. New recommendations from The International Liaison Committee on Resuscitation now recommend cooling unconscious adult patients with spontaneous circulation after out-of-hospital VF cardiac arrest to:

   A. 30°C to 32°C for 12 to 24 hours

   B. 30°C to 32°C for 24 to 36 hours

   C. 32°C to 34°C for 12 to 24 hours

   D. 32°C to 34°C for 24 to 36 hours

   E. 26°C to 28°C for 24 to 36 hours

14. Mechanical ventilation for a comatose patient after resuscitation efforts should titrate FiO_2 such that:

   A. $SpO_2 \geq 89\%$

   B. $SpO_2 \geq 92\%$

   C. $SpO_2 \geq 94\%$

   D. $SpO_2 \geq 97\%$

   E. $SpO_2 = 100\%$

ANSWERS

1. B. Since most adult cardiac arrests are due to dysrhythmias and it is critical to restore blood flow, newer AHA guidelines now recommend initiating chest compressions before attempting ventilation in an unresponsive individual if a single rescuer is present. The most common ECG pattern found in witnessed, sudden, adult cardiac arrests is ventricular fibrillation; the only consistently effective treatment is electrical defibrillation. Cardiac arrest in the operating room occurs at a rate of 7 times for every 10,000 anesthetics; approximately 4.5 of 10,000 arrests are anesthesia related. Successful resuscitation occurs in approximately 90% of anesthesia-related arrests, leading to a small (0.4 of 10,000) anesthetic mortality rate. Within the hospital, the operating room is the location where cardiopulmonary resuscitation has the highest rate of success. The principle of not interrupting chest compressions should be practiced by both healthcare practitioners and lay bystanders because blood flow ceases almost immediately when compressions are stopped, and returns only slowly when chest compressions are resumed. Rescue breaths or advanced airway support should be delayed until spontaneous circulation returns, or at least three cycles of compressions–rhythm analysis–shock are complete. Ventilation/intubation should take place while compressions are occurring. Prompt chest compressions and defibrillation (within 4 and 8 minutes, respectively) are the most important determinants of optimum survival after ventricular fibrillation. (See pages 1687: Cardiocerebral Resuscitation, 1685: Electrical Therapy, and 1673: Scope of the Problem.)

2. B. Although it frequently is given in cardiac arrest associated with asystole or slow pulseless electrical activity, there is no evidence to suggest that atropine actually improves outcomes. The most common cause of these rhythms is severe myocardial ischemia, not excessive parasympathetic activity. Therefore, the better treatment would be effective chest compressions, ventilation, and epinephrine. The half-life of vasopressin in the intact circulation is 10 to 20 minutes, and is longer than epinephrine during CPR. Current evidence suggests that vasopressin is at least as effective as epinephrine when used during CPR. Amiodarone is a pharmacologically complex drug which has sodium, potassium, calcium, and α-adrenergic and β-adrenergic blocking properties. After vasopressors, the drugs most likely to be useful during CPR are those, like amiodarone, which help suppress ectopic ventricular rhythms. Routine use of calcium during CPR is not recommended unless specific indications, such as hyperkalemia, hypocalcemia, or calcium channel blocker overdose, exist. If calcium should be given, calcium chloride is recommended over calcium gluconate because it produces higher and more consistent levels of ionized calcium than other salts. Routine use of sodium bicarbonate is also not recommended in cardiac arrest, except for arrests associated with hyperkalemia, severe pre-existing metabolic acidosis, and overdose of tricyclic antidepressants or phenobarbital. It

may also be considered for use after protracted resuscitation attempts where other modalities have been attempted and failed. (See page 1681: Pharmacologic Therapy.)

3. B. In the unconscious victim, manual dislodgement of a foreign body in the airway should be attempted only if solid material is seen. The material should be retrieved under direct visualization with an instrument, such as a Magill forceps. Blind finger sweeps or blind use of instruments is rarely successful and may damage tonsils and surrounding structures. Partial airway obstruction is characterized by rasping or wheezing respirations and coughing. Total airway obstruction is characterized by lack of air movements, inability to speak or cough, and rapid development of cyanosis. If the victim has good air movement and is able to cough forcefully, no intervention is indicated. However, if the cough weakens or cyanosis develops, the patient must be treated as if complete obstruction were present. In an awake victim, abdominal thrusts are performed in the erect position: Sitting or standing. An unconscious victim is kept supine and the rescuer kneels astride the victim and performs thrusts on the epigastrium. Sternal thrusts are a valuable alternative to abdominal thrusts in advanced pregnancy or massively obese patients. In the erect victim, the thrusts are delivered midsternum. For the unconscious, thrusts are applied from the side of the supine victim with a hand position the same as for external cardiac compression. Back blows are applied directly over the thoracic spine between the scapulae. Placing the victim in a head-down position (e.g., leaning over a chair) may help move the obstruction into the pharynx. (See page 1676: Airway Management.)

4. C. Correct doses include sodium bicarbonate: 1 mEq/kg; epinephrine: 1 mg repeated every 3 to 5 minutes; amiodarone: 300-mg rapid infusion, plus supplemental infusions of 150-mg PRN for a total daily dose of 2 g (For dysrhythmias with an intact circulation, the initial dose is 150-mg IV over 10 minutes, followed by 1 mg/min infusion for 6 hours, then 0.5 mg/min thereafter.); 10% calcium chloride: 2 to 4 mg/kg; and vasopressin: 40 units. (See page 1681: Pharmacologic Therapy.)

5. E. Partial airway obstruction by the tongue and pharyngeal tissues is a major cause for high airway pressures. Peak inspiratory airway pressures which exceed esophageal opening pressures can insufflate air into the stomach, leading to gastric distension, compromised ventilation, and increased risk of regurgitation and gastric rupture. During cardiopulmonary resuscitation (CPR) in adults and one-rescuer CPR in children, a pause for two breaths should be made after each 30 chest compressions. When there are two rescuers with a child victim, a pause for two breaths should be made after each 15 compressions. After definitive airway management is achieved with endotracheal intubation, interrupting chest compressions for breaths is unnecessary. Tidal volumes with mouth-to-mouth and mouth-to-mask ventilation are often greater than with the self-inflating resuscitation bag and mask, which may be difficult for a single rescuer to apply properly without leak. Mouth-to-mouth or mouth-to-nose ventilation provides a CO_2 concentration of 4% and an oxygen concentration of 17%. If there are two rescuers available to handle the airway, it is now recommended that one rescuer hold the mask and maintain the head position, while the other rescuer uses two hands to squeeze the bag. (See page 1677: Ventilation.)

6. C.   The critical coronary perfusion pressure associated with successful resuscitation is 15 to 25 mm Hg. Critical myocardial blood flow is associated with an aortic diastolic pressure of at least 40 mm Hg. End-tidal CO_2 has been found to be an excellent noninvasive guide to the adequacy of closed-chest compressions. An end-tidal CO_2 level less than 10 mm Hg indicates that the patient will not be resuscitated successfully. Sodium bicarbonate administration liberates CO_2 into the blood and causes a temporary increase in end-tidal CO_2. The elevation returns to baseline within 3 to 5 minutes of drug administration; end-tidal CO_2 monitoring can then be used again for monitoring effectiveness of closed-chest compressions. Similar to the beating heart, coronary perfusion during CPR occurs primarily in the relaxation phase (diastole) of chest compressions. CO_2 excretion during CPR with an endotracheal tube in place is flow dependent rather than ventilation dependent. (See page 1678: Circulation.)

7. C.   The following medications can be given through the endotracheal tube: Epinephrine, vasopressin, lidocaine, and atropine. Sodium bicarbonate should not be given endotracheally. There are no data on amiodarone administration through an endotracheal tube. Medications given via the endotracheal tube should be in doses 2 to 2.5 times larger than intravenous doses and in volumes of 5 to 10 mL to ensure proper drug delivery and systemic effect. Epinephrine's efficacy during cardiac arrest is related to its strong α-adrenergic properties. The α-adrenergic activity causes peripheral vasoconstriction, increased aortic diastolic pressure, and improved myocardial blood flow. Forty units of arginine vasopressin are currently recommended as an alternative to either the first or second dose of epinephrine. Vasopressin is a naturally occurring (antidiuretic) hormone which is a potent nonadrenergic vasoconstrictor when given in high doses. It acts by stimulating smooth muscle V1 receptors. Current evidence suggests that vasopressin is equivalent to but not better than epinephrine for use during CPR. Although the most rapid and highest drug levels occur with administration of medications through a central vein, there is poor blood flow below the diaphragm during CPR. Drugs administered through a lower extremity vein may be extremely delayed or not even reach their sites of action. (See page 1681: Pharmacologic Therapy.)

8. A.   Although CO_2 excretion is reduced during CPR, measurement of blood gases reveals an arterial respiratory alkalosis and a venous respiratory acidosis with a markedly elevated arteriovenous CO_2 difference. The primary cause

of these changes is the severely reduced cardiac output. Decreased pulmonary blood flow during CPR causes lack of perfusion to many nondependent alveoli. Consequently, mixed alveolar CO_2 (i.e., end-tidal CO_2) will be low and correlate poorly with arterial CO_2. However, end-tidal CO_2 does correlate well with cardiac output during CPR. As flow increases, more alveoli become perfused, there is less alveolar dead space, and end-tidal CO_2 measurements rise. Positioning places a critical role in successful CPR. The victim must be supine and the head level with the heart for adequate brain perfusion. The victim must be on a firm surface. The rescuer should stand or kneel next to the victim's side. Compressions are performed most effectively if the rescuer's hips are on the same level, or slightly above the level of, the victim's chest. The heel of one hand is placed on the lower sternum, and the other hand is placed on top of the first one. The sternum must be depressed at least 2 in. (5 cm) in the average adult. Occasionally, deeper compressions are necessary to generate a palpable pulse. The duration of compression should be equal to that of relaxation, and the compression rate should be at least 100 times per minute. No antiarrhythmic agent has been shown to be superior to electrical defibrillation or more effective than placebo in the treatment of VF. Consequently, defibrillation should not be withheld or delayed to establish intravenous access or to administer drugs. (See pages 1678: Circulation and 1679: Technique of Closed-chest Compression.)

9. C.   The cardiac pump mechanism assumes that sternal compression increases intraventricular pressure, thus leading to mitral and tricuspid valve closure, causing forward blood flow as intrathoracic pressure increases. The thoracic pump mechanism assumes that sternal compressions increase intrathoracic pressures in all cardiac chambers equally, that the heart is merely a passive conduit, and that forward flow during increased intrathoracic pressure is the result of backflow prevention in the venous system by the valves in the subclavian and internal jugular veins that favor flow into nondistensible arteries (i.e., aorta and carotids). Which mechanism predominates varies from victim to victim and even during the resuscitation of the same victim. Whatever the mechanism, cardiac output is reduced to 10% to 33% of normal during experimental, closed-chest, cardiac massage. During CPR, nearly all the blood flow is directed to organs above the diaphragm. Myocardial perfusion is 20% to 50% of normal, whereas cerebral perfusion is maintained at 50% to 90% of normal. Abdominal visceral and lower extremity flow is reduced to 5% of normal. (See page 1678: Circulation.)

10. C.   The fibrillation amplitude seen on any one ECG lead varies with the orientation of that lead to the vector of the fibrillatory wave. If the lead is oriented at right angles to the fibrillatory wave, a flat line can be seen. For this reason, the trace from a second lead or from a different position of paddle electrodes should always be inspected before a decision is made not to defibrillate. The AED is a device that monitors the ECG, recognizes VF, charges automatically, and gives a defibrillator shock. These devices use algorithms with nearly perfect specificity; however, sensitivity rates are somewhat lower. They sometimes have trouble recognizing low-amplitude VF and can misinterpret pacemaker spikes as QRS complexes. Unfortunately, rhythm analysis can require up to 90 seconds during which chest compressions are not being given. Low-amplitude and low-frequency fibrillatory waveforms are associated with lower rates of successful resuscitation. Although the amplitude of fibrillation waves correlates with the success of defibrillation, and α-adrenergic agonists (e.g., epinephrine) increase fibrillation amplitude, little evidence supports increased success of defibrillation after epinephrine administration. On the contrary, defibrillation should not be delayed at all when indicated. Firm paddle pressure of at least 11 kg reduces resistance by improving paddle-to-skin contact and by expelling air from the lungs. Air is a poor electrical conductor. Defibrillation is performed by current passing through a critical mass of myocardium causing simultaneous depolarization of the myofibrils. However, the output of defibrillators is indicated in energy units (joules or watt-seconds), not current (amperes). Energy (joules) = Power (watts) × Duration (seconds). Current (amperes) = Potential (volts)/Resistance (ohms). (See page 1685: Electrical Therapy.)

11. D. A higher incidence of atrioventricular block has been observed in patients receiving high-energy shocks than in patients receiving low-energy shocks. High-energy shocks may also result in myocardial damage, particularly if repeated at close intervals. Although defibrillation is less frequently needed in the pediatric age group, similar principles apply as in adults. The initial recommended starting dose is 2 J/kg (monophasic or biphasic), and can be doubled in a subsequent attempt. In adults, lower energies can be used with biphasic waveform defibrillators as compared to monophasic waveform defibrillators. Using biphasic defibrillators, an initial dose ≤200 J can be used, with studies showing comparable success to higher energy levels. Older studies using monophasic defibrillators suggested a relationship between body size and energy requirements for defibrillation, but clinical experience suggests that weight variability in adults does not have a significant impact on dosage requirements. The energy dose range for adults remains 2 to 4 J/kg. With monophasic defibrillators, a single shock of 360 J should be given with immediate resumption of chest compressions. Older recommendations (prior to 2005) for a stacked shock approach appeared to add little incremental benefit. (See pages 1685: Electrical Therapy and 1690: Pediatric Cardiopulmonary Resuscitation.)

12. E. After prolonged VF arrest, successful defibrillation almost always results in asystole or pulseless electrical activity. However, immediately resuming chest compressions after defibrillation almost always results in reversion to a perfusing rhythm. Therefore, it is recommended that one immediately resumes chest compressions after defibrillation, without pausing to check for a pulse or reanalyze the ECG rhythm Although securing a patient's airway

is crucial, rescuers must also be aware of the potentially harmful effects of positive pressure ventilation (PPV). PPV increases intrathoracic pressure, leading to decreased venous return, cardiac output, and coronary perfusion pressure. Rescuers can ameliorate these problems by strict attention to the number of breaths delivered per minute, which should not exceed ten. There is increasing awareness that there should be uniform standards in postresuscitation care to decrease mortality. For instance, cerebral autoregulation of blood flow is understood to be severely compromised after cardiac arrest. Therefore, prolonged extremes of hypotension or hypertension should be avoided. Mean arterial pressure should be maintained in the range of 90 to 110 mm Hg. Pediatric arrests, unlike adult arrests, are unlikely to be sudden events. They are more likely to be a result of progressive deterioration in respiratory and circulatory function. Asystole and PEA are the common resulting rhythms. A heart that is in ventricular fibrillation has high oxygen consumption, so high-energy phosphates in the myocardium are rapidly depleted. After approximately 4 minutes, the hemodynamic phase of cardiac arrest ensues. During this stage, ATP levels are so low as to make restoration of normal myocardial function extremely difficult. Immediate defibrillation will be counterproductive, producing asystole or pulseless electrical activity. Performing effective chest compressions first will restore myocardial blood flow, therefore restoring or at least delaying reductions in ATP levels. Therefore, after 4 minutes of ventricular fibrillation, it is important to perform chest compressions before electrical defibrillation. Of course, if an arrest is witnessed and a defibrillator or AED is available, then defibrillation should be the first priority. The first 4 to 5 minutes of arrest is the electrical phase, during which defibrillation has the greatest chance of success. (See pages 1687: Cardiocerebral Resuscitation, 1693: Postresuscitation Care, and 1690: Pediatric Cardiopulmonary Resuscitation.)

13. C. Recent studies have demonstrated improved neurologic outcome with mild therapeutic hypothermia (32°C to 34°C) when applied for 12 to 24 hours after a ventricular fibrillation victim has been resuscitated and brought to the hospital but remains comatose. These initial studies have only investigated patients who presented with VF as their initial rhythm. The International Liaison Committee on Resuscitation now recommends unconscious adult patients with spontaneous circulation after out-of-hospital cardiac arrest should be cooled to 32°C to 34°C for 12 to 24 hours when the initial rhythm was ventricular fibrillation. Such cooling may also be beneficial for other rhythms or in-hospital cardiac arrest. (See Page 1693: Postresuscitation Care.)

14. C. Mechanical ventilation after successful resuscitation should aim to avoid oxygen toxicity. FiO_2 should be titrated to maintain SpO_2 ≥94% or arterial PaO_2 greater than 100 mm Hg. Hypocapnia ($PaCO_2 < 30$ mm Hg) should also be avoided. (See Page 1693: Postresuscitation care.)